Secondary Metabolites and Their Applications in Various Diseases

Athanasios Alexiou
Novel Global Community Education Foundation, Australia

Saurabh Kumar Jha
Department of Zoology, Kalindi College, University of Delhi, India

Roma Pandey
Department of Biotechnology, IILM University, Greater Noida, India

IGI Global
Scientific Publishing
Publishing Tomorrow's Research Today

Vice President of Editorial	Melissa Wagner
Director of Acquisitions	Mikaela Felty
Director of Book Development	Jocelynn Hessler
Production Manager	Mike Brehm
Cover Design	Phillip Shickler

Published in the United States of America by
IGI Global Scientific Publishing
701 East Chocolate Avenue
Hershey, PA, 17033, USA
Tel: 717-533-8845
Fax: 717-533-7115
Website: https://www.igi-global.com E-mail: cust@igi-global.com

Library of Congress Cataloging-in-Publication Data

Library of Congress Cataloging-in-Publication Data

Names: Alexiou, Athanasios editor | Jha, Saurabh Kumar, 1989- editor | Pandey, Roma, 1989- editor
Title: Secondary metabolites and their applications in various diseases / edited by Athanasios Alexiou, Saurabh Kumar Jha, Roma Pandey.
Description: Hershey, PA : IGI Global Scientific Publishing, [2025] | Includes bibliographical references and index. | Summary: "This book will provide a comprehensive overview of secondary metabolites and their applications across various disorders including cancer, metabolic, and neurological disorders, thereby, providing a holistic view of their therapeutic potential"-- Provided by publisher.
Identifiers: LCCN 2024056690 (print) | LCCN 2024056691 (ebook) | ISBN 9798369391129 hardcover | ISBN 9798369391136 paperback | ISBN 9798369391143 ebook
Subjects: LCSH: Metabolites--Therapeutic use--Case studies | Metabolism, Secondary--Case studies
Classification: LCC QP171 .S43 2025 (print) | LCC QP171 (ebook) | DDC 612.3/9--dc23/eng/20250213
LC record available at https://lccn.loc.gov/2024056690
LC ebook record available at https://lccn.loc.gov/2024056691

British Cataloguing in Publication Data
A Cataloguing in Publication record for this book is available from the British Library.

Table of Contents

Detailed Table of Contents

Secondary metabolites are diverse, biologically active compounds that play critical roles in ecological interactions, such as defence mechanisms, signalling, and competition etc of the organism. These compounds are difficult to detect due to their low abundance and complexity but hold significant potential in unravelling biological processes. The complexity and diversity of secondary metabolites depends on innovative methods to improve detection. The study of secondary metabolites involves a wide range of analytical techniques aimed at identifying, characterizing, and quantifying these compounds. This chapter provides a comprehensive overview of various analytical methods used to study secondary metabolites, highlighting their importance in unravelling the complexity of these compounds and their bioactive potential.

Ashwagandha plant (Withania somnifera), celebrated for its therapeutic properties, is rich in secondary metabolites like withanolides, alkaloids, and flavonoids, which contribute to its medicinal value. Identifying these metabolites using traditional methods can be labor-intensive and costly. This chapter explores the transformative role of deep learning (DL) and machine learning (ML) algorithms in metabolite

methods such as machine learning (ML) and virtual screening, can improve the identification and analysis of bioactive compounds, simulate interactions between EOs and pathogens, and optimize antimicrobial formulations. By incorporating AI, researchers can accelerate discovery, identify novel metabolite combinations, and address the growing challenge of antimicrobial resistance.

Immunomodulatory drugs (IMDs) play important role in advancing therapeutic treatments across various diseases, especially autoimmune disorders, viral infections and haematological malignancies. This bibliometric review highlights the impact of immunomodulatory therapies such as immunoglobulins, antivirals, and CAR-T cell therapies, focusing on their efficacy in managing conditions like relapsed multiple myeloma (RRMM), COVID-19, and autoimmune disorders. Key findings from the Scopus database, covering a wide span of immunomodulatory treatments, are analysed to identify research trends, influential studies and collaborations. Citation analysis reveals that the United States leads in research outcomes, while countries like Belgium and the Netherlands show significantly higher citation per document, demonstrating impactful but less frequent publications. The review explores a strong trend towards the development of more effective immunotherapies, focusing on future potential in clinical applications.

Secondary metabolites, bioactive compounds from plants, fungi, and microorganisms, show significant therapeutic potential for neurodegenerative and inflammatory diseases. This chapter highlights their mechanisms of action, including antioxidant activity, modulation of inflammatory pathways, and neuroprotection, supported by preclinical and clinical evidence. Key classes like alkaloids, flavonoids, terpenoids, and polyphenols are explored for their neuroprotective and anti-inflammatory properties, alongside phytochemical sources that emphasize their drug discovery potential. However, challenges such as limited bioavailability, stability, and toxicity hinder their clinical application. Addressing these issues through novel strategies could unlock their full potential in modern medicine. This chapter bridges natural product chemistry and clinical applications, providing insights to inspire further research into secondary metabolites as essential tools for combating complex diseases.

Inflammation and immune modulation are critical for the body's defense against infection, injury, and stress, but chronic inflammation underlies many diseases, including autoimmune disorders, metabolic diseases, and neurodegenerative conditions. Secondary metabolites—bioactive compounds from plants and organisms—offer promising anti-inflammatory and immunomodulatory effects.

These include alkaloids, flavonoids, terpenoids, and polyphenols, which can inhibit pro-inflammatory cytokines, reduce oxidative stress, and modulate immune cell function. For example, compounds like curcumin, quercetin, and resveratrol target inflammatory pathways such as NF-κB and COX-2. These natural agents often have fewer side effects compared to conventional drugs, making them appealing for treating inflammation-driven diseases. The growing evidence suggests secondary metabolites could provide safer, effective alternatives to traditional anti-inflammatory treatments, offering hope for more natural therapies with broad applications.

Traditional medicine encompasses a range of ancient, culturally-rooted health practices that were developed long before modern scientific approaches were applied to healthcare. Used for centuries, these practices often involve medicinal plants, which play a role in treating cardiovascular conditions such as heart disease, cerebrovascular disorders, hypertension, and heart failure. Hypertension complicates heart function and contributes to atherosclerosis, thereby increasing the risk of heart attacks and strokes. Although numerous drugs are available to manage these conditions, many commonly used anti- hypertensive medications carry significant side effects. Medicinal herbs contain active compounds with both therapeutic and preventive properties, offering potential for the treatment of hypertension. This review provides an overview of several medicinal plants and secondary metabolites that have demonstrated hypertensive or anti-hypertensive effects.

Millet, an ancient whole grain, has a variety of health benefits. Its minerals support bone health. Incorporating millet into a healthy diet can improve overall health and provide a flexible and nutritious grain alternative. Despite its role in providing essential nutrients to the body, millet also has anticancer properties which make it an essential grain for the treatment of different types of cancer. Antioxidants of millets such as flavonoids and phenolic compounds, may help prevent oxidative stress and cellular damage, both of which have been associated with cancer formation. Its high fiber content promotes healthy digestion and intestinal regularity, potentially lowering the risk of colorectal cancer. Certain millet varieties also include lignans, which may alter hormone metabolism, potentially lowering the incidence of hormone-related malignancies such as breast cancer. This chapter will explain the role of different natural compounds and phytochemicals from varieties of millet in the treatment of these two main cancers

Secondary metabolites are highly potent organic compounds that are synthesised by plants, fungi, and bacteria as a defence mechanism against predators. Plants have been employed as traditional remedies for centuries due to their production of a diverse array of secondary metabolites. Many individuals are intrigued by the potential of food and other plant materials to serve as alternative medications due to their bioactive components, which have the ability to suppress microbial proliferation and treat it with minimal adverse effects. The critical function of these components in enhancing the therapeutic efficacy of traditional medications against a diverse array of pathogenic germs was demonstrated by their addition. Additionally, researchers have investigated the use of specific metabolites in conjunction with antimicrobial pharmacological medications to address the issues resulting from drug resistance. Therefore, this chapter examines the antimicrobial properties of secondary metabolites and their role in enhancing drug sensitivity in the presence of pathogenic organisms.

Secondary metabolites are organic compounds produced by microorganisms, higher plants, and fungi, with significant ecological and human health relevance. This chapter explores their biological activities, types, and biosynthesis, emphasizing their applications in disease prevention and control. It highlights the pharmacological properties of key compounds, including phenolics, alkaloids, flavonoids, terpenoids, glycosides, and polyketides, in treating and preventing cancer, diabetes, heart diseases, infections, mental disorders, and immune system dysfunctions. Their roles in combating aging, inflammation, oxidative stress, neurodegeneration, malaria, and modulating immunity are also discussed.

Yassine Mouniane, Laboratory of Natural Resources and Sustainable Development, Faculty of Sciences, Ibn Tofaïl University, Morocco
Yassine Kadmi, LASIRE, Equipe Physico-Chimie de l'Environnement, CNRS UMR 8516, Université Lille, France
Meryem Doubi, Faculty of Sciences, Ibn Tofail University, Kenitra, Morocco
Salma Tabi, Department of Life Sciences, Faculty of Science and Technology, Sultan Moulay Slimane University, Morocco
Issam El-Khadir, Faculty of Sciences, Ibn Tofail University, Kenitra, Morocco
Ahmed Chriqui, Faculty of Sciences, Ibn Tofail University, Kenitra, Morocco
Abdelaati Soufiani, Faculty of Sciences, Ibn Tofail University, Kenitra, Morocco
Brahim El Ouardi, Faculty of Sciences, Ibn Tofail University, Kenitra, Morocco
Khawla Rachmoune, Interdisciplinary Laboratory of Research in Bio-Resources, Environment and Materials, Higher Normal School, Cadi Ayyad University, 40000 Marrakech, Morocco
Amir Souissi, Swift Current Research and Development Centre, Agriculture and Agrifood Canada, Canada
Arpit Sharma, CHEORS, RWE, India
Shelika Joshi, Walden University, Canada
Mohammed Choukri Belkadi, Faculty of Medicine and Pharmacy, University Mohammed the First, Oujda, Morocco
Driss Hmouni, Faculty of Sciences, Ibn Tofail University, Kenitra, Morocco

Research into these bioactive compounds will allow us to better understand their contribution to health benefits. Carob (Ceratonia siliqua L.) is a Mediterranean species rich in secondary metabolites such as polyphenols, flavonoids, and other bioactive compounds. These secondary metabolites confer important antioxidants, anti-inflammatory, and antimicrobial properties to carob, offering multiple applications in the food and pharmaceutical industries. This chapter reviews the main secondary metabolites present in carob fruits and leaves and their potential applications.

The genus Origanum (Lamiaceae) encompasses a variety of species recognized for their medicinal properties. It has a wide distribution in the Northern Hemisphere, particularly in the Mediterranean Basin. The term "oregano" is used to refer to several species within the genus Origanum. Origanum species have been used in traditional medicinal practices since ancient times to treat various ailments. Secondary metabolites produced by this genus are important as they take an active role in numerous therapeutic properties and biological activities, including antibacterial, antifungal, antiviral, antioxidant, anti-inflammatory, and antitumor effects. The most prevalent secondary metabolites in this genus are carvacrol, thymol, gamma-terpinene, p-cymene, and linalool. These secondary metabolites play an important role in the therapeutic properties and biological activities of the genus. This study aims to present a comprehensive review of the traditional uses of the genus Origanum, its secondary metabolites, and their therapeutic properties.

The Salvia genus, commonly referred to as "sage", represents the largest genus within the family Lamiaceae. Approximately 1,000 species of the Salvia genus are known to grow naturally, primarily in southern Europe but also in other regions worldwide. A significant proportion of the species are utilized in traditional medicine. In vitro and in vivo studies with Salvia species have confirmed the presence of numerous secondary metabolites with various biological activities and therapeutic properties. The Salvia genus contains a variety of secondary metabolites, including sterols, flavonoids, sesquiterpenoids, sesterpenoids, diterpenoids, triterpenoids, and essential

Preface

INTRODUCTION

Secondary metabolites are bioactive compounds produced by plants, fungi, and bacteria, which have become promising in the evolving landscape of disease prevention and treatment. Over the past few decades, their unique and selective biological activities have drawn the attention of the global scientific community. These naturally occurring compounds are no longer seen merely as metabolic byproducts but are now being recognized for their significant therapeutic potential.

This edited volume, *Secondary Metabolites and Their Applications in Various Diseases*, was conceptualized to address the growing need for a comprehensive resource that thoroughly examines the role of these compounds in managing and treating a wide range of disorders. From cancer to metabolic and neurological disorders, secondary metabolites represent a rich and largely unexploited source of therapeutic potential that offers a new hope to supplement, and in some cases, even replace traditional treatment approaches. Our goal in curating this work has been to consolidate the latest scientific knowledge, explore molecular mechanisms, and present clinical relevance through the lens of modern pharmacological and biotechnological approaches.

Throughout this book, authors examine the specific roles and mechanisms of action of individual secondary metabolites, supported by recent advancements in research and clinical applications. Emphasis has been placed on the integration of cutting-edge technologies in metabolite discovery and development, offering insights into prospects and translational potential. Case studies and clinical trials included herein serve to bridge the gap between laboratory findings and real-world therapeutic applications.

This interdisciplinary approach drawing from pharmacology, molecular biology, biotechnology, and clinical medicine, ensures that the book caters to a broad academic and professional audience. Whether you are a medical graduate, a doctoral candidate, or a practicing specialist in biotechnology, biochemistry, neurology, or alternative medicine, this reference work has been designed to enrich your understanding and inspire further exploration in the field.

As editors, we are deeply grateful to the contributing authors whose expertise and scholarship have shaped this book. We also acknowledge the growing community of researchers and clinicians whose commitment to advancing the science of natural compounds continues to drive innovation and discovery in healthcare.

We hope this volume will serve as both a foundational reference and an inspiring guide for future studies, helping to unlock the full therapeutic potential of secondary metabolites in the treatment of human disease.

ORGANIZATION OF THE BOOK

This volume brings together emerging and advanced research at the intersection of natural products chemistry, biotechnology, and digital innovation, exploring the diverse roles and therapeutic potential of secondary metabolites. This book is thoughtfully structured into three distinct sections, each designed to provide a comprehensive exploration of secondary metabolites, their analysis, and their diverse applications, particularly within the field of medicinal plants.

In **Section I: Introduction and Methodological Tools**, the advanced techniques and tools employed in their analysis, offering insights into the methodologies that underpin their identification and characterization, are examined. Furthermore, it explores the cutting-edge applications of artificial intelligence, specifically deep learning and machine learning algorithms, in streamlining the identification and classification of these valuable compounds.

In *Chapter 1*, the analytical complexity and biological significance of secondary metabolites are addressed through a comprehensive review of modern detection and characterization tools. Given their low abundance yet high bioactivity, this chapter underscores the critical need for precise and innovative analytical methodologies to unravel their ecological and pharmacological roles.

In *Chapter 2*, we explore how artificial intelligence revolutionizes the identification of secondary metabolites in *Withania somnifera* (Ashwagandha). By integrating spectral imaging technologies, the chapter showcases how these computational tools not only enhance analytical precision but also pave the way for sustainable agriculture, biodiversity conservation, and personalized herbal medicine.

Chapter 3 continues this theme by examining the antimicrobial activity of secondary metabolites found in essential oils and how artificial intelligence can optimize their identification and application. The integration of AI through machine learning and virtual screening accelerates compound discovery and antimicrobial formulation design, providing novel approaches to tackle the growing challenge of antimicrobial resistance.

In *Chapter 4*, a bibliometric review captures the dynamic landscape of immunomodulatory therapies. Analyzing research trends, citation networks, and key contributors from a global perspective, the chapter identifies promising therapeutic directions, particularly in immunoglobulins, CAR-T cell therapies, and antivirals for diseases like COVID-19 and relapsed multiple myeloma.

Section II: Therapeutic Applications in Diseases transits from analytical techniques to the practical implications of secondary metabolites in addressing various health challenges. This section thoroughly examines the therapeutic roles of these compounds in the context of neurodegenerative and inflammatory diseases, elucidating their underlying mechanisms and potential applications. The section also highlights the traditional and contemporary use of medicinal plants in the treatment of hypertension and investigates the emerging role of millet, a nutrient-rich grain, in cancer therapeutics. Finally, it provides a dedicated exploration of the inherent antimicrobial properties exhibited by various secondary metabolites.

Chapter 5 focuses on the mechanisms by which secondary metabolites offer therapeutic benefits in neurodegenerative and inflammatory diseases. Alkaloids, flavonoids, terpenoids, and polyphenols are highlighted for their ability to modulate oxidative stress and inflammation. The chapter addresses pharmacokinetic challenges and proposes strategies for improving bioavailability and clinical applicability.

Building on this, *Chapter 6* delves deeper into the immunomodulatory and anti-inflammatory effects of secondary metabolites. The chapter presents compelling evidence of natural compounds such as curcumin and quercetin as potent, side-effect-sparing alternatives to conventional drugs in treating inflammation-driven conditions.

Chapter 7 shifts to cardiovascular health, offering a rich review of medicinal plants and their secondary metabolites used in the treatment of hypertension. With traditional remedies gaining scientific backing, this chapter bridges ethnopharmacology with modern therapeutic validation, discussing plant-derived alternatives to synthetic antihypertensives.

In *Chapter 8*, the ancient grain millet is recognized for its emerging role in cancer therapeutics. Rich in antioxidants, lignans, and dietary fiber, millet is presented as a multifunctional food capable of mitigating oxidative stress and hormone-related cancers, particularly colorectal and breast cancer, thus establishing its relevance in functional nutrition and preventive oncology.

Chapter 9 explores the broad antimicrobial efficacy of secondary metabolites, emphasizing their potential to both suppress pathogenic growth and enhance drug sensitivity. Thc chapter examines synergies between plant-derived compounds and conventional antimicrobials, particularly in the fight against drug-resistant infections.

Section III: Plant-Specific Case Studies offers in-depth analyses of secondary metabolites within specific plant genera and species, providing concrete examples of their therapeutic potential. This is followed by specific secondary metabolites found in the Carob Tree (*Ceratonia siliqua L.*), outlining their potential applications. Furthermore, it examines the Origanum genus, detailing its diverse array of secondary metabolites, their established therapeutic properties, and traditional uses. The medicinal applications of secondary metabolites within the Salvia genus are also thoroughly explored. Finally, this section sheds light on the often-overlooked secondary metabolites of bryophytes and thcir promising therapeutic applications, broadening our understanding of the plant medicinal resources.

Chapter 10 offers an extensive overview of the biosynthesis and pharmacological functions of key secondary metabolites across a wide disease spectrum. Their roles in combating inflammation, neurodegeneration, cancer, metabolic disorders, and immune dysfunctions are presented, highlighting the holistic and multi-targeted actions of these natural agents.

Chapter 11 turns to *Ceratonia siliqua* (carob tree), presenting its rich composition of polyphenols and flavonoids and their implications for the food and pharmaceutical sectors. This Mediterranean species is profiled for its antioxidant, anti-inflammatory, and antimicrobial effects, making it a valuable resource for natural product development.

Chapter 12 reviews the genus *Origanum*, renowned for its essential oils and widespread traditional use. The chapter comprehensively catalogs its key secondary metabolites such as carvacrol and thymol, explaining their roles in a wide array of therapeutic activities including antimicrobial, antioxidant, and anticancer effects.

Chapter 13 delves into the pharmacological richness of the Salvia genus, which is the largest genus within the Lamiaceae family. With approximately 1,000 naturally occurring species, primarily distributed in southern Europe but also found globally. Salvia has long held prominence in traditional medicine systems. The chapter highlights the genus's extensive repertoire of secondary metabolites, including sterols, flavonoids, sesquiterpenoids, diterpenoids, triterpenoids, and essential oils. In vitro and in vivo studies have substantiated the genus's therapeutic efficacy, revealing a range of biological activities such as anti-inflammatory, antimicrobial, and antioxidant effects. Through a comprehensive analysis of ethnobotanical data and pharmacological research, this chapter underscores the genus's value as a reservoir of natural compounds with promising medicinal applications.

Finally, *Chapter 14* brings attention to their unique bioactive profile, particularly their content of secondary metabolites such as steroids, alkaloids, phenols, coumarins, flavonoids, and tannins. Found in diverse terrestrial habitats, bryophytes exhibit potent therapeutic properties, including antimicrobial, antioxidant, anti-inflammatory, antidiabetic, and anticancer activities. By synthesizing ethnomedicinal knowledge with recent scientific findings, this chapter presents a compelling case for further exploration of bryophytes as a rich and underutilized source of pharmacologically active compounds.

CONCLUSION

As editors of this comprehensive volume, we are proud to present an interdisciplinary exploration of secondary metabolites and their wide-ranging applications in medicine, agriculture, biotechnology, and beyond. The chapters compiled in this book reflect the dynamic and evolving nature of natural products research, drawing from a diverse array of biological sources from well-studied angiosperms and microbial systems to the lesser known yet promising bryophytes and fungal endophytes.

Each contribution offers a unique lens into the biosynthesis, functionality, and therapeutic potential of secondary metabolites, while also emphasizing the importance of sustainable utilization and innovative technologies for their analysis and production. The depth and breadth of this collection demonstrate not only the scientific richness of secondary metabolites but also their critical relevance to global health, environmental sustainability, and industrial innovation.

We hope this book serves as a valuable resource for researchers, practitioners, and students across the life sciences and related disciplines. By integrating traditional knowledge with cutting-edge scientific inquiry, we aim to inspire continued investigation and interdisciplinary collaboration that will further unlock the potential of nature's molecular treasures.

Athanasios Alexiou
Novel Global Community Education Foundation, Australia

Saurabh Kumar Jha
Department of Zoology, Kalindi College, University of Delhi, India

Roma Pandey
IILM University, India

Chapter 1
Techniques and Tools in Secondary Metabolite Analysis

Roma Pandey
https://orcid.org/0000-0001-7090-4812
IILM University, India

Ila Ruchie
https://orcid.org/0009-0009-8074-992X
PIPRAMS, Greater Noida, India

Ranjeet Kaur
University of Delhi-South Campus, India

ABSTRACT

Secondary metabolites are diverse, biologically active compounds that play critical roles in ecological interactions, such as defence mechanisms, signalling, and competition etc of the organism. These compounds are difficult to detect due to their low abundance and complexity but hold significant potential in unravelling biological processes. The complexity and diversity of secondary metabolites depends on innovative methods to improve detection. The study of secondary metabolites involves a wide range of analytical techniques aimed at identifying, characterizing, and quantifying these compounds. This chapter provides a comprehensive overview of various analytical methods used to study secondary metabolites, highlighting their importance in unravelling the complexity of these compounds and their bioactive potential.

DOI: 10.4018/979-8-3693-9112-9.ch001

1. INTRODUCTION

1.1. Definition and Significance

Plants synthesize various types of substances which can be categorized into both primary and secondary metabolites, that are essential for the growth, development and defence of plant species (Reshi et al 2023). The metabolites directly involved in plant growth and developmental processes, and contribute towards essential cellular pathways like respiration, cell division, and photosynthesis, are categorized as the Primary metabolites. (Tariq et al 2023). On the contrary, few metabolites play diverse roles, including plant survival mechanisms against various biotic and abiotic stresses, and have been categorized as the Secondary metabolites (Chen et al 2022). Their production is primarily under the inducible control of defensive transcriptional factors, subjected to recognition of various stimuli, both internal as well as external, through plant receptors (Chen et al 2022). In addition, the secondary metabolite production is also triggered in plants during different developmental stages, physiological conditions and environmental interactions, such as mutualism, pathogenicity and herbivory (Chomel et al 2016).

1.2. Classification of Secondary Metabolites

Plant secondary metabolites have been categorized into various groups based on functional groups and chemical structure (Teoh 2016). These groups include:

1. Terpenes (including volatile compounds, sterols, and carotenoids),
2. Polysaccharides and Hydrocarbons
3. Phenolic compounds,
4. Phytoalexins (sulfur-containing compounds),
5. Alkaloids (nitrogen-containing compounds),
6. Flavonoids

However, polysaccharides mostly comprise of carbon and hydrogen as base elements, or their derivatives, hence we have included them under the single head group in the sub-sequent sections. Also, plant hormones, such as abscisic acid, gibberellic acid, jasmonic acid, polyamines, and salicylic acid, are derivatives of these above secondary metabolites.

We will discuss each of these in the following sub-sections:

1.2.1. Terpenes

Terpenes are probably one of the largest groups of plant secondary metabolites possessing a repeating five-carbon isoprene units, which forms a basic common feature for all terpenes. These include a variety of substances such as floral fragrances serving as insect attractants, pine oil, plant growth regulators, such as, gibberelic acid and abscisic acid, and some which are insecticidal. More than 30,000 terpenes have been identified so far and are further classified into seven different sub-classes based on the number of isoprene repeat units. Their structure and functional role in plants is summarized in Table 1.

Table 1. Structure and role

Type of terpene	Number of 5C isoprene repeat units	Name of the compound	Role in plant defence	Reference
Hemiterpenes	1	Pubescenoside A	Antiplatelet aggregation activity	Y.L. Powder-George, in Pharmacognosy (Second Edition), 2024
Monoterpenes	2	Geraniol, thymol, menthol	Antioxidant, anti-inflammatory, antimicrobial, antitumor, hepatoprotective, cardioprotective, and neuroprotective	Zielińska-Błajet M et al 2020
Sesquiterpenes	3	Artemesinin, Antolactone, Isoalantolactone	Antimalarial medicine, anticancer activities such as modulating nuclear factor kappa (NF-kB) activity, inhibitory action against lipid peroxidation and retarding the production of reactive oxygen & nitrogen species	Abu-Izneid T et al (2020)
Diterpenes	4	Paclitaxel	Effective against ovarian, breast, colon, non-small cell lung cancer and malignant melanoma.	Zenjanab et al 2024
Sesterterpenes	5	Leucosceptroid A and B	Antifungal and antifeedant activity (against insect attacks)	Chen et al 2021
Triterpenes	6	Triterpene saponins such as Liquorice	Antitussive (cough preventing), expectorant, analgesic, anti-inflammatory and cytotoxic effects	González-Coloma et al 2011
Carotenoids	8	Zeaxanthin, carotene	Photoprotection and pigmentation in plants	Sun et al 2022

1.2.2. Hydrocarbons and Polysaccharides

Hydrocarbons are the simplest compounds as they contain only hydrogen and carbon. They occur as straight chain aliphatic hydrocarbons or in ring forms as aromatic hydrocarbons. Hydrocarbons thus form the basic skeleton of more complex molecules, or mostly the biomolecules. These can be saturated or unsaturated with double/triple bonds. The waxy coat on leaves and fruits contains many saturated hydrocarbons which are insoluble in water. They form a protective outer coat, thereby preventing water from sticking on the surface of leaves and fruit. They also check transpiration in xerophytic plants. Olive oil also contains several saturated hydrocarbons. The gaseous plant hormone, ethylene ($H_2C=CH_2$) is an example of an unsaturated hydrocarbon. The role of ethylene is well established in ripening of fruit, abscission of leaves and fading of adjacent flowers, especially in an enclosed space which prevents dissipation of the gas.

Plant polysaccharides, including carbohydrates with beta 1–3, 1–4 or 1–6 branch-chains, are highly bioactive compounds found in herbs, such as aloe, cinnamon, gingers, and so on. Herb-derived polysaccharide compounds are widely used in medicine as tonics and anticancer agents (Cao et al 2022). They exhibit immuno-modulatory activity in vitro (Sindhu et al 2021). Other actions include an antimicrobial action (Zhou et al 2022), induction of cell differentiation (Cao et al 2022), inhibition of angiogenesis (Ren et al 2020) and an antimetastatic effect (Hoseinkhani et al 2020). Polysaccharides vary greatly in their efficacy; their greater complexity in the branch chains and higher molecular weight are directly related to higher bioactivity. Thus, plant polysaccharides have an immense potential to be used as potent medicines in human health and disease, thereby providing a greener alternative to chemical-based drugs.

1.2.3. Phenolic Compounds

Phenols and phenolic compounds comprise of one of the largest groups of secondary metabolites. On one hand, this diverse group includes simple compounds with a single aromatic ring, such as anillin, which is widely used to flavour food, while on the other hand, this group also includes complex polymers like tannins, lignins, quinones, coumarins, anthraquinones and naphthoquinones, all belong to this group of plant secondary metabolites. The ubiquitous salicylic acid is a precursor of aspirin. Denbinobin, a 1,4-phenanthrenequinone, is a potent suppressor of HIV-1 as well as several human cancer cell lines, including leukaemia, breast, lung, colorectal and stomach cancers. Phenolic compounds suppress the viral infection in plants and represses the replication of viruses through mode of actions such as damage of protein, DNA or ribose nucleic acid (RNA), inhibition of viral enzyme activities (Kumar et al 2013). Coumarins inhibit viral replication in cells by inhibition of enzymes such as protease, integrase and reverse transcriptase (Shokoohinia et al 2014).

1.2.4. Phytoalexins

Phytoalexins are low-molecular-weight compounds that play a crucial role in biotic stress tolerance in plants. These can also be classified as stilbenoids because they are derivatives of dihydrostilbenes or bibenzyls. Resveratrol is the best publicised stilbenoid. Present on the skin of grapes and playing a role in warding off attack by fungi and bacteria on the fruit, it is alleged to have many beneficial effects on plants and animals and even cytotoxic activities, but its global benefit is controversial and has never been replicated in humans. Phytoalexins are bacteriostatic and fungistatic, while being neither bactericidal nor fungicidal.

Role of phytoalexins in plant defence and human health:

Introduction of these genes encoding stilbene phytoalexins was shown to confer higher disease resistance to several plants including alfalfa, rice, barley, wheat, tomato, papaya and Arabidopsis (Jeandet et al 2014). Phytoalexins accumulate at infection sites and limit the growth of fungi and bacteria in vitro, suggesting that they could be utilised to protect plants from fungi and bacteriacaused illnesses. Phytoalexins are significantly less toxic than chemical fungicides. *Botrytis cinerea*, the pathogen that causes grey mould in grapevines, was shown to exhibit inhibition of germ-tube elongation, radial mycelial growth, and mycelia dry weight increase, when treated with resveratrol. Phytoalexins thus have immense potential to alter the physiological, morphological, and cytological characteristics of fungal cells (Sahu et al 2018).

Phytoalexins may display health-promoting effects in humans. A few of them have been reported to exert antioxidant, anticarcinogenic and cardiovascular protective activities. Maslinic acid, a natural phytoalexin-type triterpene from olives exerts a wide range of biological activities as an antitumor, antidiabetic, neuroprotective, cardioprotective, antiparasitic and growth-stimulating agent, providing evidence of the potential of this molecule as a nutraceutical [Lozano-Mena et al 2014]. Health benefit properties of Brassicaceae were attributed in part to their phytoalexins, camalexin and related indolic compounds [Jahangir et al 2009]. Camalexin is able to induce apoptosis in prostate cancer cells [Sm,ith et al 2014]. 3-deoxyanthocyanidins, flavonoid phytoalexins produced by members of the Poaceae family, are helpful in reducing the incidence of gastro-intestinal cancer [Yang et al 2009]. Moreover, other indolic phytoalexins such as brassinin and its derivative, homobrassinin, show marked antiproliferative activities in human colorectal cancer cells in vitro [Kello et al 2014].

1.2.5. Alkaloids

Alkaloids are plant-derived optically active compounds containing one or more nitrogen atoms, usually in a heterocyclic ring (an amine functional group). Like proteins, they are derived from amino acids, but they differ in being alkaline.

Role of Alkaloids in plant defence and human health:

Among their functions, alkaloids are known to play a role in germination and in protecting plants from various biotic stress agents, mostly microbes and herbivores. Many alkaloids act on the nervous system. Poppy is narcotic, caffeine and nicotine are stimulants, while cocaine is an anaesthetic, and scopolamine induces "twilight sleep." Reserpine which lowers blood pressure is an ancient Indian remedy derived from *Rauwolfia serpentina*, now totally replaced by a wide range of more potent and reliable antihypertensives. Many alkaloid stimulants (e.g. morphine, cocaine, nicotine) are addictive. Improperly applied, some stimulants and sedatives are deadly. Strychnine is used as a rat poison. Taxol which has a diterpenoid core possesses an alkaloid side chain. It is an indispensable component in the chemotherapeutic cocktail employed in the treatment of ovarian and breast cancer. Vincristine and vinblastine are two alkaloids derived from the periwinkle, *Catharanthus roseus* (not an orchid), and are also cytotoxic agents but their use is limited to late-stage cancers because of their high toxicity.

1.2.6. Flavonoids

Flavonoids are commonly popular due to their antioxidant nature. Quercetin, the most abundant dietary flavonoid (it is also present in *Dendrobium catenatum*), is a potent antioxidant with anti-allergic and anti-inflammatory properties. Some flavanoids are antibacterial, antiviral (against the common cold sore virus), anti-allergic, anti-inflammatory, antiplatelet and antineoplastic (Salem et al 2020). Anthocyanins, which impart yellow, red, mauve, pink, magenta and purple colouring to flowers, play an important role in insect mimicry.

1.3 Role in Drug Development and Natural Products Research

As already discussed in above sections, plant secondary metabolites play diverse roles in plant defence mechanisms and human health, hence they are potent targets in drug development. Researchers across the globe are targeting the analysis, extraction and in-depth examination of the multiple roles these natural products have to offer. Plant-made pharmaceuticals result from the creative application of biotechnology to plants to make drugs derived from natural products that the medical profession can employ to fight life-threatening ailments, such as asthma, influenza, cancer, tuberculosis, diabetes mellitus, coronary artery disease, and diarrhoea (Mohr et al 2015).

Developing drugs using plant-based pharmaceutical techniques offers an efficient, cost-effective, and safe alternative to conventional procedures using animal cell cultures or microbial fermentation (Chaachouay et al 2024). Therefore, drugs derived from natural compounds in plants can offer patients greater and quicker access to medications (Subramoniam et al 2014, Veeresham et al 2012). The most remarkable characteristic of natural products concerning their enduring significance in drug development is their mostly unexplored structural diversity.

2. IMPORTANCE OF ANALYTICAL TECHNIQUES IN METABOLITE STUDY

Plants have undergone robust adaptive evolutionary changes from their algal ancestors to modern day flowering plants, developing various pathways to cope with diverse types of stresses. It has become evident that plants produce a wide array of primary and secondary metabolites, which serve as chemical signals for communication with their environment for survival. These metabolites have significant physiological and ecological functions. However, the analysis of plant metabolites poses several challenges: firstly, the detection of metabolites that exhibit an extensive range, vast diversity, relatively low abundance, and dynamic nature; secondly, comprehensive data analysis and interpretation. The utilization of advanced analytical techniques has been employed to overcome these challenges, however judicious selection and careful application of the appropriate technique towards the isolation, identification and extraction of the secondary metabolite will further enhance the chances of a successful commercial production. The analysis of secondary metabolite from the parent plant requires essential steps of sample preparation and extraction.

2.1 Sample Preparation and Extraction

Importance of Sample Preparation:

Metabolite extraction is an essential stage in plant-based research that helps us understand the chemical makeup and activities of plants. However, it is crucial to properly prepare plant samples before extraction can take place. By carefully considering factors such as plant selection, sampling techniques, storage conditions, and using advanced optimization techniques, researchers can ensure that their samples are of high quality and accurately represent the metabolite profiles of the plants under study. This leads to more reliable and meaningful results in secondary metabolite analysis and study.

2.1.1 Homogenization

Homogenization is an important step in sample preparation as it helps to break down plant tissues and release metabolites. This improves extraction efficiency owing to the increased surface area, which will allow a better contact between the plant matrix and the solvent (Kim & Verpoorte 2010). Different homogenization methods can be used, such as mechanical homogenization using a blender or a mortar and pestle, or ultrasonic homogenization. Mechanical homogenization may be more suitable for larger tissue samples, while ultrasonic homogenization can be more effective for smaller samples or for samples that require gentle treatment.

2.1.2 Drying

The drying process is primarily aimed at inhibiting metabolic processes which result in stopping changes in the plant's chemical composition. This occurs by removing water from the plant material, which is necessary for plant enzymes to function properly. The lack of water and a high drying temperature contribute to the inhibition of enzymes that can break down the active ingredients. Proper drying also reduces the number of microorganisms in the final product. It significantly reduces the weight and volume of plant material, reducing the costs of packaging, transport, and storage of plant substances. Flash - freezing is a technique that rapidly freezes plant samples, minimizing the formation of ice crystals that can damage cell structures. This helps in maintaining the integrity of metabolites. Liquid nitrogen is commonly used for flash - freezing plant samples. By quickly freezing the samples, enzymatic and chemical reactions are halted, preserving the metabolite profile (Bhambere et al 2015).

2.2 Extraction of Plant Secondary Metabolite

Extraction is the separation of plant bioactive fractions by using selective solvents system and extraction procedures. Plant products are essentially liquid, semisolid, or dry powder combinations of metabolites. The nature of the bioactive chemicals being targeted is the primary determinant in the solvent system selection process. The solvents employed for extraction penetrate solid plant matter and solubilize molecules of similar polarity during the extraction process. The solvents with low boiling points and evaporation temperatures are most frequently utilized to extract analytes from solid samples. The solvents must also be chemically neutral, non-toxic, and non-flammable. They must also not negatively affect the stability of the chemicals being analysed or the instruments. Common solvents include methanol, ethanol, acetone, and ethyl acetate, as well as water-based combinations of these substances (Naczk & Shahidi 2006). Depending on their relative polarity solvents such as methanol, ethanol, or ethyl acetate are used in the extraction of hydrophilic compounds. Dichloromethane is used to extract more lipophilic compounds. Hexane is used in extraction to eliminate the chlorophyll and oil (Srivastava et al 2020). Insoluble bound complexes of phenols and phenolic acids are linked to cell wall polymers by ester and glycosidic linkages and cannot be extracted by organic solvents (Mattila et al 2007). Prior to extraction, bound phenolic acids are commonly released via base hydrolysis, acid hydrolysis, or both (Agnieszka Arceusz et al 2013). The various methods of extraction are mentioned in Figure 1.

Figure 1. Various methods of extraction used to study metabolites

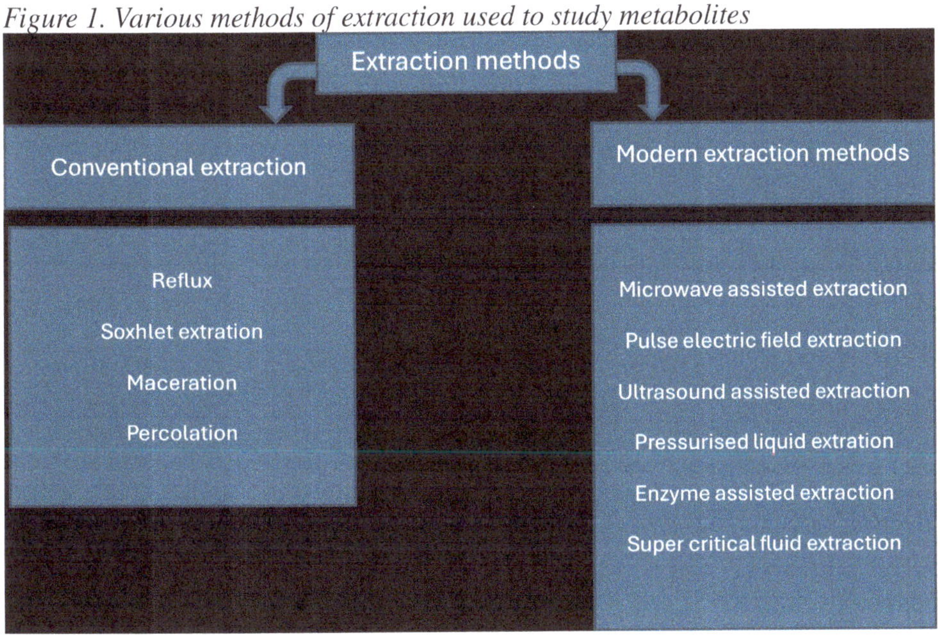

2.2.1 Conventional Extraction Methods

1. Reflux

The principle of the method is heating the solvent for a while and then allow to condense. In reflux extraction, a solution can heat in a controlled manner at a constant temperature maintaining the stability of the compound. The disadvantage of this method includes the need for more amount of solvent and a long time. However, the use of organic solvents causes environmental damage and increases the cost of operation. Because of the high equipment availability, these methods are still in use (Martínez-Ávila et al 2021).

2. Soxhlet Extraction or continuous hot extraction

Soxhlet extraction is also known as continuous hot extraction. The apparatus used for this extraction is a soxhlet extractor. This extractor setup consists of a round bottom flask, siphon tube, distillation path, expansion adapter, condenser, cooling water inlet, cooling water outlet, heat source, and thimble. The sample (dried and homogenised) is filled in a porous thimble located in the chamber. The bottom flask contains extraction solvents heated, vaporized into a sample thimble, condensed in the condenser, and dripped back. Soxhlet extraction was also used for qualitative and quantitative analysis of phenolic compounds occurring in Salvia halophila and S. virgata (Akkol et al 2008) This method is that it requires a shorter processing time but include use of toxic and flammable liquid organic solvent, which is not eco-friendly (Tzanova et al 2020).

Figure 2. Soxhlet extraction (https://alfresco-staticfiles.s3.amazonaws.com/alfresco_images/pharma/2019/08/23/b902cfb8-6438-41bb-b42e-38c70ab4b071/LCGC2_i3.jpg)

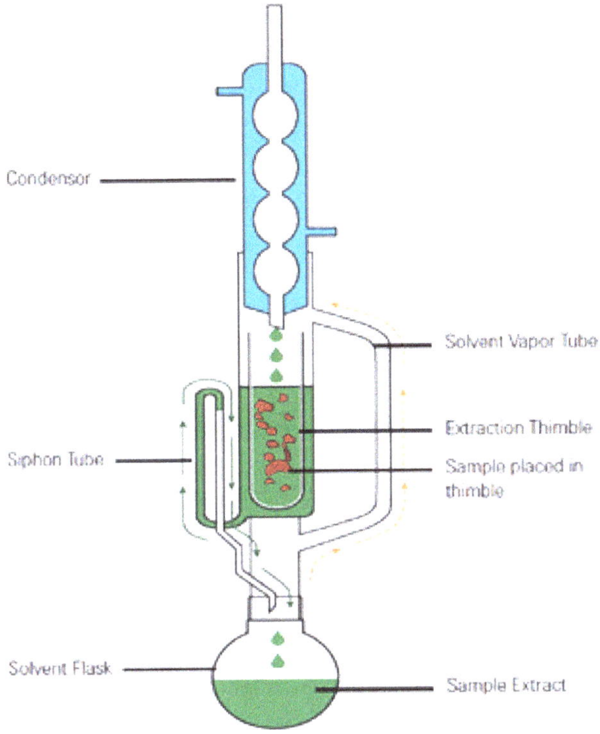

3. Maceration

The meaning of maceration is 'softening'. It is a solid-liquid extraction. The plant material is soaking in a suitable solvent for a long time with shaking. It is a cheap method but require a long time for extraction and is not an eco-friendly method (Cheok et al 2014).

4. Percolation

It is the most frequently used procedure for the extraction of active compounds. The apparatus is a percolator, and it consists of a narrow, cone-shaped vessel open at both ends. The dried and finely powdered material is mixed with solvent in a clean container and allowed to macerate for 24 hrs (Azmir et al 2013).

2.2.2 Modern Extraction Methods

1. Microwave-assisted extraction (MAE)

In this process, microwave energy is used to heat solvents and samples, promoting the partition of a compound of interest. Microwaves are electromagnetic waves and non-ionizing radiations. Their frequency range is from 300 MHz to 300 GHz. Solvent with a high dielectric constant is desirable because it will absorb more microwave energy (Llompart et al 2019). Because of the use of less solvent, it is an environment-friendly method and allows many samples to be analysed simultaneously. In MAE, extraction is possible without solvent or water (Destandau et al 2013).

2. Pulsed electric field (PEF) extraction

It is a non-thermal extraction method. The principle of this method is the disruption of the plant cell membrane by using a high electric field. This electric charge breaks interactions of membrane molecules leading to creating of pores and increasing permeability also called electroporation or electro- permeabilization. This is a desirable method for extracting thermolabile compounds (Pattnaik et al 2021). As the raw material is placed in between two electrodes inside the treatment chamber, the optimization of the process parameters, including pulse number, electric field strength, treatment temperature, and specific energy input is essential (Brito et al 2012). Luengo et al 2013, showed an increase in total phenols from 11.76 to 14.14, 26.92, 29.81, 34.80 mg Gallic acid equivalent/100 g at 1, 3, 5, 7 kV/cm, respectively on PEF treated orange peels. Similarly, Delsart et al in 2012 reported that moderate electric field treatment and shorter duration (40–100 ms) accelerated the release of phenolic compounds and anthocyanins across the cell membrane.

3. Ultrasound-Assisted Extraction (UAE)

Ultrasound extraction is one of the modern methods and the extraction of bioactive compounds. The frequency of ultrasound waves is higher than 20 kHz. This high energy creates cavitation bubbles which leads to rupture of cell membrane and release of bioactive compounds. The solvent will interact with the bioactive compounds and leads to extraction (Kumar et al 2021). The efficiency of this method is high due to some mechanisms like material fragmentation, erosion, sonicapillary effects, sonoporation, etc. (Gómez-López et al 2021).

4. Pressurized Liquid extraction (PLE)

In PLE high pressure is applied to prevent the vaporization of solvents at a higher temperature. Because of this high pressure and temperature, the solvent will effectively penetrate through the sample. This will lead to the extraction of the compound of interest. The benefits of PLE are less solvent consumption, more efficiency than classic methods, and shorter extraction time. Automation is possible in this extraction (Li et al 2012). This method is unsuitable for thermolabile compounds, and the selectivity of extraction is less (Celeste et al 2014).

5. Enzyme Assisted Extraction (EAE)

It is one of the eco-friendly methods which extract bioactive compounds by the action of enzymes on cell walls under optimum conditions. In most cases, water is used as a solvent. It requires low temperature and energy. This method is suitable for extracting phytochemicals inside the cell, like polyphenols (Lemes et al 2022).

6. Supercritical Fluid Extraction (SFE)

Supercritical fluids have temperature and pressure above the critical point. They are in mesophase because of their fluid-like and gas-like properties (Khaw et al 2017). Supercritical CO2 (SC CO2) is less expensive, nontoxic, preserves extracts from oxidation, and its critical temperature is 31.3°C. SC CO2 is used for the extraction of thermolabile compounds due to its user-friendly critical temperature (Awad et al 2021). Due to its non-polar nature, co-solvents are also required to extract polar compounds. For the extraction of anthocyanins, ethanol and methanol are co-solvents (Tena & Asuero 2022). The other properties of supercritical fluid for fast extraction are their high diffusivity and low density, viscosity, and surface tension compared to other solvents (Anticona et al 2020). Castro-Vargas HI et al in 2010 isolated phenolic components from the seeds of Psidium guajava L., family Myrtaceae, using carbon dioxide. Supercritical fluid extraction is used to remove physiologically active chemicals from plant matter, primarily those that can't be separated by a straightforward solvent extraction method (Agnieszka et al 2013).

Figure 3. Supercritical fluid extraction (https://www.researchgate.net/profile/Waseem-Gul3/publication/233604150/figure/fig1/AS:341220330098690@1458364674640/Fig-1-Supercritical-fluid-extraction-SFE-diagram.png)

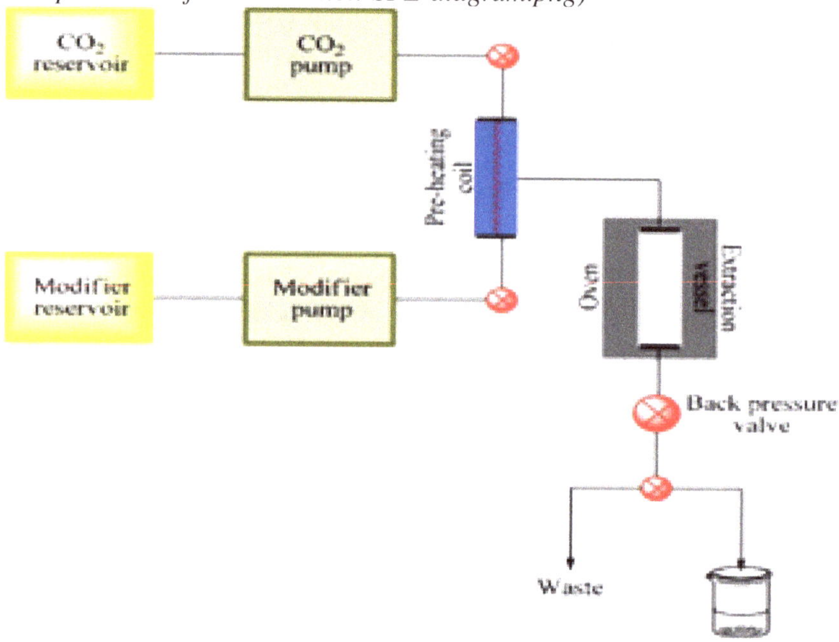

2.2.3 Fractionation, Purification and Isolation

While different techniques have evolved for the extraction of the phytoconstituents to obtain crude extracts (complex mixtures), fraction mixtures) and isolated (pure) components from natural sources.

Quantitative methods involved in isolation and detection of plant secondary metabolite

With an increasing trend towards natural product research due to many opportunities, modernization of analytical tools and availability of validated method, a wide spectrum of analytical methods has been developed for application in phytochemical research, pharmacological studies and quality control of secondary metabolites from plants. The analytical approaches can be classified as (i) the analysis of targeted compounds, i.e. specifically one compound or (ii) group-specific analysis, i.e. the analysis of several (preferably all) compounds belonging to that group, and metabolite profiling.

The following are some analytical techniques used for the study of secondary metabolites in plants.

3. CHROMATOGRAPHIC TECHNIQUES (PRINCIPLE, APPLICATION AND CASE STUDY IN PLANTS)

Chromatography is the most widely used separation technique in laboratories, where it can be explored for analysis, isolation, and purification of secondary metabolites from plant sources. Chromatography has developed over the past century from a straightforward method of pigment separation to intricate processes used to address the most challenging analytical and purification problems in separation science, such as phytochemistry (Marston 2007). Analytes move through the stationary phase at different speeds, which causes them to separate from a complex mixture. This is the fundamental idea behind the chromatographic process. The different compounds have different properties, such as absorption, solubility, ion exchange, and affinity, which can be controlled and explored through various separation mechanisms (Bellot and Condoret 1993). The primary function of the stationary phase is to retain or arrest analyte movement and that of the mobile phase is to force and hold the analyte to move from through the chromatographic system to the exit of the column (Ichi Kasai 1992).

3.1 Paper Chromatography

Paper chromatography is one of the oldest methods used for analysis of secondary metabolites since 1958, 228 flavonoids have been analysed using various solvent systems in various proportions. For the identification of secondary metabolites by paper chromatography, Whatmann, Schieicher and Schull paper and others are most often used. The solvents used are water, respectively aqueous solutions of organic acids, butanol and mixtures of organic acids, neutral mixtures of organic solvents with low polarity, water and methanol. The hydrophilic systems are used for the separation of glycosides, and the lipophilic ones for the separation of aglycones. The most used solvent systems, in various proportions like ethyl-methyl-ketone: acetone: formic acid: water; methyl isobutyl ketone: formic acid: water; chloroform: methanol: formic acid: water; and benzene: methanol: water (Chen et al 2022).

Aqueous solutions of polyvalent metals can be used for detection (lead acetate, aluminium chloride, etc. give colour reactions), solutions of sodium carbonate, methanolic sodium hydroxide, ethanolic solution of ferric chloride, Rhodamine B solution, p-Toluenesulfonic acid. For example, Flavones, such as apigenin, kaempferol, quercetin give blue or grey-blue spots, while all the corresponding glycosides give yellow to yellow brown spots (Xu et al 2022).

3.2 Thin Layer Chromatography

TLC was the most common, versatile method of choice for analysis before other instrumental chromatography methods. TLC is used as an easier method of initial screening with a semi quantitative evaluation together with other chromatographic techniques as there is relatively less change in the simple TLC separation. Thin-layer chromatography is a technique in which an analyte undergoes distribution between two phases, a stationary phase acting through adsorption and a mobile phase in the form of a liquid. The adsorbent is a relatively thin, uniform layer of dry finely powdered material applied to a glass, plastic or metal sheet or plate. Glass plates are most used. Separation may also be achieved based on the partition or a combination of partition and adsorption, depending on the support, its preparation and its use with different solvent (Gong et al 2003). Identification can be affected by observation of spots of identical Rf value and about equal magnitude obtained, respectively, with an unknown and a reference sample chromatographed on the same plate. A visual comparison of the size and intensity of the spots usually serves for semi-quantitative estimation. The approach TLC provides aesthetic effects, but it is also simple and inexpensive. Samples may be analysed in parallel, sample capability is great, and conclusions are produced quickly. TLC is adaptable, allowing for various identification. TLC bioautography can be used to test for biologically active compounds in association with microbes and other biological agents. TLC has several drawbacks, including occasional repeatability issues, and a lack of quantification precision (Kasote et al 2015).

3.3 High Performance Thin Layer Chromatography

HPTLC is a fast separation technique and flexible enough to analyse a wide variety of samples. This technique is advantageous in many means as it is simple to handle and requires a short analysis time to analyse the complex or the crude sample cleanup. HPTLC evaluates the entire chromatogram with a variety of parameters without time limits. There is a simultaneous but independent development of multiple samples and standards on each plate leading to increased reliability of results. Another advantage of HPTLC is the repeated detection (scanning) of the chromatogram with the same or different conditions (Dhalwal et al 2008). Various workers have developed HPTLC method for phytoconstituents in crude drugs or herbal formulations such as bergenin, catechine and gallic acid in Bergenia cilliata and Bergenia lingulata (Abourashed & Mossa 2004), quercetin-3-O-β-D-rhamnoside in Euphorbia hirta (Saxena et al 2000) and curcumin in herbal formulations (Scott 1995). Jug et al in 2021 used the offline multidimensional HPTLC for fractionation and isolation of flavan-3-ols, proanthocyanidins, and anthraquinones derivates from Japanese knotweed rhizome bark extract. The disadvantages of HPTLC are that it is relatively more expensive than TLC, and separation occurs only up to a certain length due to the limited plate length.

3.4 Column Chromatography

Column chromatography is one of the most useful methods for the separation and purification of both solids and liquids. This is a solid-liquid technique in which the stationary phase is solid, and the mobile phase is a liquid. The principle of column chromatography is based on differential adsorption of substance by the adsorbent. The usual adsorbents employed in column chromatography are silica, alumina, calcium carbonate, calcium phosphate, magnesia, starch, etc., selection of solvent is based on the nature of both the solvent and the adsorbent. The rate at which the components of a mixture are separated depends on the activity of the adsorbent and the polarity of the solvent. The adsorbent is made into a slurry with a suitable liquid and placed in a cylindrical tube that is plugged at the bottom by a piece of glass wool or porous disc. The mixture to be separated is dissolved in a suitable solvent and introduced at the top of the column and is allowed to pass through the column. As the mixture moves down through the column, the components are adsorbed at different regions depending on their ability for adsorption. The component with greater adsorption power will be adsorbed at the top and the other will be adsorbed at the bottom. The different components can be desorbed and collected separately by adding more solvent at the top and this process is known as elution. The weakly adsorbed component will be eluted more rapidly than the other. The different fractions are collected separately. Distillation or evaporation of the solvent from the different fractions gives the pure components. Intermolecular forces, which vary in strength according to their type, make organic molecules bind to the stationary phase. The stronger the intermolecular force, the stronger the binding to the stationary phase, therefore the longer the compound takes to go through the column (Porsch B 1994).

The following adsorbents are used: magnesol, silica gel, cellulose or polyamide powder, calcium sulfate, Sephadex LH-20, Sephadex G-10, G-25 and G-50. Methanol and ethanol are used for the elution of proanthocyanidins, and acetone for the separation of high molecular weight polyphenols. Al_2O_3 is not a good adsorbent for the separation of flavonoids, because it forms stable compounds with them. It is used for the separation of some flavonols by elution with dilute acid or acidic methanol. Polyamide is preferred, because it allows the separation of phenols and their derivatives, polyhydroxyphenols, flavones, flavanones, quinones and tannins.

The adsorbed substance is eluted by replacing it with a solvent. The most used solvents for elution are water, methanol, ethanol, acetone, dilute alkaline solutions, formamide and dimethylformamide. The detection was carried out in UV at 350 nm, and the identification of the components was done with the help of two-dimensional thin layer chromatography (Sun et al 2018).

3.5 High-Performance Liquid Chromatography (HPLC)

High Performance Liquid Chromatography HPLC is the most significant advancements in chromatography. It is a separation and purification method used to obtain compounds with a high purity. Prior to HPLC, open columns required a lot of tasting and were time-consuming, expensive, and labour-intensive. Paper chromatography and TLC could be used to analyze very small samples. However, there was still a lack of quantification, and it was difficult to determine the function of similar molecules. Using HPLC, steroids, alkaloids, and antibiotics were all examined (Costa et al 2015). HPLC can not only explore but can also isolate secondary metabolites.

Reverse-phase HPLC (RP-HPLC) is the most used HPLC mode; the stationary phase is less polar than the eluting solvent. A common RP-HPLC stationary phase is surface-modified silica. The eluent used in RP-HPLC is usually a mixture of water and a miscible organic solvent. Yingyue et al in 2020 used Sephadex column chromatography and semi-preparative RP-HPLC to purify rutin after extraction from banana leaves. After the liquid–liquid extraction process, the authors purified the fraction by using a Sephadex column. As a result, the purity of rutin was 74–84%. Then, they further purified rutin by using semi-preparative RP-HPLC. The final rutin was 98.4% pure. Based on these results, semi-preparative RP-HPLC can enhance the purity of isolated compounds (Yingyuen et al 2020). Molo et al 2021 used C18, GS-320 columns to purify phenolic compounds from a subfraction of *Chaerophyllum bulbosum* extract.

The advantages of HPLC lie in its versatility for the analysis of the secondary metabolites but the detection of non chromophoric compounds becomes difficult. Consequently, a marked increase in the use of HPLC analysis coupled with evaporative light scattering detection (ELSD) in a recent decade demonstrated that ELSD is an excellent detection method for the analysis of nonchromophoric compounds. This new detector provides a possibility for the direct HPLC analysis of many pharmacologically active secondary metabolites High performance liquid chromatography (HPLC) is a technique that offers accuracy, speed and high sensitivity.

3.6 Medium Pressure Liquid Chromatography

MPLC is one of a wide variety of preparative column chromatography techniques. Separation under pressure allows the use of smaller particle-size supports, increasing the variety of stationary phases that can be used (Hostettmann & Terreaux 2000). The instrumentation of MPLC consists of a pump for the mobile phase, a sample injection system, and a self-packed stationary phase (column). Compound separation can be followed automatically by detectors and recorders connected to the outlet of the column or monitored manually by thin-layer chromatography, then collected via a fraction collector (Hostettmann & Terreaux 2000). Although MPLC can be used to isolate a compound, it is generally used to enrich bioactive compounds (secondary metabolites) from natural products before further purification because of its low cost, high sample load, and high throughput. Six phenolic compounds (gallic acid, catechin, rutin, naringenin, quercetin and isoramnetin) were separated by this method. The operation pressure used in MPLC is 75–300 psi (Rahman 2018). The MPLC system can be applied to adsorption, partition, affinity, or ion-exchange chromatography. Dang et al 2021 purified bergenin from *Saxifraga atrata* extract. Bergenin is a compound that is derived from trihydroxybenzoic acid (phenolic acid) and has a glycoside attached to it (Salimo et al 2023). MPLC allows purification of large compound quantities Unlike open column chromatography it is faster and improved separations are obtained.

3.7 Counter Current Chromatography CCC

CCC a form of liquid–liquid partition chromatography that uses two immiscible liquids. One phase is maintained as the stationary phase in the absence of an adsorption matrix. The second phase passes through the stationary phase and is efficiently equilibrated by utilizing a hydrodynamic or turbulent mixture (Ito 2004). The difference compared with other chromatographic systems is that this method does not require solid support: the stationary phase is held in the column by gravity or centrifugal force (Shibuswa & Ito 2000). CCC is divided into hydrostatic and hydrodynamic equilibrium systems.

In general, the CCC systems have advantages compared with HPLC and MPLC: they do not require a solid column, there is low solvent consumption, there is no irreversible loss of sample because chemosorption can be avoided, there is higher sample recovery, and a high load capacity. However, CCC systems require time, especially to optimize the solvent system, and instability of the solvent system may occur (Bárcenas-Pérez et al 2021).

3.8 Hydrophilic Interaction Liquid Chromatography Hydrophilic Interaction Liquid Chromatography

or HILIC is a type of partition chromatography that uses a polar stationary phase. The partition occurs between a non-polar or organic region in the mobile phase and a polar water-enriched layer at the surface of the polar stationary phase (Hage 2018). Several stationary phases, including silanol-derivatized phases such as amino-, amide-, cyanopropyl-, carbamate-, diol-, and polyol-, have been developed for HILIC (Berlinck et al 2021). Dang et al in 2018, isolated the antioxidant phenolic compound from *Dracocephalum heterophyllum* using an offline two-dimensional reversed phase/hydrophilic interaction liquid chromatography (2D RP/HILIC) technique.

3.9 Size Exclusion Chromatography

Size-exclusion chromatography is a type of partition chromatography, used to separate molecules based on their sizes. Separation is achieved by the differential exclusion or inclusion of solutes as they pass through stationary phase consisting of heteroporous (pores of different sizes) cross linked polymeric gels or beads. The process is based upon different permeation rates of each solute molecule into the interior of gel particles. Size exclusion chromatography involves gentle interaction with the sample, enabling high retention of biomolecular activity. For the separation of biomolecules in aqueous systems, SEC is referred to as gel filtration chromatography (GFC), while the separation of organic polymers in non-aqueous systems is called gel permeation chromatography (GPC)(Werner et al 1994). Naringin a flavonoid that act as antioxidant and anticancer, has been successfully isolated from pomelo peel extract using Sephadex®LH-20 with higher purity ($95.7 \pm 0.23\%$) (Stabrauskiene et al 2021). Other phenolic compounds have also been successfully separated with Sephadex®LH-20, including quercetin and (2R)-eriodictyol in mulberry fruit extract (Xu et al 2020).

3.10 Supercritical Fluid Chromatography (SFC)

Supercritical fluid chromatography (SFC) is a separation method that uses compressed gas above the critical temperature/pressure instead of organic solvent. SFC is a green separation technique that uses mostly supercritical carbon dioxide as the mobile phase, with the eluting power controlled by the addition of organic solvent as an organic modifier. This method is known for its low operational cost and is considered an environmentally friendly alternative. This method has been applied to separate curcumin, demethoxy curcumin, and bisdemethoxycurcumin directly from turmeric on a preparative scale. After a single step of supercritical fluid chromatography separation, 20.8 mg of curcumin (97.9% purity), 7.0 mg of demethoxy curcumin (91.1%), and 4.6 mg of bisdemethoxycurcumin (94.8%) were obtained with a mean recovery of 76.6% (Song et al 2015). SFC was utilized in the first dimension to prepare the lignin fractions, while RPLC was employed in the second dimension to produce high-purity lignin compounds. This method has advantages such as high loading ability, and short time analysis (Yang et al 2017).

3.11 Gas Chromatography (GC)

GC, also known as gas-liquid chromatography (GLC), is a technique for the separation of mixtures into components by a process that depends on the distribution of the components between a stationary phase or support material in the form of a liquid, solid, or combination of both and a gaseous mobile phase. It is well-known that many pharmacologically active components in plant extract can be volatile chemical compounds. Thus, the analysis of volatile compounds by gas chromatography is very important in the analysis of volatile secondary metabolites. The first attempts to separate simple phenols by gas-liquid chromatography date back to 1968 but results regarding phenols with a more complex structure were published in 1962, when results were reported regarding the analysis of 36 flavonoids using as a phase liquid silicone polymer SE-40. This method allowed the separation, isolation and identification of milligram quantities of these compounds, but the question of the influence of methylation, acetylation and hydrogen bonds arose. Using SE-30 liquid phase, He (Helium) as gas phase, it was found that: as the number of substituents increases. Increasing the temperature brings some advantages but simultaneously increases the danger of decomposition of the injected compounds. The identification of flavonoids, especially trimethylsilyl flavonoids and their aglycones, was carried out using the OV series of silicone polymers as the liquid phase. Thus, to identify the ethers of trimethyl flavonoids, a column of silicone polymers SE-30 was used, for the identification of anthocyanidins. The flavonoids quercetin, hesperetin, kaempferol, naringenin, Wagonin and Baicalein (5,6,7-trihydroxyflavone) were identified on several types of columns (Sharifi-Rad et al 2021).

3.12 Ultra Performance Liquid Chromatography

In 2004, separation science was revolutionized with the introduction of Ultra-Performance Liquid Chromatography (UPLC). The UPLC system allows shortening of analysis time up to nine times compared to the conventional system using 5 μm particle packed analytical columns. The separation on UPLC is performed under very high pressures (up to 100 MPa is possible in the UPLC system), but it has no negative influence on the analytical column or other components of the chromatographic system. An additional benefit of UHPLC is the low consumption of the mobile phase, where it saves at least 80% compared to HPLC (Nitin Verma 2021). Advantages as enhanced separation efficiency, short analysis time and high detection sensitivity make UHPLC coupled with MS/MS an even more powerful analytical support in pharmacokinetic studies (Nitin Verma 2021).

3.13 Monolithic Chromatography

The use of a single rod monolith column is an alternative approach to the chromatographic columns packed with fine particles. The high permeability allows the use of higher flow rates and therefore shorter chromatographic runs. High flow rates may require flow splitting before entering MS. An attractive approach using monolith separation is to combine it with high flow online extraction, which allows fast extraction and separation of samples (Liu et al 1993). Current limitations in the application of these columns are the small pH range2-8, poor temperature resistance, limited column dimensions and stationary phases (C8 and C18) as well as higher costs due to higher mobile phase consumption.

Different types of chromatography undoubtedly provide thorough information about secondary plant metabolites, but they require meticulous sample preparation and take a lot of time. In situations where many samples need to be examined or where prompt identification is necessary (such as in the event of suspected forgery), techniques that minimize analysis time and expenses are sought for. To quickly evaluate sample similarity for quality control, new analytical techniques are being developed to either supplement or replace traditional methods.

4. SPECTROSCOPIC AND SPECTROMETRIC TECHNIQUES

From the variety of solutions that modern analytical techniques offered spectroscopy is one of the fast and cheap analytical technique. Spectroscopy is the branch of science dealing with the study of interaction of electromagnetic radiation with matter like atoms and molecules. The interaction of electromagnetic radiations (EMR) with matter gives rise to two types of spectra namely atomic spectra and molecular spectra. Atomic spectrum arises from the transition of electrons from one energy level to another due to changes of energy in the atom. Molecular spectrum involves transition of electrons between rotational and vibrational energy levels in addition to electronic transition. Hence molecular spectroscopy is of great use in determining the structure and constitution of compounds.

4.1 UV-Visible Spectroscopy

A spectrophotometer is an instrument which uses monochromatic light and measures the absorbance of various solutions at different wavelengths. This instrument scans the entire UV-visible regions. In a double beam spectrophotometer, radiation from hydrogen lamp or tungsten lamp enters the monochromator, which produces very narrow band widths. The beam is then passed through a reference cell and the sample cell by means of rotating mirrors. The photomultiplier tube is used as a detector which receives alternate pulses of radiation from the reference and sample beam.

The various phytochemicals including flavonoids, alkaloids, carbohydrates and protein were found to be present in the extract of *Senna Alexandrina* by the spectroscopic studies showing the characteristic peaks obtained in Ultraviolet - Visible region. the phytochemical profile showed the occurrence of peaks with in the 234-800 nm range of UV, which confirms the presence of phenolics, flavonoids and alkaloids in the leaf extract of *Senna alexandrina* (Masarrat et al 2021).

4.2 Vibrational Spectroscopy (IR Spectroscopy)

Vibrational spectroscopy is due to the interaction of matter with the Infra-red region of the electromagnetic spectrum. Quantum Approach Irradiation of sample with IR radiation brings about vibrational changes in molecules. The transition of molecule is from lower vibrational energy level to higher vibrational energy level. The transition is induced by absorption of photon of the IR radiation of appropriate frequency, which matches with energy gap between the two levels. IR absorption by molecules happens only when there is a change in the dipole moment of the molecule.

4.3 Fourier Transform Infrared Spectroscopy

Fourier transform infrared (FTIR) spectroscopy is a measurement technique that allows one to record infrared spectra. The sample is exposed to infrared light after it has passed through an interferometer (or vice versa). Infrared light that travels through the interferometer is distributed differently by a moving mirror inside the device. "Interferogram" is the term for the directly recorded signal that shows light output as a function of mirror position. A data-processing technique called Fourier transform turns this raw data into the desired result (the sample's spectrum): Light output as a function of infrared wavelength (or equivalently, wave number). However, the sample's spectrum is always compared to a reference (Nitin Verma 2021). FTIR spectrum confirmed the presence of terpenoids and polyphenols in *C. Pictus (*Jothi & Muthu 2024*).*

4.4 Raman Spectroscopy

Raman spectroscopy is an analytical technique where scattered light is used to measure the vibrational energy modes of a sample. It is named after the Indian physicist C. V. Raman who, together with his research partner K. S. Krishnan, was the first to observe Raman scattering in 1928. Raman spectroscopy can provide both chemical and structural information, as well as the identification of substances through their characteristic Raman 'fingerprint'. Raman spectroscopy extracts this information through the detection of Raman scattering from the sample. Raman spectroscopy is quick to perform and requires little pretreatment (drying) of samples (Jones 2018).

4.5 Nuclear Magnetic Resonance (NMR) Spectroscopy

Nuclear Magnetic Resonance (NMR) spectroscopy takes advantage of the magnetic properties of certain nuclei and records the absorption of energy between quantized nuclear energy levels. In an NMR experiment, the spectrometer is tuned to the frequency of a particular nucleus and the spectrum reveals all such nuclei in the molecule being investigated. The characterization of various secondary metabolites can be performed using 1D and 2D NMR experiments. Multiplicity information cannot be efficiently collected in complex mixtures or natural product extracts, due to overlapping signals. Computer-assisted structure elucidation (CASE) has been developed for chemical structure elucidation using 1D and 2D NMR data (Elyashberg & Argyropoulos 2021). Mahar et al in 2022, utilized homonuclear and heteronuclear 2D NMR experiments to identify alkaloids in the alkaloidal fraction of the different parts of *Alstonia scholaris*.

4.6 Mass Spectrometry (MS)

Mass spectrometry (MS) is an analytical chemistry technique that helps identify the amount and type of chemicals present in a sample by measuring the mass-to-charge ratio and abundance of gas-phase ions. The fundamental process of mass spectrometry involves three main steps:

i. Ionization: Conversion of sample molecules into gas-phase ions.
ii. Mass Analysis: Separation of ions based on their mass-to-charge ratio (m/z).
iii. Detection: Measurement of the quantity of ions at each m/z value.

4.6.1 Ionization

Several ionization techniques are used in mass spectrometry, each suited for different types of samples and applications.

1. **Electrospray Ionization (ESI)**: ESI is widely used for analysing large biomolecules. A solution containing the analyte is sprayed through a fine needle, creating a mist of charged droplets. As the solvent evaporates, ions are formed. Electrospray ionization is by far the preferred method for metabolite identification and quantification (Kebarle 2000). It is the most universal technique for introducing the molecules into the gas phase and it is most gentle and therefore likely to yield intact molecular ions. ESI is ideally suited for polar, ionic and thermally labile compounds. This technique requires ionization of analytes within solution prior to introduction into ion source and thus works best for fairy basic or acidic compounds. Depending on the voltage polarity, nebulised droplets trapping the ionized analyte will be positively or negatively charged. The reduction in size caused by solvent evaporation accounts for the increase in charge density in the droplet leading to its explosion when repulsive forces between charges exceed the cohesive forces of the droplet. This process occurs repeatedly until gas phase ions are produced. Ions in solution are emitted into gas phase without application of heat making ESI suitable for analysis of thermolabile compounds. Many parameters, such as analyte and solution characteristics: pKa, analyte concentration, other electrolytes in solution, dielectric constant of the solvent, affect the ion formation process (Kamel & Prakash 2006).
2. **Matrix-Assisted Laser Desorption/Ionization (MALDI)**: In MALDI, the sample is mixed with a matrix material and deposited on a target plate. A laser pulse vaporizes the matrix, transferring energy to the analyte molecules and producing ions from large molecules with minimal fragmentation. It has been used to measure the molecular weight of biomacromolecules such as peptides, proteins, nucleic acids, molecular weight distribution of polymers, and oligomer analysis. It has extended the traditional mass spectrometry technology mainly for small molecule research to analyse the range of highly polar, hardly volatile, and thermally unstable samples. Furthermore, post-translational changes, such as phosphorylation, are typically retained by ionized proteins and peptides. When using the MALDI technique, it is necessary to use a crystallising organic compound called matrix, which assists in sample ionisation under a UV laser beam (Nakashima et al 2020). When used in conjunction with MS imaging, MALDI is a quick and sensitive method that enables both the chemical analysis of metabolites and the observation of their distribution (Seaman et al 2014).

The advantage of this method is the simplicity of sample preparation without the need to isolate compounds selected for analysis from the tissue fragments

Figure 4. A schematic diagram of MALDI (Dreisewerd, K. 2014)

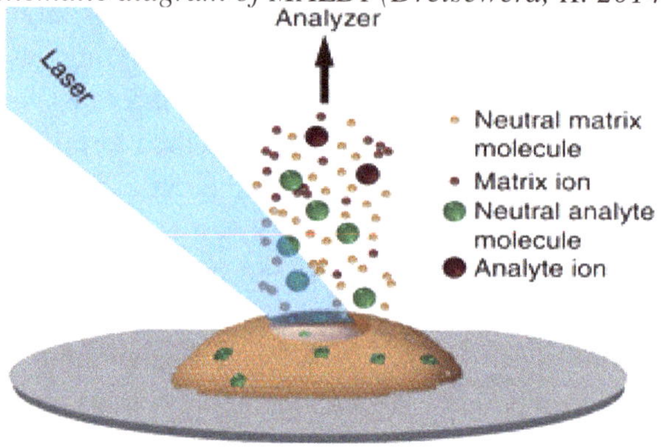

3. **Electron Ionization (EI):** EI is commonly used for small organic molecules. The sample is vaporized and bombarded with electrons, causing ionization through electron impact. In electron Impact technique molecules of the carbon compounds in the vapour state (gas phase) are bombarded with a beam of energetic electron (nearly 70ev). The molecules are ionized and broken up into many fragments. The result of this bombardment is recorded as a spectrum of positive ions separated based on m/z ratio. A parent ion results when one electron is removed from the parent molecule of the substance. The molecular ions have usually the highest m/e value in this spectrum and its m/e value is equal to the molecular mass of the compound. The molecular ion is usually not much stable and tends to fragment. The fragmentation of molecular ion produces daughter ion of definite m/e value which help in structure determination (Sharma 2010)
4. **Chemical Ionization (CI):** CI involves ion-molecule reactions, it relies on a reagent gas to assist in the ionization process of the compounds of interest. A reagent gas is ionized, and these ions subsequently ionize the sample molecules. Typical reagent gasses commonly used in CI are ammonia, methane, and isobutene. CI uses these reagent gasses as intermediates in the ionization process (Munson & Field 1966). The number molecules composing the reagent gas is far greater than the compounds of interest being detected. Initially, the reagent gas becomes ionized and through a cascade of chemical steps, ionizes the compounds of interest. This ionization transfer greatly reduces the energy

absorbed by the compounds of interest. CI is often considered a "soft ionization" because after ionization, the original molecular mass of the compound of interest is generally left intact.

4.6.2 Mass Analyzers

The function of mass analyzer is the separation of ions formed in ionization source according to their different mass-to-charge (m/z) ratios. The quality of mass separation is characterized by the degree to which close m/z values can be separated in the mass analyzer. The selection of suitable analyzer is driven by the purpose of the analysis and the instrument performance but also depends on the instrument availability and cost effectiveness. The design of modern analyzers has changed significantly in the last few years, now offering much higher accuracy, increased sensitivity, broader mass range, and the ability to give structural information. Because ionization techniques have evolved, mass analyzers have been forced to change to meet the demands of analyzing a wide range of bio-molecular ions with part per million mass accuracy and sub femtomole sensitivity (Scripps Center for Metabolomics, 2017). Mass analyzers separate ions based on their mass-to-charge ratios. Common types of mass analyzers include:

1. **Quadrupole Mass Analyzer:** Quadrupole Mass Analyzer uses oscillating electric fields to filter ions. Quadrupole mass analyzers consist of two pairs of metal rods equidistant from each other and biased at equal and opposite potentials. These twin potentials contain a fixed direct current (DC) and alternating radio frequency (RF) component, where the strength of the RF component can be varied. Any ion entering the quadrupole will have its trajectory deflected by the potential in a manner that is proportional to its m/z value. At specific RF values, only one specific m/z value will resonate with the field and be able to navigate to the end of the quadrupole and be detected. Ions with other m/z values will collide with the quadrupoles, lose their charge and not be detected (Voo et al 1997).

Figure 5. A quadruple filters charged species based on their specific charge. For a given configuration of the driving voltages and quadrupole geometry, only the particles of a certain specific charge are contained within the device and therefore transmitted (Quadrupole Mass Filters – The Velasquez Group)

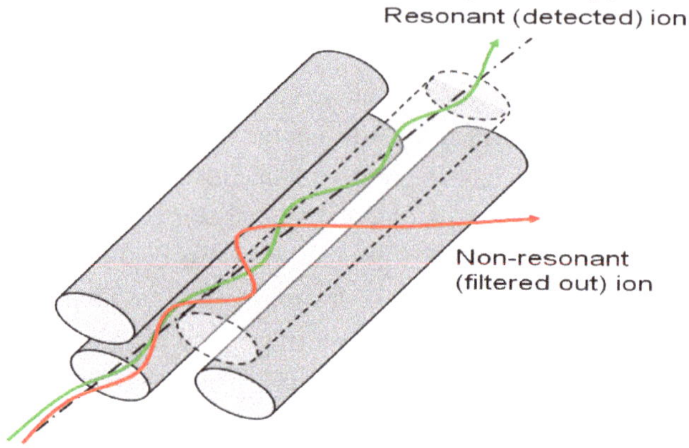

2. **Triple quadrupole instruments (QQQ)** are the most common mass spectrometers in analytical laboratories, having most often been acquired for their evident strengths in high sensitivity quantitative analysis of known analytes. In QQQ, the first quadrupole filters ions of interest, the second quadrupole also called collision cell fragments these ions and further the fragment ions are filtered by third quadrupole before reaching the mass detector. Such QQQ configuration allows performing different scans such as full scan, product ions can, precursor ion scan (PI), constant neutral loss scan (CNL), single ion monitoring (SIM) and selected reaction monitoring (SRM) or multiple reaction monitoring (MRM). PI and CNL are particularly useful in metabolite identification since both scanning modes do not require previous knowledge about the molecular weight of metabolites. High sensitivity for quantitative purposes is retained only when working in MRM mode, however, the detection sensitivity decreases dramatically when wide mass range is analyzed in a scanning mode.
3. **Time-of-Flight (TOF) Mass Analyzer**: Measures the time it takes for ions to travel a known distance. TOF analyzers provide high resolution and are frequently used with MALDI. These analyzers are the most suitable high resolution mass spectrometers for fast and cost-efficient metabolite identification. TOF are relatively simple and capable of recording all formed ions on a microsecond time scale offering high sensitivity detection. Ions are accelerated from the ion interface to a fixed kinetic energy and then pass through a field-free tube to the detector. The time needed for ion to reach the detector is proportional

to its m/z ratio. TOF strength lies in its very high detection sensitivity when acquiring wide range data, enabling the simultaneous detection of data for all metabolites of interest in one run. High mass resolution and mass accuracy (< 3-5 ppm) enable reliable and accurate identification of metabolites by determination of elemental formula of a metabolite. Additionally, the very high acquisition speed makes them ideal for fast chromatography. In the study by He et al 2022, time-of-flight secondary ion mass spectrometry (TOF-SIMS) image analysis technology was employed for the first time to investigate the distribution of metabolites in the cross-section of Coptis rhizome. This study successfully imaged and quantified the spatial distribution and content of nine active compounds, revealing an increase in these compounds with the growth years of the rhizome. Gong et al's 2023 study shed light on the spatiotemporal variations of *P. amurense* alkaloids, providing a crucial foundation for further research on the genes or enzymes involved in biosynthetic pathways and the specific functions of alkaloids in plants.

4. **Ion Trap Mass Analyzer:** Traps ions in a dynamic electric field and sequentially ejects them to a detector. Ion traps can perform multiple stages of mass spectrometry (MSn). Ion trap mass analysers are like QQQ relatively inexpensive and compatible with wide range of ionization interfaces. These analyzers utilize ion trap chamber where ions are trapped and then selectively ejected from the chamber. Additionally, the resonance excitation applied in the trap provides efficient dissociation of the precursor ions to product ions. It provides more sensitivity for structural elucidation than QQQ due to its better sensitivity in full scan mode and efficient dissociation of the precursor ions which allows multiple stages mass spectrometry (MSn).
5. **Triple quadrupole-linear ion traps (QTrap)** combine sensitive QQQ technology with high capacity of linear IT incorporating high trapping efficiencies. In this instrument, the last quadrupole of QQQ is replaced with a linear ion trap, which operates as a mass resolving quadrupole or a linear ion trap. This provides clearly increased metabolite screening capabilities compared to traditional IT or QQQ. QTrap enables high sensitivity, wide range mass scanning and MSn together with QQQ capabilities, such as PI, CNL and very high sensitive MRM data acquisition.
6. **Fourier Transform Ion Cyclotron Resonance (FT-ICR) Mass Analyzer:** Uses a magnetic field to trap ions and measures their cyclotron frequencies. FT-ICR offers ultra-high resolution and accuracy. Fourier transform-ion cyclotron resonance (FT-ICR) is the third high resolution mass analyzer. The high sensitivity, accurate mass measurements, high mass resolution and MS/MS capabilities of FT-ICR make it attractive for structural determination of ions. However, the combined requirement of ultra-high vacuum system, super conducting magnets

as well as sophisticated data system place the cost of these instruments beyond the means of most laboratories involved in drug metabolism studies.

7. **Orbitrap Mass Analyzer:** Orbitraps provide high resolution and mass accuracy, like FT-ICR. It traps ions in an electrostatic field and measures their oscillation frequencies. The Orbitrap consists of two electrically isolated cup-shaped outer electrodes facing each other and a spindle-like central electrode that holds the trap together. When voltage is applied between the outer and the central electrodes, the resulting electric field is linear along the axis, while the radial component of the field strongly attracts ions to the central electrode. Ions are injected or pulsed into the volume between the central and outer electrodes tangentially through a slot machined in one of the outer electrodes. As the electric field is increased by ramping the voltage on the inner electrode, ions get squeezed towards the inner electrode until they reach the desired orbit inside the trap. At that moment, the electric field is held constant, and the field becomes static. The injected ions will move with different rotational frequencies but with the same axial frequency. This means that ions of a specific mass-to-charge ratio spread into rings that oscillate or orbit along the inner spindle (Figure 6).

Figure 6. Schematic diagram of orbital ion trajectories in an Orbitrap and example resulting mass spectrum (Hofmann et al, 2020)

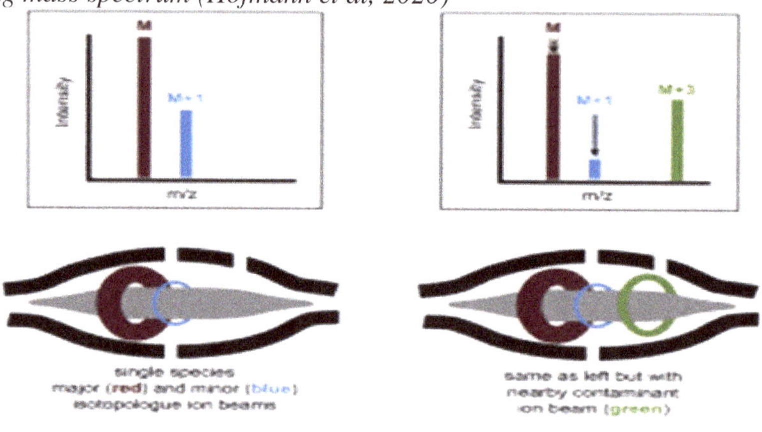

4.6.3 Detection

Ion detection is the last stage in mass spectrometry. Ion hits are transformed by detectors into electrical signals, which are further processed to provide a mass spectrum. The detector of a mass spectrometer is essential for the separated charged ions. The results are displayed as spectra that illustrate the relative abundance of the identified ions as a function of the mass-to-charge ratio. High amplification, fast time response, low noise, high collection efficiency, low cost, narrow response distribution, same response for all masses, large dynamic range, long-term stability, long life, and, if possible, the ability to be mounted outside of the vacuum are all desirable features for a detector used in a mass spectrometer (Sharad 2018). Common detectors include:

1.Ion Detectors

1.1. Electron Multiplier

Ion signals coming from a mass spectrometer's mass analyzer are detected using an electron multiplier. The function of the electron multiplier is to detect each ion of the selected mass that makes it through the mass filter. The basic physical process that allows an electron multiplier to operate is called secondary electron emission. Secondary electrons are released from atoms in the surface layer when a charged particle, such as an ion or an electron, collides with the surface (Ohring 1995). The number of secondary electrons released depends on the type of incident primary particle, its energy and characteristic of the incident surface.

1.2. Faraday Cups

The Faraday cup is named after the name of Michael Faraday who first theorized ion around 1830. An electrometer that measures the ion beam current is connected to the metal cup that is placed in the path of the beam. The basic principle is that the incident ions strike the dynode surface which emits electrons and induces a current which is amplified and recorded. In a cup the ions entered and transfer their charge to the cup (Maithal & Muralidhar 2002). Charge is usually transferred to electronics outside the vacuum system.

1.3. Photographic Plates

Photographic plate integrates the ion signals over time. The photo plates are processed by the usual photographic techniques and read with the aid of densitometer. It can detect ions of all masses simultaneously and provides reverse-geometry. This detector is generally used with radiofrequency spark instruments (Potts 1987). Despite being the simplest and oldest type of detector, it can be used in plane-focusing instruments and detect all ions. The intensity of the mark on the film is proportional to the abundance of the ions. When the ion strikes the plate, they leave the dark tracks on plate when the plate is developed (Khatri et al 2012).

1.3. **Scintillation Counter**

Scintillation Counter detects and quantifies the excitation caused by ionizing radiations. The detection and measurement of this excitation is known as scintillation and the instrument which detects the light using a photo multiplier is known as scintillation counter. The electron pulse which is detected by the photomultiplier is a result of conversion of light into electrical energy (Sharad 2018). The modern electronic scintillation counter, invented in 1944 by Sir Samual Curran counts with two different techniques: Solid Scintillation (external) counting and liquid scintillation counting (integral). In solid scintillation counting the sample is placed close to a floor crystal (crystallized silver activate zinc sulphides) for alpha emitters; sodium iodide for gamma emitters; anthracene or stilbene for beta emitters; which in turn placed adjacent to a photomultiplier. This photomultiplier is connected to a high voltage supply and a scalar. In liquid scintillation counting the radioactive sample is suspended in a scintillation system composed of solvent and appropriate scintillator. This technique is extremely useful for quantitation of soft beta emitters. The radioactive sample is dissolved or suspended in a scintillation system composed of solvent and primary and secondary scintillators. The radiation from the suspended sample molecule collides with a solvent molecule imparting a discrete amount of its energy to the solvent molecules. The solvents used in LS counting are ethanol, acetone, ethyl glycol, dimethyl ether, 1,4 dioxane, xylene, methoxybenzene (anisole) and toluene (Sharad 2018).

1.5. **Channel Electron Multipliers**

A channel multiplier is a tube of suitably resistive material, with a length which is large compared to its diameter. A vacuum potential of a few thousand volts is supplied between the ends of the multiplication channel. Electrons or other energetic particles striking the low voltage end of the channel release secondary electrons with some initial energy which carries them across the channel. The electrons are accelerated axially by the applied electric field as they move through the channel, and they collide with the wall with enough energy to release more secondary electrons. This process is repeated many times so that a very large number of electrons emerge from the output end. The pulse initiated by a single electron may in certain circumstances contain more than 10^9 electrons. Numerous factors, including the applied voltage, residual gas pressure, tube resistance and shape, and pulse repetition rate, affect the gain that can be obtained from a channel. A channel multiplier amplifies direct currents and counts energetic particles by producing corresponding pulses (Adams and Manley 1966).

2. **Conversion Dynodes**

Conversion dynode is used to increase the secondary electron emission characteristic for high mass ions and reduce the mass discrimination of the detector. It is a simple metal separate surface which can be held at a high voltage at 3 to 20kV or more. The potential of dynode serves to accelerate the ions to a point where good conversion efficiency for either electrons or secondary ions occurs. The channel electrons multipliers used to detect the secondary electrons emitted from the dynode surface. It is used to detect the positive ions, or the conversion products are thought to be the lower mass ions and electrons. The high negative potential on the dynode surface servcs to direct electrons towards the channel electrons multipliers input which is held at a low negative potential. A high positive potential on the Conversion Dynode will not produce many secondary electrons being collected by the channel electrons multipliers since the dynode will tend to recapture electrons (HEJNA 2008). They are as follows.

1. **Helium leak detectors**

This is a helium-specific partial pressure analyser. It detects the helium applied as a tracer or probe gas. It consists of a mass spectrometer tube tuned on helium. Its own vacuum system capable of 10-5 mbar in the spectrometer tube. A sensitive and stable amplifier valve and auxiliary pumps for interfacing to vacuum system. A display used for monitoring leak rates.

Sensitivity is 10-10mbar or better. A helium leak detector permits the localization of leaks and the quantitative determination of the leak rates, i.e. the gas flow through the leak. Such a leak detector is therefore a helium flow meter. In practice the leak detector performs this task by firstly evacuating the part which is to be tested so that the gas from the outside may enter through an existing leak duc to thc prcssurc difference present if there is a leak then helium can enter into the system from the leak (for example by using a spray gun). This helium flows into the leak detector and is detected (INFICON 2007).

3 Advanced Detectors

With the use of conventional electron multipliers one of the limitations of the mass spectrometry its poor efficiency with small biomolecules. To solve this problem, alternative detection schemes which works on heat pulse detection is developed. When ion strike a detector, the kinetic energy of striking ions converted into heat and then measures indirectly such heat pulse. Developing a type of cryogenic detector called superconducting tunnel junction device which produces photons when ions strike the detector (Masataka et al 2014).

4. Cryogenic Detectors

Most calorimeters used in high energy physics measure the energy loss of a particle in form of ionization (free charges) or scintillation light. However, a large fraction of the deposited energy in form of heat remains undetected. The energy resolution of these devices is therefore mainly driven by the statistical fluctuations of the number of charge carriers or photoelectrons involved in an event. In contrast, cryogenic calorimeters can measure the total deposited energy including the heat in form of phonons or quasi-particles in a superconductor. With the appropriate phonon or quasi-particle detection system much higher energy resolutions can be obtained due to the very large number of low energy quanta (meV) involved in the process. This feature makes cryogenic calorimeters very effective in the detection of very small energy deposits (eV) with resolutions more than an order of magnitude better than for example semiconductor devices (Pretzl 2020).

Multi Pixel Photon Counter

The Multi Pixel Photon counter (MPPC) is developed by HAMAMATSU PHOTONICS K. K. and it is one of the products of Si-PM (Silicon Photo multiplier) family which was originally developed in Russia. It is designed as photon counting device based on structures of a Si APD which was adopted by CERN (CMS). This device is a solid-state photon counter having Multi pixelated Geiger-mode APDs with self-quenching resistance (Zhang et al 2018). MPPC is an excellent photon counting device as it is compact, insensitive to magnetic field, High gain (~106), low bias voltage (~70V) and its low cost. Since each pixel exist in two states "Fired" and "not fired" the MPPC have multi-pixel structure. By counting number of Fired pixel one can know number of photons injected into the detector

Photonis Bipolar Maldi Tof Detector

These detectors improve the detection efficiency of very high mass of ions. It has large 250 mm^2 collection area which allows higher sensitivity without the need for higher post acceleration voltage. It consists of a highly sensitive microchannel plate, a photomultiplier and a high-speed scintillator which can detect both positive and negative ions with 30 kV isolation (Lee et al 2011). This detector has advanced design in ion source and mass spectrometry technology that Provides soft ionization in rugged design. This detector attains a new level of sample insight through speed, confirmatory analysis and high sensitivity.

The information contained in a single mass spectrum, recorded using very small amounts of sample, will often allow the unambiguous identification or structural elucidation of an unknown compound. The development of ionisation techniques that do not require the sample to be liquefied before ionisation has made mass spectrometric analysis possible for a wide range of biomedical and biological molecules. The high sensitivity and specificity of the mass spectrometer are enhanced by using a gas chromatograph as the mass spectrometer inlet (Sharad 2018).

5. HYPHENATED TECHNIQUES

The term "hyphenation" was first adapted by Hirsch Feld in 1980 to describe a possible combination of two or more instrumental analytical methods in a single run. The coupling of chromatographic techniques and spectroscopic techniques makes hyphenated techniques more attractive and widely applicable in almost all fields of science, biology, geography, engineering, agriculture, etc. While chromatographic techniques produce pure or almost pure chemical constituents in mixtures, spectroscopic techniques produce selective information to identify components using library spectra or standards. Hyphenated techniques can be double or triple techniques combined (Chinaza Godswill Awuchi et al 2023).

5.1 Advantages Of Hyphenated Technique

The ability to identify species other than the expected compounds is the main benefit of hyphenated speciation approaches (Patel et al 2010).

1. Shorter analysis time Higher degree of automation
2. Higher sample throughput
3. Better reproducibility
4. Reduction of contamination because it is a closed system
5. Enhanced combined selectivity and therefore higher degree of information.

Figure 7. Types of hyphenated techniques

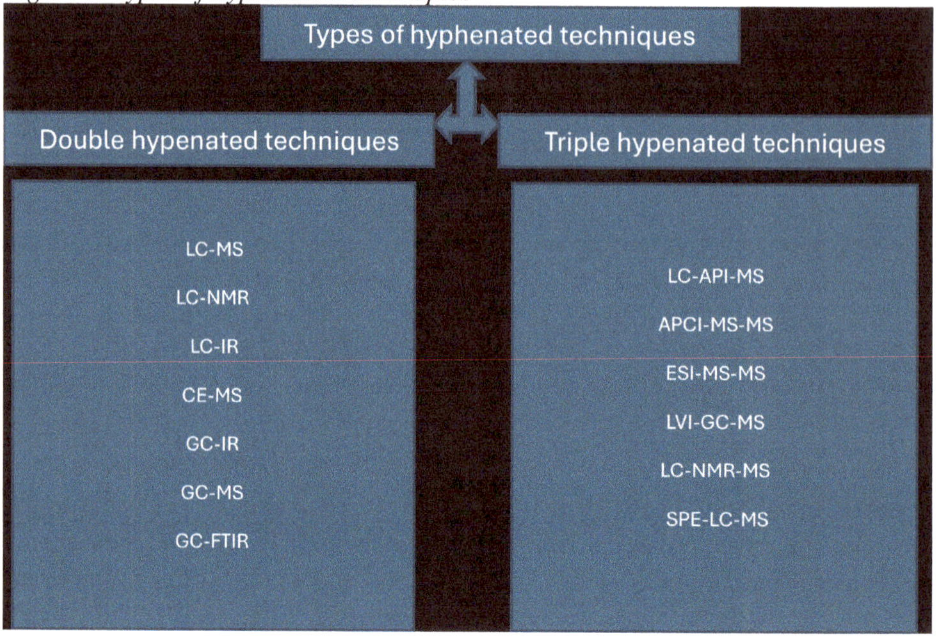

1. **Gas Chromatography-Mass Spectrometry**

Gas chromatography is a separation technique applicable to compounds which can be volatilised in a gas stream. Mass spectrometry is the most sensitive and selective method for molecular analysis and can yield information on the molecular weight as well as the structure of the molecule. Combining chromatography with mass spectrometry provides the advantage of both chromatography as a separation method and mass spectrometry as an identification method. In mass spectrometry, there is a range of methods to ionize compounds and then separate the ions. Common methods of ionization used in conjunction with gas chromatography are electron impact (EI) and electron capture ionization (ECI). GC–MS was the first successful online combination of chromatography with mass spectrometry and is widely used in the analysis of essential oil in herbal medicines. With the GC–MS, not only a chromatographic fingerprint of the essential oil of the herbal medicine can be obtained but also the information related to its most qualitative and relative quantitative composition (Kadhim et al 2016).

Instrumentation and Working

Figure 8. GC-MS (Patel et al, 2010)

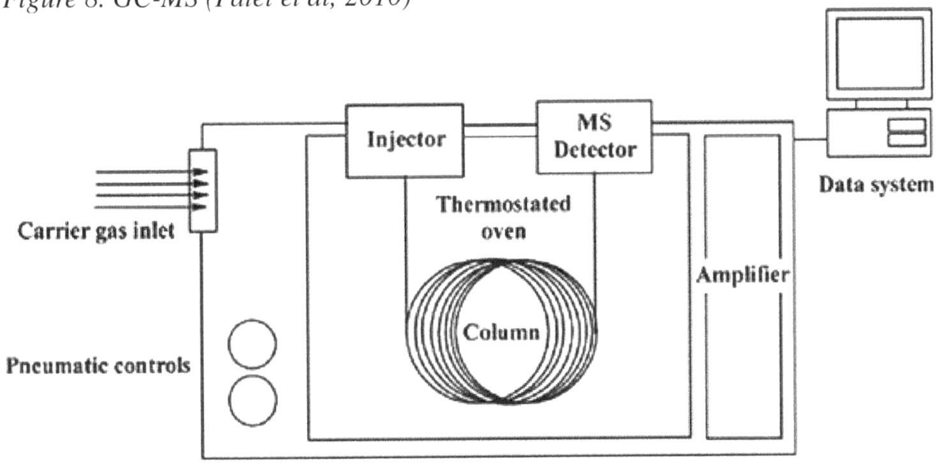

Vaporized analyse when carried through the GC column with the help of heated carrier gas the separation occurs in the column, only the carrier can also be called as the mobile phase(helium). The interactions between analyte, mobile phase, and stationary phase lead to separation of the compounds. The separation of the analyte also depends on the column's dimensions (length, diameter, and film thickness), type of carrier gas, column temperature (gradient) and the properties of the stationary phase. The sample travel through the column the difference in the boiling point and other chemical properties lead to separation of the components of the mixture. The components have differences in elution time and retention time due to their different adsorption or difference in the partition between the mobile phase and the stationary phase. This is followed by ionization, mass analysis and detection of mass-to-charge ratios of ions generated from each analyse by the mass spectrometer. An interface like effusion separator, jet/orifice separator & membrane separator can be used to connect GC with MS.

Advantages Of GC-MS

1. GC having the high-resolution power to compare other methods.
2. This method having high sensitivity when used with thermal detectors.
3. This technique having separation and analysis of sample very quickly samples with less quality is also operated.
4. This technique having relatively good accuracy and precision.

Disadvantages

1. In GC only volatile samples (or) the sample with can be made volatile and are separated by this method.

2. During injection of the gasses sample, proper attention is required (Righetti, et.al 2000).
3. **Liquid Chromatography and Nuclear Magnetic Resonance**

The combination of liquid chromatography (LC) and nuclear magnetic resonance (NMR) offers the potential of unparalleled chemical information from analytes separated from complex mixtures. Several other hyphenated NMR techniques have been developed to enhance sensitivity of this technique. LC-SPE-NMR increases the sensitivity of the instrument by utilizing a solid phase extraction device after LC column. Capillary LC-NMR also practically lowers detection limit to a nano-gram range through integration of capillary LC with NMR detection. Generally, in LC-NMR system, the LC unit comprises autosampler, LC pump, column, and a non-NMR detector (e.g., UV, DAD, EC, refractive index, or radioactivity). From this detector, the flow is guided into the LC-NMR interface, which can be equipped with additional loops for the intermediate storage of selected LC peaks. The flow from the LC-NMR interface is then guided either to the flow-cell NMR probe-head or to the waste receptacle. Following passage through the probe-head, the flow is routed to a fraction collector for recovery and further investigation of the various fractions analysed by NMR. An MS can also be attached to the system via a splitter at the output of the LC-NMR interface.

Figure 9. A typical LC-NMR system (Patel et al 2010)

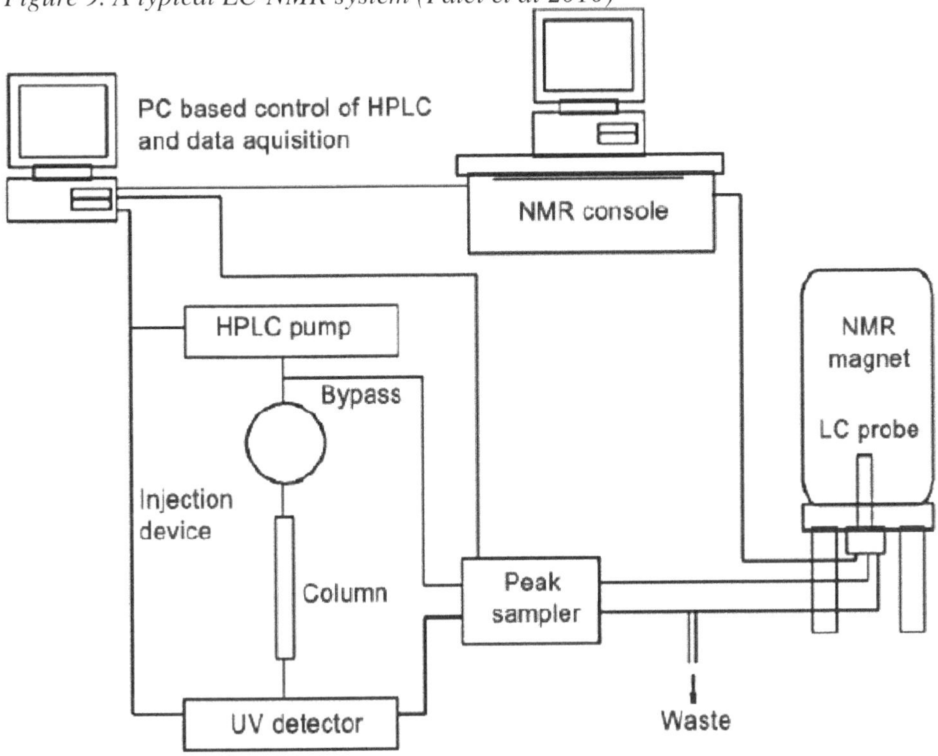

4. Liquid Chromatography- Mass Spectrometry

A typical automated LC-MS system consists of double three-way diverter in-line with an autosampler, an LC system, and the mass spectrometer. The diverter generally operates as an automatic switching valve to divert undesired portions of the eluate from the LC system to waste before the sample enters the MS. An LC-MS combines the chemical separating power of LC with the ability of an MS to selectively detect and confirm molecular identity. MS is one of the most sensitive and highly selective methods of molecular analysis and provides information on the molecular weight as well as the fragmentation pattern of the analyte molecule. LC-MS or HPLC-MS refers to the coupling of an LC with a mass spectrometer (MS) . The separated sample emerging from the column can be identified based on its mass spectral data. A switching valve can help make a working combination of the two techniques. A typical automated LC-MS system consists of double three-way diverter in-line with an autosampler, an LC system, and the mass spectrometer. The diverter generally opcrates as an automatic switching valve to divert undesired portions of the eluate from the LC system to waste before the sample enters the MS. An LC-MS combines the chemical separating power of LC with the ability of an MS to selectively detect and confirm molecular identity. MS is one of the most sensitive and highly selective methods of molecular analysis and provides information on the molecular weight as well as the fragmentation pattern of the analyte molecule. The information obtained from MS is invaluable for confirming the identities of the analyte molecules.

This qualitative analysis makes it possible to reconstruct an unknown compound from MS data. The use of LC-MS-MS is increasing rapidly. Hyphenated techniques such as HPLC coupled to UV and mass spectrometry (LC-UV-MS) have proved to be extremely useful in combination with biological screening for a rapid survey of natural products.

Figure 10. Schematic of an LC-MS (electrospray ionization interface) system (Patel et al 2010)

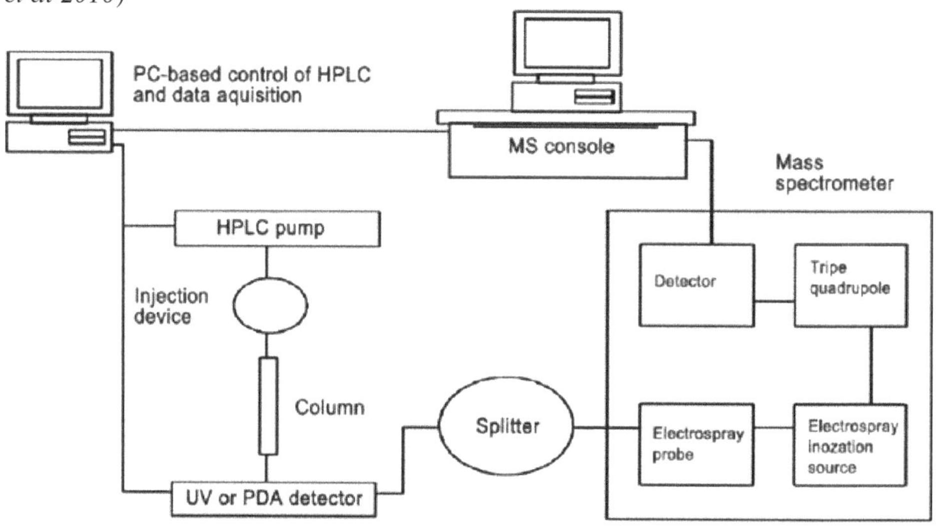

5. **Ultra-performance liquid chromatography/quadrupole time-of-flight mass spectrometry**

This application describes a novel approach to plant drug metabolism using UPLC coupled to a hybrid quadrupole orthogonal time of flight (Q-TOF) mass spectrometer. As technology progresses, better levels of detection are obtainable not only via a more sensitive assay but through better quality data. Using UPLC with QTOF-MS adds a new dimension to metabolism studies of natural products, enabling attainment of better detection limits, better throughput, and increased chromatographic resolution, which in turn will improve data quality from the mass spectrometer.

6. LC-IR (Liquid Chromatography- Infrared Spectroscopy)

The hyphenated technique developed from the coupling of an LC and the detection method infrared spectrometry (IR) or FTIR is known as LC-IR or HPLC-IR. While HPLC is one of the most powerful separation techniques available today, the IR or FTIR is a useful spectroscopic technique for the identification of organic compounds, because in the mid-IR region the structures of organic compounds have many absorption bands that are characteristic of particular functionalities, e.g., -OH, -COOH, and so on. However, a combination of HPLC and IR is difficult and the progress in this hyphenated technique is extremely slow because the hyphenated technique's 237 absorption bands of the mobile phase solvent are so huge in the mid-IR region that they often obscure the small signal generated by the sample components (Londhe 2008).

Table 2. Hyphenated techniques for secondary metabolites in plant extracts

S. No.	plant	Active component	Hyphenated techniques used	Reference
1	*Rhodolirium andicola*	Galanthamine-type alkaloids such as lycoramine, galanthaminonand 3-O-acetyl-1,2-dihidro-galanthamine, galanthamine (A), haemanthamine (B, C) and tazettine(D)	GC-MS	(Felipe Moraga-Nicolás et al 2017)
2	*Harrisia adscendens*	β-carboline alkaloid	FT-NMR	(George Luís et al 2017)
3	*Cyperus rotundus L*	alkaloids, phenols, flavonoids, and terpenes	GC-MS	Russell A.Abo-Altemen etal 2019
4	*Digitalis purpurea* (Foxglove) plant	Digitoxin and digoxin -cardiac glycosides	LC/MS/MS	(Xiaoning Lu, et al 2010)

continued on following page

Table 2. Continued

S. No.	plant	Active component	Hyphenated techniques used	Reference
5	*B. forficata* subsp. *pruinosa*	Quercetin O-glycoside derivatives	LC/ESI-MS	(Lidiane et al 2014)
6	*Moringa peregrina* (Forssk.) Fiori leaves	polyphenols steroids, alkaloid, carbohydrate glycosides, cardiac glycosides, and terpenoids	GC-MS	(Al- Owaisi et al 2014)
7	Nigella species (*Nigella arvensis, Nigella damascena, Nigella hispanica, Nigella nigellastrum, Nigella orientalis, N. sativa*)	10 flavonoids, 6 phenolics, 10 alkaloids	UPLC–MS and GC–MS	(Mohamed A. Farag et al 2014)
8	*Panax ginseng*	Ginsenosides a group of polysaccharide derivatives	UPLC-QTOF-MS/MS	Wenjing Yu et al 2022
9	*Cynodon Dactylon*	Glycosides	HPLC, LC-MS, H1-NMR, FTIR	Bagewadi et al 2014
10	Bark Extract Of *Nothapod ytes Nimmonia na*	Cardiac Glycosides (Cardenolid es), Glycosides	UV, FTIR, HPLC	Patil Anita et al 2014
11	*Corydalis* species	oxygenated protoberberine alkaloids	LC–MS and LC–NMR	Kinuko Iwasa et al 2003
12	*Paullinia cupana*	methylxanthine alkaloids	LC-MS/MS	Novaki, L. P. et al 2023
13	radish (*Raphanus sativus*)	glucosinolates and their derivatives	ultra-high-performance liquid chromatography-high-resolution tandem mass spectrometry (UHPLC-HRMS/MS) and UHPLC coupled to triple quadrupole MS (UHPLC-QQQ-MS)	Yan et al. 2023
14	*Magnolia denudata* flower	Sixteen compounds including flavonoids, phenylethanoid glycoside derivatives (PhGs), caffeoylquinic acids (CQAs)	ultra performance liquid chromatography coupled with a hybrid quadrupole orthogonal time-of-flight mass spectrometer (UPLC-Q-TOF/MS/MS)	Joo et al 2020

6. EMERGING ANALYTICAL TECHNIQUES

6.1 Metabolomics Approaches

Metabolomics represents a field of study with the identification and quantification of the metabolites present in plant systems. A Metabolome is made up of a large variety of molecules such as peptides, amino acids, nucleic acids, carbohydrates, organic acids, vitamins, flavonoids, polyphenols, alkaloids, minerals or any other chemical compound that is used, metabolized or synthesized by a cell or by a given organism. Plant metabolomics, a rapidly advancing field within plant biology, is dedicated to comprehensively exploring the intricate array of small molecules in plant systems. Several analytical methodologies utilized in plant metabolomics research can be implemented in both targeted and untargeted approaches. The targeted strategy involves precise quantification and identification of specific metabolites, employing sophisticated techniques such as Gas Chromatography-Mass Spectrometry (GC–MS), Liquid Chromatography-Mass Spectrometry (LC–MS), Capillary Electrophoresis Mass Spectrometry (CE-MS), and Ion Mobility Mass Spectrometry (IMS). These methodologies enable accurate measurement and validation of known metabolites, facilitating the elucidation of specific pathways and their regulatory mechanisms within plant systems. However, untargeted metabolomics utilizes high-throughput techniques to profile a broader spectrum of metabolites, including both known and unknown compounds (Kumar et al 2024).

A metabolomic analysis comprises three main experimental stages: (1) preparation of the sample, (2) acquisition of the data using analytical methods and (3) data mining using chemometric methods followed by compound identification.

Figure 11. Key steps of a plant metabolomics study. Additional steps can be performed or modified in certain approaches based on the analytical methods or point of interest (Salem et al 2020)

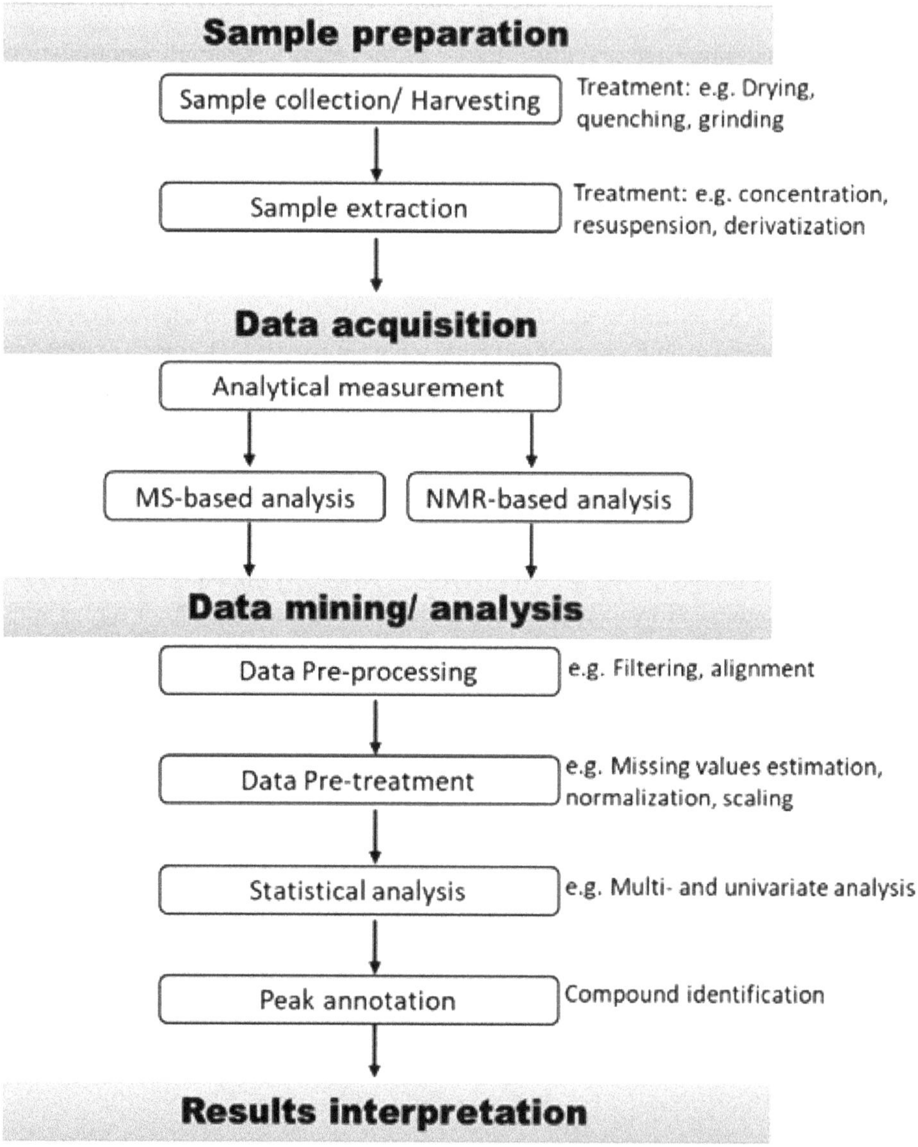

Furthermore, the complex and intricate nature of metabolomics data necessitates the application of advanced statistical and bioinformatics tools to extract valuable insights from the vast amount of generated data, uncovering patterns, correlations, and meaningful connections that help elucidate the biological context underlying the metabolomic profiles. Integration of metabolite analysis with statistical and bioinformatics methods is commonly employed by researchers to uncover the beneficial pharmacological functions of plant secondary metabolites in humans. Le Anh Minh Nguyen & Thu Huong Pham in 2024 described the volatile and non-volatile chemical profile of the dried leaves of Chinook hop grown in southern Italy through an exhaustive analysis of the metabolome performed by combining multiple analytical tools (SPME/GC–MS, PTR-ToF-MS, and NMR).

6.2 Artificial Intelligence in Data Analysis

Role of AI in Enhancing Analytical Techniques

Artificial intelligence (AI) is an exponentially expanding field poised to transform the landscape of analytical chemistry (Mousavizadegan et al 2023). Within this expansive domain, various specialized branches have emerged to confront intricate challenges. Based on type of learning, AI can be elaborated as ML (Machine Learning) and DL (Deep Learning). Machine learning (ML) empowers computers to learn and predict from large amounts of data (Big Data) (L.M. Petrick & N. Shomron 2022). ML models and algorithms are trained on the data collected in the lab and then used to make predictions on novel samples. Deep learning (DL) on the other hand is an advanced facet of ML, which harnesses artificial neural networks (ANN) inspired by the complexity of the human brain, enabling tasks such as nuanced image recognition. Other AI tools involve natural language processing (NLP), which facilitates seamless communication between computers and human languages, fuelling advancements in speech recognition and machine translation, computer vision (CV), which imparts machines with the ability to comprehend images and videos, and robotics, a pivotal arm of AI, is dedicated to the design and operation of robots, utilizing algorithms to handle tasks ranging from navigation to sophisticated manipulation. It is important to note that these branches of AI are not mutually exclusive. For example, many deep learning algorithms are also machine learning algorithms. Additionally, many AI applications use techniques from multiple branches of AI such as an open-source or commercial software, which might use DL algorithms to identify regions of interests (ROIs) contour images within the data acquired from comprehensive two-dimensional gas chromatography coupled to mass spectrometry (GC × GC-MS) (S.E. Reichenbach 2022), CV algorithms to evaluate the chromatographic fingerprint of the acquired samples images, and ML algorithms to develop supervised predictive models. Undoubtedly, the most promising application of AI in analytical chemistry is ML, whose algorithms and models are exploited for data (pre)processing, unsupervised data analysis (explorative models), supervised data analysis (classification and regression models) and design of experiment (DoE). AI algorithms serve as powerful tools, automating tasks, enhancing the precision of analytical methods, and pioneering novel techniques, especially in the -omics research. Multidimensional chromatography (MDC) techniques are powerful tools for separating and identifying these components, but it generates large and complex datasets whose interpretation can be challenging. Therefore, AI algorithms are usually exploited to ease or possibly automate the analysis of these datasets and identify patterns and trends that would be substantially impossible to detect by manual inspection (B.J. Pollo et al 2021).

6.3 Microfluidics and Lab-on-a-Chip

Miniaturization of Analytical Processes

The miniaturization of analytical methodologies reduces dimensions of conventional analytical systems. The micro-total analysis system (lab-on-a-chip, LOC), first proposed by Manz et al in 1990, has developed rapidly in recent decades as a new technology platform. As an important supporting technology of LOC, microfluidic technology is a new technology platform that uses microtubes (tens to hundreds of micrometers in size) to process or manipulate tiny fluids (nanoliters to liters in volume). The experimental platform integrating microfluidic drive, control, reaction, and detection is called microfluidic system.

Figure 12. The composition of microfluidic system and the structure of microfluidic chip (Cao & Chen 2025)

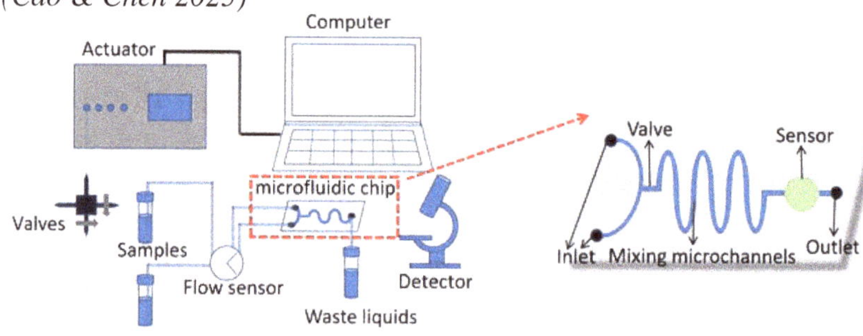

A microfluidic system is usually composed of fluid drive subsystem, process monitoring and control subsystem, microfluidic chip, and detection and analysis subsystem. Fluid drive subsystem, as the name suggests, is the part that provides driving force for the fluid to move forward in the system, usually composed of microfluidic drive pumps. Commonly used drive pumps include pressure pumps, injection pumps, and peristaltic pumps. In addition, other driving forces such as electro-osmosis, capillary force, and gravity can also drive the fluid forward. The process monitoring and control subsystem is usually composed of flow sensors and valves, which is used to achieve a variety of fluid control such as flow feedback control, sequential injection, circulation injection, and volume quantification. Common fluid control methods are electroosmotic control and microvalve control, including passive valve control and active valve control (Cao & Chen 2025). Microfluidic chip is the core of microfluidic technology, on which researchers manipulate the fluid flow and accelerate the reaction process with the help of surface tension, fluid resistance, and energy dissipation (Zhang et al 2016). These microfluidic chips made of silicon, glass, polymer materials, and paper have microchannels inside and exits/entrances connected with the outside, which can integrate the process of sample preparation, pretreatment, separation, and detection and promote the miniaturization, integration, and automation of the whole process of sample detection. The detection and analysis subsystem are used to observe, record, and analyze the reaction on the microfluidic chip and detect and amplify the signal generated by the microfluidic chip, usually with the help of high-precision equipment such as a high-speed CCD, microscope, or spectrometer. At present, the detection of microfluidic chips mainly uses spectrum, mass spectrometry, and electrochemical detectors. The entire working process of the microfluidic system is as follows. First, under the control of the pump and valve, the reagents and samples enter the microfluidic chip through the inlet to react. The signals caused by the reaction are then detected by a detector. Finally, the waste liquids are discharged through the control of the pump and valve (Cao & Chen 2025).

6.4 Biosensors

Biosensor is a general term applied to many technologies to describe a molecule, organism, or device in a biological context that couples the sensing of a specific molecule of interest (analyte) or biological process to the emission of a quantifiable signal. The term *bio* can imply a biological component of the biosensor or simply that it is incorporated into a biological system (Alford et al 2013). Idealized requirements for a sensor are that it (*a*) is highly selective for a specific analyte or biological process; (*b*) enables a quantitative readout over biologically meaningful spatial, temporal, and concentration ranges; (*c*) exhibits a high signal-to-noise ratio; and (*d*) does not perturb the biological process that it measures or the biological system in which it is integrated. Biosensors offer a nondestructive alternative to the metabolomics analysis techniques. They offer a highly sensitive, selective tool for real-time measurements of a given metabolite and as such are critical for understanding the turnover (accumulation and dynamics) of a metabolite within individual cells. This may provide valuable information towards a thorough understanding of the metabolite's mechanism of action.

7. FUTURE PERSPECTIVE

Future developments in high-throughput technology, sensitivity, automation, and computational tools will influence analytical methods used to research secondary metabolites in plants. These developments will facilitate the investigation of the intricacies of plant chemistry, improve our knowledge of the synthesis and regulation of secondary metabolites by plants, and open new avenues for medication development, crop improvement, and bioprospecting. These technologies' incorporation into agriculture, industry, and research will keep providing fresh perspectives and uses for secondary metabolites found in plants.

REFERENCES

Abo-Altemen, R., Al-Shammari, A., & Shawkat, M. (2019). GC-MS Analysis and Chemical Composition identification of Cyperus rotundus L. from Iraq. *Energy Procedia, 157*, 1462–1474. DOI: 10.1016/j.egypro.2018.11.311

Abourashed, E. A., & Mossa, J. S. (2004). HPTLC Determination of caffine in stimulant herbal products and power drinks. *Journal of Pharmaceutical and Biomedical Analysis, 36*(3), 617–620. DOI: 10.1016/j.jpba.2004.06.029 PMID: 15522538

Abu-Izneid, T., Rauf, A., Shariati, M. A., Khalil, A. A., Imran, M., Rebezov, M., & Rengasamy, K. R. (2020). Sesquiterpenes and their derivatives-natural anticancer compounds: An update. *Pharmacological Research, 161*, 105165.

Adams, J., & Manley, B. W. (1966). The mechanism of channel electron multiplication. *IEEE Transactions on Nuclear Science, 13*(3), 88–99. DOI: 10.1109/TNS.1966.4324084

Akkol, E. K., Göger, F., Koşar, M., & Başer, K. H. (2008, June 1). Phenolic composition and biological activities of Salvia halophila and Salvia virgata from Turkey. *Food Chemistry, 108*(3), 942–949. DOI: 10.1016/j.foodchem.2007.11.071 PMID: 26065756

Al-Owaisi, M., Al-Hadiwi, N., & Khan, S. A. (2014). GC- MS analysis, determination of total phenolics, flavonoid content and free radical scavenging activities of various crude extracts of Moringa peregrina (Forssk.) Fiori leaves. *Asian Pacific Journal of Tropical Biomedicine, 4*(12), 964–970. DOI: 10.12980/APJTB.4.201414B295

Alford, S. C., Wu, J., Zhao, Y., Campbell, R. E., & Knopfel, T. (2013). Optogenetic reporters. [Google Scholar]. *Biology of the Cell, 105*(1), 14–29. DOI: 10.1111/boc.201200054 PMID: 23126299

Anticona, M., Blesa, J., Frigola, A., & Esteve, M. J. (2020). High biological value compounds extraction from citruswaste with non-conventional methods. *Foods*, •••, 9. PMID: 32575685

Arceusz, A., Wesolowski, M., & Konieczynski, P. (2013). Methods for extraction and determination of phenolic acids in medicinal plants: a review. Natural product communications, 8(12), 1934578X1300801238.

Awad, A. M., Kumar, P., Ismail-Fitry, M. R., Jusoh, S., Ab Aziz, M. F., & Sazili, A. Q. (2021). Green extraction of bioactive compounds from plant biomass and their application in meat as natural antioxidant. *Antioxidants, 10*(9), 10. DOI: 10.3390/antiox10091465 PMID: 34573097

Awuchi, C. G., Twinomuhwezi, H., & Awuchi, C. G. (2022). Hyphenated techniques. In *Analytical Techniques in Biosciences* (pp. 125–145). Academic Press.

Azmir, J., Zaidul, I. S. M., Rahman, M. M., Sharif, K. M., Mohamed, A., Sahena, F., Jahurul, M. H. A., Ghafoor, K., Norulaini, N. A. N., & Omar, A. K. M. (2013). Techniques for extraction of bioactive compounds from plant materials: A review. *Journal of Food Engineering*, *117*(4), 426–436. DOI: 10.1016/j.jfoodeng.2013.01.014

Bagewadi, Z. K., Siddanagouda, R. S., & Baligar, P. G. (2014). Phytoconstituents investigation by LC-MS and evaluation of anti-microbial and anti-pyretic properties of cynodon dactylon. *International Journal of Pharmaceutical Sciences and Research*, *5*(7), 2874.

Bárcenas-Pérez, D., Lukeš, M., Hrouzek, P., Kubáč, D., Kopecký, J., Kaštánek, P., & Cheel, J. (2021). A Biorefinery Approach to Obtain Docosahexaenoic Acid and Docosapentaenoic Acid N-6 from Schizochytrium Using High Performance Countercurrent Chromatography. *Algal Research*, *55*, 102241. DOI: 10.1016/j.algal.2021.102241

Bellot, J. C., & Condoret, J. S. (1993). Modelling of liquid chromatography equilibria. *Process Biochemistry (Barking, London, England)*, *28*(6), 365–376. DOI: 10.1016/0032-9592(93)80023-A

Berlinck, R. G. S., Crnkovic, C. M., Gubiani, J. R., Bernardi, D. I., Ióca, L. P., & Quintana-Bulla, J. I. (2021). The Isolation of Water-Soluble Natural Products—Challenges, Strategies and Perspectives. *Natural Product Reports*, *39*(3), 596–669. DOI: 10.1039/D1NP00037C PMID: 34647117

Bhambere, D., Gaidhani, K., Harwalkar, M., & Nirgude, P. (2015). LYOPHILIZATION / FREEZE DRYING – A REVIEW. *World Journal of Pharmaceutical Research*, *4*, 516–543.

Bharathi, J. K., & Muthu, A. S. P. (2024). Phytochemical screening and quantitative analysis, FTIR and GC-MS analysis of Costus pictus D. Don ex Lindl. Leaf extracts – A potential therapeutic herb. *Journal of the Indian Chemical Society*, *101*(11).

Brito, P. S., Canacsinh, H., Mendes, J. P., Redondo, L. M., & Pereira, M. T. (2012). Comparison between monopolar and bipolar microsecond range pulsed electric fields in enhancement of apple juice ex-traction. *IEEE Transactions on Plasma Science*, *40*(10), 2348–2354. DOI: 10.1109/TPS.2012.2209444

Cao, Q., & Chen, X. (2025). Microfluidics Detection Technologies and Applications. In Dr. M. Oliveira, A. Prof. B. B. Holló, Dr. M. Zafar, Dr. E. H. D. A. Andrade, & Dr. M. M. Radanovic (Eds.), *Advances in Analytical and Coordination Chemistry - Applications and Innovations*. IntechOpen. DOI: 10.5772/intechopen.1008741

Cao, Y., Chen, Z., Sun, L., Lin, Y., Yang, Y., Cui, X., & Wang, C. (2022, August 15). Herb Polysaccharide-Based Drug Delivery System: Fabrication, Properties, and Applications for Immunotherapy. *Pharmaceutics*, *14*(8), 1703. DOI: 10.3390/pharmaceutics14081703 PMID: 36015329

Castro-Vargas, H. I., Rodriguez-Varela, L. I., Ferreira, S. R. S., & Parada-Alfonso, F. (2010). Extraction of phenolic fraction from guava seeds (Psidium guajava L.) using supercritical carbon dioxide and co-solvents. *The Journal of Supercritical Fluids*, *51*(3), 319–324. DOI: 10.1016/j.supflu.2009.10.012

Chaachouay, N., & Zidane, L. (2024). Plant-Derived Natural Products: A Source for Drug Discovery and Development. *Drugs and Drug Candidates*, *3*(1), 184–207. DOI: 10.3390/ddc3010011

Chen, C., Zhao, J., Chen, J., Chi, M., & Liu, Y. (2020). Separation of 3-Hydroxy-3-Methylglutaryl Flavonoid Glycosides from Oxytropis falcata Using 2D Preparative Chromatography. *Journal of Chromatographic Science*, *58*(3), 211–216. DOI: 10.1093/chromsci/bmz091 PMID: 32099992

Chen, Q., Li, J., Ma, Y., Yuan, W., Zhang, P., & Wang, G. Occurrence and biosynthesis of plant sesterterpenes (C25), a new addition to terpene diversity, Plant Communications, Volume 2, Issue 5, 2021, 100184, ISSN 2590-3462, https://doi.org/DOI: 10.1016/j.xplc.2021.100184

Cheok, C. Y., Salman, H. A. K., & Sulaiman, R. (2014). Extraction and quantification of saponins: A review. *Food Research International*, *59*, 16–40. DOI: 10.1016/j.foodres.2014.01.057

Costa, D. C., Costa, H. S., Albuquerque, T. G., Ramos, F., Castilho, M. C., & Sanches-Silva, A. (2015). Advances in phenolic compounds analysis of aromatic plants and their potential applications. *Trends in Food Science & Technology*, *45*(2), 336–354. DOI: 10.1016/j.tifs.2015.06.009

Dang, J., Ma, J., Dawa, Y., Liu, C., Ji, T., & Wang, Q. (2021). Preparative Separation of 1,1-Diphenyl-2-Picrylhydrazyl Inhibitors Originating from: Saxifraga sinomontana Employing Medium-Pressure Liquid Chromatography in Combination with Reversed-Phase Liquid Chromatography. [CrossRef] [PubMed]. *RSC Advances*, *11*(61), 38739–38749. DOI: 10.1039/D1RA05819C PMID: 35493204

Dang, J., Wang, Q., Wang, Q., Yuan, C., Li, G., & Ji, T. (2021). Preparative Isolation of Antioxidative Gallic Acid Derivatives from Saxifraga tangutica Using a Class Separation Method Based on Medium-Pressure Liquid Chromatography and Reversed-Phase Liquid Chromatography. [CrossRef] [PubMed]. *Journal of Separation Science*, *44*(20), 3734–3746. DOI: 10.1002/jssc.202100325 PMID: 34435450

De Monte, C., Carradori, S., Granese, A., Di Pierro, G. B., Leonardo, C., & De Nunzio, C. (2014). Modern extraction techniques and their impact on the pharmacological profile of Serenoa repens extracts for the treatment of lower urinary tract symptoms. *BMC Urology*, *14*, 1–11.

Delsart, C., Ghidossi, R., Poupot, C., Cholet, C., Grimi, N., Vorobiev, E., & Peuchot, M. M. (2012). Enhanced extraction of phenolic compounds from Merlot grapes by pulsed electric field treatment. *American Journal of Enology and Viticulture*, *63*(2), 205–211. DOI: 10.5344/ajev.2012.11088

Destandau, E., Michel, T., & Elfakir, C. (2013). Microwave-assisted extraction. *RSC Green Chemistry*, *c*, 113–156.

Dhalwal, K., Sindhe, V. M., Biradar, Y. S., & Mahadik, K. R. (2008). Simultaneous quantification ofbergenin, catechine, and gallic acid from Bergenia ciliate and Bergenia lingulata by using thin-layer chromatography. *Journal of Food Composition and Analysis*, *21*(6), 496–500. DOI: 10.1016/j.jfca.2008.02.008

Dias dos Santos, G. L.. (2018). Phytochemical study of Harrisia adscendens. *Revista Brasileira de Farmacognosia*, *28*(3), 298–302. DOI: 10.1016/j.bjp.2018.04.011

Dias dos Santos, G. L., Lemos, E. L., Anna, F. C. F., Vieira da Rocha, W. R., Raïssa, M. R. C., Filho, R. B., Tavares, J. F., Fechine, I. M., & Harley da Silva, A. (2018). Phytochemical study of Harrisia adscendens. *Revista Brasileira de Farmacognosia*, *28*(3), 298–302. DOI: 10.1016/j.bjp.2018.04.011

Dreisewerd, K. (2014). Recent methodological advances in MALDI mass spectrometry. *Analytical and Bioanalytical Chemistry*, *406*(9-10), 2261–2278. DOI: 10.1007/s00216-014-7646-6 PMID: 24652146

Elyashberg, M., & Argyropoulos, D. (2021). Computer Assisted Structure Elucidation (CASE): Current and Future Perspectives. [CrossRef]. *Magnetic Resonance in Chemistry*, *59*(7), 669–690. DOI: 10.1002/mrc.5115 PMID: 33197069

Gómez-López, I., Lobo-Rodrigo, G., Portillo, M. P., & Cano, M. P. (2021). Ultrasound-assisted green extraction (Uae) of antioxidant compounds (Betalains and phenolics) from opuntia stricta var. dilenii's fruits: Optimization and biological activities. *Antioxidants*, *10*(11), 10. DOI: 10.3390/antiox10111786 PMID: 34829657

Gong, F., Liang, Y. Z., Xie, P. S., & Sung, A. J. (2003). Information theory applied to chromatographic fingerprint of herbal medicine for quality control. *Journal of Chromatography. A*, *1002*(1-2), 25–40. DOI: 10.1016/S0021-9673(03)00648-4 PMID: 12885076

Gong, Q., Aoki, D., Matsushita, Y., Yoshida, M., Taniguchi, T., Endoh, K., & Fukushima, K. (2023). Microscopic distribution of alkaloids in freeze-fixed stems of Phellodendron amurense. *Frontiers in Plant Science*, *14*, 1203768.

González-Coloma, A., López-Balboa, C., Santana, O., Reina, M., & Fraga, B. M. (2011). Triterpene-based plant defenses. *Phytochemistry Reviews*, *10*(2), 245–260. DOI: 10.1007/s11101-010-9187-8

He, F., Huang, Y. F., Dai, W., Qu, X. Y., Lu, J. G., Lao, C. C., & Zhou, H. (2022). The localization of the alkaloids in Coptis chinensis rhizome by time-of-flight secondary ion mass spectrometry. *Frontiers in Plant Science*, *13*, 1092643.

Hejna, J. (2008). Application of channel electron multipliers in an electron detector for low-voltage scanning electron microscopy. *Journal of Microscopy*, *232*(2), 369–378. DOI: 10.1111/j.1365-2818.2008.02108.x PMID: 19017236

Hofmann, A. E., Chimiak, L., Dallas, B., Griep-Raming, J., Juchelka, D., Makarov, A., & Eiler, J. M. (2020). Using Orbitrap mass spectrometry to assess the isotopic compositions of individual compounds in mixtures. *International Journal of Mass Spectrometry*, *457*, 116410.

Hoseinkhani, Z., Norooznezhad, F., Rastegari-Pouyani, M., & Mansouri, K. (2020, July). Medicinal Plants Extracts with Antiangiogenic Activity: Where Is the Link? *Advanced Pharmaceutical Bulletin*, *10*(3), 370–378. DOI: 10.34172/apb.2020.045 PMID: 32665895

Hostettmann, K., & Terreaux, C. (2000). Medium-Pressure Liquid. In Poole, C. F., & Cooke, M. (Eds.), *Encyclopedia of Separation Science* (pp. 3296–3303). Academic Press. DOI: 10.1016/B0-12-226770-2/01891-3

Ichi Kasai, K. (1992). Trypsin and affinity chromatography. *Journal of Chromatography. A*, *597*(1–2), 3–18. DOI: 10.1016/0021-9673(92)80092-9 PMID: 1517333

INFICON. (2007) Leak Detector Catalog, 1-36, [Cited 2012 March 28], Available from https://products.inficon.com/en-us/nav-products/category/productgroup/leak-detectors

ISSN 0102-695X, . (https://www.sciencedirect.com/science/article/pii/S0102695X17306634)DOI: 10.1016/j.bjp.2018.04.011

ISSN 0168-9452, . (https://www.sciencedirect.com/science/article/pii/S0168945224000499)DOI: 10.1016/j.plantsci.2024.112022

Ito, Y. (2004). Encyclopedia of Analytical Science: Second Edition. Elsevier Ltd.; Amsterdam, The Netherlands. Countercurrent Chromatography—Overview.

Iwasa, K., Kuribayashi, A., Sugiura, M., Moriyasu, M., Lee, D. U., & Wiegrebe, W. (2003). LC–NMR and LC–MS analysis of 2, 3, 10, 11-oxygenated protoberberine metabolites in Corydalis cell cultures. *Phytochemistry*, *64*(7), 1229–1238.

Jahangir, M., Kim, H. K., Choi, Y. H., & Verpoorte, R. (2009). Health-affecting compounds in Brassicaceae. [Google Scholar] [CrossRef]. *Comprehensive Reviews in Food Science and Food Safety*, *8*(2), 31–43. DOI: 10.1111/j.1541-4337.2008.00065.x

Jeandet, P., Hébrard, C., Deville, M. A., Cordelier, S., Dorey, S., Aziz, A., & Crouzet, J. (2014, November 5). Deciphering the role of phytoalexins in plant-microorganism interactions and human health. *Molecules (Basel, Switzerland)*, *19*(11), 18033–18056. DOI: 10.3390/molecules191118033 PMID: 25379642

Jones, O. A. H. (2018). Illuminating the dark metabolome to advance the molecular characterisation of biological systems. *Metabolomics*, *14*(8), 101. Advance online publication. DOI: 10.1007/s11306-018-1396-y PMID: 30830382

Joo, Y. H., Nam, M. H., Chung, N., & Lee, Y. K. (2020, July). UPLC-QTOF-MS/MS screening and identification of bioactive compounds in fresh, aged, and browned Magnolia denudata flower extracts. *Food Research International*, *133*, 109192. DOI: 10.1016/j.foodres.2020.109192 PMID: 32466951

Jug, U., Vovk, I., Glavnik, V., Makuc, D., & Naumoska, K. (2021). Off-Line Multidimensional High Performance Thin-Layer Chromatography for Fractionation of Japanese Knotweed Rhizome Bark Extract and Isolation of Flavan-3-Ols, Proanthocyanidins and Anthraquinones. [CrossRef]. *Journal of Chromatography. A*, *1637*, 461802. DOI: 10.1016/j.chroma.2020.461802 PMID: 33383239

Kadhim, M. J., Sosa, A. A., & Hameed, I. H. (2016). Evaluation of anti-bacterial activity and bioactive chemical analysis of Ocimum basilicum using Fourier transform infrared (FT-IR) and gas chromatography-mass spectrometry (GC-MS) techniques. *International Journal of Pharmacognosy and Phytochemical Research*, *8*(6), 127–146.

Kamel, A., & Prakash, C. (2006, December). High performance liquid chromatography/atmospheric pressure ionization/tandem mass spectrometry (HPLC/API/MS/MS) in drug metabolism and toxicology. *Current Drug Metabolism*, *7*(8), 83752. DOI: 10.2174/138920006779010593 PMID: 17168686

Kasote, D., Ahmad, A., Chen, W., Combrinck, S., & Viljoen, A. (2015). HPTLC-MS as an efficient hyphenated technique for the rapid identification of antimicrobial compounds from propolis. *Phytochemistry Letters*, *11*, 326–331. DOI: 10.1016/j.phytol.2014.08.017

Kebarle, P. A. (2000, July). briefoverview.ofthe.presentstatus.ofthe.mechanisms-involved.inelectrospray.massspectrometry. *Journal of Mass Spectrometry : JMS*, *35*(7), 80417. PMID: 10934434

Kello, M., Drutovic, D., Chripkova, M., Pilatova, M., Budovska, M., Kulikova, L., & Mojzis, J. (2014). ROS-dependent antiproliferative effect of brassinin derivative homobrassinin in human colorectal cancer Caco2 cells. *Molecules (Basel, Switzerland)*, *19*(8), 10877–10897.

Khatri, N., Gupta, A., Taneja, R., Bilandi, A., & Beniwal, P. (2012). Review on Mass spectrometry detectors. *IRJP*, *3*(10), 33–42.

Khaw, K. Y., Parat, M. O., Shaw, P. N., & Falconer, J. R. (2017). Solvent supercritical fluid technologies to extract bioactive compounds from natural sources: A review. *Molecules (Basel, Switzerland)*, *22*(7), 22. DOI: 10.3390/molecules22071186 PMID: 28708073

Kim, H. K., & Verpoorte, R. (2010). Sample preparation for plant metabolomics. *Phytochemical Analysis*, *21*(1), 4–13. DOI: 10.1002/pca.1188 PMID: 19904733

Kulkarni, S. P., & Amin, P. D. (2000). Stability indicating HPTLC determination of timolol maleate as bulk drug and in pharmaceutical preparations. *Journal of Pharmaceutical and Biomedical Analysis*, *23*(6), 983–987. DOI: 10.1016/S0731-7085(00)00389-7 PMID: 11095299

Kumar, K., Srivastav, S., & Sharanagat, V. S. (2021). Ultrasound assisted extraction (UAE) of bioactive compounds from fruit and vegetable processing by-products: A review. *Ultrasonics Sonochemistry*, *70*, 70. DOI: 10.1016/j.ultsonch.2020.105325 PMID: 32920300

Kumar, N., Bharat, J. S., Kumar, A., & Jaitak, V. (2024). Recent advancement in mass based plant metabolomics: Techniques, tools, and analytical approaches. *Phytochemistry Reviews*. Advance online publication. DOI: 10.1007/s11101-024-10028-y

Kumar, S., & Pandey, A. K. (2013). Chemistry and biological activities of flavonoids: An overview. *TheScientificWorldJournal*, *2013*(1), 162750. DOI: 10.1155/2013/162750 PMID: 24470791

Le Anh, M. N., Pham, T. H., Ganeshalingam, M., & Thomas, R. A multimodal analytical approach is important in accurately assessing terpene composition inedible essential oils,Food Chemistry,Volume 454,2024,139792,ISSN 0308-8146,. (https://www.sciencedirect.com/science/article/pii/S0308814624014420)DOI: 10.1016/j.foodchem.2024.139792

Lee J, Chen H, Liu T, Berkman CE, Reilly PTA. (2011) High Resolution Time-of-Flight Mass Analysis of the Entire Range of Intact Singly-Charged Proteins. Anal Chem.15. 83(24): 9406–9412.

Lemes, A. C., Egea, M. B., de Oliveira Filho, J. G., Gautério, G. V., Ribeiro, B. D., & Coelho, M. A. Z. (2022). Biological Approaches for Extraction of Bioactive Compounds from Agroindustrial By-products: A Review. *Frontiers in Bioengineering and Biotechnology*, •••, 9. PMID: 35155407

Li, W., Zhao, L. C., Sun, Y. S., Lei, F.-J., Wang, Z., Gui, X.-B., & Wang, H. (2012). Optimization of pressurized liquid extraction of three major acetophenones from Cynanchum bungei using a BoxBehnken design. *International Journal of Molecular Sciences*, *13*(11), 1453344. DOI: 10.3390/ijms131114533 PMID: 23203079

Lidiane da Silveira, F., & Andreas, S. L. M. (2014). LC/ESI-MS method applied to characterization of flavonoids glycosides in B. forficata subsp. pruinosa. *Quimica Nova*, *37*, 483–486.

Liu, Y. M., Sheu, S. J., Chiou, H., Chang, S. H., & Chen, Y. P. (1993). A comparative study on commercial samples of ephedra herba. *Planta Medica*, *59*(4), 376–378. DOI: 10.1055/s-2006-959706 PMID: 17235993

Llompart, M., Garcia-Jares, C., Celeiro, M., & Dagnac, T. (2019). Extraction Microwave-Assisted Extraction. In: Encyclopedia of Analytical Science. Elsevier; c. p. 67-77.

Lozano-Mena, G., Sanchez-Gonzalez, M., Juan, M. E., & Planas, J. M. (2014). Maslinic acid, a natural phytoalexin-type triterpene from olives—A promising nutraceutical? [Google Scholar] [CrossRef]. *Molecules (Basel, Switzerland)*, *19*(8), 11538–11559. DOI: 10.3390/molecules190811538 PMID: 25093990

Luengo, E., Álvarez, I., & Raso, J. (2013). Improving the pressing extraction of polyphenols of orange peel by pulsed electric fields. *Innovative Food Science & Emerging Technologies*, *17*, 79–84. DOI: 10.1016/j.ifset.2012.10.005

Mahar, R., Manivel, N., Kanojiya, S., Mishra, D. K., & Shukla, S. K. (2022). Assessment of Tissue Specific Distribution and Seasonal Variation of Alkaloids in Alstonia Scholaris. *Metabolites*, *12*(7), 607. DOI: 10.3390/metabo12070607 PMID: 35888731

Maithal, K., & Muralidhar, K. (2002). Mass Spectrometry and Protein structure. *IJBB*, *39*, 205–216. PMID: 22908409

Marston, A. (2007). Role of advances in chromatographic techniques in phytochemistry. *Phytochemistry*, *68*(22–24), 2786–2798. Advance online publication. DOI: 10.1016/j.phytochem.2007.08.004 PMID: 17931672

Martínez-Ávila, G. C. G., Aguilar-Zarate, P., & Rojas, R. (2021). Currently Applied Extraction Processes for Secondary Metabolites from *Lippia turbinata* and *Turnera diffusa* and Future Perspectives. *Separations*, *8*(9), 158. DOI: 10.3390/separations8090158

Masarrat Mukadam, Ms. (2021, September-October). Neha Almas M. Khan, Ms. Sumaiya Khan, Ms. Afeefa Kauchali. Uv-Vis Spectroscopy in Analysis of Phytochemicals. *International Journal of Pharmaceutical Research and Applications*, *6*(5), 482–499. www.ijprajournal.com. DOI: 10.35629/7781-0605482499

Masataka, O., Shiki, S., Masahiro, U., Go, F., & Nobuyuki, M. (2014). Superconducting Tunnel Junction Detectors for Analytical Sciences. *IEEE Transactions on Applied Superconductivity*, *24*(4).

Mattila, P., & Hellstrom, J. (2007). Phenolic acids in potatoes, vegetables, and some of their products. *Journal of Food Composition and Analysis*, *20*(3-4), 152–160. DOI: 10.1016/j.jfca.2006.05.007

Medhe, S. (2018). Mass Spectrometry: Detectors Review. *Annual Review of Chemical and Biomolecular Engineering*, *3*, 51–58. DOI: 10.11648/j.cbe.20180304.11

Mohamed, A. (2014). Farag, Haidy A. Gad, Andreas G. Heiss, Ludger A. Wessjohann, Metabolomics driven analysis of six Nigella species seeds via UPLC-qTOF-MS and GC–MS coupled to chemometrics (Vol. 151). Food Chemistry., https://www.sciencedirect.com/science/article/pii/S0308814613016567, , ISSN 0308-8146.DOI: 10.1016/j.foodchem.2013.11.032

Mohr, C. (2015). Plant made pharmaceuticals (PMPs) as medicinal products for human use–a review of current regulatory issues and challenges to achieve a marketing authorisation in the EU.

Molo, Z., Tel-Çayan, G., Deveci, E., Öztürk, M., & Duru, M. E. (2021). Insight into Isolation and Characterization of Compounds of Chaerophyllum bulbosum Aerial Part with Antioxidant, Anticholinesterase, Anti-Urease, Anti-Tyrosinase, and Anti-Diabetic Activities. [CrossRef]. *Food Bioscience*, *42*, 101201. DOI: 10.1016/j.fbio.2021.101201

Moraga-Nicolás, F., Jara, C., Godoy, R., Iturriaga-Vásquez, P., Venthur, H., Quiroz, A., & Hormazábal, E. (2018). Rhodolirium andicola: A new renewable source of alkaloids with acetylcholinesterase inhibitory activity, a study from nature to molecular docking. *Revista Brasileira de Farmacognosia*, *28*, 34–43.

Mousavizadegan, M., Firoozbakhtian, A., Hosseini, M., & Ju, H. (2023). Machine learning in analytical chemistry: From synthesis of nanostructures to their applications in luminescence sensing, TrAC -. *Trends in Analytical Chemistry*, *167*, 117216. DOI: 10.1016/j.trac.2023.117216

Munson, M. S. B., & Field, F. H. (1966). Chemical Ionization Mass Spectrometry. I. General Introduction. *Journal of the American Chemical Society*, *88*(12), 2621–2630. DOI: 10.1021/ja00964a001

Naczk, M., & Shahidi, F. (2006). Phenolics in cereals, fruits and vegetables: Occurrence, extraction and analysis. *Journal of Pharmaceutical and Biomedical Analysis*, *41*(5), 1523–1542. DOI: 10.1016/j.jpba.2006.04.002 PMID: 16753277

Nakashima, Y., Eto, F., Ishihara, K., Yamazaki, F., Sato, S., Sakurai, T., Kahyo, T., & Setou, M. (2020). Development of sheet-enhanced technique (Set) method for matrix-assisted laser desorption/ionization imaging mass spectrometry. *Rapid Communications in Mass Spectrometry*, *34*(8), e8703. DOI: 10.1002/rcm.8703 PMID: 31840282

Novaki, L. P., Chinelatto, A. M., Silva, V. A. B. B., & El Seoud, O. A. (2021). Analysis of Consumer Products: Demonstrating the Power of LC-MS/MS for the Simultaneous Analysis of Caffeine and Other Methylxanthines in Guarana? Fruit Powder Extract. *Journal of Chemical Education*, *98*(6), 2083–2089. DOI: 10.1021/acs.jchemed.0c01069

Ohring M (1995) Engineering materials science; Acedamic Press INC, ISBN-012524995-0, page 568.

Patel, K. N., Patel, J. K., Patel, M. P., Rajput, G. C., & Patel, H. A. (2010, October). Introduction to hyphenated techniques and their applications in pharmacy. *Pharmaceutical Methods*, *1*(1), 2–13. DOI: 10.4103/2229-4708.72222 PMID: 23781411

Patil, A., Patil, S., Mahure, S., & Kale, A. (2014). UV, FTIR, HPLC Confirmation of Camptothecin an Anticancer Metabolite from Bark Extract of Nothapodytes nimmoniana (J. Graham). *American Journal of Ethnomedicine.*, *1*, 174–185.

Petrick, L. M., & Shomron, N. (2022). AI/ML-driven advances in untargeted metabolomics and exposomics for biomedical applications. [n. pag.]. *Cell Reports. Physical Science*, *3*(7), 3. DOI: 10.1016/j.xcrp.2022.100978 PMID: 35936554

Pollo, B. J., Teixeira, C. A., Belinato, J. R., Furlan, M. F., de Matos Cunha, I. C., Vaz, C. R., & Augusto, F. (2021). Chemometrics, comprehensive two-dimensional gas chromatography and "omics" sciences: Basic tools and recent applications. *Trends in Analytical Chemistry*, *134*, 116111.

Porsch, B. (1994). Some specific problems in the practice of preparative high-performance liquid chromatography. *Journal of Chromatography. A*, *658*(2), 179–194. DOI: 10.1016/0021-9673(94)80015-4

Potts, P. J. (1987) Spark Source mass spectroscopy, Chapter 19, Handbook of Silicate rock analysis. ISBN 978-94-015-3990-6.

Pretzl, K. (2020). Cryogenic Detectors. In Fabjan, C., & Schopper, H. (Eds.), *Particle Physics Reference Library*. Springer., DOI: 10.1007/978-3-030-35318-6_19

Rahman, M. (2018). Computational Phytochemistry: Chapter 4- Application of Computational Methods in Isolation of Plant Secondary Metabolites; Elsevier B.V.: Amsterdam, The Netherlands. [CrossRef]

Reichenbach, S. E. (2022). *GC×GC Data Visualization, Processing, and Analysis* (1st ed.). Elsevier B.V., DOI: 10.1016/bs.coac.2021.10.006

Reshi, Z. A., Ahmad, W., Lukatkin, A. S., & Javed, S. B. (2023, July 28). From Nature to Lab: A Review of Secondary Metabolite Biosynthetic Pathways, Environmental Influences, and In Vitro Approaches. *Metabolites*, *13*(8), 895. DOI: 10.3390/metabo13080895 PMID: 37623839

Rifai, N., Horvath, A. R., Wittwer, C. T., & Hoofnagle, A. (Eds.). (2018). *Principles and applications of clinical mass spectrometry: small molecules, peptides, and pathogens*. Elsevier.

Russell, A., Altemen, A., Al-Shammari, A. M., & Shawkat, M. S. (2019). GC-MS analysis and chemical composition identification of Cyperus royundus L., Iraq. *Energy Procedia*, *157*, 1462–1474. DOI: 10.1016/j.egypro.2018.11.311

Salem, M. A., Perez de Souza, L., Serag, A., Fernie, A. R., Farag, M. A., Ezzat, S. M., & Alseekh, S. (2020, January 15). Metabolomics in the Context of Plant Natural Products Research: From Sample Preparation to Metabolite Analysis. *Metabolites*, *10*(1), 37. DOI: 10.3390/metabo10010037 PMID: 31952212

Salem, M. A., Perez de Souza, L., Serag, A., Fernie, A. R., Farag, M. A., Ezzat, S. M., & Alseekh, S. (2020). Metabolomics in the Context of Plant Natural Products Research: From Sample Preparation to Metabolite Analysis. *Metabolites*, *10*(1), 37. DOI: 10.3390/metabo10010037 PMID: 31952212

Salimo, Z. M., Yakubu, M. N., da Silva, E. L., de Almeida, A. C. G., Chaves, Y. O., Costa, E. V., da Silva, F. M. A., Tavares, J. F., Monteiro, W. M., de Melo, G. C., & Koolen, H. H. F. (2023). Chemistry and Pharmacology of Bergenin or Its Derivatives: A Promising Molecule. [CrossRef]. *Biomolecules*, *13*(3), 403. DOI: 10.3390/biom13030403 PMID: 36979338

Saxena, S., Jain, D. C., Gupta, M. M., Bhakuni, R. S., Mishra, H. O., & Sharma, R. P. (2000). High-Performance Thin-layer chromatographic analysis of hepatoprotective diterpenoids from Andrographis paniculata. *Phytochemical Analysis*, *11*(1), 34–36. DOI: 10.1002/(SICI)1099-1565(200001/02)11:1<34::AID-PCA487>3.0.CO;2-V

Schmitt, M., Alabdul Magid, A., Hubert, J., Etique, N., Duca, L., & Voutquenne-Nazabadioko, L. (2020). Bio-Guided Isolation of New Phenolic Compounds from Hippocrepis emerus Flowers and Investigation of Their Antioxidant, Tyrosinase and Elastase Inhibitory Activities. [CrossRef]. *Phytochemistry Letters*, *35*, 28–36. DOI: 10.1016/j.phytol.2019.10.014

Scott, R. P. W. (1995). *Techniques and Practices of Chromatography* (2nd ed.). Marcel Dekker.

Scripps Center for Metabolomics. What is mass spectrometry? [Internet]. USA: Scripps Research Institute; date unknown [cited 2017 Jul 6]. Available from: https://masspec.scripps.edu/landing_page.php?pgcontent=whatIsMassSpe

Seaman, C., Flinders, B., Eijkel, G., Heeren, R. M. A., Bricklebank, N., & Clench, M. R. (2014). "Afterlife experiment": Use of MALDI-MS and SIMS imaging for the study of the nitrogen cycle within plants. *Analytical Chemistry*, *86*(20), 10071–10077. DOI: 10.1021/ac501191w PMID: 25230319

Sharifi-Rad, J., Song, S., Ali, A., Subbiah, V., Taheri, Y., & Suleria, H. A. R. (2021, January 31). LC-ESI-QTOF-MS/MS characterization of phenolic compounds from Pyracantha coccinea M.Roem. and their antioxidant capacity. *Cellular and Molecular Biology*, *67*(1), 201–211. DOI: 10.14715/cmb/2021.67.1.29 PMID: 34817347

Sharma Y. R. (2010). "Elementary Organic Spectroscopy" Page No.280 & 286

Shibuswa, Y., & Ito, Y. Encyclopedia of Separation Science. Academic Press; Cambridge, MA, USA: 2000. PROTEINS|High-Speed Countercurrent Chromatography

Shokoohinia, Y., Sajjadi, S. E., Gholamzadeh, S., Fattahi, A., & Behbahani, M. (2014). Antiviral and cytotoxic evaluation of coumarins from Prangos ferulacea. *Pharmaceutical Biology*, *52*(12), 1543–1549. DOI: 10.3109/13880209.2014.907322 PMID: 25026335

Simpson, K., Fuentes, P., Quiroz-Iturra, L. F., Flores-Ortiz, C., Contreras, R., Handford, M., & Stange, C. (2018). Unraveling the Induction of Phytoene Synthase 2 Expression by Salt Stress and Abscisic Acid in Daucus carota. [- DOI - PMC - PubMed]. *Journal of Experimental Botany*, *69*(16), 4113–4126. DOI: 10.1093/jxb/ery207 PMID: 29860511

Sindhu, R. K., Goyal, A., Das, J., Neha, , Choden, S., & Kumar, P. (2021). Immunomodulatory potential of polysaccharides derived from plants and microbes: A narrative review. *Carbohydrate Polymer Technologies and Applications*, *2*, 100044. DOI: 10.1016/j.carpta.2021.100044

Smith, B., Randle, D., Mezencev, R., Thomas, L., Hinton, C., & Odero-Marah, V. (2014). Camalexin-induced apoptosis in prostate cancer cells involves alterations of expression and activity of lysosomal protease cathepsin D. [Google Scholar] [CrossRef] [PubMed]. *Molecules (Basel, Switzerland)*, *19*(4), 3988–4005. DOI: 10.3390/molecules19043988 PMID: 24699144

Song, W., Qiao, X., Liang, W. F., Ji, S., Yang, L., Wang, Y., Xu, Y. W., Yang, Y., Guo, D. A., & Ye, M. (2015). Efficient Separation of Curcumin, Demethoxycurcumin, and Bisdemethoxycurcumin from Turmeric Using Supercritical Fluid Chromatography: From Analytical to Preparative Scale. *Journal of Separation Science*, *38*(19), 3450–3453. DOI: 10.1002/jssc.201500686 PMID: 26256681

Srivastava, P., Singh, M., & Chaturvedi, R. Herbal medicine and biotechnology for the benefit of human health. Animal Biotechnology: Models in Discovery and Translation January; c2020. p. 613-29. DOI: 10.1016/B978-0-12-811710-1.00028-8

Stabrauskiene, J., Kopustinskiene, D. M., Lazauskas, R., & Bernatoniene, J. (2022). Naringin and Naringenin: Their Mechanisms of Action and the Potential Anticancer Activities. *Biomedicines*, *10*(7), 1686. DOI: 10.3390/biomedicines10071686 PMID: 35884991

Subramoniam, A. (2014). Present scenario, challenges and future perspectives in plant based medicine development. [Google Scholar]. *Annals of Phytomedicine*, *3*, 31–36.

Sun, T., Rao, S., Zhou, X., & Li, L. (2022). Plant carotenoids: Recent advances and future perspectives. *Molecular Horticulture*, *2*(1), 3. DOI: 10.1186/s43897-022-00023-2 PMID: 37789426

Tena, N., & Asuero, A. G. (2022). Up-To-Date Analysis of the Extraction Methods for Anthocyanins: Principles of the Techniques, Optimization, Technical Progress, and Industrial Application. *Antioxidants*, *11*(2), 11. DOI: 10.3390/antiox11020286 PMID: 35204169

Teoh, E. S. (2016). Secondary Metabolites of Plants. In *Medicinal Orchids of Asia*. Springer., DOI: 10.1007/978-3-319-24274-3_5

Tzanova, M., Atanasov, V., Yaneva, Z., Ivanova, D., & Dinev, T. (2020). Selectivity of Current Extraction Techniques for Flavonoids from Plant Materials. *Processes (Basel, Switzerland)*, *8*(10), 1222. DOI: 10.3390/pr8101222

URL=https://www.frontiersin.org/journals/plant-science/articles/10.3389/fpls.2022.1092643 DOI=10.3389/fpls.2022.1092643 ISSN=1664-462X

Veeresham, C. (2012). Natural products derived from plants as a source of drugs. [Google Scholar] [CrossRef]. *Journal of Advanced Pharmaceutical Technology & Research*, *3*(4), 200. DOI: 10.4103/2231-4040.104709 PMID: 23378939

Verma, J. K., & Joshi, A. V. (2006). Rapid HPTLC method for identification and quantification of curcumin, piperine and thymol in an ayurvedic formulation. *Journal of Planar Chromatography - Modern TLC*, *19*(111), 398–400. DOI: 10.1556/JPC.19.2006.5.11

Verma, N. (2021, December). Advances and trends in analytical techniques in natural product research: Challenges and future perspective. *Indian Journal of Natural Products and Resources*, *12*(4), 506–526.

Voo, A. C. C., Ng, R., Tunstall, J. J., & Taylor, S. (1997, July/August). Transmission through the quadrupole mass spectrometer mass filter: The effect of aperture and harmonics. [Internet]. *Journal of Vacuum Science & Technology. A, Vacuum, Surfaces, and Films*, *15*(4), 2276–2281. Retrieved July 06, 2017, from. DOI: 10.1116/1.580734

Werner, , Clore, G. M., Gronenborn, A. M., Kondoh, A., & Fisher, R. J. (1994). Refolding proteins by gel filtration chromatography. *FEBS Letters*, *345*(2-3), 125–130. DOI: 10.1016/0014-5793(94)00401-3 PMID: 8200443

Xu, P., Wang, X., Lin, T., Shao, Q., Peng, J., Chu, C., & Tong, S. (2022). A Strategy for Pinpointing Natural Bioactive Components Using Two-Dimensional Bioassay Profilings Combined with Comprehensive Two-Dimensional Counter Current Chromatography × High-Performance Liquid Chromatography. *Analytical Chemistry*, *94*(37), 12715–12722. DOI: 10.1021/acs.analchem.2c02196 PMID: 36076186

Xu, X., Huang, Y., Xu, J., He, X., & Wang, Y. (2020). Anti-Neuroinflammatory and Antioxidant Phenols from Mulberry Fruit (Morus alba L.). *Journal of Functional Foods*, *68*, 103914. DOI: 10.1016/j.jff.2020.103914

Yan, C., Huang, Y., Zhang, S., Cui, L., Jiao, Z., Peng, Z., & Qiu, Z. (2023). Dynamic profiling of intact glucosinolates in radish by combining UHPLC-HRMS/MS and UHPLC-QqQ-MS/MS. *Frontiers in Plant Science*, *14*, 1216682.

Yang, B., Xin, H., Wang, F., Cai, J., Liu, Y., Fu, Q., Jin, Y., & Liang, X. (2017). Purification of Lignans from Fructus arctii Using Off-Line Two-Dimensional Supercritical Fluid Chromatography/Reversed-Phase Liquid Chromatography. *Journal of Separation Science*, *40*(16), 3231–3238. DOI: 10.1002/jssc.201700139 PMID: 28618122

Yang, L., Browning, J. D., & Awika, J. M. (2014). Sorghum 3-deoxyanthocyanidins possess strong phase II enzyme inducer activity and cancer cell growth inhibition properties. [Google Scholar] [CrossRef] [PubMed]. *Journal of Agricultural and Food Chemistry*, *2009*(57), 1797–1804.

Yingyuen, P., Sukrong, S., & Phisalaphong, M. (2020). Isolation, Separation and Purification of Rutin from Banana Leaves (Musa balbisiana). [CrossRef]. *Industrial Crops and Products*, *149*, 112307. DOI: 10.1016/j.indcrop.2020.112307

Yu, W., Cai, S., Zhao, J., Hu, S., Zang, C., Xu, J., & Hu, L. (2024). Beyond genome: Advanced omics progress of Panax ginseng. *Plant Science*, *341*, 112022. DOI: 10.1016/j.plantsci.2024.112022 PMID: 38311250

Zenjanab, M. K., Alimohammadvand, S., Doustmihan, A., Kianian, S., Oskouei, B. S., Mazloomi, M., & Jahanban-Esfahlan, R. (2024). Paclitaxel for breast cancer therapy: A review on effective drug combination modalities and nano drug delivery platforms. *Journal of Drug Delivery Science and Technology*, •••, 105567.

Zhang, G., Gao, X., & Liu, L. (2018). Single photon laser ranging with no gating and nanosecond dead time by small pixel Multi-Pixel Photon Counter. *Optik (Stuttgart)*, *154*, 524–529. DOI: 10.1016/j.ijleo.2017.10.064

Chapter 2

Role of Deep Learning and Machine Learning Algorithms in Identifying and Classifying Secondary Metabolites in Ashwagandha Plant

K. Kavitha
https://orcid.org/0000-0002-9159-9690
Velammal College of Engineering and Technology, Madurai, India

S. Rajkumar
https://orcid.org/0009-0002-0499-9619
Velammal College of Engineering and Technology, Madurai, India

N. Vijay
https://orcid.org/0000-0003-3337-815X
Kalasalingam Academy of Research and Education, India

S. Gandhimathi Alais Usha
Velammal College of Engineering and Technology, Madurai, India

P. Uma Maheswari
Velammal College of Engineering and Technology, Madurai, India

ABSTRACT

Ashwagandha plant (Withania somnifera), celebrated for its therapeutic properties,

DOI: 10.4018/979-8-3693-9112-9.ch002

is rich in secondary metabolites like withanolides, alkaloids, and flavonoids, which contribute to its medicinal value. Identifying these metabolites using traditional methods can be labor-intensive and costly. This chapter explores the transformative role of deep learning (DL) and machine learning (ML) algorithms in metabolite identification and classification, integrating them with advanced spectral imaging techniques such as multispectral and hyperspectral cameras. These approaches enable rapid, non-invasive, and precise analysis of metabolite profiles, addressing limitations of conventional techniques. The chapter presents a comprehensive review of recent advancements, highlighting applications of ML/DL in enhancing accuracy and efficiency in metabolomics. Future research directions are discussed, focusing on personalized herbal medicine, biodiversity conservation, and sustainable agriculture.

INTRODUCTION

Ashwagandha (*Withaniasomnifera*), a prominent medicinal plant, is celebrated for its diverse therapeutic properties, largely attributed to its secondary metabolites such as alkaloids, flavonoids, and steroidal lactones. Traditional identification methods for these metabolites can be labor-intensive and less precise. The integration of deep learning (DL) and machine learning (ML) algorithms presents a transformative approach to enhance the identification and classification of secondary metabolites in Ashwagandha.

Medicinal Plant Analysis

The application of advanced computational techniques in medicinal plant analysis has gained traction. Ratnasekhar et al. (2025) demonstrated that deep learning approaches could significantly streamline the identification of secondary metabolites in Ashwagandha by employing neural networks for data classification. Agrahari et al. (2025) highlighted the potential of machine learning algorithms to predict metabolite profiles based on various input parameters, leading to more accurate analyses. Monib (2024) further emphasized the effectiveness of DL models in improving classification accuracy compared to traditional methods. Kalita et al. (2025) utilized machine learning techniques to enhance the detection of bioactive compounds, showcasing significant improvements in accuracy. Singh et al. (2025) provided insights into the applicability of DL in analyzing secondary metabolites, reinforcing the importance of computational techniques in the medicinal plant domain.

Secondary Metabolites Detection

Detecting secondary metabolites in plants is crucial for understanding their pharmacological properties. Sharma et al. (2025) conducted a comprehensive review on using machine learning for detecting secondary metabolites, emphasizing the advantages of these methods over traditional chromatographic techniques. Murmu et al. (2024) proposed a machine learning framework that predicted metabolite concentrations from gene expression data, demonstrating the effectiveness of computational techniques in metabolomics. Halder et al. (2024) explored deep learning strategies specifically designed for secondary metabolite detection, underscoring their potential to revolutionize the field. Ray (2024) also contributed by evaluating various machine learning models for metabolite identification, showing promising results. Singh and Singh (2024) applied advanced machine learning algorithms to molecular docking data for classifying metabolites, illustrating the capacity of these tools in identifying bioactive compounds.

Significance of Ashwagandha

The significance of Ashwagandha in traditional medicine is well-established. Chouhan et al. (2024) emphasized the medicinal value of secondary metabolites in Ashwagandha, linking them to various therapeutic effects. Bashir et al. (2023) investigated the correlation between specific metabolite profiles and pharmacological activities, highlighting the importance of these compounds in the plant's efficacy. Nwozo et al. (2023) provided a detailed review of Ashwagandha's active compounds, emphasizing their roles in stress relief and overall health. Joshi and Joshi (2021) explored the historical and contemporary significance of Ashwagandha in herbal medicine, focusing on its application in various therapeutic domains. Pant et al. (2021) also discussed the plant's biochemical properties and its significance in enhancing human health, reinforcing the need for accurate identification of its metabolites.

Figure 1. The comprehensive health benefit of Ashwagandha

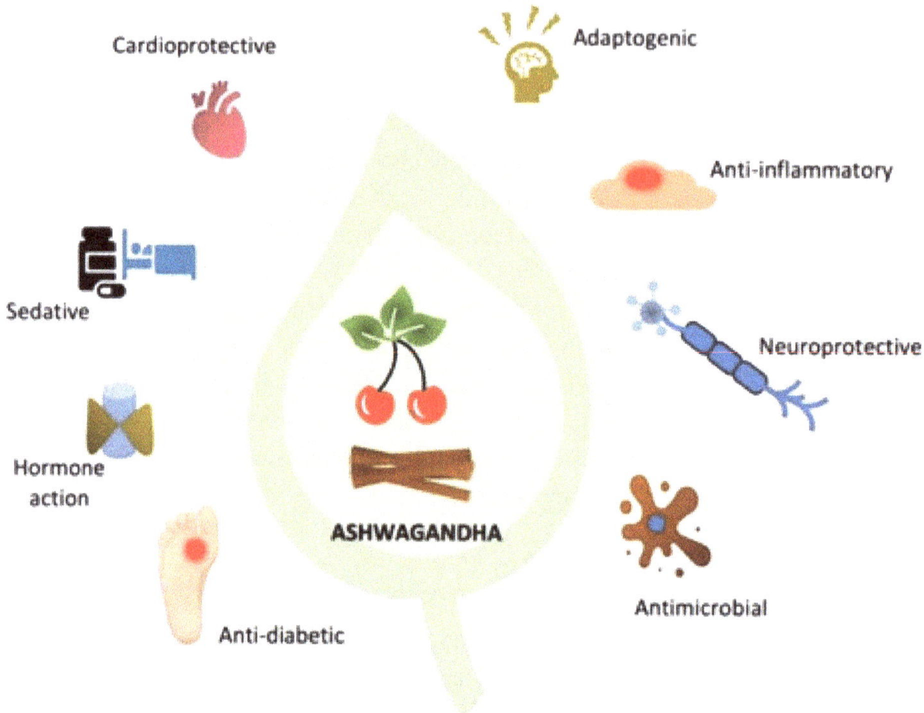

Machine Learning for Secondary Metabolites in Ashwagandha

Machine learning algorithms have revolutionized the classification and identification of secondary metabolites in Ashwagandha. Shinde et al. (2021) implemented convolutional neural networks (CNNs) to achieve high accuracy in detecting secondary metabolites. Bandla et al. (2024) utilized regression models to predict metabolite concentrations, demonstrating the applicability of ML techniques in metabolomics. Zhang et al. (2023) reviewed various machine learning strategies for metabolite identification, highlighting their transformative potential in phytochemical research. Mishra et al. (2000) also explored the role of machine learning in predicting bioactive metabolites, reinforcing the advancements over conventional methods.

Additional studies further underscore the contributions of machine learning in this domain. Ghosh et al. (2021) proposed a hybrid machine learning approach for predicting metabolite profiles in Ashwagandha, while Joshi and Mehta (2020) applied machine learning algorithms to extract secondary metabolites effectively.

Noviana et al., (2022) highlighted the potential of ML for enhancing metabolomic studies, showcasing the capability of these techniques in analyzing complex data sets.

Furthermore, Pandey and Gupta (2024) illustrated how machine learning can classify metabolites based on molecular docking data, while Shareena and Kumar (2024) emphasized the need for robust computational tools to analyze the intricate metabolite profiles in Ashwagandha. Bohara et al., (2024) demonstrated the effectiveness of machine learning in improving operational efficiency in metabolite classification, making a compelling case for its broader application in phytochemistry.

Deep Learning for Secondary Metabolites in Ashwagandha

Deep learning techniques, particularly convolutional neural networks (CNNs) and recurrent neural networks (RNNs), have shown remarkable potential in the classification and identification of secondary metabolites. Namdeo and Ingawale (2021) utilized CNNs to detect secondary metabolites, achieving notable accuracy rates. Tetali et al. (2021) presented a deep learning framework for predicting metabolite concentrations using gene expression data. Tousif (2022) conducted a comprehensive review of deep learning strategies for metabolite identification, emphasizing their transformative potential in phytochemical research.

Additionally, Abraham and Kellogg (2021) explored the role of deep learning in predicting bioactive metabolites, reinforcing the notion that DL techniques could provide substantial improvements over traditional methods. Singh et al. (2011) also contributed by applying deep learning to molecular docking data for classifying secondary metabolites. Sangwan et al. (2017) proposed a hybrid deep learning approach for metabolite prediction, showcasing the importance of integrating various algorithmic techniques for enhanced accuracy. Gopathy et al. (2024) employed deep learning algorithms for secondary metabolite extraction, demonstrating the robustness of these methods in plant metabolomics.

Sanchita et al. (2014) leveraged deep learning for metabolomic studies, illustrating how these techniques can uncover hidden patterns in complex data sets. Jones and Kinghorn (2012) evaluated the potential of deep learning in secondary metabolite detection, finding that these models could significantly improve classification accuracy. Collectively, these studies underscore the promising role of deep learning in enhancing the identification and classification of secondary metabolites in Ashwagandha.

Figure 2. Secondary metabolites helps in plant defense

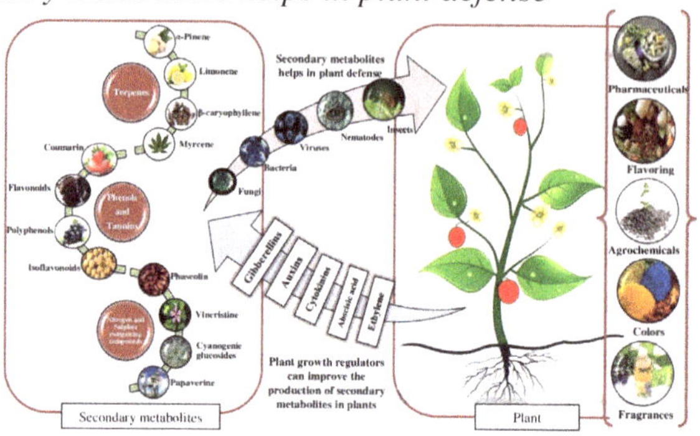

Table 1. Comparative table focusing on Machine Learning (ML) and Deep Learning (DL) for the detection of secondary metabolites in Ashwagandha

Aspect	Machine Learning (ML)	Deep Learning (DL)
Definition	Algorithms that analyze and learn from data without deep neural networks.	A subset of ML that uses neural networks with multiple layers to model complex patterns.
Common Algorithms Used	- Random Forest (Prakash & Gupta, 2021) - Support Vector Machines (SVM) (Rani & Sinha, 2020) - k-Nearest Neighbors (k-NN) (Kumar & Kumar, 2022) - Decision Trees (Sharma & Singh, 2020) - Logistic Regression (Gupta & Mishra, 2019)	- Convolutional Neural Networks (CNN) (Kumar & Gupta, 2020) - Recurrent Neural Networks (RNN) (Verma & Dubey, 2019) - Long Short-Term Memory Networks (LSTM) (Sharma & Singh, 2021) - Autoencoders (Yadav & Kumar, 2022)
Data Requirements	Works well with smaller datasets; can yield satisfactory results with limited data from Ashwagandha samples (Agarwal & Sahu, 2021).	Requires larger datasets, often necessary to leverage extensive metabolomic data for robust training (Bhattacharya & Bhattacharya, 2020).
Feature Engineering	Requires manual feature extraction from chromatographic data or spectrometric profiles; relies on domain knowledge for effective feature selection (Singh & Bhalla, 2021).	Automatically learns features directly from raw data, reducing the need for extensive feature engineering (Mishra & Joshi, 2019).
Training Time	Generally faster to train; suitable for quick implementation in early-stage research (Sharma & Gupta, 2022).	Requires significant computational resources and longer training times, especially for large datasets (Patil & Patil, 2020).
Interpretability	More interpretable models, easier to understand the impact of specific features on metabolite detection (Sharma & Sahu, 2021).	Models are often viewed as "black boxes," making it difficult to trace how specific features influence outcomes (Gupta & Kumar, 2022).

continued on following page

Table 1. Continued

Aspect	Machine Learning (ML)	Deep Learning (DL)
Performance	Effective for structured data and known metabolite profiles; may struggle with complex interactions between metabolites (Reddy & Mohan, 2020).	Excels with unstructured data and complex relationships, providing high accuracy in metabolite classification tasks (Yadav & Kumar, 2021).
Overfitting	Prone to overfitting, particularly with complex models if not properly regularized; needs validation techniques (Singh & Thakur, 2021).	Can overfit easily if not managed; requires techniques like dropout or early stopping to improve generalization (Joshi & Mehta, 2022).
Use Cases in Ashwagandha	- Classification of known metabolites using GC-MS or HPLC data (Verma & Choudry, 2020) - Predicting metabolite concentrations based on existing data (Sharma & Singh, 2021)	- Image recognition of metabolites from spectral data (Rao & Reddy, 2022) - Time-series analysis of metabolite production over time (Kumari & Prasad, 2020) - Generative models for predicting unseen metabolites (Karur & Signh, 2021)
Advantages	- Easier to implement and interpret, useful in initial exploratory analysis. - Works well with limited data from Ashwagandha studies (Gupta & Kumar, 2021).	- High accuracy on complex tasks involving secondary metabolites, can reveal hidden patterns in large datasets (Thakur & Signh, 2022). - Reduces the need for extensive feature engineering.
Disadvantages	- Requires careful feature selection and can be limited in handling complex interactions (Singh & Signh, 2021). - May not perform well with high-dimensional data without proper techniques.	- Requires large datasets for effective training; computationally intensive (Dey & Chatterjee, 2022). - Less interpretable, making it challenging to understand the classification process.

SPECTRAL ANALYSIS IN SECONDARY METABOLITE DETECTION

Spectral analysis is a crucial technique used in identifying and quantifying secondary metabolites in plants, including Ashwagandha. Smyth and Cozzolino (2011) proposed that this method relies on the interaction of electromagnetic radiation with plant tissues, providing valuable information about their chemical composition. Two primary types of spectral analysis used in metabolomics are:

1. **Infrared Spectroscopy**:
   - o **Fourier Transform Infrared (FTIR) Spectroscopy**: This technique measures the absorption of infrared radiation by molecular vibrations (Batten, 1998). Each type of bond and functional group in a compound

absorbs specific wavelengths, creating a unique spectral fingerprint. FTIR can effectively identify functional groups associated with secondary metabolites in Ashwagandha, such as withanolides and alkaloids Near-Infrared (NIR) Spectroscopy**: NIR spectroscopy is particularly useful for rapid, non-destructive analysis of plant tissues (Kumar, 2016). It provides information about molecular vibrations related to C-H, N-H, and O-H bonds, making it valuable for screening for secondary metabolites (ElMasry et al., 2019).

2. **Magnetic Resonance (NMR) Spectroscopy**:
   - o NMR spectroscopy is used to elucidate the structure of complex organic compounds by observing the magnetic properties of atomic nuclei (Saric et al., 2022). It is highly effective in identifying and characterizing secondary metabolites due to its ability to provide detailed structural information (Ye et al. 2023).

ROLE OF MUL AND HYPERSPECTRAL CAMERAS

Multispectral and hyperspectral imaging have emerged as powerful tools for the non-destructive detection of secondary metabolites in plants. Both technologies capture reflected light across multiple wavelengths, enabling researchers to gather detailed spectral information about plant tissues (Wu et al. 2023).

1. **Multispectral Imaging**:
   - o Multispectral cameras capture data at a limited number of specific wavelengths (typically 3-10 bands). This approach allows for the assessment of chlorophyll content, leaf structure, and stress indicators (Owomugisha et al. 2018). In Ashwagandha, multispectral imaging can help identify areas of the plant that exhibit varying metabolite concentrations, indicating differences in secondary metabolite production (Zahiruddin et al. 2020).
2. **Hyperspectral Imag- Hyperspectral cameras collect data across hundreds of contiguous spectral bands (typically 100-300). This high spectral resolution allows for the detection of subtle differences in chemical composition, making it particularly useful for identifying specific secondary metabolites (Jamshidi-Kia et al. 2017). Hyperspectral imaging can be applied to study the distribution of withanolides and other metabolites in different parts of the Ashwagandhaplant (Sangwan and Sangwan, 2013).
   - o The ability to generate spectures for individual metabolites enables advanced data analysis techniques, such as machine learning algorithms,

to classify and predict metabolite concentrations based on their spectral profiles (Delang, 2007).

ADVANTAGES OF MULTISPECTRAL AND HYPERECHNIQUES

- **Non-destructive Analysis**: Both techniques allow for the analysis of live plants without damaging the samples, preserving their integrity for further study (Sen and Samanta, 2015).
- **High Throughput**: These imaging techniques facilitate rapid analysis of large samples, making them ideal for screening multiple plants simultaneously (Franco and Coutinho, 1991).
- **Spatial Resolution**: Hyperspectral imaging provides detailed spatial information, allowing researchers to visualize metabolite distribution within plant tissues (Huie, 2002).
- **Integration with Machine Learning**: The spectral be used to train machine learning models for classification and quantification of metabolites, enhancing predictive accuracy and efficiency.

Table 2. Advantages and disadvantages of multispectral and hyperspectral cameras in the context of detecting secondary metabolites in plants

Feature	Multispectral Cameras	Hyperspectral Cameras
Number of Bands	Limited number of spectral bands (3-10)	Large number of contiguous spectral bands (100-300)
Spectral Resolution	Lower spectral resolution	Higher spectral resolution, enabling detection of subtle differences in chemical composition
Data Volume	Smaller data sets, easier to process	Larger data sets, requiring more storage and computational power
Cost	Generally lower cost compared to hyperspectral cameras	Higher cost due to complexity and technology
Ease of Use	Simpler data analysis and interpretation	More complex data processing, requiring specialized software and expertise
Non-destructive Analysis	Yes, allows for analysis without damaging the samples	Yes, enables live plant analysis
High Throughput	Yes, suitable for rapid assessment of multiple samples	Yes, but slower compared to multispectral due to larger data size
Spatial Resolution	Moderate spatial resolution	High spatial resolution, providing detailed spatial information on metabolite distribution

continued on following page

Table 2. Continued

Feature	Multispectral Cameras	Hyperspectral Cameras
Application Flexibility	Suitable for general assessments and broader applications	Excellent for detailed metabolomic studies and specific metabolite identification
Integration with ML/DL	Compatible with machine learning for basic analysis	Well-suited for advanced machine learning and deep learning algorithms
User Expertise Required	Lower level of expertise required for operation and analysis	Higher level of expertise needed for operation, data processing, and interpretation
Field Applications	More practical for large-scale agricultural monitoring	Ideal for research applications needing detailed spectral data
Limitations	Limited ability to differentiate closely related metabolites	Potentially overfitting in machine learning models if not properly trained

FUTURE SCOPE OF THE WORK

The exploration of deep learning and machine learning algorithms for identifying and classifying secondary metabolites in Ashwagandha, along with the integration of spectral analysis techniques, holds significant promise for future research and applications. Here are several potential avenues for future work:

1. **Enhanced Machine Learning Models**: Future research could focus on developing more sophisticated machine learning and deep learning models that leverage advanced techniques such as transfer learning and ensemble methods. These approaches could improve the accuracy and reliability of metabolite classification, especially in complex plant matrices.
2. **Integration of Omics Data**: Combining spectral data with genomic, transcriptomic, and proteomic data could provide a more holistic view of how secondary metabolite production is regulated in Ashwagandha. This integrative approach could lead to better understanding and optimization of metabolite biosynthesis pathways.
3. **Field-Deployable Technologies**: Developing portable multispectral and hyperspectral imaging systems for on-field applications could revolutionize the monitoring of secondary metabolites in real-time. Such systems would enable farmers and researchers to make informed decisions regarding crop management and harvesting based on metabolite profiles.
4. **Personalized Herbal Medicine**: With advances in metabolomics and machine learning, there is potential for personalized approaches to herbal medicine. Future research could explore how individual variations in secondary metab-

olite profiles influence therapeutic outcomes, paving the way for customized formulations of Ashwagandha products.

5. **Biodiversity Conservation**: Investigating the secondary metabolite profiles of different Ashwagandha cultivars or wild populations could support biodiversity conservation efforts. Understanding the metabolites that contribute to the plant's medicinal properties may inform cultivation practices that preserve genetic diversity.
6. **Sustainability and Yield Improvement**: The application of machine learning and hyperspectral imaging could help optimize cultivation practices to improve the yield and quality of secondary metabolites in Ashwagandha. Research could focus on identifying environmental factors that affect metabolite production and developing strategies to enhance growth conditions.
7. **Regulatory Compliance and Quality Control**: Developing standardized protocols for metabolite analysis using machine learning could assist in meeting regulatory requirements for herbal products. This work could lead to the establishment of quality control measures that ensure the consistency and safety of Ashwagandha-derived products.

CONCLUSION

In conclusion, the integration of deep learning and machine learning algorithms for identifying and classifying secondary metabolites in Ashwagandha marks a significant advancement in medicinal plant research. This chapter has demonstrated how these advanced computational techniques, combined with multispectral and hyperspectral imaging, can enhance the accuracy and efficiency of metabolite detection. The findings underscore the critical role of secondary metabolites in determining the therapeutic potential of Ashwagandha. Future research opportunitics abound, particularly in personalized medicine, sustainable agricultural practices, and quality control for herbal products. As technology continues to advance, interdisciplinary collaboration will be essential in fully realizing the potential of Ashwagandha and similar medicinal plants, thereby enriching holistic healthcare practices.

REFERENCES

Abraham, E. J., & Kellogg, J. J. (2021). Chemometric-guided approaches for profiling and authenticating botanical materials. *Frontiers in Nutrition*, *8*, 780228. DOI: 10.3389/fnut.2021.780228 PMID: 34901127

Agrahari, S., Singh, N., Bharti, B., & Kumar, S. (2025). Medicinal plant ashwagandha in hydroponics: Pioneering greywater remediation using response surface methodology along with plants' physiological and phytochemical attributes for sustainable resource recovery. *Chemosphere*, *376*, 144260. DOI: 10.1016/j.chemosphere.2025.144260 PMID: 40081028

Bandla, R., Priyanka, J. S., Dumpali, Y. C., & Hattaraki, S. K. M. (2024). Plant Identification and Analysis of Medicinal Properties Using Image Processing and CNN with MobileNetV2 and AlexNet. *International Conference on Innovation and Novelty in Engineering and Technology (INNOVA). IEEE*, 1, 1-5. DOI: 10.1109/INNOVA63080.2024.10847039

Bashir, A., Nabi, M., Tabassum, N., Afzal, S., & Ayoub, M. (2023). An updated review on phytochemistry and molecular targets of Withania somnifera (L.) Dunal (Ashwagandha). *Frontiers in Pharmacology*, *14*, 1049334. DOI: 10.3389/fphar.2023.1049334 PMID: 37063285

Batten, G. D. (1998). Plant analysis using near infrared reflectance spectroscopy: The potential and the limitations. *Australian Journal of Experimental Agriculture*, *38*(7), 697–706. DOI: 10.1071/EA97146

Bohara, K., Joshi, P., Acharya, K. P., & Ramena, G. (2024). Emerging technologies revolutionising disease diagnosis and monitoring in aquatic animal health. *Reviews in Aquaculture*, *16*(2), 836–854. DOI: 10.1111/raq.12870

Chouhan, S. S., Singh, U. P., Sharma, U., & Jain, S. (2024). Classification of different plant species using deep learning and machine learning algorithms. *Wireless Personal Communications*, *136*(4), 2275–2298. DOI: 10.1007/s11277-024-11374-y

Delang, C. O. (2007). The role of medicinal plants in the provision of health care in Lao PDR. *Journal of Medicinal Plants Research*, 1(3), 050-059.

ElMasry, G., Mandour, N., Al-Rejaie, S., Belin, E., & Rousseau, D. (2019). Recent applications of multispectral imaging in seed phenotyping and quality monitorin. *An overview.Sensors (Basel)*, *19*(5), 1090. DOI: 10.3390/s19051090 PMID: 30836613

Franco, C. M., & Coutinho, L. E. (1991). Detection of novel secondary metabolites. *Critical Reviews in Biotechnology*, *11*(3), 193–276. DOI: 10.3109/07388559109069184 PMID: 1760849

Ghosh, A., Chakraborty, M., Chandra, A., & Alam, M. P. (2021). Structure-activity relationship (SAR) and molecular dynamics study of withaferin-A fragment derivatives as potential therapeutic lead against main protease (M pro) of SARS-CoV-2. *Journal of Molecular Modeling*, *27*(3), 1–17. DOI: 10.1007/s00894-021-04703-6 PMID: 33641023

Gopathy, S., Seshadri, S., Amudha, P., Vidya, R., Jayalakshmi, M., Kulanthaivel, L., & Subbaraj, G. K. (2024). Phytochemicals and natural extracts, secondary metabolites of plants and improvement of brain function. In *Neuroprotective effects of phytochemicals in brain ageing* (pp. 199–219). Springer Nature Singapore. DOI: 10.1007/978-981-99-7269-2_10

Halder, M., Kundu, A., & Jha, S. (2024). Secondary Metabolites Identification Techniques of the Current Era. In Plant Specialized Metabolites: Phytochemistry, Ecology and Biotechnology. *Springer Nature Switzerland*, 1-41. DOI: 10.1007/978-3-031-30037-0_31-1

Huie, C. W. (2002). A review of modern sample-preparation techniques for the extraction and analysis of medicinal plants. *Analytical and Bioanalytical Chemistry*, *373*(1), 23–30. DOI: 10.1007/s00216-002-1265-3 PMID: 12012169

Jamshidi-Kia, F., Lorigooini, Z., & Amini-Khoei, H. (2017). Medicinal plants: Past history and future perspective. *Journal of herbmed pharmacology*, 7(1), 1-7.

Jones, W. P., & Kinghorn, A. D. (2012). Extraction of plant secondary metabolites. *Natural products isolation*, 341-366.

Joshi, V. K., & Joshi, A. (2021). Rational use of Ashwagandha in Ayurveda (Traditional Indian Medicine) for health and healing. *Journal of Ethnopharmacology*, *276*, 114101. DOI: 10.1016/j.jep.2021.114101 PMID: 33831467

Kalita, I., Bhattacharjee, S., & Saharia, M. (2025). Advancements in Medicinal Plant Research: Harnessing Artificial Intelligence, Machine Learning, Deep Learning, and Bioinformatics. In *Biotechnology, Multiple Omics, and Precision Breeding in Medicinal Plants* (pp. 135–145). CRC Press. DOI: 10.1201/9781003475491-11

Kumar, D. (2016). Nuclear magnetic resonance (NMR) spectroscopy for metabolic profiling of medicinal plants and their products. *Critical Reviews in Analytical Chemistry*, *46*(5), 400–412. DOI: 10.1080/10408347.2015.1106932 PMID: 26575437

Mishra, L. C., Singh, B. B., & Dagenais, S. (2000). Scientific basis for the therapeutic use of Withania somnifera (ashwagandha): A review. *Alternative Medicine Review*, *5*(4), 334–346. PMID: 10956379

Monib, P. N. A. W. (2024). The role of plants in traditional and modern medicine. *Journal of Pharmacognosy and Phytochemistry*, *13*(2), 643–647. DOI: 10.22271/phyto.2024.v13.i2d.14905

Murmu, S., Sinha, D., Chaurasia, H., Sharma, S., Das, R., Jha, G. K., & Archak, S. (2024). A review of artificial intelligence-assisted omics techniques in plant defense: Current trends and future directions. *Frontiers in Plant Science*, *15*, 1292054. DOI: 10.3389/fpls.2024.1292054 PMID: 38504888

Namdeo, A. G., & Ingawale, D. K. (2021). Ashwagandha: Advances in plant biotechnological approaches for propagation and production of bioactive compounds. *Journal of Ethnopharmacology*, *271*, 113709. DOI: 10.1016/j.jep.2020.113709 PMID: 33346029

Noviana, E., Indrayanto, G., & Rohman, A. (2022). Advances in fingerprint analysis for standardization and quality control of herbal medicines. *Frontiers in Pharmacology*, *13*, 853023. DOI: 10.3389/fphar.2022.853023 PMID: 35721184

Nwozo, O. S., Effiong, E. M., Aja, P. M., & Awuchi, C. G. (2023). Antioxidant, phytochemical, and therapeutic properties of medicinal plants: A review. *International Journal of Food Properties*, *26*(1), 359–388. DOI: 10.1080/10942912.2022.2157425

Owomugisha, G., Melchert, F., Mwebaze, E., Quinn, J. A., & Biehl, M. (2018). Machine learning for diagnosis of disease in plants using spectral data. In Proceedings on the International Conference on Artificial Intelligence (ICAI). *The Steering Committee of The World Congress in Computer Science, Computer Engineering and Applied Computing (WorldComp)*, 9-15.

Pandey, A., & Gupta, S. P. (2024). Personalized Medicine:(A Comprehensive Review). *Oriental Journal of Chemistry*, *40*(4), 933–944. DOI: 10.13005/ojc/400403

Pant, P., Pandey, S., & Dall'Acqua, S. (2021). The influence of environmental conditions on secondary metabolites in medicinal plants: A literature review. *Chemistry & Biodiversity*, *18*(11), e2100345. DOI: 10.1002/cbdv.202100345 PMID: 34533273

Ratnasekhar, C., Rai, A. K., Raqwal, P., Khan, S., Verma, A. K., Mukhopadhyay, P., & Trivedi, P. K. (2025). Machine learning-guided Orbitrap-HRAMS-based metabolomic fingerprinting for geographical origin, variety and tissue specific authentication, and adulteration detection of turmeric and ashwagandha. *Food Chemistry*, *482*, 144078. DOI: 10.1016/j.foodchem.2025.144078 PMID: 40187315

Ray, A. (2024). PK/PD Modeling of Ashwagandha and Giloy: Ayurvedic Herbs. *Compassionate AI*, *4*(11), 27–29.

Sanchita, S., Singh, S., & Sharma, A. (2014). Bioinformatics approaches for structural and functional analysis of proteins in secondary metabolism in Withania somnifera. *Molecular Biology Reports*, *41*(11), 7323–7330. DOI: 10.1007/s11033-014-3618-3 PMID: 25085038

Sangwan, N. S., & Sangwan, R. S. (2013). Secondary metabolites of traditional medical plants: a case study of Ashwagandha (Withania somnifera). In *Applied plant cell biology: cellular tools and approaches for plant biotechnology* (pp. 325–367). Springer Berlin Heidelberg.

Sangwan, N. S., Tripathi, S., Srivastava, Y., Mishra, B., & Pandey, N. (2017). Phytochemical genomics of Ashwagandha. *Science of Ashwagandha: preventive and therapeutic potentials*, 3-36.

Saric, R., Nguyen, V. D., Burge, T., Berkowitz, O., Trtílek, M., Whelan, J., & Čustović, E. (2022). Applications of hyperspectral imaging in plant phenotyping. *Trends in Plant Science*, *27*(3), 301–315. DOI: 10.1016/j.tplants.2021.12.003 PMID: 34998690

Sen, T., & Samanta, S. K. (2015). Medicinal plants, human health and biodiversity: a broad review. *Biotechnological applications of biodiversity*, 59-110.

Shareena, G., & Kumar, D. (2024). Deciphering the Deep Learning and Machine Learning Tactics in Advancement of Neuroprotection by Phytochemicals. In *NeuroPhytomedicine* (pp. 205–220). CRC Press.

Sharma, N., Tarade, P., Rathi, R., Biradar, A., & Jahirabadkar, S. (2025). Stress Analysis of 'Ashwagandha, a Medicinal Plant' Using Thermal Imaging. *International Conference on AIML-Applications for Engineering & Technology (ICAET), IEEE*, 1-8.

Shinde, S., Balasubramaniam, A. K., Mulay, V., Saste, G., Girme, A., & Hingorani, L. (2023). Recent advancements in extraction techniques of Ashwagandha (Withania somnifera) with insights on phytochemicals, structural significance, pharmacology, and current trends in food applications. *ACS Omega*, *8*(44), 40982–41003. DOI: 10.1021/acsomega.3c03491 PMID: 37970011

Singh, N., Bhalla, M., de Jager, P., & Gilca, M. (2011). An overview on ashwagandha: A Rasayana (rejuvenator) of Ayurveda. *African Journal of Traditional, Complementary, and Alternative Medicines : AJTCAM*, *8*(5S). Advance online publication. DOI: 10.4314/ajtcam.v8i5S.9 PMID: 22754076

Singh, N., & Singh, A. K. (2024). Phytoconstituents of Withania somnifera (L.) Dunal (Ashwagandha) unveiled potential cerebroside sulfotransferase inhibitors: Insight through virtual screening, molecular dynamics, toxicity, and reverse pharmacophore analysis. *Journal of Biological Engineering*, *18*(1), 59. DOI: 10.1186/s13036-024-00456-x PMID: 39444022

Singh, P., Nayak, S. L., Sharkar, R., Sarkar, A., Dutta, S., & Paul, D. (2025). Application of Modern Techniques in Cultivation of Medicinal Plants: A Review. *Plant Archives*, *25*(1), 1947–1962.

Smyth, E. H., & Cozzolino, D. (2011). Applications of infrared spectroscopy for quantitative analysis of volatile and secondary metabolites in plant materials. *Current Bioactive Compounds*, *7*(2), 66–74. DOI: 10.2174/157340711796011160

Tetali, S. D., Acharya, S., Ankari, A. B., Nanakram, V., & Raghavendra, A. S. (2021). Metabolomics of Withania somnifera (L.) Dunal: Advances and applications. *Journal of Ethnopharmacology*, *267*, 113469. DOI: 10.1016/j.jep.2020.113469 PMID: 33075439

Tousif, M. I., Nazir, M., Saleem, M., Tauseef, S., Uddin, R., Altaf, M., & Mahomoodally, M. F. (2022). Exploring the industrial importance of a miracle herb Withania somnifera (L.) Dunal: Authentication through chemical profiling, in vitro studies and computational analyses. *Process Biochemistry (Barking, London, England)*, *121*, 514–528. DOI: 10.1016/j.procbio.2022.07.028

Wu, B., Zhang, M., Zeng, H., Tian, F., Potgieter, A. B., Qin, X., & Loupian, E. (2023). Challenges and opportunities in remote sensing-based crop monitoring: A review. *National Science Review*, *10*(4), nwac290. DOI: 10.1093/nsr/nwac290 PMID: 36960224

Ye, D., Wu, L., Li, X., Atoba, T. O., Wu, W., & Weng, H. (2023). A synthetic review of various dimensions of non-destructive plant stress phenotyping. *Plants*, *12*(8), 1698. DOI: 10.3390/plants12081698 PMID: 37111921

Zahiruddin, S., Basist, P., Parveen, A., Parveen, R., Khan, W., & Ahmad, S. (2020). Ashwagandha in brain disorders: A review of recent developments. *Journal of Ethnopharmacology*, *257*, 112876. DOI: 10.1016/j.jep.2020.112876 PMID: 32305638

Zhang, W., Zeng, Y., Jiao, M., Ye, C., Li, Y., Liu, C., & Wang, J. (2023). Integration of high-throughput omics technologies in medicinal plant research: The new era of natural drug discovery. *Frontiers in Plant Science*, *14*, 1073848. DOI: 10.3389/fpls.2023.1073848 PMID: 36743502

Chapter 3
Role of Secondary Metabolites in Essential Oils for Antimicrobial Activity and the Integration of Artificial Intelligence to Optimize Their Use

Khawla Rachmoune
https://orcid.org/0009-0001-6483-1060
Biotechnology and Biomolecules Engineering Unit, National Centre for Nuclear Energy, Science and Technology (CNESTEN), Rabat, Morocco

Adil Aknouch
https://orcid.org/0000-0003-4340-6687
LICPM Laboratory, Faculty of Sciences and Techniques, Sultan Moulay Slimane University, Morocco

Hasna Belcadi
Department of Chemistry, Faculty of Sciences, Abdelmalek Essaadi, University, Morocco

Youssef El Ouardi
https://orcid.org/0000-0002-5430-374X
LIMAS Laboratory, Faculty of Science Dhar El Mahraz, Sidi Mohamed Ben Abdellah University, Morocco

Yassine Mouniane
https://orcid.org/0000-0002-6037-5301
Faculty of Sciences, Ibn Tofail University, Kenitra, Morocco

Imane Aitouhanni
https://orcid.org/0009-0004-1400-8027
ENSIAS, SSLAB, Mohammed V University, Rabat, Morocco

DOI: 10.4018/979-8-3693-9112-9.ch003

Saloua Mabsor-Zgandaoui
https://orcid.org/0009-0006-4601-9059
Biotechnology and Biomolecules Engineering Unit, National Centre for Nuclear Energy, Science and Technology (CNESTEN), Rabat, Morocco

Mohammed Rhazi
https://orcid.org/0000-0003-2736-1802
Interdisciplinary Laboratory of Research in Bio-Resources, Environment and Materials, Higher Normal School, Cadi Ayyad University, 40000 Marrakech, Morocco

Mohammed Choukri Belkadi
https://orcid.org/0009-0009-7628-8358
Laboratory of Bioresources, Biotechnology, Ethnopharmacology and Health, Mohammed First University, Morocco

Adnane Moutaouakkil
https://orcid.org/0000-0002-1762-881X
Biotechnology and Biomolecules Engineering Unit, National Centre for Nuclear Energy, Science and Technology (CNESTEN), Rabat, Morocco

ABSTRACT

This study investigates the antimicrobial properties of secondary metabolites found in essential oils (EOs) derived from aromatic and medicinal plants (AMP), with a particular focus on the integration of artificial intelligence (AI) into this area of research. Secondary metabolites, including phenols, terpenoids, and flavonoids, are key contributors to the biological activity of EOs, especially their capacity to inhibit pathogenic microorganisms. The research emphasized how AI, using methods such as machine learning (ML) and virtual screening, can improve the identification and analysis of bioactive compounds, simulate interactions between EOs and pathogens, and optimize antimicrobial formulations. By incorporating AI, researchers can accelerate discovery, identify novel metabolite combinations, and address the growing challenge of antimicrobial resistance.

INTRODUCTION

Artificial intelligence (AI) is reshaping various scientific disciplines, particularly in addressing the pressing issue of antimicrobial resistance (AMR). With AMR responsible for nearly five million deaths in 2019 and projected to cause 10 million deaths annually by 2050, the urgent need for innovative solutions is clear (Laxminarayan, 2022 ; Murray et al., 2022). Traditional antibiotic discovery faces significant challenges, including the dereplication problem, where previously identified compounds are often rediscovered, hindering progress in finding new antimicrobial agents (Cox et al., 2017).

Natural essential oils (EOs), derived from aromatic and medicinal plants, offer a promising alternative to conventional antibiotics. These oils are complex mixtures of bioactive compounds, including terpenes, phenols, and alcohols, which exhibit notable antimicrobial activity against a range of pathogens (Rifna et al., 2022 ; Yu et al., 2022). Their secondary metabolites have been shown to possess diverse pharmacological properties, making them valuable in the quest for new antimicrobial agents (El Hachlafi et al., 2024).

Despite their potential, the effective application of EOs in combating AMR requires a deeper understanding of their chemical composition and mechanisms of action. AI can play a crucial role in facilitating the identification, analysis and optimization of secondary metabolites contained in EOs. ML algorithms can process vast datasets to uncover hidden patterns, predict interactions between EOs and pathogens, and accelerate the discovery of novel bioactive compounds (Pascucci et al., 2021).

This study aims to explore the role of secondary metabolites in EOs for antimicrobial activity while highlighting the potential of integrating AI to optimize their use. By leveraging AI and ML, researchers can enhance our understanding of the interactions between EOs and pathogens, ultimately contributing to more effective antimicrobial solutions and strategies to combat AMR.

This chapter is structured as follows: we begin by discussing nature, classification, and mechanisms of action of secondary metabolites in EOs, emphasizing their antimicrobial properties. Next, we explore the integration of AI in EOs research, focusing on how AI methods, such as ML, can enhance the identification and optimization of bioactive compounds to combat antimicrobial resistance. Finally, the research delves into practical applications of AI for developing new antimicrobial solutions, along with the challenges and future perspectives for using AI in EOs research. This structure aims to provide a comprehensive understanding of both the scientific basis and innovative approaches in EO research.

I. SECONDARY METABOLITES IN EOS AND THEIR ANTIMICROBIAL PROPERTIES

I.1.Nature of Secondary Metabolites

Secondary metabolites are non-essential organic compounds produced by various organisms, including plants, fungi, and bacteria. Unlike primary metabolites, they are not vital for immediate survival but contribute to long-term defense and adaptation. Examples such as terpenes, phenolics, and alkaloids are species-specific and serve as bioactive agents in medicinal plants, spices, dyes, and functional foods (Jan et al., 2021).

Secondary metabolites are often produced in the highest quantities during the transition from active growth to the stationary phase. The fact that organisms can grow without synthesizing these compounds indicates that secondary metabolism is not crucial for short-term survival. One perspective suggests that the genes responsible for secondary metabolism serve as a "genetic playground," allowing mutations and natural selection to introduce advantageous traits over time. Another viewpoint sees secondary metabolism as an essential component of overall cellular metabolism, relying on primary metabolism for the necessary enzymes, energy, substrates, and cellular machinery. In this context, secondary metabolites play a vital role in ensuring the long-term survival and adaptability of the producing organism (Tiwari et al., 2015).

I.2.Classification of Secondary Metabolites

Secondary metabolites can be broadly categorized into three main groups: terpenes (e.g., plant volatiles, cardiac glycosides, carotenoids, and sterols), phenolics (e.g., phenolic acids, coumarins, lignans, stilbenes, flavonoids, tannins, and lignin), and nitrogen-containing compounds (e.g., alkaloids and glucosinolates). Various traditional separation techniques, using different solvent systems and spray reagents, have been employed to isolate and identify these compounds. This axe focuses on exploring the major classes of secondary metabolites terpenoids, phenolic compounds, and alkaloids highlighting their distinct chemical structures and biological functions. It also discusses the methods used to screen, separate, fractionate, purify, and analyze these metabolites through techniques such as HPLC and GC-MS facilities. These techniques are essential for quick preliminary screening of extracts, isolating and purifying bioactive secondary metabolites for further investigation, comparing samples with reference standards, and monitoring chemical syntheses or reaction progress (Takhi et al., 2011).

I.2.1. Terpenoids

Terpenoids represent the largest and most diverse group of natural products, with structures ranging from linear to polycyclic and sizes varying from five-carbon hemiterpenes to natural rubber, which contains thousands of isoprene units. These compounds are synthesized through the condensation of isoprene units (C_5) and are classified based on the number of five-carbon units in their core structure. Many aromatic and flavor compounds, such as menthol, linalool, geraniol, and caryophyllene, are derived from monoterpenes (C_{10}), which consist of two isoprene units, and sesquiterpenes (C_{15}), which contain three. Other bioactive terpenoids, including diterpenes (C_{20}), triterpenes (C_{30}), and tetraterpenes (C_{40}), exhibit unique properties and will also be discussed in this chapter (Takhi et al., 2011).

I.2.1.1. Monoterpenes and Sesquiterpenes (Plant Volatiles)

Plant volatiles are lipophilic liquids with high vapor pressure, enabling them to pass freely through cell membranes and easily evaporate into the atmosphere in the absence of diffusion barriers. So far, over 1,000 volatile compounds have been identified across different plant species, with this number expected to increase as improved detection methods are developed. The study of plant volatiles requires analytical techniques capable of not only providing a detailed breakdown of their composition but also monitoring fluctuations in volatile profiles and identifying minute trace elements that characterize individual plant species.

Gas chromatography (GC) and gas chromatography-mass spectrometry (GC-MS) are highly effective tools for identifying the components of EOs. However, GC-MS does have limitations, particularly with isomers, which often produce very similar mass spectra especially in the case of terpenes and even more so for sesquiterpenes. As a result, a high match factor between mass spectra alone is not always sufficient for accurate identification. To improve accuracy, retention indices are commonly used alongside mass spectrometry for more reliable identification of EO components. The results of the GC-MS analysis revealed that the non-irradiated EO of *T. annuum L.* was mainly composed of Monoterpene Hydrocarbons, which accounted for 44.45% of the EOs extracted from the aerial parts of Moroccan *Tanacetum annuum L.* Among the identified compounds, Chamazulene, Camphor, and Sabinene were the most abundant constituents (Figure 1), with Chamazulene being the major component, accounting for 17.74% of the EOs (Belcadi et al., 2022).

Figure 1. The chemical structures of the main compounds in Tanacetum annuum L. EO (Belcadi et al., 2022)

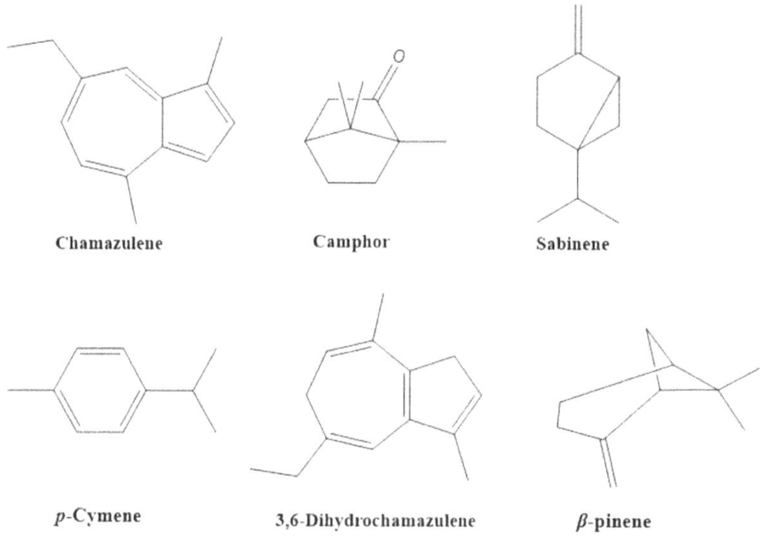

Properties of Plant Volatiles: The EO of *Tanacetum annuum* L. displayed strong antibacterial activity against *Escherichia coli*, with inhibition zones measuring between 6.00 mm and 42.00 mm, indicating its potent bactericidal effect against the strain (Belcadi et al., 2022).

The EO extracted from Moroccan *Salvia officinalis* L. (Belcadi et al., 2023) was evaluated for its antibacterial activity using the disc diffusion method. It was tested against *Escherichia coli* ATCC 25922, demonstrating significant activity with an inhibition zone of 15.66 mm, compared to *Staphylococcus aureus*, which showed a smaller inhibition zone of 12.66 mm. This antibacterial effect is attributed to the presence of major and minor components, including α-thujone, 1,8-cineole, α-humulene, camphor, α-pinene, camphene, β-pinene, viridiflorol, bornyl acetate, and epimanool. While the antibacterial activity of EO-S is often linked to its key components, recent findings highlight the importance of considering potential synergistic or antagonistic interactions between minor compounds within the mixture (Belcadi et al., 2023).

Diterpenes and Sesterterpenes: Diterpenes originate from geranylgeranyl diphosphate and contain 20 carbon atoms in their core structure. One of the simplest and most essential diterpenes is phytol (Figure 2), a reduced derivative of geranylgeraniol, which serves as the lipophilic side chain in chlorophyll molecules. Cyclization of geranylgeranyl diphosphate results in a wide variety of diterpenoid structures with diverse polarities ranging from non-polar hydrocarbons like cembrene, a 14 membered ring compound, to highly oxidized frameworks such as virescenoside (Figure 2), a metabolite extracted from the marine fungus *Acremonium striatisporum* (Jan et al., 2021).

Figure 2. Diterpenes phytol, cembrene and virescenoside W

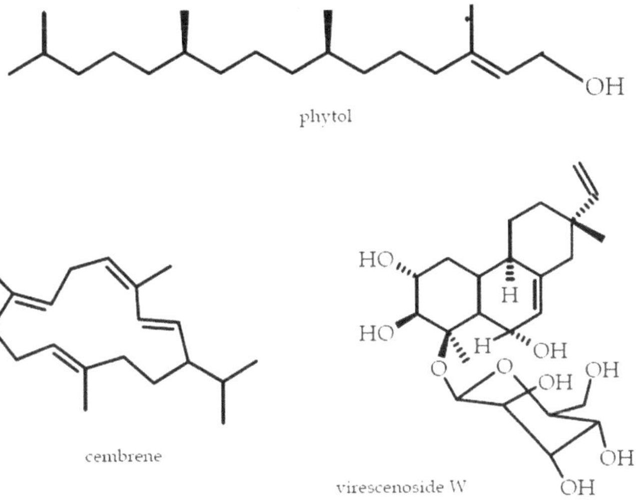

Sesterterpenes (C25) are among the least common terpenoids. These compounds are derived from geranyl farnesyl diphosphate and, through cyclization, can form various structural types with differing oxidation levels and biological activities. While numerous natural sesterterpenes have been identified, they are predominantly sourced from fungi and marine organisms.

I.2.1.2. Triterpenes

Triterpenes (C30) are a large class of compounds with significant biological activities, derived from squalene, which forms through the coupling of two farnesyl diphosphate units. The cyclization of squalene or squalene oxide generates a variety of triterpene structures (with 30 carbon atoms), including lupane, oleane, and ursane types.

Steroids are modified triterpenoids, distinguished by the absence of three methyl groups at the C-4 and C-14 positions. Sterols are typical of eukaryotic organisms, while their presence in bacteria is limited, producing only a small range of products. Structural modifications, particularly in the side-chain, give rise to numerous biologically important compounds, such as sterols, steroidal saponins, cardioactive glycosides, bile acids, corticosteroids, and sex hormones in mammals. Saponins, a group of natural compounds, consist of triterpenoid or steroidal aglycones (called genin or sapogenin) covalently linked to one or more sugar molecules (Tiwari et al., 2015).

I.2.1.4. Tetraterpenes (Carotenoids)

Over 650 carotenoids (C40) are present in nature, making them the largest group of natural dyes. Carotenoids possess unique properties that are not found in other substances, which underlie their diverse functions and actions across various living organisms. Plants, algae, fungi, yeasts, and bacteria synthesize these compounds (Tiwari et al., 2015).

Carotenoids are isoprenoid compounds formed through the tail-to-tail linkage of two geranylgeranyl diphosphate molecules, resulting in a parent C40 carbon skeleton from which all variations are derived. This skeleton can be modified in several ways:

a) By cyclization at one or both ends of the molecule to create seven different end groups
b) By altering the level of hydrogenation
c) By adding oxygen-containing functional groups

I.2.2. Phenolic Compounds

Phenolic compounds are abundantly found in nature and exhibit a wide range of chemical structures. They can include simple phenols (C6), such as hydrobenzoic acid derivatives and catechols, as well as high molecular weight polymers like catechol melanins $(C6)_6$, lignins (C6-C3) , and condensed tannins (C6-C3-C6) . Stilbenes (C6-C2-C6) and flavonoids (C6-C3-C6) are phenolic compounds with intermediate molecular weights that exhibit various pharmacological and biological activities (Jan et al., 2021). Flavonoids, which encompass anthocyanins, flavonols (including quercetin and myricetin), and isoflavones (such as daidzein and genistein), are derived from multiple biosynthetic pathways that originate from chalcone (Tiwari et al., 2015).

I.2.3. Alkaloids

Alkaloids are defined as basic compounds produced by living organisms, characterized by the presence of one or more heterocyclic nitrogen atoms. They are typically derived from amino acids, though there are some exceptions, and are known for their pharmacological activity. The name of this class stems from the fact that nearly all alkaloids are alkaline compounds. Alkaloids represent a vast group of secondary metabolites, with over 12,000 distinct substances having been isolated.

This group is marked by a wide variety of structural formulas arising from different biosynthetic pathways and exhibiting a diverse range of pharmacological activities.

Alkaloids are linked to a variety of pharmacological activities. Many of them are toxic and can be lethal, even in small doses. Some possess antibiotic properties, while others affect behavior, including antidepressants like reserpine and hallucinogens such as mescaline. The role of alkaloids in plants and animals appears to be associated with defense mechanisms, as their toxicity serves as an effective means to deter predators, such as herbivores (Tiwari et al., 2015).

I.3. Mechanisms of Action of EOs on Microorganisms

Plants produce a diverse array of secondary metabolites that primarily serve to protect against predators and microbes, functioning according to the toxic nature of these threats to deter both microbes and herbivores. Some of these secondary metabolites also aid in communication with other organisms, while others protect from abiotic stressors, such as UV-B radiation. Thus, secondary metabolites are crucial for plant growth and development. The three main categories of secondary metabolites produced in plants are phenolics, terpenes, and nitrogen/sulfur-containing compounds. Terpenes, which have a basic unit of 5-carbon isoprene, act as toxins and deter herbivores. The shikimic acid pathway yields products that form phenolics, enhancing the plant's defensive capabilities. Nitrogen and sulfur-containing compounds are primarily synthesized from amino acids. The defensive roles of secondary metabolites in plants have been confirmed through in vitro studies, where their expression was modified using modern techniques. The formation of these metabolites is the result of millions of years of interaction between plants and pathogens, with over 100,000 metabolites identified as part of the plant defense system; however, many aspects remain unclear. While it is believed that plants with higher concentrations of secondary metabolites are more resistant to biotic and abiotic stresses, the production of these compounds is thought to be resource-intensive for plant growth and reproduction. The functions and structures of plant secondary metabolites illustrate why plants have developed induced defenses, characterized by increased concentrations in response to stress. Numerous studies have revealed that hundreds of plant compounds play ecological and chemical defensive roles, leading to a new area of research known as ecological biochemistry (Jan et al., 2021).

I.4. Secondary Metabolites in Plant Interactions With Pathogens

For a long time, secondary metabolites have been recognized for their interactions with pathogenic organisms. Among the earliest studies of plant immune responses is the investigation of secondary metabolites in the context of plant-pathogen interactions (Figure 3). Decades of research have established that many secondary metabolites play a significant role in the plant defense response to pathogens. Although these compounds exhibit high structural diversity, their functions are largely organized within a conserved framework, while several biosynthetic pathways remain non-conserved across the plant kingdom. The production and activation of these compounds, like other conserved plant defense mechanisms, are triggered by microbial detection through defense proteins or the recognition of microbe-associated molecular patterns (MAMPs) by pattern recognition receptors. Due to the diversity of these secondary metabolites in plant immunity, various classification criteria have been proposed, including common precursors, core structures, and mechanisms of action. Common classifications are based on the synthesis and accumulation of defense-related phytochemicals. Metabolites produced de novo in response to infection are referred to as phytoalexins, while phytoanticipins are those defense-related metabolites that are produced and stored within plant tissues (Maurya, 2020).

Figure 3. Schematic classification of secondary metabolites that may play a role in the defense mechanisms of species against microbial fungi and viruses (Zaynab et al., 2018)

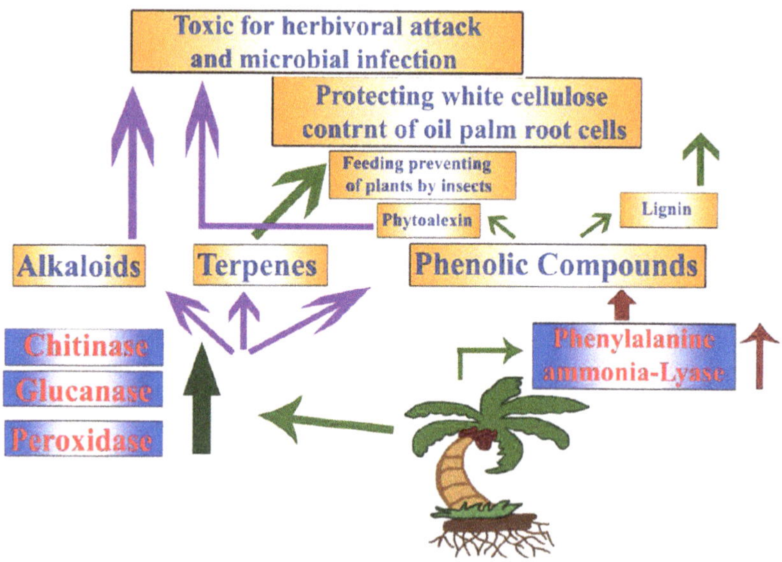

I.5. Mode of Action of Secondary Metabolites

Phenylpropanoids and flavonoids are widespread plant defense compounds with diverse actions, including enzyme inhibition and disruption of pathogen reproduction. Their phenolic hydroxyl groups form hydrogen and ionic bonds with proteins, leading to astringency and denaturation. By altering protein structure through interactions with thiol, hydroxyl, or amino groups, these secondary metabolites can impair protein function and stability, notably via covalent and strong non-covalent bonds, as seen with polyphenols. The formation of these weak non-covalent bonds can simultaneously affect protein flexibility, leading to protein inactivation. The polar nature of phenols generally makes them less toxic, as their absorption is lower after oral intake. An experiment was conducted to investigate the effects of resveratrol and pinosylvin (stilbene compounds) on fungal growth using wood decay tests with aspen and birch samples impregnated with stilbene. The plate experiment indicated that at concentrations sufficient to inhibit fungal growth, pinosylvin was effective, whereas resveratrol enhanced fungal growth (Zaynab et al., 2018).

I.5.1. Secondary Metabolites Against Plant Insects

Secondary metabolites do not inhibit the growth and development of plants; rather, they impact the fodder value of the tissues where they are produced. These metabolites can either be induced in response to attacks from microbes and insects (phytoalexins) or stored in inactive forms (phytoanticipins) (Figure 4). During herbivory, the activation of phytoanticipins by β-glucosidase leads to the release of biocidal aglycones. A classic example of phytoanticipins is the hydrolysis of glucosinolates by myrosinases during tissue disruption. Benzoxazinoids (BXs), found in the Poaceae family, serve as another example of phytoanticipins; when tissue is damaged, their hydrolysis by plastid-targeted β-glucosidase produces biocidal aglycone BXs that act as insect repellents. In contrast, phytoalexins including alkaloids, terpenoids, and isoflavonoids negatively affect herbivore performance. In addition to providing defense, secondary metabolites enhance the overall fitness of plants (Zaynab et al., 2018).

Figure 4. Overview of plant secondary metabolites and their roles in the plant defense system (Zaynab et al., 2018)

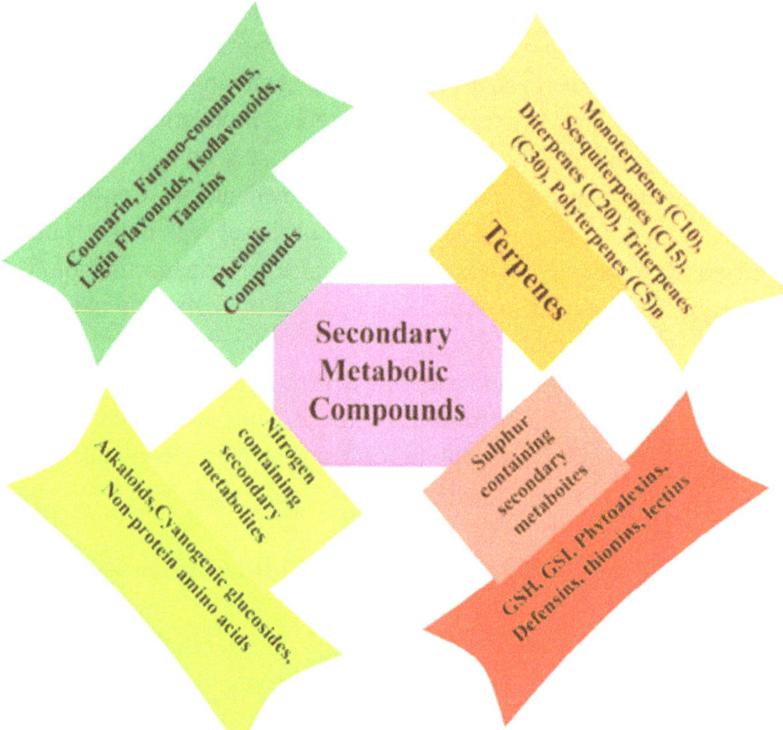

I.5.2. Secondary Metabolites Against Plant Viruses

Various secondary metabolites in plants, such as alkaloids, phenolics, and flavonoids, exhibit antiviral properties. Alkaloids, with their diverse structures, encompass many biologically active compounds that affect living organisms. Research has identified approximately 18,000 alkaloids in ancient Chinese herbs known for their antiviral effects. One notable example is 7-deoxy-trans-dihydronarciclasine, derived from plantain lilies (Hosta plantaginea), which demonstrates anti-Tobacco Mosaic Virus (TMV) activity with a low IC_{50} value of 1.80 μM. Similarly, Bruceine-D, found in the extract of Brassica japonica, shows inhibitory effects against Potato Virus Y (PVY), Cucumber Mosaic Virus (CMV), and TMV (Raut and Karuppayil, 2014).

II. INTEGRATION OF AI FOR ENHANCING THE ANTIMICROBIAL ACTIVITY OF EOS

AI is defined as the set of methods that enable machines (computers, robots, etc.) to imitate behaviors similar to those of humans. These behaviors include problem-solving, decision-making, and learning. AI encompasses several subfields, with the two most widely applied being ML and Deep Learning (DL). DL is a branch of ML (Talat and Khan, 2023; Zhu, 2020).

ML enables machines to learn from data without being explicitly programmed. It includes three types of learning: supervised (where data is labeled), unsupervised, and reinforcement learning. Supervised and unsupervised learning are the most commonly applied in chemistry and biology. In supervised learning, algorithms learn from labeled data, meaning the training data comes with expected output results. The model aims to find a function that links inputs to outputs. Algorithms or models used in this type of learning include linear and logistic regression, decision trees and random forests, support vector machines (SVM), and k-nearest neighbors (K-NN). Unsupervised learning, on the other hand, uses unlabeled training data and groups data based on similarities or reduces data dimensionality to simplify it. Clustering algorithms (such as k-means and hierarchical clustering) and dimensionality reduction algorithms (such as Principal Component Analysis) are used in this type of learning (Talat and Khan., 2023; Sarker, 2021; Alzubaidi et al., 2021)

DL relies on deep neural networks (with multiple layers) to extract complex features from data. Neural networks are computational models inspired by the human brain, consisting of layers of interconnected artificial neurons where each neuron takes inputs and generates an output. Types of neural networks used in DL include convolutional neural networks (CNNs), recurrent neural networks (RNNs), and artificial neural networks (ANNs). DL can use the three types of learning mentioned above. Figure 5 provides a summary of AI and its branches (Murcia-Soler et al., 2004).

Figure 5. ML, branches and methods commonly used

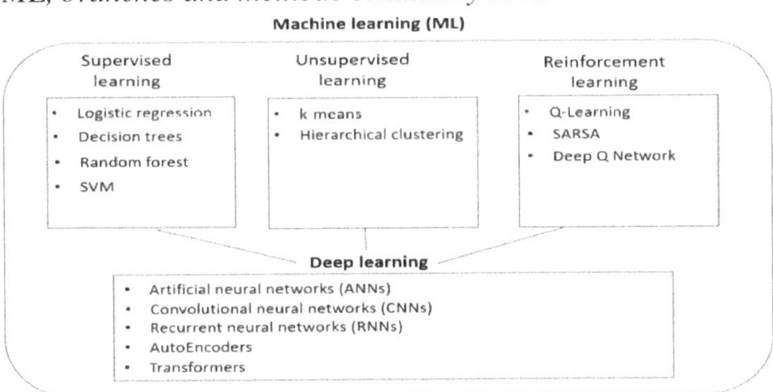

Due to its ability to analyze massive datasets, learn autonomously, and predict outcomes, AI is applied in numerous areas of human life, such as industry, medicine, chemistry, and biology, among others. In medicine, AI is used for early disease detection, clinical trial management, and personalized treatment. For example, using medical images, ML algorithms can diagnose diseases such as cancer (Blasiak et al., 2020). Indeed, based on data in the form of medical images (such as X-rays, mammograms, MRIs, etc.), a set of ML models (particularly DL) can be used for anomaly detection. In the case of cancers, they can even determine the location and stage of the tumor. Among the most commonly used algorithms in this context are CNNs, ResNet (Residual Network), and VGG (Visual Geometry Group).

AI plays a pivotal role in biology and chemistry by employing ML and DL techniques to analyze structure–activity relationships and predict molecular interactions with biological targets. These approaches facilitate the identification of compounds with optimized properties (e.g., activity, toxicity), thereby reducing both the time and cost associated with drug and compound development. In fact, AI accelerates the drug discovery process by reducing the number of compounds that need to be tested experimentally. In addition, AI is used to accurately predict the outcomes of chemical reactions by considering conditions and reaction parameters as they are in reality (pressure, temperature, and concentration of reactants, etc.). Indeed, it helps to minimize the number of experimental tests, errors related to experimental methods, and also reduces the traditional techniques used in laboratories to understand reaction mechanisms. AI also helps biologists understand the processes of interactions between biological molecules, such as proteins and nucleic acids nucléiques (Blasiak et al., 2020; Hosny et al., 2018).

II.1. Analysis of Bioactive Compounds with AI

Antimicrobial activity of EOs is due to the presence of various secondary metabolites like phenols, aldehydes and alcohols. Bioactive analysis of EOs means characterization of the compounds that exert this anti-microbial action. However, this process is experimentally complicated given the chemical diversity of EOs. Bioactive analysis may be explained as a method or process whereby molecules with particular biological activities (e.g: antimicrobial and antioxidant) are investigated (Soni et al., 2023).

Bioactive analysis processes are enhanced, and automated into faster processes using AI. Depending on bioactive, there are several techniques being involved in analysis such as ML and DL. These methods take advantage of large datasets of past experiments and from chemical and biological databases, thus allowing to correlate between the chemical structure of compounds and their biological activity, and to then optimize and predict the most active compounds (Papa et al. 2020).

After collecting data from various sources, they are preprocessed to increase their quality and ensure their compliance with exploratory analysis methods and algorithms. During the data preprocessing step, several techniques are applied, such as cleaning, normalization, feature selection, and transformation. Together, these preprocessing steps improve the quality of the data, making it suitable for effective modeling and analysis. After the data preprocessing operation, by clustering techniques such as K-means and hierarchical clustering, an exploratory analysis is applied allowing a grouping of compounds according to their chemical or biological similarities (structural characteristics, activity, etc.). Indeed, these clustering methods identify and provide information on the relationships between different EO compounds and their biological activities (Yabuuchi et al., 2023).

The third step is to build predictive models using ML learning methods. The goal of these models is to predict the biological activity of compounds based on their chemical characteristics. After the modeling phase, the chemical structures are refined to improve their effectiveness using optimization techniques. These techniques allow us to test the effectiveness of different structural modifications of the molecules and choose the best molecular structures before proceeding to experimental testing. Figure 6 illustrates the process of bioactive analysis using AI.

Figure 6. Bioactive analysis process using AI

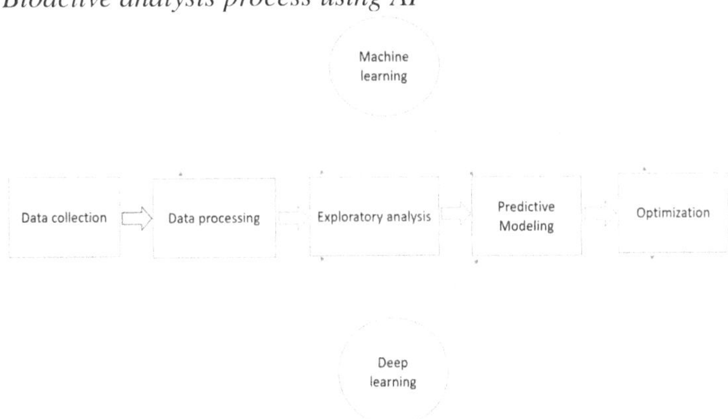

II.2. Optimization of EOs Formulations

AI assisted EOs optimization include, lab method used to select EOs combinations with maximum antimicrobial potential. In contrast to the bioactive compounds analysis which aims to identify the values of individual properties of components, optimization refers to obtaining a new and more active compounds formulations by means of adjusting the levels of individual components, taking into consideration the interactions between the different components and their combined effects on pathogens (Xiang et al., 2012). In this context, AI helps evaluating a large number of possible compounds formulations without the need to conduct experimental trials for each one. This significantly reduces the time and resources required to obtain optimal combinations.

The optimization process begins with collecting data on EOs (their properties, including their effectiveness in different possible formulations) by exploring databases, either chemical or biological, or other data resources. AI, through prediction and ML methods, is then used to model the relationships between the components and the desired results (Papa et al., 2020; Mihaylova et al., 2024). Multivariate regression algorithms and DL is used for the optimization of EOs formulations. With these techniques, it is possible to predict the expected results for new formulations taking out the data from previous combinations. Notably, DL has the capacity to study complicated molecular architecture and discern complex nonlinear interactions between individual EO components. AI models can subsequently provide new combinations of these which, while maximizing antibacterial effect, also minimizes host adverse reactions or production costs (Xiang et al. 2012; Smith et al. 2020). Clustering algorithms can also be used for optimization by grouping EOs whose chemical and biological properties are similar. This enables new blends to be identified, as it can help determine potentially successful formulations based on results of similar groups (Smith et al., 2020; Mihaylova et al., 2024).

The last of these steps is to experimentally validate the optimized formulations predicted. The AI-derived models are validated in the lab to assure that they over-deliver and meet pre-determined performance metrics (antimicrobial, safety, etc.). Changes can be made depending the results of the experiment, if needed. So, AI allows us to automate the optimization of EOs which will lead to better and faster formulations. Figure 7 illustrates this formulation optimization process, showing the various steps from data collection to the validation of the optimized formulations.

Figure 7. Process of optimizing EOs formulations using AI

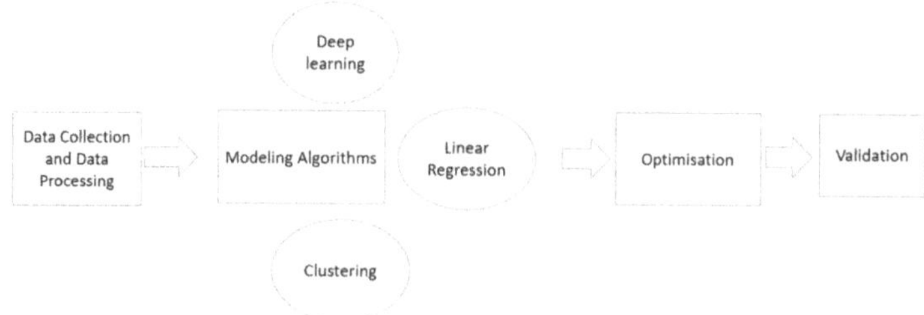

III. PRACTICAL APPLICATION OF AI IN DEVELOPING ANTIMICROBIAL SOLUTIONS

The growing application of AI for the development of antimicrobial solutions represents a whole new chapter in public health and agri-food research and innovation. The alarming emergence of antibiotic-resistant bacteria has been recognized as a major threat to global health. AI is now emerging as a key tool for accelerating the discovery of new drugs and optimizing existing formulations. The use of ML algorithms and predictive modeling techniques, together with the screening of large databases of molecules, enable the rapid identification of new bioactive molecules with antimicrobial activity (Branda and Scarpa, 2024).

AMR is becoming a challenge for our medical treatments and food safety, which is why AI is helping not only to find new antimicrobial agents, but also to provide stable formulations. The development of predictive modeling makes it possible not only to design compounds with the desired activity, but also those with reduced toxicity, which is crucial for the treatment of multidrug-resistant infections (Ahmed et al., 2024). In addition, AI meets the stringent regulatory requirements of the medical and agri-food sectors to ensure the safety and efficacy of the products developed (Ikram et al., 2024). Consequently, the implication of AI application in this field is not limited to the discovery of new treatments, but also to the iterative design of formulations for specific applications notably with regard to infection prevention and the improvement of natural preservatives (Visan and Negut, 2024).

This dynamic opens new perspectives for research in microbiology and pharmacology, reinforcing the importance of AI in the development of innovative antimicrobial solutions adapted to contemporary challenges.

III.1. The Role of AI in Antibiotic Discovery

The discovery of new antibiotics is becoming increasingly difficult. Natural product discovery faces the dereplication problem, where the same molecules are frequently rediscovered (Cox et al., 2017). Additionally, the rapid expansion of accessible chemical spaces through the derivatization of complex scaffolds (Ortholand and Ganesan, 2004) has resulted in more failures than successes when engineering next-generation versions of existing antibiotics. As a result, many antibiotic discovery programs have shifted to screening large synthetic chemical libraries (Tommasi et al., 2015). However, these libraries, which can contain hundreds of thousands to millions of molecules, are often prohibitively expensive to curate, limited in chemical diversity, and do not adequately represent the inherent chemistry of antibiotic molecules (Brown et al., 2014). Since the advent of high-throughput screening in the 1980s, no new clinical antibiotics have been discovered using this method.

To enhance the identification rate of new antibiotics while reducing the associated costs, novel approaches are essential. Recent advancements in ML (Camacho et al., 2018) open the door for algorithmic solutions in molecular property prediction, enabling the identification of new structural classes of antibiotics. By adopting methodologies that allow early drug discovery to be conducted primarily in silico, researchers can explore vast chemical spaces that current experimental approaches cannot access.

ML models offer a flexible way to simulate and predict complex pathogen-host interactions, crucial for understanding diseases (Nguyen et al., 2019). AI provides innovative strategies to tackle antibiotic resistance crises. For instance, AI can analyze genomic data to detect resistance markers early, facilitating timely interventions. Moreover, AI-driven decision support systems can optimize antibiotic use by recommending effective treatments based on patient data and local resistance patterns. AI can expedite drug discovery by predicting the efficacy of new compounds and identifying potential antibacterial agents.

One promising approach is the computational design of new antibiotics (Mak et al., 2023). As larger genomic collections become available, studies utilize ML algorithms to predict susceptible and resistant phenotypes (Nguyen et al., 2018). AI-based diagnostic tools can efficiently analyze vast data volumes, often outperforming human accuracy, enabling faster, targeted diagnoses. Notably, ML algorithms can be trained to recognize specific features in microscopic images of bacterial cultures indicative of antibiotic resistance. For instance, a study by Hayashi et al. employed Convolutional Neural Networks (CNNs) to identify drug-resistant bacterial cells in transmission electron microscope (TEM) images without the need for antibiotic exposure (Hayashi et al., 2021).

DL algorithms also play a significant role in rapidly analyzing antibiotic susceptibility testing (AST), reducing the time to determine resistance from days to hours. Recurrent Neural Networks (RNNs) are crucial in this domain, with Arango-Argoty et al. 2018 developing DeepARG, a DL approach designed to predict antibiotic resistance genes (ARGs) from metagenomic data, incorporating two models tailored for different annotation strategies.

Overall, the application of AI, particularly ML and DL, is expanding across various fields, including healthcare (Wang et al., 2022; Joshi et al., 2024). AI is being harnessed to design new antibiotics and generate synergistic combinations of drugs (Nava et al., 2019). ML algorithms analyze patterns in antimicrobial use and resistance, enabling healthcare providers to make informed decisions about drug usage. Furthermore, ML models are employed for monitoring antimicrobial resistance, analyzing large datasets to identify emerging resistance patterns and hotspots, thus helping public health authorities respond to resistant infection outbreaks more efficiently.

In terms of antimicrobial stewardship, ML can optimize antimicrobial use in healthcare settings, identifying the best drug combinations for specific infections or predicting which patients are at risk of developing resistant infections (Javaid et al., 2022).

III.2. Use of Predictive Algorithms to Determine Optimal Doses and Minimize Adverse Effects

Optimizing drug dosages is a significant challenge in healthcare, as inappropriate dosing can lead to serious adverse effects and diminish therapeutic efficacy. Predictive algorithms emerge as a promising solution by integrating patient data, pharmacokinetic characteristics, and individual factors. These algorithms analyze large datasets to provide personalized dosing recommendations that account for interindividual variability. Consequently, the application of such technologies can substantially enhance treatment safety and optimize clinical outcomes (Olatunji et al., 2024).

Table 1 illustrates key factors influencing drug dosage optimization through predictive algorithms. Each factor—patient data, pharmacokinetics, disease state, and data qualityaffects the precision of dosing recommendations, enhancing therapeutic effectiveness and minimizing adverse effects. For instance, integrating genetic and health history data allows algorithms to provide personalized recommendations by accounting for individual variability. Pharmacokinetic characteristics, such as enzyme activity, help adjust dosages to accommodate differences in drug metabolism, improving efficacy and reducing side effects. Additionally, considering disease state allows dosing to adapt as conditions progress, a critical feature for managing chronic diseases. High-quality and extensive datasets further bolster these algorithms by enabling robust and data-driven clinical decision-making. Together, these components underscore the importance of leveraging comprehensive data and advanced AI techniques to optimize patient outcomes in dosage management.

Table 1. Factors and solutions in drug dosage optimization using predictive algorithms

Factor	Impact on Dosage	Predictive Algorithm Application	Outcome
Patient Data	Identifies individual needs	Integrates genetic and health history data	Personalized dosing recommendations
Pharmacokinetic Characteristics	Variability in drug metabolism	Adjusts for enzyme activity levels	Reduces adverse effects, increases efficacy
Disease State	Alters response to drugs	Accounts for progression of disease	Adaptive dosing in chronic disease management
Data Volume and Quality	Affects accuracy of predictions	Uses large datasets with ML models	Optimizes clinical decision-making

III.3. Optimization of Time in Diagnosis and AMR Detection

III.3.1. Traditional Diagnostics Challenges and Advancements

Classic antimicrobial diagnostics are often slow and complex, with current susceptibility tests taking over 24 hours and requiring expert interpretation of extensive whole-genome sequencing data (Ma et al., 2023). Recent studies have focused on reducing diagnosis time, achieving results as quickly as 3 hours through techniques like flow cytometry combined with ML (Inglis et al., 2020). AI-based solutions have been developed to enhance the efficiency of genome data management (Wattam et al., 2014) and establish optimal antibiotic use strategies in sepsis treatment (Tsoukalas et al., 2023). These AI approaches can identify suitable actions and predict patient outcomes with high accuracy, addressing the urgency of timely interventions in critical conditions like sepsis, where delays can significantly impact mortality (Zasowski et al.,2020).

III.3.2. AI in Antimicrobial Susceptibility Testing (AST)

To improve AST methods, Inglis et al. introduced a combined flowcytometer antimicrobial susceptibility testing (FAST) method integrated with supervised ML (Mulroney et al., 2017), achieving reliable results in under 3 hours (Inglis et al., 2020). Similarly, Lechowicz et al. developed an IR-spectrometer method that reduced AST duration from 24 hours to 30 minutes by utilizing infrared (IR) spectroscopy and artificial neural networks (Lechowicz et al., 2013).

III.3.3. Whole-Genome Sequencing for AMR (WGS-AST)

Current studies on WGS-AST predominantly rely on k-mer analysis derived from whole-genome samples (Arango et al., 2018). However, the size and redundancy of k-mer datasets present challenges for direct AI applications. To overcame this by converting k-mer data into a binary matrix via rapid annotation using subsystem technology (RAST) (Overbeek et al., 2014). Mahé et al. further optimized the predictive models by employing stability selection to generate a smaller, more manageable subset of k-mer data, enhancing interpretability (Mahé et al., 2018).

III.4. Optimization of Drug Dosage Using AI

III.4.1. Importance of Optimized Dosage

Optimizing drug dosage is crucial to ensuring patient safety, maximizing treatment efficacy and reducing healthcare costs. Indeed, conventional dosing methods, although fundamental, may not meet individual patient needs, particularly due to metabolic variations (Ekechukwu, 2021; Maha et al., 2024). It is essential to take these differences into account in order to avoid undesirable effects and potential inefficiencies. This opens up a debate on the need for a more precise and individualized approach, which could be facilitated by advanced technologies such as AI.

III.4.2. Role of AI in Dosage Optimization

AI represents a promising advance in overcoming the limitations of traditional methods, as it can analyze a multitude of patient data such as genetic information, physiological parameters and medical history. This ability to adapt to the specifics of each patient enables treatment personalization and a significant reduction in the risk of adverse effects (Amajuoyi et al., 2024). This transition to adaptive dosing strategies could transform the way treatments are designed and administered, raising questions about the place of the human in the management of these technologies.

III.4.3. Addressing Variability in Drug Response

Standardized dosing methods are often based on population averages, which can lead to limited efficacy in some individuals. In comparison, AI algorithms can analyze a wide range of variables to tailor the drug regimen, making treatment more effective and safer (Amajuoyi et al., 2024; Kwakye et al., 2024). This personalization is particularly important in the face of variability in pharmacokinetic responses between patients, underscoring the need for healthcare systems that embrace data-driven solutions to ensure optimized treatments.

III.5. Enhancing Food Safety With AI-Driven Encapsulation of EOs in Antimicrobial Packaging

Food contamination from spoilage and pathogenic microbes poses significant risks to public health, food security, and sustainability. Consequently, EOs have gained popularity due to their antioxidant and antimicrobial properties, which help prevent food spoilage (Mukurumbira et al., 2022). However, their effectiveness is often limited by their chemical instability and hydrophobic nature. To address these challenges, encapsulation technologies are being explored to stabilize EOs, mask their odors, and potentially enhance their antimicrobial efficacy through sustained release.

AI and ML are revolutionizing science and technology, drawing significant interest for their diverse applications. With AI's capacity to simulate human reasoning through algorithms, researchers can now generate hypotheses, plan experiments, and analyze large datasets efficiently, an ability enhanced by platforms like ChatGPT. In food science, AI plays a crucial role in optimizing nanoemulsions for food preservation by enhancing the stability, release kinetics, and antimicrobial efficacy of EOs. Integrating mathematical modeling with AI provides insights into nanoemulsion formulation, preparation methods, and stability factors, facilitating a controlled release of EOs and their bioactive components, thus improving food preservation systems.

Researchers are delving into sophisticated ML techniques—such as artificial neural networks (ANNs), genetic algorithms (GA), support vector machines (SVM), random forest, K-means clustering, and decision trees—to innovate food-delivery systems. These approaches aim to develop more effective and consistent release mechanisms for food preservation applications, resulting in higher efficiency and targeted delivery within various food systems.

IV. CHALLENGES AND PERSPECTIVES OF USING AI IN EO RESEARCH

The use of AI in fundamental investigations on EOs, especially related to their antimicrobial properties, has great potential and is a very complicated challenge at the same time. We will explore the scientific, technology, ethical, regulation and safety issues involved and look toward the best potential future directions for leveraging AI in this arena (Lai et al., 2020; Hannan et al.2021; Abdalla et al.2021).

IV.1. Technological and Scientific Challenges

IV.1.1. Limitations of Current Databases on Metabolites

The absence of diverse databases regarding secondary metabolites with a significant number of compounds and high-quality standards is one of the main obstacles for the use of AI in this field, particularly to design new antimicrobial EOs. These metabolites are the most important bioactive compounds in EOs, giving them their antimicrobial, antiviral and antifungal properties. Nevertheless, existing databases are mostly non-standardized, incomplete, and fragmented with respect to integrated data on the chemical structures, biological activity and interactions of these compounds. The lack of data diminishes the predictive power of AI models which need high-quality datasets to predict the antimicrobial activity of EOs (Machireddy et al., 2021).

A solution to this issue might be a concerted effort toward developing larger and more elaborate metabolite databases as shown in Table 2. This implies integrating chemical information, biological activity records, and molecular interactions to provide a sound basis for AI systems to generate reliable predictions (Aldoseri et al., 2023).

Table 2. Limitations and proposed solutions for metabolite databases

Limitation	Proposed Solution
Lack of standardization	Develop internationally standardized metabolite databases
Incomplete data	Expand the collection of chemical and biological activity data
Lack of molecular interaction information	Integrate detailed molecular interaction records

IV.1.2. Difficulties in Modeling Complex Molecular Interactions

The secondary metabolites of EOs have a synergistic effect where the combined impact is different (and usually more potent) than their individual actions. AI has a big task ahead of it in modeling these convoluted molecular interactions. However, for EOs the chemical environments can be more complex and dynamic which would prove difficult in simulating with ML and DL models that have shown promise in other fields (Sarkar et al., 2023).

Irrespective of the degree to which chemical similarity has been employed in drug-discovery AI, multi-layered modeling approaches are required to have a complete understanding of the ways that such compounds interact with bacterial or fungal targets to inhibit growth something that arguably remains beyond the reach of current AI tools. Furthermore, EOs may target multiple biological pathways, so even the most advanced AI algorithms may not be able to determine a single mechanism of action (Bender and Cortes-Ciriano, 2021).

So, a new study revealed that the convolutional neural networks (CNN) combined with smartphone-captured images can predict bergamot EOs contents in some cultivars at an accuracy of 0.797. But the spectrally closest match cameras limit their ability to resolve with the lack of non-visible spectral bands (NIR or SWIR). The study further noticed that cultivar-specific models outperform the general model. The final step to achieving the use of this technology in Agriculture 4.0 is being able to directly and constantly apply it within the field (Anello et al., 2024).

IV.2. Ethical, Regulatory, and Safety Aspects of Using AI

IV.2.1. Issues Related to the Acceptability of AI-Developed Solutions

With AI systems having impacts on research results and the decision-making regarding, for example, the use of EOs in antimicrobial applications, their acceptability is called into question. Regulatory agencies, researchers, and consumers alike may not want to trust results or formulations generated by AI — particularly when human knowledge is partially (or totally) replaced. It is important to develop trust in AI solutions (Table 3) through openness of the approaches used, the data sources referred to and decisions made by AI systems (Trunk et al., 2020; Sarker, 2022).

Moreover, the branch of EOs frequently overlaps into traditional medicine where a long-standing tradition of empirical knowledge may contradict AI predicted recommendations. Cultural sensitivities such as these will need to be effectively engaged to ensure the widespread acceptability of AI-optimized EOs (Robinson, 2020; Kim and Lee, 2024).

Table 3. Challenges and solutions in AI-optimized EOs

Challenges	Proposed Solutions
Incomplete metabolite databases	Development of more sophisticated and comprehensive databases
Complexity of molecular interactions	Advanced AI models and multi-layered simulation techniques
Ethical concerns	Transparency and cultural sensitivity in AI applications
Regulatory uncertainty	Creation of international standards and guidelines

IV.2.2. Regulation and Standardization of AI-Optimized Eos

A major other challenge is concerned with regulation and standardization of the developed solutions using AI techniques. Growing interest in the involvement of AI technology for optimizing EOs formulations emphasizes developing international standards for assessing the efficacy, safety and quality of such automated AI-based products. The science behind this approach, however—like the regulatory framework ahead of it—is not ready for AI. As a result, EOs produced using such approaches might struggle to gain approval for medicinal or industrial use (Jurado et al., 2024).

It may be worth considering the establishment of guidelines as they relate to the development and regulation of these AI-optimized EOs. This would involve standards for the calibration of AI algorithms, mechanisms to guarantee the safety and consistency of end output, frameworks for post-market surveillance regarding harmful implications or safety signals (Outeda, 2024).

IV.3. Future Perspectives and Recommendations

IV.3.1. The Potential of AI in Combating Antimicrobial Resistance

This is reflected in one of the most promising future perspectives of AI in EOs research: to help in overcoming AMR. As traditional antibiotics become ineffective against resistant bacterial strains, the use of antimicrobial properties of EOs may provide alternatives in therapy. AI can also prove to be a hotshot by enabling us to quickly screen and select those EOs or their metabolites that are most effective against resistant microbes.

In addition, antibiogram based research under the influence of AI could explore the synergistic combinations between EOs and common antibiotics to minimize resistance induction and improve overall antimicrobial activity alone or together. Such an approach may result in new therapies to combat the increasing issue of AMR.

IV.3.2. New Research Directions for Using EOs in Medicine and Industry

AI unveils more possibilities, in terms of medicine and also industry, on how to apply EOs, AI could generate new therapeutic uses of EOs in medicine from chronic diseases, cancer, and inflammatory conditions. With its ability to parse vast quantities of biological and chemical data, AI can identify new properties for EOs that may allow them to be used in precision medicine (Sabzi-Nojadeh et al., 2021).

AI could improve the industrial production of EOs by predicting optimal plant cultivation, extraction methods and formulations to obtain maximum yield and potency. It could make production processes more sustainable and resource use lower. Moreover, AI may be applied to devise EOs mixtures for specific industrial uses including cosmetic or food applications or as natural pesticides (Niazian and Niedbała., 2020).

CONCLUSION

This chapter illustrates the power of AI in the research of secondary metabolites of EOs and their application as antimicrobial agents. The extensive analytical capabilities of AI, such as ML and virtual screening, enable researchers to explore the underlying complex interactions of bioactive compounds with pathogens. Such tools can expedite the identification and characterization of potent anti-microbial agents and assist in devising combinations that exhibit synergy to obtain a more potent functionality of EOs, respectively. This AI integration is a crucial answer to the growing threat of antimicrobial resistance, paving the way for a new generation of sustainable solutions with the potential to replace or supplement conventional antibiotics.

This research will have far-reaching consequences in the use of AI to change the very nature of how we study natural compounds, with applications that extend beyond just antimicrobials. AI allows researchers to sift through massive data sets more quickly and discover hidden patterns and correlations that they might never find otherwise. This enables the study of previously less studied metabolites, discovery of new anti-microbial compounds, and the designing of EO formulations according to medical and industry specific requirements.

As future work, the further development of AI in EOs research may bring several major changes. With the rise of advanced AI technologies, we see more targeted and scalable EO applications, making EOs potentially attractive for wider medical and industrial applications. In medicine, and particularly for infections, AI may propel the potential for personalized antimicrobial therapies, with EOs customized to target infections by various bacterial strains or to meet a particular health need unique to an individual patient. Such individualized work could result in novel efficient and environmentally sustainable therapies especially with the burgeoning resistance of microorganisms to conventional therapeutics.

REFERENCES

Abdalla, A. N., Nazir, M. S., Tao, H., Cao, S., Ji, R., Jiang, M., & Yao, L. (2021). Integration of energy storage system and renewable energy sources based on artificial intelligence: An overview. *Journal of Energy Storage*, *40*, 102811. DOI: 10.1016/j.est.2021.102811

Ahmed, S. K., Hussein, S., Qurbani, K., Ibrahim, R. H., Fareeq, A., Mahmood, K. A., & Mohamed, M. G. (2024). Antimicrobial resistance: Impacts, challenges, and future prospects. *Journal of Medicine, Surgery, and Public Health*, *2*, 100081. DOI: 10.1016/j.glmedi.2024.100081

Aldoseri, A., Al-Khalifa, K. N., & Hamouda, A. M. (2023). Re-thinking data strategy and integration for artificial intelligence: Concepts, opportunities, and challenges. *Applied Sciences (Basel, Switzerland)*, *13*(12), 7082. DOI: 10.3390/app13127082

Amajuoyi, P., Benjamin, L. B., & Adeus, K. B. (2024). Agile methodologies: Adapting product management to rapidly changing market conditions. *GSC Advanced Research and Reviews*, *19*(2), 249–267. DOI: 10.30574/gscarr.2024.19.2.0181

Anello, M., Mateo, F., Bernardi, B., Giuffre, A. M., Blasco, J., & Gómez-Sanchis, J. (2024). Convolutional neural networks to assess bergamot essential oil content in the field from smartphone images. *Industrial Crops and Products*, *220*, 119233. DOI: 10.1016/j.indcrop.2024.119233

Arango-Argoty, G., Garner, E., Pruden, A., Heath, L. S., Vikesland, P., & Zhang, L. (2018). DeepARG: A deep learning approach for predicting antibiotic resistance genes from metagenomic data. *Microbiome*, *6*(1), 1–15. DOI: 10.1186/s40168-018-0401-z PMID: 29391044

Belcadi, H., Aknouch, A., El Amrani, S., Chraka, A., Lachkar, M., Mouhib, M., Zantar, S., & Ibnmansour, A. (2023). Gamma-irradiation effect on the chemical composition and antibacterial activity of the moroccan tanacetum annuum L. essential oil. *Heliyon*, *9*(6), e16625. Advance online publication. DOI: 10.1016/j.heliyon.2023.e16625 PMID: 37292271

Belcadi, H., Aknouch, A., El Amrani, S., Chraka, A., Lachkar, M., Mouhib, M., Zantar, S., & Ibnmansour, A. (2023). Gamma-irradiation effect on the chemical composition and antibacterial activity of the moroccan tanacetum annuum L. essential oil. *Heliyon*, *9*(6), e16625. DOI: 10.1016/j.heliyon.2023.e16625 PMID: 37292271

Bender, A., & Cortes-Ciriano, I. (2021). Artificial intelligence in drug discovery: what is realistic, what are illusions? Part 2: a discussion of chemical and biological data. *Drug Discovery Today*, *26*(4), 1040–1052. DOI: 10.1016/j.drudis.2020.11.037 PMID: 33508423

Branda, F., & Scarpa, F. (2024). Implications of Artificial Intelligence in Addressing Antimicrobial Resistance: Innovations, Global Challenges, and Healthcare's Future. *Antibiotics (Basel, Switzerland)*, *13*(6), 502. DOI: 10.3390/antibiotics13060502 PMID: 38927169

Brown, D. G., May-Dracka, T. L., Gagnon, M. M., & Tommasi, R. (2014). Trends and exceptions of physical properties on antibacterial activity for Gram-positive and Gram-negative pathogens. *Journal of Medicinal Chemistry*, *57*(23), 10144–10161. DOI: 10.1021/jm501552x PMID: 25402200

Camacho, D. M., Collins, K. M., Powers, R. K., Costello, J. C., & Collins, J. J. (2018). Next-generation machine learning for biological networks. *Cell*, *173*(7), 1581–1592. DOI: 10.1016/j.cell.2018.05.015 PMID: 29887378

Cox, G., Sieron, A., King, A. M., De Pascale, G., Pawlowski, A. C., Koteva, K., & Wright, G. D. (2017). A common platform for antibiotic dereplication and adjuvant discovery. *Cell Chemical Biology*, *24*(1), 98–109. DOI: 10.1016/j.chembiol.2016.11.011 PMID: 28017602

Cox, G., Sieron, A., King, A. M., De Pascale, G., Pawlowski, A. C., Koteva, K., & Wright, G. D. (2017). A common platform for antibiotic dereplication and adjuvant discovery. *Cell Chemical Biology*, *24*(1), 98–109. DOI: 10.1016/j.chembiol.2016.11.011 PMID: 28017602

Ekechukwu, D. E. (2021). Overview of sustainable sourcing strategies in global value chains: A pathway to responsible business practices. International Journal of Multidisciplinary Research in Science. *Technology and Innovation*, *3*(1), 1–12.

El Hachlafi, N., Fikri-Benbrahim, K., Al-Mijalli, S. H., Elbouzidi, A., Jeddi, M., Abdallah, E. M., Assaggaf, H., Bouyahya, A., Alnasser, S. M., Attar, A., Goh, K. W., Ming, L. C., Ong, S.-K., Mrabti, H. N., & Chahdi, F. O. (2024). Tetraclinis articulata (Vahl) Mast. essential oil as a promising source of bioactive compounds with antimicrobial, antioxidant, anti-inflammatory and dermatoprotective properties: In vitro and in silico evidence. *Heliyon*, *10*(1), e23084. DOI: 10.1016/j.heliyon.2023.e23084 PMID: 38169772

Hannan, M. A., Al-Shetwi, A. Q., Ker, P. J., Begum, R. A., Mansor, M., Rahman, S. A., Dong, Z. Y., Tiong, S. K., Mahlia, T. M. I., & Muttaqi, K. M. (2021). Impact of renewable energy utilization and artificial intelligence in achieving sustainable development goals. *Energy Reports*, *7*, 5359–5373. DOI: 10.1016/j.egyr.2021.08.172

Hayashi-Nishino, M., Aoki, K., Kishimoto, A., Takeuchi, Y., Fukushima, A., Uchida, K., Echigo, T., Yagi, Y., Hirose, M., Iwasaki, K., Shin'ya, E., Washio, T., Furusawa, C., & Nishino, K. (2022). Identification of bacterial drug-resistant cells by the convolutional neural network in transmission electron microscope images. *Frontiers in Microbiology*, *13*, 839718. DOI: 10.3389/fmicb.2022.839718 PMID: 35369486

Ikram, A., Mehmood, H., Arshad, M. T., Rasheed, A., Noreen, S., & Gnedeka, K. T. (2024). Applications of artificial intelligence (AI) in managing food quality and ensuring global food security. *CYTA: Journal of Food*, *22*(1), 2393287. DOI: 10.1080/19476337.2024.2393287

Inglis, T. J., Paton, T. F., Kopczyk, M. K., Mulroney, K. T., & Carson, C. F. (2020). Same-day antimicrobial susceptibility test using acoustic-enhanced flow cytometry visualized with supervised machine learning. *Journal of Medical Microbiology*, *69*(5), 657–669. DOI: 10.1099/jmm.0.001092 PMID: 31665100

Jan, R., Asaf, S., Numan, M., Lubna, , & Kim, K.-M. (2021). Plant secondary metabolite biosynthesis and transcriptional regulation in response to biotic and abiotic stress conditions. *Agronomy (Basel)*, *11*(5), 968. DOI: 10.3390/agronomy11050968

Javaid, M., Haleem, A., Singh, R. P., Suman, R., & Rab, S. (2022). Significance of machine learning in healthcare: Features, pillars and applications. *International Journal of Intelligent Networks*, *3*, 58–73. DOI: 10.1016/j.ijin.2022.05.002

Joshi, G., Jain, A., Araveeti, S. R., Adhikari, S., Garg, H., & Bhandari, M. (2024). FDA-approved artificial intelligence and machine learning (AI/ML)-enabled medical devices: An updated landscape. *Electronics (Basel)*, *13*(3), 498. DOI: 10.3390/electronics13030498

Jurado, R. D. A., Ye, X., Plaza, V. O., Suárez, M. Z., Moreno, F. P., & Valdés, R. M. A. (2024). An introduction to the current state of standardization and certification on military AI applications. *Journal of Air Transport Management*, *121*, 102685. DOI: 10.1016/j.jairtraman.2024.102685

Kim, S. W., & Lee, Y. (2024). Investigation into the influence of socio-cultural factors on attitudes toward artificial intelligence. *Education and Information Technologies*, *29*(8), 9907–9935. DOI: 10.1007/s10639-023-12172-y

Kwakye, J. M., Ekechukwu, D. E., & Ogundipe, O. B. (2024). Systematic review of the economic impacts of bioenergy on agricultural markets. *International Journal of Advanced Economics*, *6*(7), 306–318. DOI: 10.51594/ijae.v6i7.1342

Lai, J. P., Chang, Y. M., Chen, C. H., & Pai, P. F. (2020). A survey of machine learning models in renewable energy predictions. *Applied Sciences (Basel, Switzerland)*, *10*(17), 5975. DOI: 10.3390/app10175975

Laxminarayan, R. (2022). The overlooked pandemic of antimicrobial resistance. *Lancet*, *399*(10325), 606–607. DOI: 10.1016/S0140-6736(22)00087-3 PMID: 35065701

Lechowicz, Ł., Urbaniak, M., Adamus-Białek, W., & Kaca, W. (2013). The use of infrared spectroscopy and artificial neural networks for detection of uropathogenic Escherichia coli strains' susceptibility to cephalothin. *Acta Biochimica Polonica*, *60*(4), 713–718. DOI: 10.18388/abp.2013_2046 PMID: 24432322

Ma, L., Yi, J., Wisuthiphaet, N., Earles, M., & Nitin, N. (2023). Accelerating the detection of bacteria in food using artificial intelligence and optical imaging. *Applied and Environmental Microbiology*, *89*(1), e01828–e22. DOI: 10.1128/aem.01828-22 PMID: 36533914

Machireddy, J. R., Rachakatla, S. K., & Ravichandran, P. (2021). AI-Driven Business Analytics for Financial Forecasting: Integrating Data Warehousing with Predictive Models. *Journal of Machine Learning in Pharmaceutical Research*, *1*(2), 1–24.

Maha, C. C., Kolawole, T. O., & Abdul, S. (2024). Empowering healthy lifestyles: Preventing non-communicable diseases through cohort studies in the US and Africa. *International Journal of Applied Research in Social Sciences*, *6*(6), 1068–1083. DOI: 10.51594/ijarss.v6i6.1172

Mahé, P., & Tournoud, M. (2018). Predicting bacterial resistance from whole-genome sequences using k-mers and stability selection. *BMC Bioinformatics*, *19*(1), 1–11. DOI: 10.1186/s12859-018-2403-z PMID: 30332990

Mak, K. K., Wong, Y. H., & Pichika, M. R. (2023). Artificial intelligence in drug discovery and development. Drug Discovery and Evaluation: Safety and Pharmacokinetic Assays, 1-38. DOI: 10.1007/978-3-030-73317-9_92-1

Mak, K. K., Wong, Y. H., & Pichika, M. R. (2024). Artificial intelligence in drug discovery and development. Drug discovery and evaluation: safety and pharmacokinetic assays, 1461-1498. DOI: 10.1016/j.drudis.2020.10.010

Maurya, A. K. (2020). Role of plant volatile organic compounds (VOCS) in seed priming and plant-herbivore interactions. https://doi.org/.DOI: 10.18297/etd/3404

Mukurumbira, A. R., Shellie, R. A., Keast, R., Palombo, E. A., & Jadhav, S. R. (2022). Encapsulation of essential oils and their application in antimicrobial active packaging. *Food Control, 136*, 108883. DOI: 10.1016/j.foodcont.2022.108883

Mullowney, M. W., Duncan, K. R., Elsayed, S. S., Garg, N., van der Hooft, J. J., Martin, N. I., Meijer, D., Terlouw, B. R., Biermann, F., Blin, K., Durairaj, J., Gorostiola González, M., Helfrich, E. J. N., Huber, F., Leopold-Messer, S., Rajan, K., de Rond, T., van Santen, J. A., Sorokina, M., & Medema, M. H. (2023). Artificial intelligence for natural product drug discovery. *Nature Reviews. Drug Discovery, 22*(11), 895–916. DOI: 10.1038/s41573-023-00774-7 PMID: 37697042

Mulroney, K. T., Hall, J. M., Huang, X., Turnbull, E., Bzdyl, N. M., Chakera, A., Naseer, U., Corea, E. M., Ellington, M. J., Hopkins, K. L., Wester, A. L., Ekelund, O., Woodford, N., & Inglis, T. J. J. (2017). Rapid susceptibility profiling of carbapenem-resistant Klebsiella pneumoniae. *Scientific Reports, 7*(1), 1903. DOI: 10.1038/s41598-017-02009-3 PMID: 28507322

Murray, C. J., Ikuta, K. S., Sharara, F., Swetschinski, L., Aguilar, G. R., Gray, A., & Tasak, N. (2022). Global burden of bacterial antimicrobial resistance in 2019: A systematic analysis. *Lancet, 399*(10325), 629–655. DOI: 10.1016/S0140-6736(21)02724-0 PMID: 35065702

Nava Lara, R. A., Aguilera-Mendoza, L., Brizuela, C. A., Peña, A., & Del Rio, G. (2019). Heterologous machine learning for the identification of antimicrobial activity in Human-Targeted drugs. *Molecules (Basel, Switzerland), 24*(7), 1258. DOI: 10.3390/molecules24071258 PMID: 30935109

Nguyen, M., Brettin, T., Long, S. W., Musser, J. M., Olsen, R. J., Olson, R., Shukla, M., Stevens, R. L., Xia, F., Yoo, H., & Davis, J. J. (2018). Developing an in silico minimum inhibitory concentration panel test for Klebsiella pneumoniae. *Scientific Reports, 8*(1), 421. DOI: 10.1038/s41598-017-18972-w PMID: 29323230

Nguyen, M., Long, S. W., McDermott, P. F., Olsen, R. J., Olson, R., Stevens, R. L., Tyson, G. H., Zhao, S., & Davis, J. J. (2019). Using machine learning to predict antimicrobial MICs and associated genomic features for nontyphoidal Salmonella. *Journal of Clinical Microbiology, 57*(2), 10–1128. DOI: 10.1128/JCM.01260-18 PMID: 30333126

Niazian, M., & Niedbała, G. (2020). Machine learning for plant breeding and biotechnology. *Agriculture, 10*(10), 436. DOI: 10.3390/agriculture10100436

Olatunji, A. O., Olaboye, J. A., Maha, C. C., Kolawole, T. O., & Abdul, S. (2024). Next-Generation strategies to combat antimicrobial resistance: Integrating genomics, CRISPR, and novel therapeutics for effective treatment. *Engineering Science & Technology Journal*, *5*(7), 2284–2303. DOI: 10.51594/estj.v5i7.1344

Ortholand, J. Y., & Ganesan, A. (2004). Natural products and combinatorial chemistry: Back to the future. *Current Opinion in Chemical Biology*, *8*(3), 271–280. DOI: 10.1016/j.cbpa.2004.04.011 PMID: 15183325

Outeda, C. C. (2024). The EU's AI act: A framework for collaborative governance. *Internet of Things : Engineering Cyber Physical Human Systems*, *27*, 101291. DOI: 10.1016/j.iot.2024.101291

Overbeek, R., Olson, R., Pusch, G. D., Olsen, G. J., Davis, J. J., Disz, T., Edwards, R. A., Gerdes, S., Parrello, B., Shukla, M., Vonstein, V., Wattam, A. R., Xia, F., & Stevens, R. (2014). The SEED and the Rapid Annotation of microbial genomes using Subsystems Technology (RAST). *Nucleic Acids Research*, *42*(D1), D206–D214. DOI: 10.1093/nar/gkt1226 PMID: 24293654

Pascucci, M., Royer, G., Adamek, J., Asmar, M. A., Aristizabal, D., Blanche, L., Bezzarga, A., Boniface-Chang, G., Brunner, A., Curel, C., Dulac-Arnold, G., Fakhri, R. M., Malou, N., Nordon, C., Runge, V., Samson, F., Sebastian, E., Soukieh, D., Vert, J.-P., & Madoui, M.-A. (2021). AI-based mobile application to fight antibiotic resistance. *Nature Communications*, *12*(1), 1–10. DOI: 10.1038/s41467-021-21187-3 PMID: 33608509

Raut, J. S., & Karuppayil, S. M. (2014). A status review on the medicinal properties of essential oils. *Industrial Crops and Products*, *62*, 250–264. DOI: 10.1016/j.indcrop.2014.05.055

Rifna, E. J., Pandiselvam, R., Kothakota, A., Rao, K. S., Dwivedi, M., Kumar, M., & Ramesh, S. V. (2022). Advanced process analytical tools for identification of adulterants in edible oils–A review. *Food Chemistry*, *369*, 130898. DOI: 10.1016/j.foodchem.2021.130898 PMID: 34455326

Robinson, S. C. (2020). Trust, transparency, and openness: How inclusion of cultural values shapes Nordic national public policy strategies for artificial intelligence (AI). *Technology in Society*, *63*, 101421. DOI: 10.1016/j.techsoc.2020.101421

Sabzi-Nojadeh, M., Niedbała, G., Younessi-Hamzekhanlu, M., Aharizad, S., Esmaeilpour, M., Abdipour, M., Kujawa, S., & Niazian, M. (2021). Modeling the Essential Oil and Trans-Anethole Yield of Fennel (Foeniculum vulgare Mill. var. vulgare) by Application Artificial Neural Network and Multiple Linear Regression Methods. *Agriculture*, *11*(12), 1191. DOI: 10.3390/agriculture11121191

Sarkar, C., Das, B., Rawat, V. S., Wahlang, J. B., Nongpiur, A., Tiewsoh, I., Lyngdoh, N. M., Das, D., Bidarolli, M., & Sony, H. T. (2023). Artificial intelligence and machine learning technology driven modern drug discovery and development. *International Journal of Molecular Sciences*, *24*(3), 2026. DOI: 10.3390/ijms24032026 PMID: 36768346

Sarker, I. H. (2022). AI-based modeling: Techniques, applications and research issues towards automation, intelligent and smart systems. *SN Computer Science*, *3*(2), 158. DOI: 10.1007/s42979-022-01043-x PMID: 35194580

Stokes, J. M., Yang, K., Swanson, K., Jin, W., Cubillos-Ruiz, A., Donghia, N. M., MacNair, C. R., French, S., Carfrae, L. A., Bloom-Ackermann, Z., Tran, V. M., Chiappino-Pepe, A., Badran, A. H., Andrews, I. W., Chory, E. J., Church, G. M., Brown, E. D., Jaakkola, T. S., Barzilay, R., & Collins, J. J. (2020). A deep learning approach to antibiotic discovery. *Cell*, *180*(4), 688–702. DOI: 10.1016/j.cell.2020.01.021 PMID: 32084340

Takhi, D., Ouinten, M., & Yousfi, M. (2011). Study of antimicrobial activity of secondary metabolites extracted from spontaneous plants from the area of Laghouat, Algeria. *Advances in Environmental Biology*, 469–477.

Talat, A., & Khan, A. U. (2023). Artificial intelligence as a smart approach to develop antimicrobial drug molecules: A paradigm to combat drug-resistant infections. *Drug Discovery Today*, *28*(4), 103491. DOI: 10.1016/j.drudis.2023.103491 PMID: 36646245

Tiwari, R., & Rana, C. S. (2015). Plant secondary metabolites: A review. *International Journal of Engineering Research and General Science*, *3*(5), 661–670.

Tommasi, R., Brown, D. G., Walkup, G. K., Manchester, J. I., & Miller, A. A. (2015). ESKAPEing the labyrinth of antibacterial discovery. *Nature Reviews. Drug Discovery*, *14*(8), 529–542. DOI: 10.1038/nrd4572 PMID: 26139286

Trunk, A., Birkel, H., & Hartmann, E. (2020). On the current state of combining human and artificial intelligence for strategic organizational decision making. *Business Research*, *13*(3), 875–919. DOI: 10.1007/s40685-020-00133-x

Tsoukalas, A., Albertson, T., & Tagkopoulos, I. (2015). From data to optimal decision making: A data-driven, probabilistic machine learning approach to decision support for patients with sepsis. *JMIR Medical Informatics*, *3*(1), e3445. DOI: 10.2196/medinform.3445 PMID: 25710907

Visan, A. I., & Negut, I. (2024). Integrating Artificial Intelligence for Drug Discovery in the Context of Revolutionizing Drug Delivery. *Life (Chicago, Ill.)*, *14*(2), 233. DOI: 10.3390/life14020233 PMID: 38398742

Wang, G., Badal, A., Jia, X., Maltz, J. S., Mueller, K., Myers, K. J., Niu, C., Vannier, M., Yan, P., Yu, Z., & Zeng, R. (2022). Development of metaverse for intelligent healthcare. *Nature Machine Intelligence*, *4*(11), 922–929. DOI: 10.1038/s42256-022-00549-6 PMID: 36935774

Wattam, A. R., Abraham, D., Dalay, O., Disz, T. L., Driscoll, T., Gabbard, J. L., Gillespie, J. J., Gough, R., Hix, D., Kenyon, R., Machi, D., Mao, C., Nordberg, E. K., Olson, R., Overbeek, R., Pusch, G. D., Shukla, M., Schulman, J., Stevens, R. L., & Sobral, B. W. (2014). PATRIC, the bacterial bioinformatics database and analysis resource. *Nucleic Acids Research*, *42*(D1), D581–D591. DOI: 10.1093/nar/gkt1099 PMID: 24225323

Yu, S., Long, Y., Li, D., Shi, A., Deng, J., Ma, Y., Wen, J., Li, X., Zhang, Y., Liu, S., Wan, J., Li, N., & Guo, J. (2022). Natural essential oils efficacious in internal organs fibrosis treatment: Mechanisms of action and application perspectives. *Pharmacological Research*, *182*, 106339. DOI: 10.1016/j.phrs.2022.106339 PMID: 35792297

Zasowski, E. J., Bassetti, M., Blasi, F., Goossens, H., Rello, J., Sotgiu, G., & Aliberti, S. (2020). A systematic review of the effect of delayed appropriate antibiotic treatment on the outcomes of patients with severe bacterial infections. *Chest*, *158*(3), 929–938. DOI: 10.1016/j.chest.2020.03.087 PMID: 32446623

Zaynab, M., Fatima, M., Abbas, S., Sharif, Y., Umair, M., Zafar, M. H., & Bahadar, K. (2018). Role of secondary metabolites in plant defense against pathogens. *Microbial Pathogenesis*, *124*, 198–202. DOI: 10.1016/j.micpath.2018.08.034 PMID: 30145251

Chapter 4

Novel Healthcare Trends:
A Bibliometric Exploration of Immunomodulatory Therapies

Pragya Karnwal
https://orcid.org/0009-0003-2820-2333
Graphic Era University, India

Madhav Chaudhary
https://orcid.org/0009-0009-5840-2057
Graphic Era University, India

Shweta Bajaj
https://orcid.org/0000-0002-1177-6352
Graphic Era University, India

Rajesh Tiwari
https://orcid.org/0000-0002-5345-2508
Graphic Era University, India

ABSTRACT

Immunomodulatory drugs (IMDs) play important role in advancing therapeutic treatments across various diseases, especially autoimmune disorders, viral infections and haematological malignancies. This bibliometric review highlights the impact of immunomodulatory therapies such as immunoglobulins, antivirals, and CAR-T cell therapies, focusing on their efficacy in managing conditions like relapsed multiple myeloma (RRMM), COVID-19, and autoimmune disorders. Key findings from the Scopus database, covering a wide span of immunomodulatory treatments, are analysed to identify research trends, influential studies and collaborations. Citation analysis reveals that the United States leads in research outcomes, while countries like Belgium and the Netherlands show significantly higher citation per document,

DOI: 10.4018/979-8-3693-9112-9.ch004

demonstrating impactful but less frequent publications. The review explores a strong trend towards the development of more effective immunotherapies, focusing on future potential in clinical applications.

INTRODUCTION

Focusing on novel therapeutic approaches, the study highlights into haematological malignancies in multiple myeloma, showcasing significant progress in immunotherapy (Moreau et al., 2022). Cilta-cel therapy demonstrated a high overall response rate of 97.9% in refractory multiple myeloma, with 82.5% of patients attaining stringent complete responses at 28 months median flow up (Martin et al., 2023). Novel SARS-CoV-2 variants highlights diagnostic and therapeutic challenges. The advancements in antiviral drugs, vaccines and their mechanisms have been reviewed (Fernandes et al 2022). Updated CIDP guidelines simplifies diagnostic criteria and classifies CIDP variants as distinct entities. IVIg or corticosteroids remain first-line treatments, with additional strategies like plasma exchange and immunosuppressants (Van et al., 2021).

Therapeutic advancements for COVID-19 have resulted in approved antiviral and immunomodulatory treatments, including antiviral agents like remdesivir and immunomodulators such as baricitinib (Li et al., 2023). The updated CIDP guidelines differentiates between typical CIDP and well-characterized variants, redefining diagnostic certainty levels to “CIDP” and “possible CIDP” (Van et al., 2021). The Loco-Motion study demonstrated limited efficacy of SOC in patients with triple-class exposed RRMM patients, achieving 29.8% response rate, with median progression-free survival of 4.6 months and median overall survival of 12.4 months (Mateos et al., 2022). The 13-month follow-up of DREAMM-2 demonstrated sustained efficacy of belantamab mafadotin belamaf), achieving a 32% overall response rate in patients with heavily pretreated RRMM, within a median response duration of 11 months (Lonial et al., 2021). Cilta-cel, an anti-BCMA CAR-T therapy, demonstrated favourable outcomes in heavily pretreated relapsed/ multiple myeloma patients, achieving a 60% overall response rate and 35% MRD negativity (Cohen et al., 2023).

MPB-BA a mesoporous Prussian blue (MPB)-based nanoplatform, combining anti-inflammatory, antioxidant, and antibacterial properties modulates the Nrf2/ NF-$_{K}$B signalling pathway to effectively treat periodontitis (Tian et al., 2022). The POLARIS phase 1 trial identified that GPRC5D-targeted CAR T-cell therapy showed high efficacy and safety in relapsed multiple myeloma with a 100% overall response rate (Zhang et al., 2023). Both general and specific immunomodulatory therapies (e.g., methotrexate and TNF-alpha inhibitors respectively) have demonstrated promising results in reducing blood pressure and organ protection in hypertension (Murray et al., 2021).

Primary central nervous system lymphoma (PCNSL) is a rare malignancy that majorly affects the brain, spinal cord, and other parts of the CNS. Emerging therapies targeting aberrant tumour pathways, like obrutinib and immunomodulatory drugs, shows results in relapsed cases (Schaff et al., 2022). Autoimmune hepatitis is a liver inflammation characterised by immune-mediated inflammation, progressing to cirrhosis if untreated. Early treatment with corticosteroids and immunomodulatory drugs can induce remission and may reverse liver failure (Muratori et al., 2023). ABBV-383, a B-cell maturation antigen x CD3 T-cell engaging bispecific antibody, demonstrated a 57% overall response rate and promising safety in treating relapsed multiple myeloma (RRMM) (D'souza et al., 2022).

I. METHOD

The Scopus database was used. The keyword used were "immunomodulatory drugs" AND "immunoglobulins". The date of search was 20th November 2024. The documents were examined based on inclusion criteria. The first inclusion criteria were language. Only English language documents were included. 934 documents were retained. The next level of exclusion was done based on type of document. Retracted documents (4) were excluded. 930 documents were retained. 930 documents were used for the bibliometric analysis. The bibliometric analysis was done using VOS viewer.

II. RESULTS

A. Citation Analysis

The prominent cited countries are depicted in Table 1. The high number of documents, 293, and citations, 4306, by United States would have a relatively low citation per document at 15, indicated to be very large but of lesser impact. Belgium has the highest citation per document at 66, suggesting that the work done here is highly impactful although fewer publications are done. Netherlands and Canada have 45 and 35 citations per document, respectively, indicating powerful academic impacts. Canada is one with a high output and has a relatively low citation per document of 9; meaning that its work is significant in volume but probably less visible.

Table 1. Prominent cited countries

S. No	Country	Documents	Citations	Total link strength	Citations per document
1	United states	293	4306	495	15
2	Germany	91	2346	313	26
3	United Kingdom	79	2098	218	27
4	Belgium	29	1939	193	67
5	Spain	56	1587	259	29
6	Italy	88	1557	200	18
7	Netherlands	35	1549	133	45
8	France	61	1471	228	25
9	China	130	1114	36	9
10	Canada	29	1012	193	35

B. Co-Citation Analysis

The prominent papers are, Berdeja et al., (2021), Gandhi et al., (2019), and Munshi et al. (2021), which are usually co-cited because of their foundational role in treating RRMM. Indeed, these works are coarsely huddled together in a single co-citation cluster and include therapies like CAR T-cell therapy, immunomodulatory drugs. The very high total link strength of these papers suggests that the authors are well-academically connected and implies that, for example, immunomodulatory drugs and therapies are tightly linked with other success stories in this area-medication or treatment for RRMM.

Table 2. Prominent co-cited references

S. No	Cited Reference	Citations	Total Link Strength
1	"berdeja j.g., madduri d., usmani s.z., et al., ciltacabtagene autoleucel, a b-cell maturation antigen-directed chimeric antigen receptor t-cell therapy in patients with relapsed or refractory multiple myeloma (cartitude-1): a phase 1b/2 open-label study, lancet, 398, pp. 314-324, (2021)"	20	83
2	"gandhi u.h., cornell r.f., lakshman a., et al., outcomes of patients with multiple myeloma refractory to cd38-targeted monoclonal antibody therapy, leukemia, 33, pp. 2266-2275, (2019)"	15	53
3	"munshi n.c., anderson l.d., shah n., et al., idecabtagene vicleucel in relapsed and refractory multiple myeloma, n engl j med, 384, pp. 705-716, (2021)"	14	57
4	"munshi n.c., anderson l.d., shah n., et al., idecabtagene vicleucel in relapsed and refractory multiple myeloma, n engl j med, 384, 8, pp. 705-716, (2021)"	13	90
5	"ito t., ando h., suzuki t., ogura t., hotta k., imamura y., yamaguchi y., handa h., identification of a primary target of thalidomide teratogenicity, science, 327, pp. 1345-1350, (2010)"	12	25

continued on following page

Table 2. Continued

S. No	Cited Reference	Citations	Total Link Strength
6	"kumar s., paiva b., anderson k.c., et al., international myeloma working group consensus criteria for response and minimal residual disease assessment in multiple myeloma, lancet oncol, 17, pp. e328-e346, (2016)"	11	29
7	"rajkumar s.v., multiple myeloma: 2020 update on diagnosis, risk-stratification and management, am j hematol, 95, 5, pp. 548-567, (2020)"	11	39
8	"kronke j., udeshi n.d., narla a., grauman p., hurst s.n., mcconkey m., svinkina t., heckl d., comer e., li x., et al., lenalidomide causes selective degradation of ikzf1 and ikzf3 in multiple myeloma cells, science, 343, pp. 301-305, (2014)"	10	22
9	"lonial s., lee h.c., badros a., et al., belantamab mafodotin for relapsed or refractory multiple myeloma (dreamm-2): a two-arm, randomised, open-label, phase 2 study, lancet oncol, 21, 2, pp. 207-221, (2020)"	10	50
10	"facon t., kumar s., plesner t., et al., daratumumab plus lenalidomide and dexamethasone for untreated myeloma, n engl j med, 380, 22, pp. 2104-2115, (2019)"	9	61

C. Co-Authorship

United States leads the co-authorship with link strength of 371, as well as the research output of 293 documents, despite having a relatively low citation per document, suggesting that while there is wealth, individual contributions were perhaps less influential than those of other countries. In the United Kingdom, link strength is modestly strong at 217, reflecting research co-authorship, with moderate citation per document indicating it has good influences in research with global collaborative efforts. Italy (175 link strength) and Spain (178 link strength) both show moderate collaboration, which suggests increasing research output, but not so much in international co-authorship as in the case of the U.S or the U.K. Belgium, China and Canada display relatively weak links, indicating more localized or more minor collaboration groups.

Table 3. Prominent countries by co-authorship

S. No	Country	Documents	Citations	Total link strength
1	United States	293	4306	371
2	Germany	91	2346	216
3	United Kingdom	79	2098	224
4	Belgium	29	1939	116
5	Spain	56	1587	178
6	Italy	88	1557	175
7	Netherlands	35	1549	120
8	France	61	1471	170

S. No	Country	Documents	Citations	Total link strength
9	China	130	1114	52
10	Canada	29	1012	75

D. Co-Occurrence

The term with the highest occurrence is human, with 729 and the highest link strength at 22,004. It proves that this term played a prominent central role in most immunological results. Multiple Myeloma was also of immense importance, with an occurrence of 309 and a link strength of 10,693. Controlled study, with an occurrence of 278, had a link strength of 9009. Key words immunomodulating agents, aged, adults, appear with a frequency of 233, 176, and 268 while having a relatively high strength of links; that is, they indicate a robust medical research base. Examples of medical vocabulary include lenalidomide which appears 230 times with a link strength of 8854 and dexamethasone occurs 170 times with a link strength of 7106, indicating the niche applications of immunotherapy and immunomodulating techniques respectively. Overall, there is a very strong trend in the data toward immunomodulatory drugs and paying increasing attention to certain applications in medical therapies.

Table 4. Frequently occurring keywords

S.No	keyword	occurrences	total link strength
1	human	729	22004
2	humans	506	16295
3	article	479	15629
4	multiple myeloma	309	10693
5	male	306	10677
6	female	300	10502
7	controlled study	278	9009
8	adult	268	9387
9	review	244	7060
10	immunomodulating agent	233	7285
11	lenalidomide	230	8854
12	nonhuman	226	6941
13	aged	176	6695
14	dexamethasone	170	7106

E. Bibliographic Coupling

Cluster I: Treatment Progress

Schaff et al., (2020) argued that high-dose methotrexate improves progress in treatment for primary central nervous system lymphoma (PCSNL), significantly improving survival rates, though relapse remains a challenge. 13-monyh follow-up data from DREAMM-2 trial reveals that belantamab mafodotin provides an overall response rate of 31.3% in relapsed multiple myeloma patients, showing complete response in a subset of patients, ocular toxicities remain a concern (Lonial et al., 2021). A CRISPR screen identified a molecular glue-like degrader that targets bromodomain-containing proteins BRD2 and BRD4, by engaging DCAF16, a ubiquitin ligase adapter, effectively suppressing cancel cell proliferation (Shergalis et al., 2023). A novel proximity biotinylating method was used to map dynamic interactions between target proteins and E3 ligases triggered by PROTACs and molecular glues (Yamanaka et al., 2022).

Cluster II: Relapsed Case Treatment

Teclistamab, a bispecific antibody targeting BCMA (B-cell maturation antigen), showed a 63% ORR and significant efficacy in heavily pretreated patients with relapsed multiple myeloma (RRMM), with manageable Cytokine release syndrome (CRS) and hematologic side effects (Moreau et al., 2022). The 2-year follow-up data for CARTITUDE-1 trial demonstrates cilta-cel's high efficacy about 98% ORR and long-lastingresponses. However, immune and neurologic side effects are key challenges (Martin et al., 2023). Mateos et al., (2023) revealed limited efficacy of current therapies for treating relapsed myeloma, with a response rate of 31.5%, median progression-free survival of 4.6 months, and overall survival of 13.8 months, underlining the urgent need for improved therapies. Cohen et al., 2023 demonstrated that cilta-cel achieved notable efficacy with 60% overall response rate and 9,1 months of progression free survival in multiple myeloma patients treated with anti-BMCA agents, alongside manageable safety concerns. OriCAR-017, a GPRC5D-targeted CAR T-cell therapy, evaluated by POLARIS phase 1 trial. Showed a 100% overall response rate, in 10 RRMM patients, with 60% showing complete remission and 40% achieving partial remission, making it promising for patients post-BCMA therapies.

Cluster III: Severe Case Survival

Significant progress in COVID-19 therapies, including antivirals and immunomodulators, offers relief for severe COVID-19, enhancing survival in severe cases (Li et al., 2023). Emerging variants of COVID-19, particularly those with spike protein mutations, reduces vaccine efficacy and diagnostic accuracy, underscoring the importance of next-gen solutions for future pandemics (Fernandes et al., 2022). Meta-analysis on hydroxychloroquine (HCQ) demonstrated no efficacy as prophylaxis or in preventing COVID-19, offering no clinical advantage (Martins-Filho et al., 2021). The current landscape for COViD-19 therapeutics now include antivirals and monoclonal antibodies to reduce severe disease with updated WHO recommendations informing treatments based on patient conditions (Toussi et al., 2023).

Cluster IV: Sustainability of Treatment

Single-agent Belantamab mafodotin (belamaf) demonstrated sustained efficacy in patients with RRMM after a 13-month follow-up, with 32% overall response rates (ORR) and 35% for the 2.5 mg/kg and 3.4 mg/kg dosing groups, with median PFS of 2.8 to 3.9 months (Lonial et al., 2021). Ramasamy et al., (2021) discusses advancements and emerging treatment options for relapsed multiple myeloma, including the combinations of monoclonal and bispecific antibodies, CAR-T cell therapies, and celmod agents, to overcome drug resistance. The International Myeloma Working Group (IMWG) emphasizes early and aggressive intervention for multiple myeloma (MM) related renal impairment (RI), focusing on reduction of monoclonal free light chains (FLCs) through therapies such as bortezomib-based regimens, self-care such as hydration, and avoiding nephrotoxic agents (Dimopoulos et al., 2023).

B-cell maturation antigen (BCMA) is a vital therapeutic target in multiple myeloma, with BMCA-directed antibody-drug conjugates (ADCs), chimeric antigen receptor (CAR) T-cell therapies, and bispecific T-cell engagers (BiTEs), showing significant efficacy in refractory cases (Kleber et al., 2021). Cho et al., (2021) discusses emerging antigens targets like GPRC5D, FcRH5, and SLAMF7 in multiple myeloma (MM) immunotherapy, demonstrating distinct expression patterns on myeloma cells, fuelling innovations in CAR T-cell therapies and ADCs, showing potential for overcoming BMCA limitations (Nicol et al., 2022).

Cluster V: Tailor Made Treatment

The multicentre phase 1/2a study highlighted the potential of Indatuximab ravtansine (BT062), an antibody-drug conjugate targeting CD138 in combination with dexamethasone and lenalidomide, improving outcomes in heavily pretreated

RRMM patients (Kelly et al., 2021). Immune checkpoint inhibitors and CAR T-cell therapies demonstrates promising results in treating certain cancers during pregnancy but also carries potential risks to both the mother and foetus, leading to complications such as preterm labour, foetal loss, or immune-related adverse effects (Borgers et al., 2021). Costa et al., (2022), highlights cilta-cel's significant advantages in achieving higher overall response rates (ORR) and longer progression-free survival (PFS), and manageable CRS-related toxicity. Systemic amyloidosis, a rare condition illustrated by abnormal protein deposition presents a paradox of thromboembolic and bleeding risks, emphasizing the need of specific tailored therapeutic approaches (Borgers et al., 2021).

III. CONCLUSION

Immunomodulatory drugs have shown significant progress in distinct therapeutic areas, specifically in haematological malignancies and autoimmune disorders. The study demonstrates the growing impact of CAR T-cell therapies, immunoglobulins and antiviral agents in clinical settings. The bibliometric analysis also underpins the significance of collaboration across countries and research groups in enhancing the understanding and applications of these therapies. As research evolution continues, the development of more targeted and efficient immunomodulatory treatments holds efficacy for improving patient outcomes across a span of diseases, with CAR T-cell therapies and immunotherapies at the forefront of these immunological advancements.

REFERENCES

Augsberger, C., Hänel, G., Xu, W., Pulko, V., Hanisch, L. J., Augustin, A., Challier, J., Hunt, K., Vick, B., Rovatti, P. E., Krupka, C., Rothe, M., Schönle, A., Sam, J., Lezan, E., Ducret, A., Ortiz-Franyuti, D., Walz, A.-C., Benz, J., & Subklewe, M. (2021). Targeting intracellular WT1 in AML with a novel RMF-peptide-MHC-specific T-cell bispecific antibody. *Blood*, *138*(25), 2655–2669. DOI: 10.1182/blood.2020010477 PMID: 34280257

Borgers, J. S., Heimovaara, J. H., Cardonick, E., Dierickx, D., Lambertini, M., Haanen, J. B., & Amant, F. (2021). Immunotherapy for cancer treatment during pregnancy. *The Lancet. Oncology*, *22*(12), e550–e561. DOI: 10.1016/S1470-2045(21)00525-8 PMID: 34856152

Cho, S. F., Xing, L., Anderson, K. C., & Tai, Y. T. (2021). Promising antigens for the new frontier of targeted immunotherapy in multiple myeloma. *Cancers (Basel)*, *13*(23), 6136. DOI: 10.3390/cancers13236136 PMID: 34885245

Cohen, A. D., Mateos, M. V., Cohen, Y. C., Rodriguez-Otero, P., Paiva, B., van de Donk, N. W., Martin, T., Suvannasankha, A., De Braganca, K. C., Corsale, C., Schecter, J. M., Varsos, H., Deraedt, W., Wang, L., Vogel, M., Roccia, T., Xu, X., Mistry, P., Zudaire, E., & San-Miguel, J. (2023). Efficacy and safety of cilta-cel in patients with progressive multiple myeloma after exposure to other BCMA-targeting agents. *Blood*, *141*(3), 219–230. DOI: 10.1182/blood.2022015526 PMID: 36095849

D'souza, A., Shah, N., Rodriguez, C., Voorhees, P. M., Weisel, K., Bueno, O. F., Pothacamury, R. K., Freise, K. J., Yue, S., Ross, J. A., Polepally, A. R., Talati, C., Lee, S., Jin, Z., Buelow, B., Vij, R., & Kumar, S. (2022). A phase I first-in-human study of ABBV-383, a B-cell maturation antigen× CD3 bispecific T-cell redirecting antibody, in patients with relapsed/refractory multiple myeloma. *Journal of Clinical Oncology*, *40*(31), 3576–3586. DOI: 10.1200/JCO.22.01504 PMID: 36029527

Dimopoulos, M. A., Merlini, G., Bridoux, F., Leung, N., Mikhael, J., Harrison, S. J., Kastritis, E., Garderet, L., Gozzetti, A., van de Donk, N. W. C. J., Weisel, K. C., Badros, A. Z., Beksac, M., Hillengass, J., Mohty, M., Ho, P. J., Ntanasis-Stathopoulos, I., Mateos, M.-V., Richardson, P., & Terpos, E. (2023). Management of multiple myeloma-related renal impairment: Recommendations from the International Myeloma Working Group. *The Lancet. Oncology*, *24*(7), e293–e311. DOI: 10.1016/S1470-2045(23)00223-1 PMID: 37414019

Fernandes, Q., Inchakalody, V. P., Merhi, M., Mestiri, S., Taib, N., Moustafa Abo El-Ella, D., Bedhiafi, T., Raza, A., Al-Zaidan, L., Mohsen, M. O., Yousuf Al-Nesf, M. A., Hssain, A. A., Yassine, H. M., Bachmann, M. F., Uddin, S., & Dermime, S. (2022). Emerging COVID-19 variants and their impact on SARS-CoV-2 diagnosis, therapeutics and vaccines. *Annals of Medicine*, *54*(1), 524–540. DOI: 10.1080/07853890.2022.2031274 PMID: 35132910

Kelly, K. R., Ailawadhi, S., Siegel, D. S., Heffner, L. T., Somlo, G., Jagannath, S., Zimmerman, T. M., Munshi, N. C., Madan, S., Chanan-Khan, A., Lonial, S., Chandwani, S., Minasyan, A., Ruehle, M., Barmaki-Rad, F., Abdolzade-Bavil, A., Rharbaoui, F., Herrmann-Keiner, E., Haeder, T., & Anderson, K. C. (2021). Indatuximab ravtansine plus dexamethasone with lenalidomide or pomalidomide in relapsed or refractory multiple myeloma: A multicentre, phase 1/2a study. *The Lancet. Haematology*, *8*(11), e794–e807. DOI: 10.1016/S2352-3026(21)00208-8 PMID: 34529955

Kleber, M., Ntanasis-Stathopoulos, I., & Terpos, E. (2021). BCMA in multiple myeloma—A promising key to therapy. *Journal of Clinical Medicine*, *10*(18), 4088. DOI: 10.3390/jcm10184088 PMID: 34575199

Li, G., Hilgenfeld, R., Whitley, R., & De Clercq, E. (2023). Therapeutic strategies for COVID-19: Progress and lessons learned. *Nature Reviews. Drug Discovery*, *22*(6), 449–475. DOI: 10.1038/s41573-023-00672-y PMID: 37076602

Lonial, S., Lee, H. C., Badros, A., Trudel, S., Nooka, A. K., Chari, A., Abdallah, A.-O., Callander, N., Sborov, D., Suvannasankha, A., Weisel, K., Voorhees, P. M., Womersley, L., Baron, J., Piontek, T., Lewis, E., Opalinska, J., Gupta, I., & Cohen, A. D. (2021). Longer term outcomes with single-agent belantamab mafodotin in patients with relapsed or refractory multiple myeloma: 13-month follow-up from the pivotal DREAMM-2 study. *Cancer*, *127*(22), 4198–4212. DOI: 10.1002/cncr.33809 PMID: 34314018

Martin, T., Usmani, S. Z., Berdeja, J. G., Agha, M., Cohen, A. D., Hari, P., Avigan, D., Deol, A., Htut, M., Lesokhin, A., Munshi, N. C., O'Donnell, E., Stewart, A. K., Schecter, J. M., Goldberg, J. D., Jackson, C. C., Yeh, T.-M., Banerjee, A., Allred, A., & Jagannath, S. (2023). Ciltacabtagene autoleucel, an anti–B-cell maturation antigen chimeric antigen receptor T-cell therapy, for relapsed/refractory multiple myeloma: CARTITUDE-1 2-year follow-up. *Journal of Clinical Oncology*, *41*(6), 1265–1274. DOI: 10.1200/JCO.22.00842 PMID: 35658469

Martins-Filho, P. R., Ferreira, L. C., Heimfarth, L., de Souza Araújo, A. A., & Quintans-Júnior, L. J. (2021). Efficacy and safety of hydroxychloroquine as pre-and post-exposure prophylaxis and treatment of COVID-19: A systematic review and meta-analysis of blinded, placebo-controlled, randomized clinical trials. *Lancet Regional Health. Americas*, *2*, 2. DOI: 10.1016/j.lana.2021.100062 PMID: 34485970

Mateos, M. V., Weisel, K., De Stefano, V., Goldschmidt, H., Delforge, M., Mohty, M., Cavo, M., Vij, R., Lindsey-Hill, J., Dytfeld, D., Angelucci, E., Perrot, A., Benjamin, R., van de Donk, N. W. C. J., Ocio, E. M., Scheid, C., Gay, F., Roeloffzen, W., Rodriguez-Otero, P., & Moreau, P. (2022). LocoMMotion: A prospective, non-interventional, multinational study of real-life current standards of care in patients with relapsed and/or refractory multiple myeloma. *Leukemia*, *36*(5), 1371–1376. DOI: 10.1038/s41375-022-01531-2 PMID: 35332278

Moreau, P., Garfall, A. L., van de Donk, N. W., Nahi, H., San-Miguel, J. F., Oriol, A., Nooka, A. K., Martin, T., Rosinol, L., Chari, A., Karlin, L., Benboubker, L., Mateos, M.-V., Bahlis, N., Popat, R., Besemer, B., Martínez-López, J., Sidana, S., Delforge, M., & Usmani, S. Z. (2022). Teclistamab in relapsed or refractory multiple myeloma. *The New England Journal of Medicine*, *387*(6), 495–505. DOI: 10.1056/NEJMoa2203478 PMID: 35661166

Muratori, L., Lohse, A. W., & Lenzi, M. (2023). Diagnosis and management of autoimmune hepatitis. *bmj, 380.*

Murray, E. C., Nosalski, R., MacRitchie, N., Tomaszewski, M., Maffia, P., Harrison, D. G., & Guzik, T. J. (2021). Therapeutic targeting of inflammation in hypertension: From novel mechanisms to translational perspective. *Cardiovascular Research*, *117*(13), 2589–2609. DOI: 10.1093/cvr/cvab330 PMID: 34698811

Nicol, M., Siguret, V., Vergaro, G., Aimo, A., Emdin, M., Dillinger, J. G., Baudet, M., Cohen-Solal, A., Villesuzanne, C., Harel, S., Royer, B., Arnulf, B., & Logeart, D. (2022). Thromboembolism and bleeding in systemic amyloidosis: A review. *ESC Heart Failure*, *9*(1), 11–20. DOI: 10.1002/ehf2.13701 PMID: 34784656

Ramasamy, K., Gay, F., Weisel, K., Zweegman, S., Mateos, M. V., & Richardson, P. (2021). Improving outcomes for patients with relapsed multiple myeloma: Challenges and considerations of current and emerging treatment options. *Blood Reviews*, *49*, 100808. DOI: 10.1016/j.blre.2021.100808 PMID: 33863601

Schaff, L. R., & Grommes, C. (2022). Primary central nervous system lymphoma. *Blood*, *140*(9), 971–979. DOI: 10.1182/blood.2020008377 PMID: 34699590

Shergalis, A. G., Marin, V. L., Rhee, D. Y., Senaweera, S., McCloud, R. L., Ronau, J. A., Hutchins, C. W., McLoughlin, S., Woller, K. R., Warder, S. E., Vasudevan, A., & Reitsma, J. M. (2023). CRISPR screen reveals BRD2/4 molecular glue-like degrader via recruitment of DCAF16. *ACS Chemical Biology*, *18*(2), 331–339. DOI: 10.1021/acschembio.2c00747 PMID: 36656921

Tian, Y., Li, Y., Liu, J., Lin, Y., Jiao, J., Chen, B., Wang, W., Wu, S., & Li, C. (2022). Photothermal therapy with regulated Nrf2/NF-κB signaling pathway for treating bacteria-induced periodontitis. *Bioactive Materials*, *9*, 428–445. DOI: 10.1016/j.bioactmat.2021.07.033 PMID: 34820581

Toussi, S. S., Hammond, J. L., Gerstenberger, B. S., & Anderson, A. S. (2023). Therapeutics for COVID-19. *Nature Microbiology*, *8*(5), 771–786. DOI: 10.1038/s41564-023-01356-4 PMID: 37142688

Van den Bergh, P. Y., van Doorn, P. A., Hadden, R. D., Avau, B., Vankrunkelsven, P., Allen, J. A., Attarian, S., Blomkwist-Markens, P. H., Cornblath, D. R., Eftimov, F., Goedee, H. S., Harbo, T., Kuwabara, S., Lewis, R. A., Lunn, M. P., Nobile-Orazio, E., Querol, L., Rajabally, Y. A., Sommer, C., & Topaloglu, H. A. (2021). European Academy of Neurology/Peripheral Nerve Society guideline on diagnosis and treatment of chronic inflammatory demyelinating polyradiculoneuropathy: Report of a joint Task Force—Second revision. *Journal of the Peripheral Nervous System*, *26*(3), 242–268. DOI: 10.1111/jns.12455 PMID: 34085743

Yamanaka, S., Horiuchi, Y., Matsuoka, S., Kido, K., Nishino, K., Maeno, M., Shibata, N., Kosako, H., & Sawasaki, T. (2022). A proximity biotinylation-based approach to identify protein-E3 ligase interactions induced by PROTACs and molecular glues. *Nature Communications*, *13*(1), 183. DOI: 10.1038/s41467-021-27818-z PMID: 35013300

Zhang, M., Wei, G., Zhou, L., Zhou, J., Chen, S., Zhang, W., Wang, D., Luo, X., Cui, J., Huang, S., Fu, S., Zhou, X., Tang, Y., Ding, X., Kuang, J., He, X. P., Hu, Y., & Huang, H. (2023). GPRC5D CAR T cells (OriCAR-017) in patients with relapsed or refractory multiple myeloma (POLARIS): A first-in-human, single-centre, single-arm, phase 1 trial. *The Lancet. Haematology*, *10*(2), e107–e116. DOI: 10.1016/S2352-3026(22)00372-6 PMID: 36725117

Chapter 5

The Therapeutic Role of Secondary Metabolites in Neurodegenerative and Inflammatory Diseases, Mechanisms, and Potential Applications

Jawad Laadraoui
https://orcid.org/0000-0002-9784-1265
Faculty of Sciences, Aïn Chock, Hassan II University, Casablanca, Morocco

Hamid Kabdy
https://orcid.org/0009-0004-7438-3638
Faculty of Sciences Semlalia, University Cadi Ayyad, Marrakech, Morocco

Sara Oufquir
Faculty of Sciences Semlalia, University Cadi Ayyad, Marrakech, Morocco

Mehdi Aitlarradia
Ministry of Health and Social Protection, Beni Mellal, Morocco

Fatimzahra Agouram
https://orcid.org/0000-0002-8073-2126
Faculty of Sciences Semlalia, University Cadi Ayyad, Marrakech, Morocco

Abdelfatah Ait Baba
https://orcid.org/0000-0002-5650-3868
Faculty of Sciences Semlalia, University Cadi Ayyad, Marrakech, Morocco

Khadija Oubella
https://orcid.org/0000-0003-1943-9454
Faculty of Sciences Semlalia, University Cadi Ayyad, Marrakech, Morocco

Bilal El-Mansoury
https://orcid.org/0000-0002-2583-7515
Royal College of Surgeons in Ireland, University of Medicine and Health Sciences, Dublin, Ireland

DOI: 10.4018/979-8-3693-9112-9.ch005

ABSTRACT

Secondary metabolites, bioactive compounds from plants, fungi, and microorganisms, show significant therapeutic potential for neurodegenerative and inflammatory diseases. This chapter highlights their mechanisms of action, including antioxidant activity, modulation of inflammatory pathways, and neuroprotection, supported by preclinical and clinical evidence. Key classes like alkaloids, flavonoids, terpenoids, and polyphenols are explored for their neuroprotective and anti-inflammatory properties, alongside phytochemical sources that emphasize their drug discovery potential. However, challenges such as limited bioavailability, stability, and toxicity hinder their clinical application. Addressing these issues through novel strategies could unlock their full potential in modern medicine. This chapter bridges natural product chemistry and clinical applications, providing insights to inspire further research into secondary metabolites as essential tools for combating complex diseases.

1. INTRODUCTION

Secondary metabolites are a diverse class of bioactive compounds synthesized by various organisms, including plants, microorganisms, and certain marine species, (Bills & Gloer, 2016) (Jain, Khatana, & Vijayvergia, 2019). While not essential for primary metabolic processes, these molecules play critical roles in environmental adaptation, biological defense, and interspecies interactions, (Mérillon & Ramawat, 2020) (Kumar *et al.,* 2023). Specialized metabolic pathways, resulting in a broad chemical diversity that includes alkaloids, polyphenols, flavonoids, and terpenoids, drive their biosynthesis. These compounds, often specific to particular species or families, represent valuable sources for the discovery of novel bioactive molecules, (Laadraoui *et al.,* 2018) (Guerriero *et al.,* 2018). Medicinal plants, in particular, serve as a major source, while microorganisms and aquatic organisms offer emerging opportunities in this field, (Luckner, 2013). The diversity of these natural products highlights their potential for uncovering new therapeutic agents, (Yang *et al.,* 2025).

Beyond their ecological roles, secondary metabolites have significant industrial relevance, (Azizan *et al.,* 2016). They play a crucial role in pharmaceutical research and production due to their ability to modulate biological processes in humans and animals, (Bourgaud *et al.,* 2001) (Bafor, 2017). Furthermore, their applications extend to other industries, including cosmetics, nutrition, and the manufacturing of industrial goods such as dyes, fragrances, flavors, and dietary supplements, (Bermudez-Torres *et al.,* 2013) (Gainche, 2020). This wide range of uses underscores their economic and scientific importance.

Secondary metabolites are crucial in the development of novel therapeutic strategies. Historically, these compounds have served as prototypes or precursors for the synthesis of widely used pharmaceuticals. Prominent examples include morphine, quinine, and taxol, which are derived from natural sources and remain fundamental therapeutic agents, (Alamgir, 2017) (Egbuna *et al.,* 2019). These molecules are distinguished by their ability to selectively interact with biological targets, (Najmi *et al.,* 2022), imparting a range of pharmacological activities, such as anti-inflammatory, antioxidant, antimicrobial, and anticancer effects, (Choudhary *et al.,* 2021). Their application in modern medicine is facilitated by their favorable bioavailability, reduced side effects, and potential for use in combination therapies, (Rao & Ravishankar, 2002) (Alminger *et al.,* 2014), thus providing new avenues for more effective and better-tolerated treatments.

Recent advances in the understanding of complex diseases, such as neurodegenerative and inflammatory disorders, have underscored the critical involvement of secondary metabolites in regulating pathophysiological processes, (Merecx-Sadowska *et al.,* 20023) (Pilipović *et al.,* 2023). Neurodegenerative diseases, such as Alzheimer's disease and Parkinson's disease, are characterized by progressive neuronal degeneration, often accompanied by oxidative stress, chronic inflammation, and the accumulation of misfolded proteins, (Knezevic et al., 2023) (Tchekalarova & Tzoneva, 2023) (Carardonna *et al.,* 2024). Various secondary metabolites, including polyphenols such as flavonoids (quercetin) and resveratrol, have demonstrated neuroprotective effects by modulating oxidative stress, regulating inflammatory pathways, and inhibiting neuronal apoptosis, (Grewal *et al.,* 2021) (Miguel *et al.,* 2021). Similarly, chronic inflammatory diseases, such as rheumatoid arthritis and inflammatory bowel diseases, benefit from the anti-inflammatory properties of secondary metabolites. Compounds such as curcuminoids from turmeric and plant-derived terpenoids function by inhibiting the production of inflammatory mediators, including tumor necrosis factor-alpha (TNF-α) and pro-inflammatory interleukins, (Azeez & Lunghar, 2021) (Ge *et al.,* 2022). These mechanisms of action confer substantial therapeutic potential for managing these diseases.

This chapter aims to explore the molecular mechanisms through which secondary metabolites exert their therapeutic effects in neurodegenerative and inflammatory diseases. By analyzing their interactions with biological pathways involved in oxidative stress, inflammation, and cellular degeneration, this chapter highlights their potential as innovative therapeutic agents. Such an analysis could pave the way for the development of targeted therapies for these complex conditions, while expanding the role of secondary metabolites in contemporary medicine.

2. NEURODEGENERATIVE DISEASES AND INFLAMMATION: A BRIEF OVERVIEW

2.1. Pathophysiological Mechanisms of Neurodegenerative Diseases

Neurodegenerative diseases (NDDs) represent a heterogeneous group of neurological disorders that severely impact the quality of life for millions of individuals worldwide. These pathologies are characterized by the progressive degeneration of neurons within the CNS or the peripheral nervous system. The deterioration of neuronal network structure and function, combined with the irreversible loss of neurons unable to regenerate effectively due to their terminal differentiation leads to the disruption of fundamental communication circuits, (Erkkinen, Kim, & Geschwind, 2018) (El-Mansoury *et al.,* 2023). This results in a wide range of impairments, including memory, cognition, behavior, sensory, and motor functions.

These conditions encompass a wide array of disorders, including Alzheimer's disease (AD), (Long & Holtzman, 2019) (Jawad *et al.,* 2024), Parkinson's disease (PD) (Poewe *et al.,* 2017), primary tauopathies, frontotemporal dementia (FTD), amyotrophic lateral sclerosis (ALS) (Kiernan *et al.,* 2011), synucleinopathies (e.g., dementia with Lewy bodies (DLB) and multiple system atrophy (MSA), Huntington's disease (HD), and related polyglutamine (polyQ) diseases (including spinocerebellar ataxias (SCAs), prion diseases (PrDs), traumatic brain injury (TBI), chronic traumatic encephalopathy (CTE), stroke, spinal cord injury (SCI), and multiple sclerosis (MS), (Dugger & Dickson, 2017). The epidemiology, clinical manifestations, genetic basis, and pathological hallmarks of these specific neurodegenerative disorders have been extensively and elegantly reviewed in prior studies, (Butt, De La Rocha, & Rivera, 2019).

Although the clinical manifestations of NDDs vary some primarily affecting memory and cognitive functions, while others impair motor abilities, speech, or respiratory functions these disorders share several common pathological hallmarks. These include pathological protein aggregation, synaptic and neuronal network dysfunction, aberrant proteostasis, cytoskeletal abnormalities, disruption of energy homeostasis, DNA and RNA defects, chronic inflammation, and neuronal cell death (Wilson *et al.,* 2023) (Figure 1).

In addition to these shared mechanisms, the genetic basis of NDDs reveals the intricate interplay of underlying cellular and molecular processes. A non-exhaustive list of high-risk causal and associated genes highlights the aggregation-prone proteins implicated in these disorders. These include Aβ peptides formed by cleavage of amyloid precursor protein (APP; APP gene) (Tanzi, 2012), tau protein (MAPT gene), alpha-synuclein (SNCA gene), TAR DNA-binding protein 43 (TDP-43;

TARDBP gene), superoxide dismutase [Cu-Zn] (SOD1; SOD1 gene), dipeptide repeat proteins (DPRs; C9orf72 gene), RNA-binding protein FUS (FUS gene), huntingtin (PolyQ; HTT gene), PolyQ proteins, and cellular prion protein (PrP^C; PRNP gene), (Goedert, 2015).

The interrelations among these molecular and genetic contributors emphasize the complexity of NDD pathophysiology. Understanding these intricate mechanisms is crucial to devising effective therapeutic strategies, which remain an urgent need in combating these debilitating disorders, (Aimrane *et al.,* 2023) (Abeliovich & Gitler, 2016).

Figure 1. Hallmarks of neurodegenerative diseases

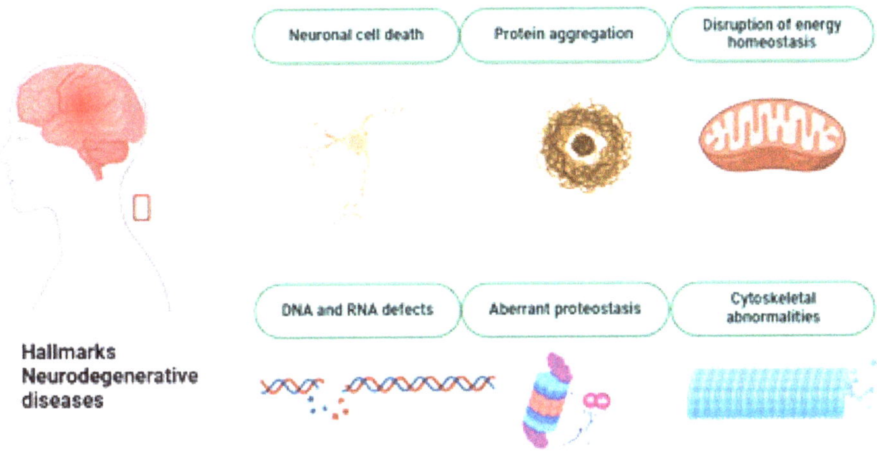

A fundamental approach to elucidating the pathophysiology of a disease involves the establishment of model systems that accurately replicate its defining characteristics. Robust experimental models, including widely utilized organisms such as mice, Drosophila melanogaster, Caenorhabditis elegans, and even Saccharomyces cerevisiae, have long served as invaluable tools in the investigation of neurodegenerative disorders. These models have yielded critical insights into the molecular and cellular mechanisms underpinning disease progression, thereby advancing our understanding of these complex pathologies, (Schöll *et al.,* 2019).

2.2. Role of Inflammation in the Progression of Chronic Diseases

Inflammasomes are cytosolic multiprotein complexes that play a pivotal role in activating the pro-inflammatory caspase-1, which is responsible for the maturation and secretion of the cytokines IL-1β and IL-18, as well as the induction of pyroptosis, a form of pro-inflammatory cell death, (Orlando & Mainous, 2024). The activation of inflammasomes is initiated by specific stimuli that trigger the oligomerization of pattern recognition receptor (PRR) proteins. This process leads to the recruitment and autoactivation of procaspase-1 within the complex, producing its active form, (Mahad, Trapp, & Lassmann, 2015).

Active caspase-1 cleaves the inactive pro-peptides, pro-IL-1β and pro-IL-18, converting them into their mature forms, which are then secreted to mediate inflammatory responses. In addition to cytokine maturation, caspase-1 also induces pyroptosis by activating gasdermin D (GSDMD). Upon cleavage by caspase-1 (or caspase-11 in mice and caspase-4/5 in humans), the amino-terminal domain of GSDMD oligomerizes and forms pores in the plasma membrane, (Voet *et al.,* 2019a). This leads to cell swelling, membrane rupture, and the release of intracellular contents, further amplifying the inflammatory response. This dual function of inflammasomes cytokine maturation and induction of pyroptosis highlights their central role in both promoting inflammation and modulating immune responses, with implications for various inflammatory and pathological conditions.

Inflammation is a central factor in the development and progression of NDDs, including Alzheimer's disease, PD, ALS, HD, and MS. At the core of this process lies neuroinflammation, driven by the activation of microglia and astrocytes, the primary immune and support cells of the CNS. Microglia respond to damage or stress by releasing inflammatory cytokines, performing phagocytosis, and generating reactive oxygen species (ROS). While these responses are protective in acute conditions, their prolonged activation results in chronic inflammation, which exacerbates neuronal damage and dysfunction. Similarly, reactive astrocytes contribute to neuroinflammation by impairing glutamate homeostasis and disrupting synaptic networks, thereby accelerating neurodegeneration, (Voet *et al.,* 2019b).

Key inflammatory mediators such as interleukins IL-1β and IL-18 play dual roles in the CNS. While they are involved in essential cognitive functions, including learning and memory, their elevated levels during CNS infection, injury, or NDDs contribute to inflammatory signaling cascades that promote neuronal injury and cell death. These processes are often associated with pyroptosis, apoptosis, and necroptosis cell death pathways that amplify inflammation and exacerbate neurodegeneration, (Alboni *et al.,* 2010).

Inflammasome activation, primarily attributed to microglia, is a critical mechanism in CNS inflammation. However, neurons, astrocytes, and other CNS cell types also express inflammasome components, indicating a broader involvement in NDD pathology. The persistence of inflammasome activation, driven by danger signals like protein aggregates, misfolded proteins, and mitochondrial ROS, underscores its role in sustaining chronic inflammation in NDDs. Despite the association of inflammasome components and inflammatory markers with NDDs, further research is needed to delineate their specific contributions and to develop CNS-targeted therapies (Baecher-Allan, Kaskow, & Weiner, 2018) (Figure 2).

This interplay between neuroinflammation, inflammasome activation, and other pathological features of NDDs, such as protein aggregation and oxidative stress, highlights the need for targeted therapeutic strategies. By addressing both the inflammatory response and the underlying molecular mechanisms, there is potential to mitigate disease progression and improve patient outcomes, (Alboni *et al.*, 2010).

Figure 2. Inflammasome activation in neurodegenerative diseases

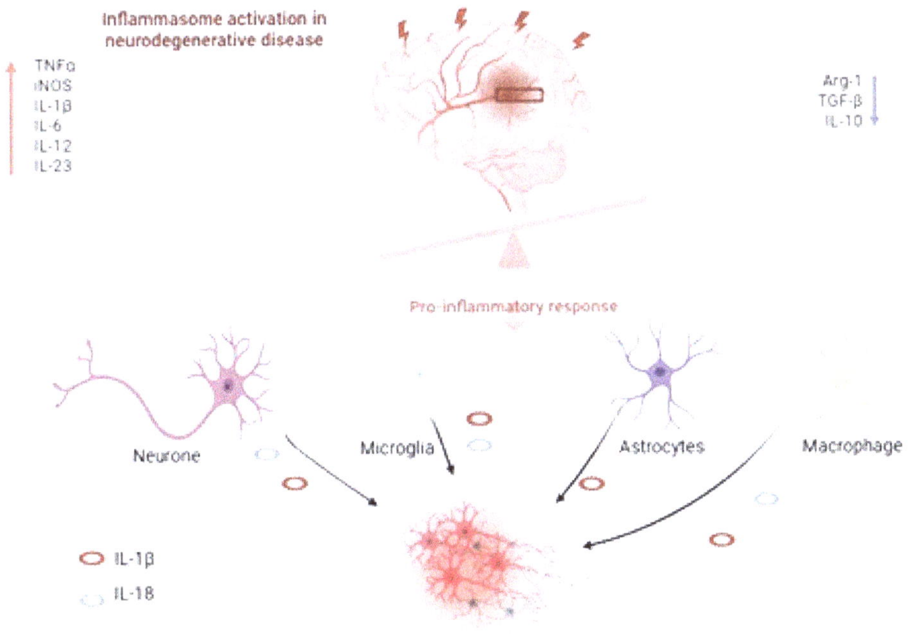

2.2.1 Alzheimer's Disease: Neuroinflammation

Alzheimer's disease is the most common neurodegenerative disorder in the elderly, characterized by progressive memory loss and cognitive decline. According to the amyloid hypothesis, the pathology of AD is primarily driven by the extracellular accumulation of misfolded beta-amyloid (Aβ) plaques, which are believed to initiate the disease. However, neuroinflammation is increasingly recognized as a key factor that actively contributes to the progression of AD, (Jawad *et al.,* 2024) (Sala Frigerio & De Strooper, 2016). This neuroinflammatory response is primarily driven by microglia, resident cells in the CNS Although microglia can play a beneficial role in clearing Aβ deposits through phagocytosis, excessive accumulation of Aβ sensitizes microglia, promoting their activation and the release of inflammatory mediators. Over time, this prolonged activation impairs their ability to clear Aβ efficiently, leading to synaptic dysfunction and neuronal damage, (Sala Frigerio & De Strooper, 2016).

Recent studies have highlighted the crucial role of inflammasomes in AD development. Elevated expression of interleukin-1β (IL-1β) has been observed in microglia surrounding Aβ plaques. Gene expression analyses have revealed increased levels of inflammasome components, including NLRP3, ASC, caspase-1, and caspase-5, as well as cytokines IL-1β and IL-18, in peripheral blood mononuclear cells (PBMCs) from AD patients. Increased levels of NLRC4 and ASC have also been detected in brain samples from certain sporadic AD patients. Additionally, genetic variants of NLRP1 have been associated with an increased risk of AD, and a higher number of NLRP1-positive neurons have been observed in the brains of AD patients, (Sarlus & Heneka, 2017) (Shi & Holtzman, 2017).

In vitro studies have demonstrated that fibrillar Aβ activates the NLRP3 inflammasome when phagocytosed by microglia, leading to the activation of caspase-1 and the release of IL-1β. NLRP3 activation has also been documented in vivo in the APP/PS1 transgenic mouse model of AD. Deletion of NLRP3 in these models resulted in significant improvements in spatial memory deficits and hyperactive behaviors, accompanied by reduced Aβ deposits in the hippocampus and cortex, smaller plaque volumes, decreased pro-inflammatory cytokine levels, and enhanced microglial phagocytic ability. Similar results were obtained in APP/PS1 mice deficient in caspase-1, (Tzeng *et al.,* 2018).

Pharmacological inhibition of the NLRP3 inflammasome, such as with MCC950/CRID3, promoted Aβ clearance and improved cognitive function in mouse models. Indirect inhibition using non-steroidal anti-inflammatory drugs targeting cyclooxygenase enzymes and volume-regulated anion channels (VRAC) also reduced neuroglial inflammation and memory loss in 3×TgAD mice. Additionally, caspase-1 inhibition by VX-765 reduced Aβ accumulation, brain inflammation, and cognitive impairment, (Flores *et al.,* 2020).

These findings suggest that misfolded Aβ activates the NLRP3 inflammasome in microglia, triggering the release of pro-inflammatory factors that perpetuate a chronic neuroinflammatory environment and exacerbate AD pathology. Furthermore, NLRP3 activation results in the extracellular release of ASC particles, which act as danger signals to activate surrounding macrophages. These ASC specks physically bind to Aβ, promoting its aggregation and plaque formation in a prion-like process, (Venegas & Heneka, 2017).

The pathogenic role of IL-1β in AD has been demonstrated in mice deficient in IL-1 receptor antagonist (IL-1ra), which exhibited increased vulnerability after intracerebroventricular injection of human oligomeric Aβ1–42. Another study showed that IL-1β injection in the cerebral hemisphere increased Aβ-APP protein levels in wild-type mice. However, sustained hippocampal IL-1β overexpression in APP/PS1 mice reduced plaque pathology, which may be attributed to increased microglial and macrophage phagocytic activity. Similar observations were made in 3×TgAD mice, although tau phosphorylation was also increased, highlighting the complex role of IL-1 signaling in AD. Conversely, IL-1R1 deficiency in mice did not affect Aβ deposition in Tg2567 mice. Likewise, IL-18 deletion did not provide protective effects in APP/PS1 mice, although these mice showed increased susceptibility to grand-mal seizures and altered synaptic proteins, leading to heightened excitatory synaptic transmission. Thus, IL-18 may play an unexpected role in controlling neuronal activity, (Alfei & Zuccari, 2025). While the focus has been on NLRP3 in AD, other inflammasomes have also been studied. The AIM2 inflammasome has been shown to increase Aβ deposition, microglial activation, and cytokine production, but it does not affect behavior or memory in transgenic 5xFAD mice. Knockdown of NLRP1 in APP/PS1 mice resulted in significantly reduced neuronal pyroptosis and improved cognitive impairments. Finally, the NLRC4 inflammasomc was shown to increase neuronal Aβ levels via activated pro-inflammatory astrocytes, (Alfei & Zuccari, 2025).

2.2.2 Parkinson's Disease: Neuroinflammation

PD is a progressive neurodegenerative disorder characterized by the loss of dopaminergic neurons in the substantia nigra pars compacta. One of the pathological features of PD is the presence of Lewy bodies, which are primarily composed of intracellular aggregates of fibrillar α-synuclein, (Przedborski, 2017). Studies of serum samples from PD patients have revealed elevated levels of IL-1β and caspase-1 (Zhou *et al.,* 2016), and increased IL-1β levels have also been found in the striata of PD patients, (Mogi *et al.*, 1994). In the A53T transgenic mouse model of PD, which overexpresses mutant human A53T α-synuclein, there is also an increase in IL-1β levels in the midbrain, (Zhou *et al.*, 2016). Chronic expression of IL-1β in the substantia nigra of rats, via a recombinant adenovirus, has been shown to induce progressive death of dopaminergic neurons and result in motor impairments, (Ferrari *et al.*, 2006). However, most of the evidence linking PD to inflammasome signaling comes from in vitro studies, and the role of inflammasomes in PD remains not fully understood. α-Synuclein has been shown to activate the NLRP3 inflammasome in human monocytes and BV2 microglial cells, (Zhou *et al.*, 2016) (Li *et al.*, 2021) (Boza-Serrano *et al.*, 2014), although it did not trigger inflammasome activation in primary microglia, (Gustin *et al.*, 2015). In vivo, microinjection of the caspase-1 inhibitor Ac-YVAD-CMK has been found to reduce NLRP3 inflammasome signaling proteins and improve the survival of dopaminergic neurons in LPS-induced and 6-hydroxydopamine-induced PD in rats, (Yang *et al.*, 2020). Consistent with this, NLRP3 knockout mice were resistant to the loss of dopaminergic neurons induced by the neurotoxin 1-methyl-4-phenyl-1,2,3,6-tetrahydropyridine (MPTP), with a reduction in caspase-1 activation and secretion of IL-1β and IL-18, (Yan *et al.*, 2015). Additionally, caspase-1 was shown to cleave α-synuclein in vitro, producing an aggregation-prone form of the protein that was toxic to cultured neurons, (Wang *et al.*, 2016).

Mutations in the Parkin, PARK2, PARK6, and PINK1 genes have been linked to early-onset, autosomal recessive PD. Microglia and macrophages from PARK2 and PINK1 knockout mice, as well as from patients with PARK2 mutations, have exhibited an exacerbated NLRP3 inflammasome response. This response is thought to result from impaired expression of the anti-inflammatory protein A20, which negatively regulates NLRP3 activation, (Mouton-Liger *et al.*, 2018).

3. SECONDARY METABOLITES WITH NEUROPROTECTIVE AND ANTI-INFLAMMATORY PROPERTIES

The term "secondary metabolite" is employed to describe an extensive array of chemical compounds in plants that are responsible for a variety of peripheral functions, many of which are indirectly essential to the sustenance of life. Such functions include intercellular communication, the defense mechanisms of the plant, and the regulation of catalytic cycles. Secondary metabolites (also referred to as 'natural products') are organic molecules that are not directly involved in the process of an organism's development or reproductive capacity. Their absence does not result in immediate death, but may potentially limit the survival, fecundity, or appearance of an organism. Alternatively, their absence may have no discernible effect.

Secondary metabolites are primarily responsible for enhancing the competitive advantage of the organism that biosynthesizes them. In essence, secondary metabolites provide the organism with a distinct advantage over other biological entities. Secondary metabolites, however, have biological functions that can prove essential. For example, isoprenoid pigments and fragrances (volatile isoprenoids) of plants attract pollinating insects (which are essential for reproduction). They also serve as means of defense against biotic and abiotic aggressions. Furthermore, they facilitate communication between plants, microorganisms or animals (hormones, pheromones, etc.).

3.1. Classifications of Secondary Metabolites

It is postulated that there exists a plethora of secondary metabolites, numbering several hundred thousand, exhibiting a vast array of structural and functional diversities. Consequently, a multitude of classifications has been proposed, with varying sources of origin. The most fundamental classification of secondary metabolites can be divided into the following main compounds:

3.1.1 Alkaloids

Alkaloids are produced by a large variety of organisms, such as bacteria, fungi, animals but mostly by plants as secondary metabolites. To date, more than 27,000 different alkaloids have been identified. 21,000 of these come from different plant species. Alkaloids are a group of secondary metabolites containing basic nitrogen atoms. Alkaloids also include some related compounds with neutral and weak acid properties. Besides carbon, hydrogen and nitrogen, this group can contain oxygen, sulphur and rarely other elements like chlorine, bromine and phosphorus, (Nolaou, Chen, & Corey, 2011). It is the nitrogen atoms that give the alkaloids their basic properties and allow them to exist as water soluble salts after interaction with acids. In addition, alkaloids possessing quaternary nitrogen atoms can be identified in nature, (Setyorini & Antarlina, 2022). Even in instances wherein a standardized categorization for alkaloids is absent, a plethora of standards has been employed for the purpose of organizing them. These standards encompass the following criteria: their biosynthetic origin, the existence of a fundamental heterocyclic nucleus within their structure, their pharmacological attributes, and their distribution among various plant families, (Chawla *et al.*, 2013). The occurrence of alkaloids can be evidenced in a variety of plant components, including foliage, branches, bark, and seeds. The majority of naturally occurring alkaloids have been demonstrated to elicit specific physiological responses. While certain alkaloids are toxic, others are of significant medicinal value, (Bhambhani, Kondhare, & Giri, 2021).

3.1.2 Phenolic Compounds

Phenolic compounds are present in a number of by-products of the winemaking process, namely in the seeds, skins, stems and pomace of grapes. They constitute a highly diverse collection of secondary metabolites, which are defined as substances that possess both an aromatic hydrocarbon and a hydroxyl group bonded to them. From a chemical perspective, the most fundamental member of this class is phenol, (Velderrain- Rodríguez *et al*., 2014). The classification of plant phenolics is based on the number of hydroxylic groups present. Accordingly, they may be classified as monohydroxy, dihydroxy, and polyatomic phenols. Phenolic compounds containing more than one OH group in an aromatic ring are classified as polyphenols. The chemical composition of these compounds can be further categorized as mono-, di-, oligo- and polyphenols. Additionally, the number of aromatic rings and carbon atoms in the side chain can be used to distinguish between different polyphenol subgroups. In accordance with the aforementioned principle, phenolic compounds are subdivided into four principal categories: those with a single aromatic ring, those with two aromatic rings, quinones, and polymers.

To current knowledge, there are in excess of 8,000 different polyphenolic compounds that have been identified. This is the reason why the terminology and classification of polyphenols is intricate and perplexing. Despite the fact that all polyphenols possess analogous chemical structures, there are nevertheless some distinctive differences. In accordance with these differentiating characteristics, polyphenols can be classified into two principal categories: flavonoids and non-flavonoids, which include tannins, (Subhan *et al.,* 2024).

3.1.3 Flavonoids

Flavonoids represent a group of significant secondary metabolites that are pervasively distributed in a multitude of fruits, vegetables, herbs, stems, cereals, nuts, flowers, and seeds, (Malik *et al.,* 2020). To date, over 10,000 flavonoid compounds have been isolated and identified. Flavonoids are predominantly located within plant cell vacuoles, predominantly in the form of C-glycosides or O-glycosides, (Johnson *et al.,* 20210. The fundamental molecular structure of flavonoids is based on a C6–C3–C6 skeleton. The classification of flavonoids is based on modifications to their basic skeletons, which can be divided into seven subclasses. These subclasses include flavones, flavanones, isoflavones, flavonols, chalcones, flavanols, and anthocyanins, (Bulea *et al.,* 2015).

3.1.4 Flavones

Flavones represent one of the prevailing classes of flavonoids, comprising 4H-chromen-4-one derivatives bearing a phenyl substituent at the 2 positions. Flavones are predominantly present as 7-O-glycosides, which are identified in celery, parsley, red pepper, chamomile, mint, and ginkgo, (Luca *et al.*, 2020). Apigenin and luteolin constitute two of the most prevalent flavones.

3.1.5 Flavonols

Flavonols are a class of flavonoids that possess a ketone group. They serve as the fundamental constituents of proanthocyanidins. Flavonols are widely distributed in a diverse range of fruits and vegetables. In comparison to flavones, flavonols possess a hydroxyl group in position 3 of the C ring, which may also undergo glycosylation. Similarly, flavonols exhibit a high degree of diversity in methylation and hydroxylation patterns. When considering the various glycosylation patterns, it can be posited that they represent the most prevalent and expansive subgroup of flavonoids in fruits and vegetables. For example, quercetin is a common flavonoid found in a wide variety of plant foods, (Iwashina, 2013).

3.1.6 Isoflavone

Isoflavonoids are distinctive metabolites of leguminous plants, as evidenced by studies conducted by Hummelova *et al.* (2015) and Lim *et al.* (2020). Isoflavones possess a B-ring at the C3 position of the heterocyclic C-ring of the diphenylpropane (C6–C3–C6) backbone, which distinguishes them from other flavonoids in terms of their chemical structure, (Kopečná-Zapletalová *et al.*, 2017). The most prevalent isoflavones are genistein, daidzein, glycitein, and formononetin.

3.1.7 Anthocyanins

A total of over 650 anthocyanins have been identified across a range of plant species, (Khoo *et al.*, 2017). These can be grouped into five main categories: cyanidin, delphinidin, malvidin, pelargonidin, and peonidin, along with their corresponding derivatives, (Chaves-Silva *et al.*, 2018). As glycosylated polyphenolic compounds, anthocyanins constitute a group of soluble vacuolar pigments that exhibit a range of colors, from orange, red, and purple to blue, contingent on the pH of the micro-environment of the flowers, seeds, fruits, and vegetative tissues, (Fang, 2015). Furthermore, anthocyanins are frequently employed as food colorants.

3.1.8 Terpenes

Terpenes, which are the constituents of essential oils, represent a vast array of organic chemical compounds and are among the most heterogeneous natural products found in plants, particularly with regard to their structural composition. A substantial proportion of plant species synthesize terpenes, which are characterized by their aromatic properties and high volatility. The fundamental structural unit of terpenes is derived from isoprene (2-methyl-1,3-butadiene), which is a relatively straightforward hydrocarbon molecule and is also prevalent among numerous other secondary metabolites in plants. Terpenoids are similar to terpenes, but with a notable difference: they are the by-products of terpenes that have undergone denaturation through oxidation, resulting in the addition of an oxygen atom to their chemical structure. The terpenoid family of phytoconstituents exhibits a paucity of functional and structural commonalities. Examples of this diverse family of compounds include steroids, carotenoids, and gibberellic acid. They are composed of the most important group of active compounds in plants, with over 23,000 known structures. They are polymeric isoprene derivatives, synthesized from acetate via the mevalonic acid pathway. During the formation of these compounds, the isoprene units are attached in a head-to-tail configuration. The total number of units incorporated into a particular terpene is used as a fundamental basis for their classification.

3.2. Pharmacological Activities and Mechanisms of Action

3.2.1. The Anti-Inflammatory Properties of Secondary Metabolites

The process of inflammation is a complex pathophysiological phenomenon, which is mediated by a variety of signaling molecules. These are produced by a number of different cell types, including leukocytes, macrophages and mast cells. In addition, the activation of complement factors also plays a role in the formation of edema. This occurs as a result of the extravasation of fluid and proteins, as well as the accumulation of leukocytes at the site of the inflammatory response, (Galvão *et al.*, 2018). The inflammatory response is, in general, protective and ultimately eliminates both the cause and consequences of tissue injury that can accompany host defense, (Doyle & Godson, 2022). The phenomenon of inflammation, as a fundamental biological response to injury, has been recognized for millennia. Anti-inflammatory drugs are broadly classified into two categories: These can be further classified as either steroidal or non-steroidal anti-inflammatory agents (NSAIDs). Steroidal drugs exert their effects on inflammatory cells and inflammatory mediators. Non-steroidal anti-inflammatory drugs (NSAIDs) exert their effects by inhibiting the activity of cyclooxygenase 1 and 2 (COX-1 and COX-2), (Doyle & Godson,

2022). Secondary metabolites from plants have constituted an essential source of pharmaceuticals since antiquity, with approximately half of all currently utilised drugs derived from natural sources.

3.2.1.1 Alkaloids

The pharmacological activity of alkaloids is typified by their capacity to act as competitive antagonists of muscarinic acetylcholine receptors, exerting anti-cholinergic effects and exhibiting anti-myopia properties, (Singh *et al.,* 2020). The source of berberine is the Berberis genus. Evidence has been presented which demonstrates the anti-inflammatory, antibacterial and antiviral properties of the compound in question. Moreover, it has been demonstrated that nicotine Solanaceae plants, which belong to the Solanaceae family, and quinine from *Cinchona succirubra, C. calisya, C. ledgeriana,* plants of Rubiaceae family, possess anti-inflammatory properties.

It is established that certain alkaloids, including isoquinoline, indole and diterpene, possess notable anti-inflammatory properties. Seven distinct types of isoquinoline alkaloids were identified in the roots, barks, and branches of Turkish Berberis species. These included protoberberine (berberine, palmatine, jatrorrhizine, and columbamine), bisbenzylisoquinoline (berbamine, oxyacanthine, and aromoline), and aporphine (magnoflorine) types. It is well documented that inflammation plays a role in the progression of numerous diseases, including NDDs, (Zhang *et al.,* 2023). Therefore, anti-inflammatory treatment is beneficial in the management of these related disorders. In 2017, Leonoudakis *et al.* reported the anti-inflammatory activity of securinine at concentrations of 2.5–10 μM in BV2 cells, whereby NF-κB and MAPK were inhibited. Furthermore, securinine has been demonstrated to inhibit the production of nitric oxide in response to interferon-γ (IFN-γ) and the expression of the enzyme iNOS mRNA, suggesting a potential for its use in the treatment of NDDs associated with neuroinflammation.

3.2.1.2 Phenolic Compounds

Phenolic compounds possess significant pharmacological value, with some demonstrating anti-inflammatory properties. A variety of phenolic compounds, including flavonoids, condensed tannins, and gallotannins, have been demonstrated to impede the activity of specific molecular targets associated with pro-inflammatory mediators in the context of inflammatory responses, (Pannucci *et al.,* 2023). It has been demonstrated by researchers that polyphenol-rich extracts and fractions have the capacity to inhibit the production of NO (Nitric Oxide) and the expression of iNOS (inducible nitric oxide synthase) in macrophages that have been stimulated with LPS (lipopolysaccharide) and in dendritic cells, (Figueirinha *et al.,* 2010). In consequence, a number of phenolic compounds have been documented to exert an influence on the synthesis of iNOS protein and the production of NO. The mRNA levels of iNOS could be reduced by tyrosol, 6-shogaol, verbascoside, curcumin, and resveratrol. Furthermore, additional studies have identified apigenin, (Mushtaq *et al.,* 2023), ochnaflavone (Dutta *et al.,* 2024) and quercetin (Bıçakcıoğlu *et al.,* 2023) as compounds capable of inhibiting iNOS transcriptional activity. Additionally, arctigenin has been reported to possess similar inhibitory effects on iNOS activity, (Balkrishna *et al.,* 2024). Phenolic compounds have the capacity to modulate the expression of various cytokines, thereby exerting an anti-inflammatory effect. The mRNA levels of TNF-α are decreased by quercetin, while the protein levels are reduced by caffeic acid, verbascoside, curcumin, the lignan arctigenin, glabridin, kurarinone and kuraridin. Luteolin, genistein, quercetin, isoquercetin, rutin, icariin derivatives, EGCG, cyanidin-3-O-glucoside, scopoletin and chrysophanol, (Andleeb *et al.,* 2024).

3.2.1.3 Flavonoids

Apigenin, a flavonoid, has been demonstrated to reduce the steady-state mRNA levels induced by TNF-α and to downregulate the expression of intercellular adhesion molecule-1 (ICAM-1), E-selectin, and vascular cell adhesion molecule-1 (VCAM-1) in endothelial cells. Yang et al. (2020) reported that numerous flavonoids were observed to reduce the expression of pro-inflammatory cytokines (e.g., TNF-α, IL-1β, IL-8, IL-6, and monocyte chemoattractant protein-1 (MCP-1)) in Jurkat T cells, as well as in peripheral blood mononuclear cells and RAW macrophages, (Yang & Huang, 2020). The combined inhibition of TNF-α and IL-1β by quercetin and catechins has been demonstrated to increase IL-10 production, (Yahfoufi *et al.,* 2018). A number of flavonoids have been demonstrated to reduce the production of arachidonic acid and inhibit the activities of phospholipase A2, cyclooxygenase, and NOS. This results in a further reduction in the production of key inflammatory substances (prostaglandins, leukotrienes, and NO), (Al-Khayri *et al.,* 2022).

Additionally, flavonoids have been demonstrated to inhibit the production of arachidonic acid metabolites and chemokines, thereby reducing leukocyte infiltration and edema, (Tunon *et al.,* 2009). Furthermore, flavonoids have the potential to chelate metal iron, suppress the activation of the complement system, and reduce inflammation. Naringenin has been demonstrated to possess anti-inflammatory properties, as evidenced by its ability to inhibit pro-inflammatory cytokines and reduce leukocyte infiltration. A number of chalcones (including trans-chalcone, hesperidin and methyl chalcone) have been observed to exhibit inhibitory activity against pro-inflammatory cytokines.

3.2.1.4 Terpene

Due to their redox properties and ability to act as antioxidants, secondary metabolites can further be used as anti-inflammatory agents. Inflammation is a typical response of live tissue triggered by cellular injury and involves a cascade of biochemical reactions to protect the body from harmful stimuli. Although a defensive mechanism to protect the body from harmful stimuli, chronic inflammation can lead to variety of health problems. In such cases, compounds with anti-inflammatory properties. According to researchers, molecular basis of the anti-inflammatory action of diterpenoids is presented with special emphasis on their ability to modulate critical cell signaling pathways involved in the inflammatory response of the body such as nuclear transcription factor-kappaB (NF-κB) activation. NF-κB plays an important role in the regulation of immune and inflammatory responses. Indeed, deregulated NF-κB expression is a characteristic phenomenon in several inflammatory diseases and NF-κB has become a major target in drug discovery, (Hortelano, 2009).

Ursolic acid, a vibenstone-type (diterpenoid), has been demonstrated to reduce the production of various biogenic amines, including histamine, bradykinin, serotonin, and prostaglandins (PGs). Additionally, it has been shown to inhibit the expression of several key inflammatory mediators, including interleukin-6 (IL-6), tumor necrosis factor-α (TNF-α), inducible nitric oxide synthase (iNOS), nuclear factor kappa-light-chain-enhancer of activated B cells (NF-κB), and cyclooxygenase-2 (COX-2), (Wu *et al.*, 2021). Moreover, terpenes (phytol) have been demonstrated to markedly diminish paw oedema by impeding the COX and 5-LOX pathways, (Jigam *et al.*, 2020).

3.2.2. The Neuroprotective Properties of Secondary Metabolites

3.2.2.1 Phenolic Compounds

The interest in phenolic compounds in foods has grown significantly since the 1990s, driven by mounting evidence of their beneficial impact on human health. The evidence from in vitro, in vivo studies and clinical trials indicates that polyphenols from apple, grape and citrus fruit juices demonstrate a greater neuroprotective effect than antioxidant vitamins. The interest in phenolic compounds in foods has grown significantly since the 1990s, driven by the mounting evidence of their beneficial impact on human health. The evidence from in vitro, in vivo studies and clinical trials suggests that polyphenols from apple, grape and citrus fruit juices may offer a more pronounced neuroprotective benefit than antioxidant vitamins. The phenolic compounds (catechins and epicatechins) present in green tea have been demonstrated to possess neuroprotective properties. These compounds have been shown to safeguard neurons against a range of oxidative and metabolic insults. This includes the protection of dopaminergic neurons from damage induced by 6-hydroxydopamine in a rat model of PD (Guo *et al.,* 2007), the safeguarding of retinal neurons against ischemia reperfusion injury, and the reduction of mutant huntingtin misfolding and neurotoxicity in Huntington's disease models, (Zhang *et al.,* 2007) (Ehrnhoefer *et al.,* 2006).

Catechins are a type of polyphenol that have been observed to exhibit neuro-protective activities. These effects are at least partly mediated by the activation of protein kinase C (PKC) and transcription factors, which induce the expression of genes involved in cellular survival, (Mandel *et al.,* 2005). It has been postulated that catechins may prove efficacious in the suppression of the pathogenesis of Alzheimer's disease and in the protection of neurons against the processes of Alzheimer's disease. It has been demonstrated that catechins and their metabolites activate a number of signaling pathways that can exert cell-survival and anti-inflammatory actions. These include the alteration of the expression of pro-apoptotic and anti-apoptotic proteins, as well as the upregulation of antioxidant defenses, (Sutherland, Rahman, & Appleton, 2006).

3.2.2.2 Flavonoids

Flavonoids have been demonstrated to have a positive preventative effect on cardiovascular and neurodegenerative events. The flavonoid family is classified into six groups. Of these, flavones and flavonols, based on the 2-phenylchromen-4-one (2-phenyl-1-benzopyran-4-one) skeleton, are the most commonly encountered in families and genera of higher plants, (Khan *et al.,* 2021). A substantial body of evidence from scientific studies indicates that flavones, such as luteolin, and flavonols, including kaempferol and quercetin, possess neuroprotective properties in experimental models of neurodegeneration, (Calis, Mogulkoc, & Baltaci, 2020) (Hasan *et al.,* 2023). As posited by Dajas *et al.* (2013), neuroprotection appears to be linked to specific structural motifs that extend beyond those involved in antioxidation. When employed as standalone agents or as templates for the synthesis of novel compounds, flavones and flavonols demonstrate promise as multifaceted therapeutic agents for the protection of the brain. A substantial body of scientific evidence substantiates the assertion that the antidepressant and neuroprotective effects of flavonoids represent a multifaceted influence on the nervous system. These effects are mediated by a range of molecular targets that are integral to the pathogenesis of neuropathology (Rushendran *et al.,* 2024), a complex process encompassing oxidative stress, cytotoxicity, and inflammation. These biochemical mechanisms are implicated in the development of neuropathological conditions.

3.2.2.3 Terpene

A multitude of terpenes, primarily derived from essential oils and plant extracts, along with forest bathing, have been documented to demonstrate a vast array of crucial bioactivities, encompassing antioxidant, anti-inflammatory, and anticancer properties, as well as neuroprotective capabilities, (Zeng *et al.*, 2023). Consequently, a various terpenes have been investigated for their neuroprotective effects through:

Inhibition of Aβ production represents a promising avenue for the development of novel therapeutic strategies for Alzheimer's disease (AD). BACE1 plays a pivotal role in the formation of Aβ plaques, which are a hallmark of Alzheimer's disease (AD) pathogenesis. As previously outlined, BACE1 acts as a rate-limiting enzyme in this process. Consequently, the inhibition of this enzyme reduces the load of Aβ plaques in neuronal cells by slowing or reversing the process, (Naija *et al.*, 2021). It is also important to note that terpene compounds are characterized by low molecular weight and high hydrophobicity. This enables them to cross cellular membranes and the blood-brain barrier (BBB), which is an essential attribute for BACE1 inhibition in vivo, (Somova *et al.*, 2003).

The inhibition of NFT formation is a key objective in this field of research. Diterpenes have been identified as a potential source of inhibitors for NFT formation. In addition to inhibiting BACE1, the norditerpenes gracilins (3–6) also inhibit tau phosphorylation, (Lima & Medeiros, 2024).

The inhibition of pro-inflammatory factors represents a key mechanism of action. Monoterpene: The production of ROS in AD flies that were fed (+)-limonene (44) was found to be significantly reduced, indicating that (+)-limonene (44) possesses antioxidant activity both in vitro and in vivo. The antioxidant activity of (+)-limonene (44) has been demonstrated to have anti-inflammatory effects, resulting in a reduction in the inflammatory response observed in this Drosophila model of AD following ingestion of the compound, (Hadipour, Shahangian, & Mashayekhi, 2024).

3.3. Studies of Specific Metabolites in Disease Models

3.3.1 Diabetes Mellitus

Diabetes mellitus represents a significant global health burden, responsible for an estimated 4.2 million deaths and a further economic cost of 760 million US dollars in healthcare expenditure in 2019, (Kengene & Ramachandran, 2024). The latest data on diabetes from the International Diabetes Federation (IDF) indicates that approximately 463 million adults between the ages of 20 and 79 are affected, with the majority residing in low- and middle-income countries, (Harding *et al.*, 2024).

A prenyl flavonoid (8-prenylnaringenin), namely a xanthohumol metabolite. It is present in the Rutaceae family of plants (Li *et al.,* 2024) more precisely the genus Citrus, and is found only in trace amounts in citrus fruits such as oranges, lemons, grapefruits, and tangerines, (Marino, 2023). Previous studies have indicated that 8-prenylnaringenin exerts a protective effect on menopausal and postmenopausal symptoms. Additionally, it has been demonstrated to possess anticancer properties, including the induction of autophagy and the modulation of the cell cycle, which collectively suppress tumor growth. These findings have been substantiated in diverse in vitro experimental model systems, (Bartmańska *et al.,* 2018) (Wang *et al.*, 2023). It demonstrated the capacity to diminish oxidative stress, inflammatory processes, and the secretion of angiogenic factors. Additionally, it demonstrated efficacy in regulating vascularization processes, including angiogenesis, (Wang *et al.,* 2024).

In a mouse model of type 2 diabetes mellitus induced by a high-fat diet (HFD), a study demonstrated that 8-prenylnaringenin normalized the expression of galectin-3 (Gal3), a protein overexpressed during the diabetic state and was markedly correlated with oxidative stress in the liver and kidneys of diabetic mice. Furthermore, it diminished 3-nitrotyrosine (a marker of cellular damage), inflammatory responses, and nitric oxide production, while enhancing the generation of advanced glycation end products, (Asahi *et al.*, 2000).

The flavonoid rhoifolin, with the molecular formula $C_{27}H_{30}O_{14}$, is one of the most prevalent flavonoids and is employed extensively in preclinical studies to investigate its pharmacological effects in a diverse range of chronic diseases, including diabetes and obesity. It is present in a number of citrus fruits, including bitter oranges, grapefruits, lemons, and unripe grapes, (Suri, Singh, & Nema, 2023). Previous studies have demonstrated that rhoifolin exerts a range of biological activities, including antioxidant, anti-inflammatory, hepatoprotective, and anticancer effects. Additionally, rhoifolin was extracted from the leaves of the *Citrus grandis* (L.) Osbeck plant, and its insulin-mimetic properties were documented by Rao et al. in an in vitro investigation utilizing differentiated 3T3-L1 adipocytes. It was demonstrated that rhoifolin exerts its effects by promoting the secretion of adiponectin, the phosphorylation of IR-β, and the translocation of GLUT4, which are considered to be critically involved in the development of diabetic complications. The action of rhoifolin against these genes may provide novel targets for combating insulin-resistance-associated diseases, (Samanta *et al.*, 2023).

Rutin, also known as quercetin 3-rutinoside, is a glycosidic flavonoid that can be commonly found in dietary sources. The primary citrus fruits that contain rutin are oranges, grapefruits, lemons, and limes. In a study, the potential benefits of rutin treatment for biochemical alterations associated with experimental diabetes in animals were investigated. The administration of rutin resulted in a reduction in blood glucose levels and an improvement in the lipid profile. Furthermore, it was observed that the administration of rutin prevented alterations in the activities of ALT, AST, and LDH in the serum, liver, and heart, thereby indicating the protective effect of the molecule against hepatic and cardiac toxicity in diabetic rats, (Fernandes *et al.*, 2010).

3.3.2 Cancer

The use of plants for the development of new anticancer molecules represents an approach to cancer therapy that has been the basis for the discovery of several chemotherapy drugs. Despite conventional medicine remaining the dominant field in this area, it should be noted that this strategy is worthy of further investigation. In contrast to lengthy chemical research processes, this approach proposes molecular models for use as is or through hemisynthesis. Natural products derived from plants, marine organisms, and microorganisms represent over 60% of the currently utilized anticancer agents, with approximately 25% derived from plants and another 25% derived from plants, (Khalif *et al.,* 2019) (Chaachouay & Zidane, 2024). This research presents a detailed account of the secondary metabolites derived from plants that have demonstrated anti-cancer properties.

A number of phenolic compounds have been demonstrated to possess a range of interesting pharmacological properties, including antioxidant, anti-inflammatory, neuroprotective and anticancer properties, (Rodrigues *et al.*, 2024). A number of studies have investigated the anti-colorectal cancer effects of phenolic compounds. These studies have employed animal models and have revealed the in vivo colorectal activity of the compounds under investigation. In this paper, we have selected a number of relatively well-studied compounds in order to provide further insight into their anti-colorectal cancer activities. Apigenin is derived from parsley, wheat, onions, and apples. The compound has been observed to induce apoptosis of CRC cells, as well as to upregulate FADD expression and its phosphorylation, (Sung, Chung, & Kim, 2016). Additionally, other studies have employed a model of CF-1 mice induced by AOM and Min mice carrying the mutant APC gene, (Shankar *et al.,* 2017). Moreover, the compound Aciculatin was investigated in an animal model comprising SCID mice with a tumor xenograft induced by HCT116. The study demonstrated that the compound suppressed tumor growth without causing weight loss, upregulated p53 expression and downregulated Ki-67 expression, induced apoptosis and arrested cells in the sub-G1 phase. Additionally, Oufquir et al., (2024) provide evidence from an in vivo study that the extract contains phenolic compounds and flavonoids with high antioxidant potential. Consequently, it can be inferred that *A. muricata* may have therapeutic benefits in managing the adverse effects of keratocanthoma development (skin cancer) using a model of dba2 mice, (Oufquir *et al.*, 2024).

Moreover, Matrine, a quinolizidine alkaloid, has been isolated from plants in the Sophora genus, including Sophora flavescens (Leguminosae). It has a variety of pharmacological effects, including anti-cancer properties demonstrated in vitro. *In vivo* studies in mice have demonstrated that matrine significantly reduces the volume of tumors artificially induced with the Eca-109 cell line at a dose of 5 mg/kg after 15 days of treatment. The induction of apoptosis in ESCC cells by matrine is accompanied by an increase of reactive oxygen species and an inhibition of Bid-mediated mitochondrial function, (Ying Jie *et al.,* 2018).

4. MOLECULAR MECHANISMS UNDERPINNING THERAPEUTIC EFFECTS

NDDs affect approximately 50 million people worldwide, posing a significant challenge to modern medicine. Statistical projections indicate that the global aging population (60 years and older) will rise from 703 million (9%) in 2019 to 1.5 billion (16%) by 2050, suggesting a substantial increase in the prevalence of NDDs in the coming decades, (Gadhave *et al.,* 2024). Currently, therapeutic options for these conditions are extremely limited, and existing treatments show relatively low success rates. This urgent situation underscores the need for the clinical and scientific communities to develop novel and effective therapies. Existing therapies fail to slow or halt the progression of NDDs, primarily due to significant challenges such as the limited permeability of the BBB and numerous undesirable side effects. These obstacles contribute to low survival rates among patients, (Pooviah *et al.*, 2018). Recent research has highlighted the potential of nanoscale strategies for addressing CNS disorders, including NDDs, (Chhabra, Tosi, & Grabrucker, 2015). Emerging studies suggest that biomaterials offer remarkable selectivity and efficacy, enabling molecular detection, targeted drug delivery, therapeutic monitoring, and enhanced diagnostic capabilities for NDDs (138–140) (Figure 3).

Figure 3. Treatment for neurodegenerative diseases.

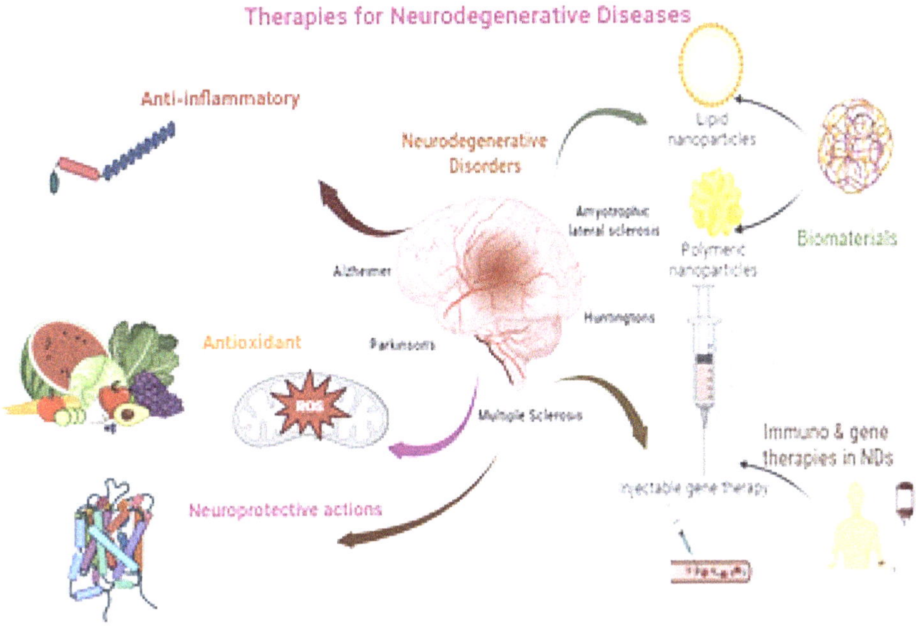

4.1. Gene Therapy

Gene therapy is emerging as a promising approach to treat NDDs due to its potential to correct genetic deficits and deliver active therapeutic proteins, (Gowing, Svendsen, & Svendsen, 2017). This strategy targets diseases such as Alzheimer's, Parkinson's, and Huntington's diseases, (Chen, Hu, & Ju, 2020). Methods include direct gene delivery using plasmids or viral vectors, as well as in vitro genetic modification followed by the transplantation of modified cells, (Deverman *et al.*, 2018). These approaches aim to restore lost cellular functions using efficient viral vectors, such as adeno-associated vectors (AAV) and lentiviral vectors (LV), (Piguet *et al.*, 2017).

Two main modalities of gene therapy are utilized: in vivo and ex vivo. In in vivo therapy, therapeutic genes are administered directly to the brain, often through stereotactic injections targeting specific regions to treat conditions like PD and HD, (Piguet *et al.*, 2017). In contrast, ex vivo therapy involves the modification of cells (typically hematopoietic stem cells) outside the body, followed by autologous transplantation. This technique allows for the sustained production of active therapeutic proteins within the CNS, (Piguet *et al.*, 2017).

4.2. Immunotherapy

Current therapeutic approaches for NDDs remain largely symptomatic, failing to address the underlying causes of these diseases. In this regard, immunotherapy has emerged as a promising strategy, targeting protein aggregates and misfolded substances associated with NDDs, (Mortada *et al.*, 2021). For example, monoclonal antibodies targeting the aggregation and propagation of alpha-synuclein in PD show potential in slowing disease progression, (Whone, 2022). Aducanumab, a human monoclonal antibody, was recently approved by the FDA as a disease-modifying treatment for Alzheimer's disease, highlighting progress in this field, (Diniz, 2024). However, challenges persist, such as the limited permeability of the BBB and the side effects of antibody-based therapies, including high costs and the need for frequent administration, (Mortada *et al.*, 2021). Solutions like nanocarriers or surface modifications provide ways to overcome these limitations and improve the delivery of therapeutic compounds to the brain, (Sharma & Dang, 2023). Finally, while early clinical trials using monoclonal antibodies, such as prasinezumab (Phase II) and BIIB054, have shown encouraging results, further research is needed to optimize immunogen particle types, delivery methods, and mechanisms of action for immunotherapies, (Jankovic et al., 2018) (Hanif *et al.,* 2020).

4.3. Biomaterials for Neurodegenerative Disease Treatment

Due to the limitations of symptomatic treatments for NDDs, biomaterials are gaining increasing interest as advanced solutions to enhance drug delivery and explore the pathogenesis of these disorders, (Bordoni *et al.,* 2020). These materials, defined by their biocompatibility, biodegradability, and bio-inert functionality, include nanoparticles, hydrogels, nanofibers, and nanoemulsions, and are being studied for their unique properties in managing NDDs, (Bordoni *et al.,* 2020).

Nano-biomatériaux, characterized by nanostructures ranging from 1 to 100 nm, presents a promising solution to overcome the BBB in the treatment of NDDs, (Mittal *et al.,* 2022). For example, cerium, manganese, or iron oxide nanoparticles have demonstrated their role as antioxidants and enzyme mimetics, helping reduce oxidative stress in NDDs, (Eleftheriadou *et al.,* 2020). Furthermore, metallic nanoparticles such as gold and silver exhibit antimicrobial and regenerative effects, while quantum dots have applications in imaging and diagnostics, (Kumar *et al.,* 2022). Recent examples include lipid nanocarriers, which are used to efficiently deliver therapeutic compounds. For instance, lipid nanoparticles conjugated with an anti-Fas ligand antibody have been successfully targeted to an ischemic brain region in mice, (Cacciatore *et al.,* 2016). These materials enable controlled drug release, promote treatment personalization, and cater to the needs of personalized medicine. However, significant challenges remain, such as the efficient crossing of the BBB, concerns regarding toxicity (immunotoxicity and cytotoxicity), and undesirable immune responses, (Bordoni *et al.,* 2020). Overcoming these obstacles is crucial to maximizing the potential of biomaterials in the treatment of NDDs.

4.4. Antioxidant and Anti-Inflammatory Pathways

NDDs are characterized by distinct causal factors and pathological features. A common hallmark among these disorders is oxidative stress (OS), which results from the excessive production of reactive oxygen species during disease progression, (Niedzielska *et al.,* 2016). Additionally, the pathological features of NDDs, such as elevated levels of protein aggregates, can trigger chronic inflammation through microglial activation.

Carotenoids (CTs), naturally occurring pigments, have demonstrated significant potential in mitigating brain disorders. Found abundantly in plants, microorganisms, and animals, more than 750 CTs have been identified in nature, (Wagner & Elmadfa, 2003). These pigments are responsible for the red, yellow, and orange hues in various organisms, with each color reflecting the presence of specific types of CTs, (Manochkumar *et al.,* 2021). Due to their unique structure, CTs exhibit various bioactive properties, particularly their anti-inflammatory and antioxidant effects, (Kabir *et al.*, 2022) (Rasmus & Kozlowska, 2023). β-carotene, for example, serves as an essential source of vitamin A and plays a vital role in maintaining human health, (Miller, Coronel, & Amengual, 2020). These protective attributes have established a strong link between CT levels in the human body and the prevention or treatment of various diseases, including NDDs, (Gandla *et al.,* 2023). Their benefits in addressing OS and neuroinflammation make CTs a promising component in managing these conditions.

4.5. Neuroprotective Actions (Inhibition of β-Amyloid Aggregation, Dopaminergic Neuron Preservation)

Neuroprotection, by definition, refers to effects that promote the preservation, recovery, or regeneration of the nervous system, its cells, structure, and function, (Olney, 1969). It is believed that a variety of neurochemical modulators influence nervous system damage. In the case of epilepsy, excessive glutamate-mediated neurotransmission, dysfunction of voltage-sensitive sodium and calcium channels, impaired GABA-mediated inhibition, and disturbances in acid-base balance can initiate a cascade of events leading to neuronal damage and cell death, (Barker-Haliski & White, 2015). Glutamate-induced retinal degeneration in neonatal mice has been observed, demonstrating the potential for excitotoxicity-induced damage to neurons, (Olney, 1969). Both acute and chronic damage to the nervous system in response to an insult can led to immediate or delayed neuronal death, apoptotic cell death, neuronal degeneration, injury, and gliosis. The neuropathogenesis of mitochondrial diseases also underscores the critical role of excitotoxicity and its long-term effects on neuronal survival, (Brown & Squier, 1996). After injury, cell death in the CNS can occur through apoptosis, necrosis, or a combination of both. Neurotoxic mechanisms involving NO-related species and mitochondrial dysfunction further complicate neuronal damage, (Martin, 2010). Generally, excitotoxic injury mediated by NMDA and non-NMDA receptors results in neurodegeneration along a continuum of apoptosis and necrosis, (Martin *et al.*, 1998). The role of excitotoxicity in ALS has been examined, highlighting its contribution to the progression of the disease, (Van Den Bosch *et al.*, 2006). The extent of neuronal injury depends on factors such as the maturity of the brain and the site of the lesion. There is evidence supporting the idea that neuroprotection could be a realistic and achievable goal using existing drugs, which are currently limited to specific indications. Early intervention with these drugs might significantly reduce the need for developing new medications, which would require extensive evaluation in animal studies and human clinical trials. The efficacy and cellular actions of various anticonvulsant and antiepileptic drugs have been studied, showing their potential in modulating excitotoxic damage, (Scheffer *et al.*, 1995) (White, 1999). Furthermore, new drugs must be shown to be safe, physiologically compatible with humans, and free of idiosyncratic adverse effects.

5. CLINICAL AND PRECLINICAL APPLICATIONS

Plant-based compounds belonging to the most varied chemical families have already shown a high level of anti-inflammatory activity, (Fialho *et al.*, 2018). These include alkaloids, terpenes, (Bi *et al.*, 2016) (Mondal *et al.*, 2019) (Hussein & El-Anssary, 2019) (Singh & Sharma, 2015), and phenolic compounds such tannins, lignanes, coumarines, saponines, and most notably flavonoids, (Hussein & El-Anssary, 2019) (Singh & Sharma, 2015) (Gorlenko *et al.*, 2020) (Muthukrishnan & Subramaniyan, 2012) (Mitra, Saha, & Roy, 2010) (Rex, Muthukumar, & Selvakumar, 2018).

Flavonoids have significant anti-inflammatory properties, mainly by modulating the arachidonic acid pathway and inhibiting enzymes such as cyclooxygenase, lipoxygenase, and NADH oxidase. For example, luteolin, with a catecholic oxygenation pattern on the B ring and hydroxylation at the 5-position of the A ring, shows strong inhibition of NO and TNF-α, (Aravindaram & Yang, 2010). Quercetin, present in high concentrations in plants such as Allium cepa and Camellia sinensis, significantly reduces the volume of oedema, with an efficacy comparable to phenylbutazone, (Azab, Nassar, & Azab, 2016). However, glycosylation of flavonoids may attenuate their anti-inflammatory activity, although some glycosides retain an inhibitory effect depending on their degree of glycosylation, (Szeja, Grynkiewicz, & Rusin, 2017). Quercetin has been the subject of numerous clinical studies. For example, it decreases CRP, GM-CSF, and various interleukins (IL-1β, IL-6, IL-8) in several trials, (Kondrad *et al.*, 2011).

However, its efficacy depends on the conditions. Although studies show significant reductions in TNF-α in patients with rheumatoid arthritis (Javadi *et al.*, 2017), others have not observed an impact in healthy subjects, (Abbey & Rankin, 2011). Furthermore, gallic acid (15 mg/day) reduced CRP by 39% in diabetic patients (Ferk *et al.*, 2018), while ferulic acid attenuated TNF-α by 13% and CRP by 32% in hyper lipidemic patients, (Bumrungpert *et al.*, 2018). Other bioactive compounds, such as tannins and terpenes, also show anti-inflammatory properties. Tannins, by forming complexes with metal ions or proteins, contribute to the treatment of inflammatory diseases, (Xie, Roto, & Bolling, 2012). Terpenes, such as triterpenes present in plants such as *Thymus serpyllum* and *Rosmarinus officinalis*, reduce oedema in a manner comparable to hydrocortisone, (Azab, Nassar, & Zab, 2016). In addition, plant antioxidants, by reducing ROS and lipid peroxidation, prevent cellular damage associated with chronic inflammatory pathologies such as arthritis and cancer, (Ali *et al.*, 2008). Finally, inflammatory processes are closely linked to oxidative stress, which unbalances antioxidant defenses and promotes the formation of free radicals. The modulation of these radicals by bioactive compounds could explain the traditional use of plants in the treatment of various inflammatory and oxidative diseases, (Halliwell, 2009).

One of the main factors contributing to neuronal damage in neurological disorders is inflammation. Neurons in the brain deteriorate as a result of persistent inflammation. Because they produce pro-inflammatory mediators that cause neurodegeneration, resident brain cells called microglia are essential in causing and sustaining neuroinflammation. Prostaglandins, leukotrienes, free radicals, inflammatory cytokines including IL-1b, IL-6, and tumor necrosis factor alpha are some examples of these mediators, (Gomez-Nicola *et al.*, 2013). All these steps of the inflammatory response pathway are targeted and inhibited by phytochemicals for neuroprotection. All of these molecules in the inflammatory response pathway are targeted and inhibited by phytochemicals for neuroprotection.

Flavonoids play a vital role in maintaining CNS homeostasis. They act as anxiolytics and anticonvulsants, modulating neuronal oxidative metabolism and neurotransmitters while targeting signaling cascades such as MAPK and P13/Akt to reduce oxidative damage and prevent neuronal death. Their unique functional groups make them potent inhibitors of neurodegenerative enzymes, scavenging ROS, (Salińska, Danysz, &

Łazarewicz, 2005) (Kumar & Khanum, 2012). Alkaloids, although neurotoxic in some cases, also have therapeutic benefits, serving as antidepressants and powerful analgesics by stimulating nicotinic receptors and inhibiting cholinesterase activity, (Kumar & Khanum, 2012) (Dey & Mukherjee, 2018).

Terpenes and terpenoids enhance nervous system function by binding to GABA(B) receptors and exhibit anti-inflammatory, antioxidant, and anti-apoptotic properties, promoting neuronal survival against degenerative mechanisms, (Kumar & Khanum, 2012). Polysaccharides, traditionally recognized for structural roles, are now known to provide neuroprotection through the Nrf2/HO-1 pathway, NFkB interference, and activation of neurotrophic pathways, shielding neurons from neurodegenerative processes, (Gao *et al.*, 2018). Fatty acids, particularly omega-3 and omega-6, are critical for neuronal membrane fluidity, restoring aging membranes and maintaining synaptic plasticity, thus supporting neuronal homeostasis, (Lo Van *et al.*, 2019) (Nobre *et al.*, 2016).

Specific phytochemicals like apigenin, a flavone found in various fruits and vegetables, protect against kainite-induced excitotoxicity and Ab toxicity through antioxidant mechanisms, reducing neuronal hyperexcitability and improving spatial memory, (Zhao *et al.*, 2013) (Zhao *et al.*, 2011). Quercetin, a flavonol, mitigates Ab-induced cytotoxicity, enhances antioxidant enzyme activity, and reduces tau and ROS levels, demonstrating efficacy in Alzheimer's, Parkinson's, and Huntington's diseases models, (Bao *et al.*, 2017) (Ansari *et al.*, 2009). Epigallocatechin gallate (EGCG), a green tea flavanol, lowers Ab levels, protects dopaminergic neurons, and stabilizes signaling pathways, showing neuroprotective effects in various neurodegenerative disease models, (Xu *et al.*, 2006) (Rezai-Zadeh *et al.*, 2008) (Koh *et al.*, 2004).

Huperzine A, a sesquiterpene alkaloid, inhibits acetylcholinesterase (AChE), reduces glutamate excitotoxicity, and exhibits anti-inflammatory effects. It is currently in phase III clinical trials for ALS and MS, (Xing *et al.*, 2014) (Hemendinger *et al.*, 2008). Galantamine, derived from Galanthus species, is FDA-approved for AD treatment, enhancing cholinergic neurotransmission, (Aarsland, Hutchinson, & Larsen, 2003) (Loy & Schneider, 2006). Rivastigmine, a derivative of physostigmine, is used to improve memory and cognition in PD, ALS, and MS, (Shaygannejad *et al.*, 2008) (Birks & Evans, 2015).

Finally, ginkgolides, terpenoids from Ginkgo biloba, increase cholinergic transmission, protect against neurotoxic damage, and exhibit anti-inflammatory and antioxidant properties in PD and AD models, (Kavitha *et al.*, 2020). These advancements underscore the potential of natural compounds in neuroprotection, although further research is needed to optimize their therapeutic applications.

However, despite their promising neuroprotective and anti-inflammatory activities against neurodegenerative and inflammatory diseases in the preclinical setting, translation of promising preclinical neuroprotective and anti-inflammatory research to clinical application has proven to be challenging as there is a contradiction in the results of human clinical trials on these pathologies. Natural products and their isolated natural compounds present some challenges and limitations that could affect their clinical efficacy, namely their low bioavailability and limited water solubility, physicochemical instability, rapid metabolism. Several natural compounds, for example tea catechins (Cascella *et al.,* 2017) (Hodgson, Randell, & Jeukendrup, 2013), resveratrol (Renaud & Martinoli, 2019), and curcumin, (Hu *et al.,* 2015) (Begum *et al.,* 2008) (Rakotoarisoa & Angelova, 2019), exhibit low bioavailability and limited stability because these natural compounds are susceptible to degradation or transformation into inactive derivatives, (Shoji & Nakashima, 2004) (Coimbra *et al.,* 2011).

Given the complexity of phenolic compounds absorption, various innovative techniques have been developed to limit interactions that limit their efficacy, while promoting their chemical protection and targeted delivery, (Souza, Gurak, & Marczak, 2017) (de Souza *et al.,* 2020) (López de Dicastillo *et al.*, 2019) (Mansour, Salah, & Xu, 2020) (Rashidinejad *et al.,* 2016) (Luo *et al.*, 2011). Nanoencapsulation approaches using customized wall materials appear to be the most promising for protecting polyphenols from metabolic degradation and targeting specific tissues.

6. PHYTOCHEMICAL SOURCES OF SECONDARY METABOLITES

Plant-derived compounds have emerged as promising neuroprotective agents due to their diverse mechanisms of action and therapeutic potential. Numerous studies have demonstrated their effectiveness in protecting against neurodegenerative disorders such as AD, PD, and HD, (Elufioye, Berida, & Habtemariam, 2017). These compounds exhibit antioxidant, anti-inflammatory, anti-aggregative, anti-cholinesterase, and anti-apoptotic properties, which contribute to preserving neuronal structure and function, (Rabie *et al.*, 2023). With their varied mechanisms and ability to mitigate neurodegenerative processes, they stand out as promising candidates for the development of novel neuroprotective therapies, (Fridzadeh *et al.,* 2022).

6.1. Phyto-Cannabinoids

Cannabis has drawn significant attention for its potential therapeutic role in NDDs owing to its diverse bioactive compounds, including cannabinoids, terpenes, and flavonoids, (Jin *et al.*, 2020). Among these, delta-9-tetrahydrocannabinol (THC) and cannabidiol (CBD) are the most studied, demonstrating promising pharmacological effects in countering the mechanisms underlying neurodegeneration, (Al-Khazaleh *et al.*, 2024) (Figure 4). Recent evidence highlights not only their individual benefits but also the synergistic interactions between cannabis constituents, amplifying its overall therapeutic potential. Cannabinoids exhibit anti-inflammatory, antioxidant, and neuroprotective properties that help mitigate the progressive neuronal damage characteristic of disorders such as AD, PD, and MS. Specifically, cannabinoids regulate microglial activation, a pivotal factor in neuroinflammation, and protect neurons by reducing ROS, a major driver of oxidative stress. Additionally, both THC and CBD modulate critical molecular pathways, including MAPK and NF-κB, which are involved in cellular survival and inflammatory responses, (Al-Khazaleh *et al.*, 2024).

Several specific mechanisms have been proposed to explain the neuroprotective effects of cannabis-derived secondary metabolites. For instance, cannabinoids may function as dopamine regulators in PD, potentially alleviating motor symptoms, (Al Mansouri *et al.*, 2014). In Alzheimer's disease, they inhibit the aggregation of β-amyloid peptides, a key pathological hallmark, (Gertsch *et al.*, 2008). Furthermore, cannabinoids exert anti-inflammatory, antineuroinflammatory, and antioxidant effects, all of which address known drivers of neurodegenerative processes, (Al-Khazaleh *et al.*, 2024).

Terpenes, the aromatic components of cannabis, enhance these effects by increasing the bioavailability and activity of cannabinoids. Additionally, they display intrinsic therapeutic properties, such as anti-inflammatory and sedative effects, which may help manage symptoms like pain and sleep disorders commonly associated with neurodegeneration, (Abd Rashed, Abd Rahman, & Rathi, 2021). Similarly, flavonoids contribute by neutralizing oxidative stress and reducing inflammation, further preserving neuronal integrity, (Erridge *et al.*, 2020).

Treatment optimization, based on exploiting the full spectrum of cannabis compounds, could improve therapeutic outcomes while reducing side effects. The figure summarizes some of the mechanisms involved in the therapeutic effects of cannabis on NDDs (Figure 4).

Figure 4. Mechanisms involved in the therapeutic effects of cannabis on neurodegenerative diseases

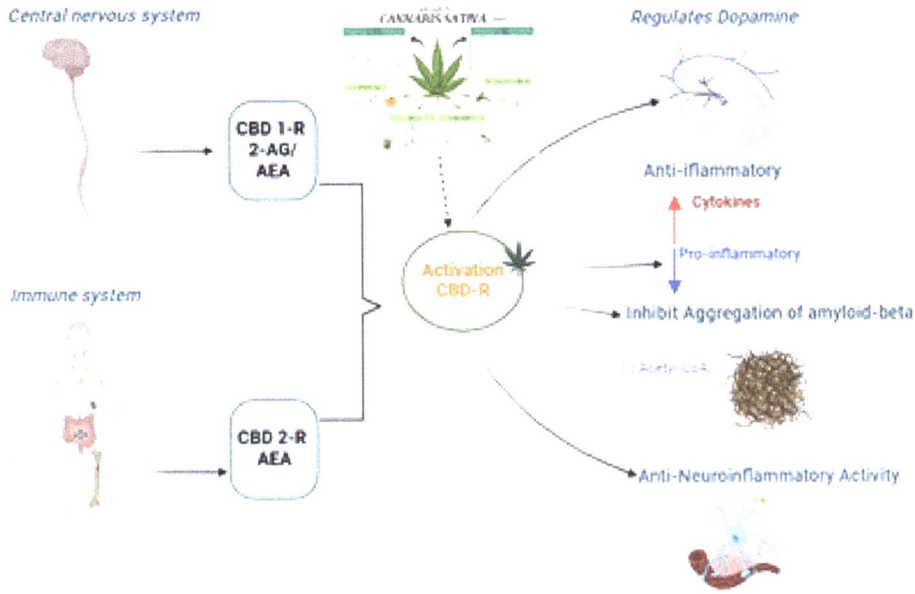

6.2. Carotenoids

Carotenoids (TC) are part of the tetraterpenoid family, (Kopsell & Kopsell, 2006). They are divided into two main categories: hydrocarbon TC and xanthophylls (Armstrong & Hearst, 1996), derived from aquatic plants or animals. Hydrocarbon TC, which are naturally non-polar, include phytofluene, phytoene, lycopene, along with α-, β-, and γ-carotene. These compounds are responsible for the red, yellow, and orange pigmentation observed in various animals and plants, with each color typically corresponding to specific TC types, (Irwandi Jaswari, 2011). TC exhibit diverse bioactive properties due to their distinctive molecular structure. Often referred to as "molecular rivets," they have a length similar to the phospholipid bilayer, enhancing membrane rigidity, stability, and overall organismal integrity, (Zia-Ul-Haq, 2021). Most TC are lipophilic, which enables them to cross the BBB, (Guest & Grant, 2016). These metabolites appear to be involved in various molecular mechanisms with therapeutic potential. Carotenoids have demonstrated their ability to slow the onset of NDDs through multiple mechanisms that may act simultaneously, (Miller, Coronel, & Amengual, 2020). In addition to their role in the red, yellow, and orange pigmentation of numerous plants and animals, CT are notable for their potent bioactive properties, including anti-inflammatory and antioxidant effects, (Miller, Coronel, & Amengual, 2020). These protective attributes explain the strong association between CT levels in the human body and the prevention or treatment of various diseases, including NDDs. This axis explores the relationship between oxidative stress, neuroinflammation, and NDDs, while highlighting the antioxidant and anti-inflammatory properties of CT in their therapeutic management, (Guest & Grant, 2016) (Table 1).

Table 1. Summary of in vitro and in vivo studies on the effects of carotenoids on neurodegenerative diseases

Carotenoids	*Source*	*Properties*	*NDDs*	*References*
Lutein	Vegetal Animal	Antioxidant and anti-neuroinflammatory	AD and PD	(Guest & Grant, 2016); (Miller *et al.*, 1996)
Zeaxanthin	Vegetal	Antioxidant and anti-neuroinflammatory	AD	(Prakash & Kumar, 2014); (Kesse-Guyot *et al.*, 2014)
β-Carotene	Vegetal	Antioxidant	PD, AD and ALS	(Guest & Grant, 2016)
α-Carotene	Vegetal Animal	Antioxidant	AD and ALS	(Kim *et al.*, 2016); (Isonaka *et al.*, 2011)
Astaxanthin	Vegetal Animal Aquatic	Antioxidant and anti-neuroinflammatory	AD and PD	(Miller *et al.*, 1996); (Guest & Grant, 2016)

6.3. Polyphenols

Polyphenols are plant-derived chemical compounds characterized by multiple phenolic groups in their structure, and are abundantly found in fruits and vegetables, (Li *et al.*, 2009). These compounds have shown therapeutic potential for various diseases, including NDDs, cardiovascular diseases, and cancer. Their neuroprotective effect is primarily attributed to their ability to cross the blood-brain barrier, (Potì *et al.*, 2019a). One of the most studied properties of polyphenols is their antioxidant activity, which can be direct (by eliminating free radicals) and/or indirect (by activating endogenous antioxidant pathways). This effect is likely responsible for the neuroprotective efficacy observed for certain flavonoids, (Potì *et al.*, 2019a).

Recent research suggests that polyphenols, particularly flavonoids, influence key processes associated with the onset of NDDs. These effects include the reduction of neuropathological protein accumulation and the improvement of synaptic plasticity, (Freyssin *et al.*, 2018). Anti-inflammatory mechanisms have also been observed in glial and neuronal cells exposed to high concentrations of flavonoids. Additionally, some clinical studies have shown that flavonoids can reduce plasma levels of several inflammatory markers. Anthocyanins inhibit the activation of nuclear factor κB in monocytes and reduce plasma concentrations of pro-inflammatory mediators, (Karlsen *et al.,* 2007).

Furthermore, polyphenols increase the levels of neurotrophic factors and interact directly with their membrane receptors, thereby modulating and activating signaling cascades that promote neuronal plasticity, survival, proliferation, and growth of nerve cells. These effects contribute to improvements in memory, learning, and cognition, (Schmatz *et al.,* 2009). Finally, polyphenols pose no significant risk of severe side effects when consumed, (Potì *et al.,* 2019b).

7. FUTURE PERSPECTIVES AND CHALLENGES

Neurodegenerative and inflammatory diseases remain significant global health challenges due to their complex pathophysiology and the lack of curative treatments, driving interest in neuroprotection and the therapeutic potential of natural compounds. Despite promising neuroprotective effects observed in preclinical studies, clinical translation remains difficult, as evidenced by inconsistent outcomes in trials for AD and PD, attributed to methodological heterogeneity and limited understanding of pharmacological mechanisms, (Hendrickz *et al.,* 2020).

Additionally, natural compounds such as resveratrol and curcumin face challenges like low bioavailability, rapid metabolic transformation, and limited blood-brain barrier penetration, which hinder their therapeutic efficacy, (Rahman *et al.,* 2021) (Xu *et al.,* 2015). Nanotechnology offers potential solutions through advanced delivery systems, such as polymeric nanoparticles and liposomes, which improve the stability and solubility of compounds, as demonstrated in studies using curcumin and epigallocatechin gallate for neurodegenerative disorders, (Sun *et al.,* 2012) (Riccardi *et al.,* 2021). Secondary metabolites also present opportunities for developing combination therapies and personalized medicine approaches, enhancing treatment efficacy by targeting complementary pathways and tailoring therapies to genetic profiles, (Gupta *et al.,* 2020) (Aware *et al.*, 2022) (Muscolo *et al.*, 2024). However, clinical development is impeded by regulatory constraints, such as the need for standardization of natural extracts, which vary by source and extraction method, and the requirement for robust safety and efficacy data to classify these compounds as drugs rather than dietary supplements, (Kunle, Egharevba, & Ahmadu, 2012) (Brown, 2017).

8. CONCLUSION

Secondary metabolites represent a treasure trove of bioactive compounds with remarkable therapeutic potential. Their diverse biological activities, including antioxidant, anti-inflammatory, antimicrobial, and neuroprotective properties, have been widely recognized in the treatment of various diseases, particularly neurodegenerative and inflammatory disorders. These compounds, derived from plants, fungi, and microorganisms, have the potential to address some of the critical gaps in current therapeutic approaches, offering natural, cost-effective, and efficient alternatives to synthetic drugs. However, the journey from identifying bioactive metabolites to their clinical application is fraught with challenges. Issues such as limited bioavailability, instability, and potential toxicity have often hindered their broader adoption in modern medicine. Furthermore, the complexity of their mechanisms of action requires deeper exploration to optimize their therapeutic effects while minimizing adverse outcomes. These challenges underscore the need for innovative solutions and advanced technologies to bridge the gap between natural product chemistry and clinical practice.

To fully harness the potential of secondary metabolites, a multidisciplinary approach is essential. Collaborative efforts between pharmacologists, chemists, biotechnologists, and clinicians can enable comprehensive research into their pharmacokinetics, safety profiles, and efficacy. Advanced tools such as high-throughput screening, bioinformatics, and nanotechnology can further enhance the development and delivery of secondary metabolite-based therapies. Additionally, integrating traditional knowledge of medicinal plants with modern scientific techniques can unlock new opportunities for drug discovery.

Moreover, addressing global health challenges with sustainable and accessible treatment options demands strategic partnerships between academia, industry, and healthcare systems. Such collaboration will not only accelerate the development of secondary metabolite-based therapeutics but also ensure equitable access to these innovations. In conclusion, secondary metabolites hold immense promise as a cornerstone for future therapeutic strategies. By fostering multidisciplinary research and leveraging cutting-edge technologies, we can unlock their full potential, transforming them into viable solutions for complex and challenging diseases. This approach will not only advance medical science but also contribute to a more sustainable and integrative healthcare system.

REFERENCES

Aarsland, D., Hutchinson, M., & Larsen, J. P. (2003). Cognitive, psychiatric, and motor response to galantamine in Parkinson's disease with dementia. *International Journal of Geriatric Psychiatry, 18*(10), 937–941. DOI: 10.1002/gps.949 PMID: 14533126

Abbey, E. L., & Rankin, J. W. (2011). Effect of quercetin supplementation on repeated-sprint performance, xanthine oxidase activity, and inflammation. *International Journal of Sport Nutrition and Exercise Metabolism, 21*(2), 91–96. DOI: 10.1123/ijsnem.21.2.91 PMID: 21558570

Abd Rashed, A., Abd Rahman, A. Z., & Rathi, D. N. G. (2021). Essential oils as a potential neuroprotective remedy for age-related neurodegenerative diseases: A review. *Molecules (Basel, Switzerland), 26*(4), 1107. DOI: 10.3390/molecules26041107 PMID: 33669787

Abeliovich, A., & Gitler, A. D. (2016). Defects in trafficking bridge Parkinson's disease pathology and genetics. *Nature, 539*(7628), 207–216. DOI: 10.1038/nature20414 PMID: 27830778

Aimrane, A., Sabir, E. S., Laadraoui, J., El-Mansoury, B., Smimih, K., Khanouchi, M., & Ibrahimi, A. (2023). An overview of the genetics of Parkinson's disease. In *Experimental and Clinical Evidence of the Neuropathology of Parkinson's Disease* (pp. 164–181). Springer., DOI: 10.4018/978-1-6684-5156-4.ch010

Al-Khayri, J. M., Sahana, G. R., Nagella, P., Joseph, B. V., Alessa, F. M., & Al-Mssallem, M. Q. (2022). Flavonoids as potential anti-inflammatory molecules: A review. *Molecules (Basel, Switzerland), 27*(9), 2901. DOI: 10.3390/molecules27092901 PMID: 35566252

Al-Khazaleh, A. K., Zhou, X., Bhuyan, D. J., Münch, G. W., Al-Dalabeeh, E. A., Jaye, K., & Chang, D. (2024). The neurotherapeutic arsenal in *Cannabis sativa*: Insights into anti-neuroinflammatory and neuroprotective activity and potential entourage effects. *Molecules (Basel, Switzerland), 29*(2), 410. DOI: 10.3390/molecules29020410 PMID: 38257323

Al Mansouri, S., Ojha, S., Al Maamari, E., Al Ameri, M., Nurulain, S. M., & Bahi, A. (2014). The cannabinoid receptor 2 agonist, β-caryophyllene, reduced voluntary alcohol intake and attenuated ethanol-induced place preference and sensitivity in mice. *Pharmacology, Biochemistry, and Behavior, 124*, 260–268. DOI: 10.1016/j.pbb.2014.06.025 PMID: 24999220

Alamgir, A. N. M. (2017). Drugs: Their natural, synthetic, and biosynthetic sources. In *Therapeutic use of medicinal plants and their extracts: Volume 1* (pp. 105–123). Springer. DOI: 10.1007/978-3-319-63862-1_4

Alboni, S., Cervia, D., Sugama, S., & Conti, B. (2010). Interleukin 18 in the CNS. *Journal of Neuroinflammation*, *7*(1), 9. DOI: 10.1186/1742-2094-7-9 PMID: 20113500

Alfei, S., & Zuccari, G. (2025). Ellagic acid (EA): A green multi-target weapon reducing oxidative stress and inflammation thus preventing and ameliorating Alzheimer disease (AD) condition. *International Journal of Molecular Sciences*, *26*, 844. DOI: 10.3390/ijms26020844 PMID: 39859559

Ali, S. S., Kasoju, N., Luthra, A., Singh, A., Sharanabasava, H., Sahu, A., & Bora, U. (2008). Indian medicinal herbs as sources of antioxidants. *Food Research International*, *41*(1), 1–15. DOI: 10.1016/j.foodres.2007.10.001

Alminger, M., Aura, A.-M., Bohn, T., Dufour, C., El, S. N., Gomes, A., Karakaya, S., Martínez-Cuesta, M. C., McDougall, G. J., Requena, T., & Santos, C. N. (2014). In vitro models for studying secondary plant metabolite digestion and bioaccessibility. *Comprehensive Reviews in Food Science and Food Safety*, *13*(4), 413–436. DOI: 10.1111/1541-4337.12081 PMID: 33412708

Andleeb, F., Elsadek, M. F., Asif, M., Al-Numair, K. S., Chaudhry, S. R., Saleem, M., & Yehya, A. H. S. (2024). Down-regulation of NF-κB signalling by methanolic extract of *Viola odorata* (L.) attenuated in vivo inflammatory and angiogenic responses. *Inflammopharmacology*, *32*(5), 3521–3535. DOI: 10.1007/s10787-024-01505-z PMID: 39030451

Ansari, M. A., Abdul, H. M., Joshi, G., Opii, W. O., & Butterfield, D. A. (2009). Protective effect of quercetin in primary neurons against Aβ (1–42): Relevance to Alzheimer's disease. *The Journal of Nutritional Biochemistry*, *20*(4), 269–275. DOI: 10.1016/j.jnutbio.2008.03.002 PMID: 18602817

Aravindaram, K., & Yang, N. S. (2010). Anti-inflammatory plant natural products for cancer therapy. *Planta Medica*, *76*(11), 1103–1117. DOI: 10.1055/s-0030-1249859 PMID: 20432202

Armstrong, G. A., & Hearst, J. E. (1996). Genetics and molecular biology of carotenoid pigment biosynthesis. *The FASEB Journal*, *10*(2), 228–237. DOI: 10.1096/fasebj.10.2.8641556 PMID: 8641556

Asahi, K., Ichimori, K., Nakazawa, H., Izuhara, Y., Inagi, R., Watanabe, T., Miyata, T., & Kurokawa, K. (2000). Nitric oxide inhibits the formation of advanced glycation end products. *Kidney International, 58*(4), 1780–1787. DOI: 10.1111/j.1523-1755.2000.00340.x PMID: 11012913

Aware, C. B., Patil, D. N., Suryawanshi, S. S., Mali, P. R., Rane, M. R., Gurav, R. G., et al. (2022). Natural bioactive products as promising therapeutics: A review of natural product-based drug development. *South African Journal of Botany, 151*, 512-528. DOI: 10.1016/j.sajb.2022.06.011

Azab, A., Nassar, A., & Azab, A. N. (2016). Anti-inflammatory activity of natural products. *Molecules (Basel, Switzerland), 21*(10), 1321. DOI: 10.3390/molecules21101321 PMID: 27706084

Azeez, T. B., & Lunghar, J. (2021). Antiinflammatory effects of turmeric (*Curcuma longa*) and ginger (*Zingiber officinale*). In *Inflammation and Natural Products* (pp. 83–102).

Azizan, M. S., Zamani, A. I., Stahmann, K. P., & Ng, C. L. (2016). Fungal metabolites and their industrial importance: A brief review. *Malaysian Journal of Biochemistry and Molecular Biology, 19*, 15–23.

Baecher-Allan, C., Kaskow, B. J., & Weiner, H. L. (2018). Multiple sclerosis: Mechanisms and immunotherapy. *Neuron, 97*(4), 742–768. DOI: 10.1016/j.neuron.2018.01.021 PMID: 29470968

Bafor, E. E. (2017). Editorial: Potentials for use of medicinal plants in female reproductive disorders – The way forward. *African Journal of Reproductive Health, 21*(4), 9–16. DOI: 10.29063/ajrh2017/v21i4.1 PMID: 29624946

Balkrishna, A., Rana, M., Mishra, S., Rajput, S. K., & Dhanasekaran, M. (2024). Arctigenin: Harnessing nature's power as an anti-inflammatory agent. *Current Research in Complementary & Alternative Medicine, 8*(255), 2577–2201. DOI: 10.54085/crcam.2024.8.255

Bao, D., Wang, J., Pang, X., & Liu, H. (2017). Protective effect of quercetin against oxidative stress-induced cytotoxicity in rat pheochromocytoma (PC-12) cells. *Molecules (Basel, Switzerland), 22*(7), 1122. DOI: 10.3390/molecules22071122 PMID: 28684704

Barker-Haliski, M., & White, H. S. (2015). Glutamatergic mechanisms associated with seizures and epilepsy. *Cold Spring Harbor Perspectives in Medicine, 5*(8), a022863. DOI: 10.1101/cshperspect.a022863 PMID: 26101204

Bartmańska, A., Tronina, T., Popłoński, J., Milczarek, M., Filip-Psurska, B., & Wietrzyk, J. (2018). Highly cancer selective antiproliferative activity of natural prenylated flavonoids. *Molecules (Basel, Switzerland)*, *23*(11), 2922. DOI: 10.3390/molecules23112922 PMID: 30423918

Begum, A. N., Jones, M. R., Lim, G. P., Morihara, T., Kim, P., Heath, D. D., & Galasko, D. (2008). Curcumin structure-function, bioavailability, and efficacy in models of neuroinflammation and Alzheimer's disease. *The Journal of Pharmacology and Experimental Therapeutics*, *326*(1), 196–208. DOI: 10.1124/jpet.108.137455 PMID: 18417733

Bermudez-Torres, K., Ortega-Castro, J., Quiñones-Maldonado, M., Acevedo-Rivera, D., Torres-Rivera, D., & Rivera-Echevarría, M.. (2013). The industrial applications of secondary metabolites: A review. *Journal of Industrial Biotechnology*, *8*(2), 75–86.

Bhambhani, S., Kondhare, K. R., & Giri, A. P. (2021). Diversity in chemical structures and biological properties of plant alkaloids. *Molecules (Basel, Switzerland)*, *26*(11), 3374. DOI: 10.3390/molecules26113374 PMID: 34204857

Bi, W., Bi, Y., Gao, X., Yan, X., Zhang, Y., Xue, P., Bammert, C. E., Legalley, T. D., Michael Gibson, K., Bi, L., & Wang, J.-X. (2016). Anti-inflammatory, analgesic and antioxidant activities of novel kyotorphin-nitroxide hybrid molecules. *Bioorganic & Medicinal Chemistry Letters*, *26*(8), 2005–2013. DOI: 10.1016/j.bmcl.2016.02.086 PMID: 26961795

Bıçakcıoğlu, M., Doğukan, M., Duran, M., Doğan, Z., & Türk, B. A. (2023). The effect of quercetin, a flavonoid, on lung injury caused by sepsis. *Journal of Surgery & Medicine*, *7*(9), 618–622. Advance online publication. DOI: 10.28982/josam.7926

Bills, G. F., & Gloer, J. B. (2016). Biologically active secondary metabolites from the fungi. In Heitman, J., Howlett, B. J., & Stukenbrock, E. H. (Eds.), *Microbiology Spectrum, 4(6), 4.6.01.*, DOI: 10.1128/microbiolspec.FUNK-0009-2016

Birks, J. S., & Evans, J. G. (2015). Rivastigmine for Alzheimer's disease. *Cochrane Database of Systematic Reviews, 2015*(4). DOI: 10.1002/14651858.CD001191.pub3

Bordoni, M., Scarian, E., Rey, F., Gagliardi, S., Carelli, S., Pansarasa, O., et al. (2020). Biomaterials in neurodegenerative disorders: A promising therapeutic approach. *International Journal of Molecular Sciences, 21*(9), 3243. DOI: 10.3390/ijms21093243

Bourgaud, F., Gravot, A., Milesi, S., & Gontier, E. (2001). Production of plant secondary metabolites: A historical perspective. *Plant Science*, *161*(5), 839–851. DOI: 10.1016/S0168-9452(01)00490-3

Boza-Serrano, A., Reyes, J. F., Rey, N. L., Leffler, H., Bousset, L., Nilsson, U., & Deierborg, T. (2014). The role of Galectin-3 in α-synuclein-induced microglial activation. *Acta Neuropathologica Communications*, *2*(1), 156. DOI: 10.1186/s40478-014-0156-9 PMID: 25387690

Brown, A. C. (2017). An overview of herb and dietary supplement efficacy, safety, and government regulations in the United States with suggested improvements. Part 1 of 5 series. *Food and Chemical Toxicology, 107*, 449-471. DOI: 10.1016/j.fct.2017.06.003

Brown, G. K., & Squier, M. V. (1996). Neuropathology and pathogenesis of mitochondrial diseases. *Journal of Inherited Metabolic Disease*, *19*(4), 553–572. DOI: 10.1007/BF01799116 PMID: 8884579

Bulea, M., Khan, F., & Niaz, D. (2015). Flavonoids (flavones, flavonols, flavanones, flavanonols, flavanols or flavan-3-ols, isoflavones, anthocyanins, chalcones/coumestans). In *Recent advances in natural products analysis* (pp. 42–56).

Bumrungpert, A., Lilitchan, S., Tuntipopipat, S., Tirawanchai, N., & Komindr, S. (2018). Ferulic acid supplementation improves lipid profiles, oxidative stress, and inflammatory status in hyperlipidemic subjects: A randomized, double-blind, placebo-controlled clinical trial. *Nutrients*, *10*(6), 713. DOI: 10.3390/nu10060713 PMID: 29865227

Butt, A. M., De La Rocha, I. C., & Rivera, A. (2019). Oligodendroglial cells in Alzheimer's disease. In *Neuroglia in neurodegenerative diseases* (pp. 325–333). Academic Press., DOI: 10.1007/978-981-13-9913-8_12

Cacciatore, I., Ciulla, M., Fornasari, E., Marinelli, L., & Di Stefano, A. (2016). Solid lipid nanoparticles as a drug delivery system for the treatment of neurodegenerative diseases. *Expert Opinion on Drug Delivery, 13*(8), 1121–1131. https://doi.org/DOI: 10.1080/17425247.2016.1160243

Calis, Z., Mogulkoc, R., & Baltaci, A. K. (2020). The roles of flavonols/flavonoids in neurodegeneration and neuroinflammation. *Mini-Reviews in Medicinal Chemistry*, *20*(15), 1475–1488. DOI: 10.2174/1389557519666190617150051 PMID: 31288717

Caradonna, E., Nemni, R., Bifone, A., Gandolfo, P., Costantino, L., Giordano, L., Mormone, E., Macula, A., Cuomo, M., Difruscolo, R., Vanoli, C., Vanoli, E., & Ferrara, F. (2024). The brain–gut axis, an important player in Alzheimer and Parkinson disease: A narrative review. *Journal of Clinical Medicine*, *13*(14), 4130. DOI: 10.3390/jcm13144130 PMID: 39064171

Cascella, M., Bimonte, S., Muzio, M. R., Schiavone, V., & Cuomo, A. (2017). The efficacy of epigallocatechin-3-gallate (green tea) in the treatment of Alzheimer's disease: An overview of pre-clinical studies and translational perspectives in clinical practice. *Infectious Agents and Cancer*, *12*(1), 36. DOI: 10.1186/s13027-017-0145-6 PMID: 28642806

Chaachouay, N., & Zidane, L. (2024). Plant-derived natural products: A source for drug discovery and development. *Drugs and Drug Candidates*, *3*(1), 184–207. DOI: 10.3390/ddc3010011

Chaves-Silva, S., Dos Santos, A. L., Chalfun-Júnior, A., Zhao, J., Peres, L. E., & Benedito, V. A. (2018). Understanding the genetic regulation of anthocyanin biosynthesis in plants – Tools for breeding purple varieties of fruits and vegetables. *Phytochemistry*, *153*, 11–27. DOI: 10.1016/j.phytochem.2018.05.013 PMID: 29803860

Chawla, R., Thakur, P., Chowdhry, A., Jaiswal, S., Sharma, A., Goel, R., Sharma, J., Priyadarshi, S. S., Kumar, V., Sharma, R. K., & Arora, R. (2013). Evidence-based herbal drug standardization approach in coping with challenges of holistic management of diabetes: A dreadful lifestyle disorder of 21st century. *Journal of Diabetes and Metabolic Disorders*, *12*(1), 35. DOI: 10.1186/2251-6581-12-35 PMID: 23822656

Chen, W., Hu, Y., & Ju, D. (2020). Gene therapy for neurodegenerative disorders: Advances, insights and prospects. *Acta Pharmaceutica Sinica B, 10*(8), 1347–1359. https://doi.org/DOI: 10.1016/j.apsb.2020.05.013

Chhabra, R., Tosi, G., & Grabrucker, A. M. (2015). Emerging use of nanotechnology in the treatment of neurological disorders. *Current Pharmaceutical Design, 21*(22), 3111–3130. https://doi.org/DOI: 10.2174/1381612821666151112165304

Choudhary, S., Zehra, A., Mukarram, M., Wani, K. I., Naeem, M., & Hakeem, K. R.. (2021). Potential uses of bioactive compounds of medicinal plants and their mode of action in several human diseases. In Aftab, T., & Hakeem, K. R. (Eds.), *Medicinal and aromatic plants* (pp. 143–158). Springer., DOI: 10.1007/978-3-030-58975-2_5

Coimbra, M., Isacchi, B., van Bloois, L., Torano, J. S., Ket, A., Wu, X., & Aderjan, R. (2011). Improving solubility and chemical stability of natural compounds for medicinal use by incorporation into liposomes. *International Journal of Pharmaceutics*, *416*(2), 433–442. DOI: 10.1016/j.ijpharm.2011.01.056 PMID: 21291975

Dajas, F., Juan Andres, C. A., Florencia, A., Carolina, E., & Felicia, R. M. (2013). Neuroprotective actions of flavones and flavonols: Mechanisms and relationship to flavonoid structural features. *Central Nervous System Agents in Medicinal Chemistry*, *13*(1), 30–35. DOI: 10.2174/1871524911313010005 PMID: 23092407 de Souza, V. B., Thomazini, M., Chaves, I. E., Ferro-Furtado, R., & Favaro-Trindade, C. S. (2020). Microencapsulation by complex coacervation as a tool to protect bioactive compounds and to reduce astringency and strong flavor of vegetable extracts. *Food Hydrocolloids*, *98*, 105244. DOI: 10.1016/j.foodhyd.2019.105244

Deverman, B. E., Ravina, B. M., Bankiewicz, K. S., Paul, S. M., & Sah, D. W. (2018). Gene therapy for neurological disorders: Progress and prospects. *Nature Reviews Drug Discovery, 17*(9), 641–659. https://doi.org/DOI: 10.1038/s41573-018-0002-9

Dey, A., & Mukherjee, A. (2018). Plant-derived alkaloids: A promising window for neuroprotective drug discovery. In *Discovery and development of neuroprotective agents from natural products* (pp. 237–320). Elsevier., DOI: 10.1016/B978-0-12-809593-5.00006-9

Diniz, B. S. (2024). Immunotherapy in Alzheimer's disease: From the bench to the bedside. *The American Journal of Geriatric Psychiatry, 32*(5), 584–585. https://doi.org/DOI: 10.1016/j.jagp.2024.01.009

Doyle, R., & Godson, C. (2022). Endogenous anti-inflammatory and pro-resolving lipid mediators in renal disease. In *Regenerative Nephrology* (pp. 55–67). Elsevier., https://www.sciencedirect.com/science/article/pii/B9780128233184000093 DOI: 10.1016/B978-0-12-823318-4.00009-3

Dugger, B. N., & Dickson, D. W. (2017). Pathology of neurodegenerative diseases. *Cold Spring Harbor Perspectives in Biology*, *9*(7), a028035. DOI: 10.1101/cshperspect.a028035 PMID: 28062563

Dutta, S., Nishad, K., Usha, T., Ramesh, N., & Middha, S. K. (2024). In-vitro scientific validation of anti-inflammatory activity of *Punica granatum* L. on leukemia monocytic cell line. *African Health Sciences*, *24*(4), 240–249. DOI: 10.4314/ahs.v24i4.31 PMID: 40190537

Egbuna, C., Ezzat, S. M., Tijjani, H., & Srivastav, V. K. (2019). Synthetic analogs of phytochemicals. In Kumar, S., & Egbuna, C. (Eds.), *Phytochemistry: An in-silico and in-vitro update* (pp. 23–55). Springer., DOI: 10.1007/978-981-13-6920-9_2

Ehrnhoefer, D. E., Duennwald, M., Markovic, P., Wacker, J. L., Engemann, S., Roark, M., Legleiter, J., Marsh, J. L., Thompson, L. M., Lindquist, S., Muchowski, P. J., & Wanker, E. E. (2006). Green tea (-)-epigallocatechin-gallate modulates early events in huntingtin misfolding and reduces toxicity in Huntington's disease models. *Human Molecular Genetics*, *15*(18), 2743–2751. DOI: 10.1093/hmg/ddl210 PMID: 16893904

El-Mansoury, B., Laadraoui, J., El Khiat, A., El Hiba, O., Jayakumar, A. R., Ferssiwi, A., ... (2023). Ataxia in multiple sclerosis: From current understanding to therapy. In *Ataxia – Practice essentials and interventions*. IntechOpen. https://www.intechopen.com/chapters/87486

Eleftheriadou, D., Kesidou, D., Moura, F., Felli, E., & Song, W. (2020). Redox-responsive nanobiomaterials-based therapeutics for neurodegenerative diseases. *Small, 16*(43), 1907308. DOI: 10.1002/smll.201907308

Elufioye, T. O., Berida, T. I., & Habtemariam, S. (2017). Plants-Derived neuroprotective agents: Cutting the cycle of cell death through multiple mechanisms. *Evidence-Based Complementary and Alternative Medicine : eCAM, 3574012*(1), 3574012. Advance online publication. DOI: 10.1155/2017/3574012 PMID: 28904554

Erkkinen, M. G., Kim, M. O., & Geschwind, M. D. (2018). Clinical neurology and epidemiology of the major neurodegenerative diseases. *Cold Spring Harbor Perspectives in Biology, 10*(4), a033118. DOI: 10.1101/cshperspect.a033118 PMID: 28716886

Erridge, S., Mangal, N., Salazar, O., Pacchetti, B., & Sodergren, M. H. (2020). Cannflavins – From plant to patient: A scoping review. *Fitoterapia, 146*, 104712. DOI: 10.1016/j.fitote.2020.104712 PMID: 32858172

Fang, J. (2015). Classification of fruits based on anthocyanin types and relevance to their health effects. *Nutrition (Burbank, Los Angeles County, Calif.), 31*(11–12), 1301–1306. DOI: 10.1016/j.nut.2015.04.015 PMID: 26250485

Faridzadeh, A., Salimi, Y., Ghasemirad, H., Kargar, M., Rashtchian, A., Mahmoudvand, G., Karimi, M. A., Zerangian, N., Jahani, N., Masoudi, A., Sadeghian Dastjerdi, B., Salavatizadeh, M., Sadeghsalehi, H., & Deravi, N. (2022). Neuroprotective potential of aromatic herbs: Rosemary, sage, and lavender. *Frontiers in Neuroscience, 16*, 909833. DOI: 10.3389/fnins.2022.909833 PMID: 35873824

Ferk, F., Kundi, M., Brath, H., Szekeres, T., Al-Serori, H., Mišík, M., Saiko, P., Marculescu, R., Wagner, K.-H., & Knasmueller, S. (2018). Gallic acid improves health-associated biochemical parameters and prevents oxidative damage of DNA in type 2 diabetes patients: Results of a placebo-controlled pilot study. *Molecular Nutrition & Food Research, 62*(4), 1700482. DOI: 10.1002/mnfr.201700482 PMID: 29193677

Fernandes, A. A. H., Novelli, E. L. B., Okoshi, K., Okoshi, M. P., Di Muzio, B. P., & Guimarães, J. F. C.. (2010). Influence of rutin treatment on biochemical alterations in experimental diabetes. *Biomedicine and Pharmacotherapy, 64*(3), 214–219. DOI: 10.1016/j.biopha.2009.08.007 PMID: 19932588

Ferrari, D., Pizzirani, C., Adinolfi, E., Lemoli, R. M., Curti, A., Idzko, M., Panther, E., & Di Virgilio, F. (2006). The P2X7 receptor: A key player in IL-1 processing and release. *The Journal of Immunology : Official Journal of the American Association of Immunologists, 176*(7), 3877–3883. DOI: 10.4049/jimmunol.176.7.3877 PMID: 16547218

Fialho, L., Santa-Maria, A. F., Madureira, F. A., & Iglesias, A. C. (2018). Comparative study of systemic early postoperative inflammatory response among elderly and non-elderly patients undergoing laparoscopic cholecystectomy. *Revista do Colégio Brasileiro de Cirurgiões, 45*(1), e1586. DOI: 10.1590/0100-6991e-20181586 PMID: 29590237

Figueirinha, A., Cruz, M. T., Francisco, V., Lopes, M. C., & Batista, M. T. (2010). Anti-inflammatory activity of *Cymbopogon citratus* leaf infusion in lipopolysaccharide-stimulated dendritic cells: Contribution of the polyphenols. *Journal of Medicinal Food, 13*(3), 681–690. DOI: 10.1089/jmf.2009.0115 PMID: 20438326

Flores, J., Noël, A., Foveau, B., Beauchet, O., & LeBlanc, A. C. (2020). Presymptomatic Caspase-1 inhibitor delays cognitive decline in a mouse model of Alzheimer disease and aging. *Nature Communications, 11*(1), 4571. DOI: 10.1038/s41467-020-18405-9 PMID: 32917871

Freyssin, A., Page, G., Fauconneau, B., & Rioux Bilan, A. (2018). Natural polyphenols effects on protein aggregates in Alzheimer's and Parkinson's prion-like diseases. *Neural Regeneration Research, 13*(6), 955. https://doi.org/DOI: 10.4103/1673-5374.234199

Gadhave, D. G., Sugandhi, V. V., Jha, S. K., Nangare, S. N., Gupta, G., Singh, S. K., et al. (2024). Neurodegenerative disorders: Mechanisms of degeneration and therapeutic approaches with their clinical relevance. *Ageing Research Reviews, 102357*. DOI: 10.1016/j.arr.2024.102357

Gadhave, D. G., Sugandhi, V. V., & Kokare, C. R. (2024). Potential biomaterials and experimental animal models for inventing new drug delivery approaches in the neurodegenerative disorder: Multiple sclerosis. *Brain Research, 1822*, 148674. https://doi.org/DOI: 10.1016/j.brainres.2024.148674

Gainche, M. (2020). *Études phytochimiques et activités anti-inflammatoires de plantes médicinales auvergnates* [Doctoral dissertation, Université Clermont Auvergne].

Galvão, I., Sugimoto, M. A., Vago, J. P., Machado, M. G., & Sousa, L. P. (2018). Mediators of inflammation. In Riccardi, C., Levi-Schaffer, F., & Tiligada, E. (Eds.), *Immunopharmacology and inflammation* (pp. 3–32). Springer., DOI: 10.1007/978-3-319-77658-3_1

Gandla, K., Babu, A. K., Unnisa, A., Sharma, I., Singh, L. P., Haque, M. A., Dashputre, N. L., Baig, S., Siddiqui, F. A., Khandaker, M. U., Almujally, A., Tamam, N., Sulieman, A., Khan, S. L., & Emran, T. B. (2023). Carotenoids: Role in neurodegenerative diseases remediation. *Brain Sciences*, *13*(3), 457. DOI: 10.3390/brainsci13030457 PMID: 36979267

Gao, Q. H., Fu, X., Zhang, R., Wang, Z., & Guo, M. (2018). Neuroprotective effects of plant polysaccharides: A review of the mechanisms. *International Journal of Biological Macromolecules*, *106*, 749–754. DOI: 10.1016/j.ijbiomac.2017.08.075 PMID: 28818727

Ge, J., Liu, Z., Zhong, Z., Wang, L., Zhuo, X., Li, J., Jiang, X., Ye, X.-Y., Xie, T., & Bai, R. (2022). Natural terpenoids with anti-inflammatory activities: Potential leads for anti-inflammatory drug discovery. *Bioorganic Chemistry*, *124*, 105817. DOI: 10.1016/j.bioorg.2022.105817 PMID: 35490583

Gertsch, J., Leonti, M., Raduner, S., Racz, I., Chen, J. Z., Xie, X. Q., Altmann, K.-H., Karsak, M., & Zimmer, A. (2008). Beta-caryophyllene is a dietary cannabinoid. *Proceedings of the National Academy of Sciences of the United States of America*, *105*(26), 9099–9104. DOI: 10.1073/pnas.0803601105 PMID: 18574142

Goedert, M. (2015). Alzheimer's and Parkinson's diseases: The prion concept in relation to assembled Aβ, tau, and α-synuclein. *Science*, *349*(6248), 1255555. DOI: 10.1126/science.1255555 PMID: 26250687

Gomez-Nicola, D., Teeling, J., Guaza, C., Godbout, J. P., & Taub, D. D. (2013). The role of inflammatory mediators in immune-to-brain communication during health and disease. *Mediators of Inflammation*, *429231*, 1–3. Advance online publication. DOI: 10.1155/2013/429231 PMID: 24109163

Gorlenko, C. L., Kiselev, H. Y., Budanova, E. V., Zamyatnin, A. A.Jr, & Ikryannikova, L. N. (2020). Plant secondary metabolites in the battle of drugs and drug-resistant bacteria: New heroes or worse clones of antibiotics? *Antibiotics (Basel, Switzerland)*, *9*(4), 170. DOI: 10.3390/antibiotics9040170 PMID: 32290036

Gowing, G., Svendsen, S., & Svendsen, C. N. (2017). *Ex vivo gene therapy for the treatment of neurological disorders* (Vol. 230). Progress in Brain Research, DOI: 10.1016/bs.pbr.2016.11.003

Grewal, A. K., Singh, T. G., Sharma, D., Sharma, V., Singh, M., Rahman, H. H., Najda, A., Walasek-Janusz, M., Kamel, M., Albadrani, G. M., Akhtar, M. F., Saleem, A., & Abdel-Daim, M. M. (2021). Mechanistic insights and perspectives involved in neuroprotective action of quercetin. *Biomedicine and Pharmacotherapy*, *140*, 111729. DOI: 10.1016/j.biopha.2021.111729 PMID: 34044274

Guerriero, G., Berni, R., Muñoz-Sanchez, J. A., Apone, F., Abdel-Salam, E. M., Qahtan, A. A., Alatar, A. A., Cantini, C., Cai, G., Hausman, J.-F., Siddiqui, K. S., Hernández-Sotomayor, S. M. T., & Faisal, M. (2018). Production of plant secondary metabolites: Examples, tips and suggestions for biotechnologists. *Genes*, *9*(6), 309. DOI: 10.3390/genes9060309 PMID: 29925808

Guest, J., & Grant, R. (2016). Carotenoids and neurobiological health. In Essa, M. M., Akbar, M., & Guillemin, G. (Eds.), *The benefits of natural products for neurodegenerative diseases* (pp. 199–228). Springer International Publishing., DOI: 10.1007/978-3-319-28383-8_11

Guo, S., Yan, J., Yang, T., Yang, X., Bezard, E., & Zhao, B. (2007). Protective effects of green tea polyphenols in the 6-OHDA rat model of Parkinson's disease through inhibition of ROS-NO pathway. *Biological Psychiatry*, *62*(12), 1353–1362. DOI: 10.1016/j.biopsych.2007.04.020 PMID: 17624318

Gupta, N., Verma, K., Nalla, S., Kulshreshtha, A., Lall, R., & Prasad, S. (2020). Free radicals as a double-edged sword: The cancer preventive and therapeutic roles of curcumin. *Molecules, 25*(22), 5390. DOI: 10.3390/molecules25225390

Gustin, A., Kirchmeyer, M., Koncina, E., Felten, P., Losciuto, S., Heurtaux, T., & Michelucci, A. (2015). NLRP3 inflammasome is expressed and functional in mouse brain microglia but not in astrocytes. *PLoS One*, *10*(6), e0130624. DOI: 10.1371/journal.pone.0130624 PMID: 26091541

Hadipour, E., Shahangian, S. S., & Mashayekhi, F. (2024). Monoterpenes and diterpenes in combating Alzheimer disease, mechanisms, and clinical insights: A comprehensive review. *Caspian Journal of Neurological Sciences*, *10*(1), 1–19. DOI: 10.32598/CJNS.10.36.460.1

Halliwell, B. (2009). The wanderings of a free radical. *Free Radical Biology & Medicine*, *46*(5), 531–542. DOI: 10.1016/j.freeradbiomed.2008.11.008 PMID: 19111608

Hanif, S., Muhammad, P., Chesworth, R., Rehman, F. U., Qian, R. J., Zheng, M., et al. (2020). Nanomedicine-based immunotherapy for central nervous system disorders. *Acta Pharmacologica Sinica, 41*(7), 936–953. https://doi.org/DOI: 10.1038/s41401-020-00441-6

Harding, J. L., Weber, M. B., & Shaw, J. E. (2024). The global burden of diabetes. In Holt, R. I. G., & Flyvbjerg, A. (Eds.), *Textbook of diabetes* (1st ed., pp. 28–40). Wiley., https://onlinelibrary.wiley.com/doi/10.1002/9781119697473.ch3 DOI: 10.1002/9781119697473.ch3

Hasan, S., Khatri, N., Rahman, Z. N., Menezes, A. A., Martini, J., Shehjar, F., Mujeeb, N., & Shah, Z. A. (2023). Neuroprotective potential of flavonoids in brain disorders. *Brain Sciences*, *13*(9), 1258. DOI: 10.3390/brainsci13091258 PMID: 37759859

Hemendinger, R. A., Armstrong, E. J., Persinski, R., Todd, J., Mougeot, J. L., Volvovitz, F., & Barres, B. A. (2008). Huperzine A provides neuroprotection against several cell death inducers using in vitro model systems of motor neuron cell death. *Neurotoxicity Research*, *13*(1), 49–61. DOI: 10.1007/BF03033367 PMID: 18367440

Hendrickx, J. O., van Gastel, J., Leysen, H., Martin, B., & Maudsley, S. (2020). High-dimensionality data analysis of pharmacological systems associated with complex diseases. *Pharmacological Reviews, 72*(1), 191-217. https://doi.org/ DOI: 10.1124/pr.120.020022

Hodgson, A. B., Randell, R. K., & Jeukendrup, A. E. (2013). The effect of green tea extract on fat oxidation at rest and during exercise: Evidence of efficacy and proposed mechanisms. *Advances in Nutrition*, *4*(2), 129–140. DOI: 10.3945/an.112.003269 PMID: 23493529

Hortelano, S. (2009). Molecular basis of the anti-inflammatory effects of terpenoids. *Inflammation & Allergy Drug Targets*, *8*(1), 28–39. DOI: 10.2174/187152809787582534 PMID: 19275691

Hu, S., Maiti, P., Ma, Q., Zuo, X., Jones, M. R., Cole, G. M., & Lutz, C. (2015). Clinical development of curcumin in neurodegenerative disease. *Expert Review of Neurotherapeutics*, *15*(6), 629–637. DOI: 10.1586/14737175.2015.1044981 PMID: 26035622

Hummelova, J., Rondevaldova, J., Balastikova, A., Lapcik, O., & Kokoska, L. (2015). The relationship between structure and in vitro antibacterial activity of selected isoflavones and their metabolites with special focus on antistaphylococcal effect of demethyltexasin. *Letters in Applied Microbiology*, *60*(3), 242–247. DOI: 10.1111/lam.12361 PMID: 25421722

Hussein, R. A., & El-Anssary, A. A. (2019). Plants secondary metabolites: The key drivers of the pharmacological actions of medicinal plants. *Herbal Medicine*, *1*(3), 11–30. DOI: 10.5772/intechopen.76139

Isonaka, R., Hiruma, H., Katakura, T., & Kawakami, T. (2011). Inhibition of superoxide dismutase selectively suppresses growth of rat spinal motor neurons: Comparison with phosphorylated neurofilament-containing spinal neurons. *Brain Research, 1425*, 13-19. DOI: 10.1016/j.brainres.2011.09.013

Iwashina, T. (2013). Flavonoid properties of five families newly incorporated into the order Caryophyllales. *Bulletin of the National Museum of Nature and Science, 39*(1), 25–51.

Jain, C., Khatana, S., & Vijayvergia, R. (2019). Bioactivity of secondary metabolites of various plants: A review. *International Journal of Pharmaceutical Sciences and Research, 10*(2), 494–504. DOI: 10.13040/IJPSR.0975-8232.10(2).494-04

Jankovic, J., Goodman, I., Safirstein, B., Marmon, T. K., Schenk, D. B., Koller, M., et al. (2018). Safety and tolerability of multiple ascending doses of PRX002/RG7935, an anti–α-synuclein monoclonal antibody, in patients with Parkinson disease: A randomized clinical trial. *JAMA Neurology, 75*(10), 1206–1214. https://doi.org/DOI: 10.1001/jamaneurol.2018.1947

Jaswir, I. (2011). Carotenoids: Sources, medicinal properties and their application in food and nutraceutical industry. *Journal of Medicinal Plants Research, 5*(33), 7090–7098. DOI: 10.5897/JMPR11.1019

Javadi, F., Ahmadzadeh, A., Eghtesadi, S., Aryaeian, N., Zabihiyeganeh, M., Rahimi Foroushani, A., & Jazayeri, S. (2017). The effect of quercetin on inflammatory factors and clinical symptoms in women with rheumatoid arthritis: A double-blind, randomized controlled trial. *Journal of the American College of Nutrition, 36*(1), 9–15. DOI: 10.1080/07315724.2016.1140093 PMID: 27710596

Jawad, L., Kabdy, H., Azraida, H., Abdelmohcine, A., & Smimih, K. (2024). Glial cell biology and their multifaceted functions in Alzheimer's disease: New therapeutic prospects. In *Physiology and function of glial cells in health and disease* (pp. 280–312). IGI Global., https://www.igi-global.com/chapter/glial-cell-biology-and-their-multifaceted-functions-in-alzheimers-disease/335248

Jigam, A. A., Musa, R., Abdullahi, A., & Lawal, B. (2020). Characterization of anti-plasmodial, analgesic and anti-inflammatory fraction of *Maytenus senegalensis* (Lam.) Exell leaf extract in mice. *Clinical Phytoscience, 6*(1), 56. DOI: 10.1186/s40816-020-00201-z

Jin, D., Dai, K., Xie, Z., & Chen, J. (2020). Secondary metabolites profiled in cannabis inflorescences, leaves, stem barks, and roots for medicinal purposes. *Scientific Reports, 10*(1), 3309. DOI: 10.1038/s41598-020-60172-6 PMID: 32094454

Johnson, J. B., Mani, J. S., Broszczak, D., Prasad, S. S., Ekanayake, C. P., Strappe, P., Valeris, P., & Naiker, M. (2021). Hitting the sweet spot: A systematic review of the bioactivity and health benefits of phenolic glycosides from medicinally used plants. *Phytotherapy Research, 35*(7), 3484–3508. DOI: 10.1002/ptr.7042 PMID: 33615599

Kabir, M. T., Rahman, M. H., Shah, M., Jamiruddin, M. R., Basak, D., Al-Harrasi, A., et al. (2022). Therapeutic promise of carotenoids as antioxidants and anti-inflammatory agents in neurodegenerative disorders. *Biomedicine & Pharmacotherapy, 146*, 112610. DOI: 10.1016/j.biopha.2021.112610

Karlsen, A., Retterstøl, L., Laake, P., Paur, I., Kjølsrud-Bøhn, S., Sandvik, L., et al. (2007). Anthocyanins inhibit nuclear factor-κB activation in monocytes and reduce plasma concentrations of pro-inflammatory mediators in healthy adults. *The Journal of Nutrition, 137*(8), 1951-1954. DOI: 10.1093/jn/137.8.1951

Kavitha, R. V., Kumar, J. R., Egbuna, C., & Ifemeje, J. C. (2020). Phytochemicals as therapeutic interventions in neurodegenerative diseases. In *Phytochemicals as lead compounds for new drug discovery* (pp. 161–178). Elsevier., DOI: 10.1016/B978-0-12-817890-4.00010-X

Kengne, A. P., & Ramachandran, A. (2024). Feasibility of prevention of type 2 diabetes in low- and middle-income countries. *Diabetologia, 67*(5), 763–772. DOI: 10.1007/s00125-023-06085-1 PMID: 38355989

Kesse-Guyot, E., Andreeva, V. A., Ducros, V., Jeandel, C., Julia, C., Hercberg, S., et al. (2014). Carotenoid-rich dietary patterns during midlife and subsequent cognitive function. *British Journal of Nutrition, 111*(5), 915-923. https://doi.org/DOI: 10.1017/S000711451300347X

Khalifa, S. A., Elias, N., Farag, M. A., Chen, L., Saeed, A., Hegazy, M. E. F., Moustafa, M. S., Abd El-Wahed, A., Al-Mousawi, S. M., Musharraf, S. G., Chang, F.-R., Iwasaki, A., Suenaga, K., Alajlani, M., Göransson, U., & El-Seedi, H. R. (2019). Marine natural products: A source of novel anticancer drugs. *Marine Drugs, 17*(9), 491. DOI: 10.3390/md17090491 PMID: 31443597

Khan, A. U., Dagur, H. S., Khan, M., Malik, N., Alam, M., & Mushtaque, M. D. (2021). Therapeutic role of flavonoids and flavones in cancer prevention: Current trends and future perspectives. *European Journal of Medicinal Chemistry Reports, 3*, 100010. DOI: 10.1016/j.ejmcr.2021.100010

Khoo, H. E., Azlan, A., Tang, S. T., & Lim, S. M. (2017). Anthocyanidins and anthocyanins: Colored pigments as food, pharmaceutical ingredients, and the potential health benefits. *Food & Nutrition Research, 61*(1), 1361779. DOI: 10.1080/16546628.2017.1361779 PMID: 28970777

Kiernan, M. C., Vucic, S., Cheah, B. C., Turner, M. R., Eisen, A., Hardiman, O., Burrell, J. R., & Zoing, M. C. (2011). Amyotrophic lateral sclerosis. *Lancet, 377*(9769), 942–955. DOI: 10.1016/S0140-6736(10)61156-7 PMID: 21296405

Kim, J. H., Hwang, J., Shim, E., Chung, E. J., Jang, S. H., & Koh, S. B. (2016). Association of serum carotenoid, retinol, and tocopherol concentrations with the progression of Parkinson's disease. *Nutritional Research and Practice, 11*(2), 114-120. DOI: 10.4162/nrp.2017.11.2.114

Knezevic, E., Nenic, K., Milanovic, V., & Knezevic, N. N. (2023). The role of cortisol in chronic stress, neurodegenerative diseases, and psychological disorders. *Cells*, *12*(23), 2726. DOI: 10.3390/cells12232726 PMID: 38067154

Koh, S. H., Kim, S. H., Kwon, H., Kim, J. G., Kim, J. H., Yang, K. H., & Lee, W. (2004). Phosphatidylinositol-3 kinase/Akt and GSK-3 mediated cytoprotective effect of epigallocatechin gallate on oxidative stress-injured neuronal-differentiated N18D3 cells. *Neurotoxicology*, *25*(5), 793–802. DOI: 10.1016/j.neuro.2004.02.001 PMID: 15288510

Konrad, M., Nieman, D. C., Henson, D. A., Kennerly, K. M., Jin, F., & Wallner-Liebmann, S. J. (2011). The acute effect of ingesting a quercetin-based supplement on exercise-induced inflammation and immune changes in runners. *International Journal of Sport Nutrition and Exercise Metabolism*, *21*(4), 338–346. DOI: 10.1123/ijsnem.21.4.338 PMID: 21813917

Kopečná-Zapletalová, M., Krasulová, K., Anzenbacher, P., Hodek, P., & Anzenbacherová, E. (2017). Interaction of isoflavonoids with human liver microsomal cytochromes P450: Inhibition of CYP enzyme activities. *Xenobiotica*, *47*(4), 324–331. DOI: 10.1080/00498254.2016.1195028 PMID: 27312150

Kopsell, D. A., & Kopsell, D. E. (2006). Accumulation and bioavailability of dietary carotenoids in vegetable crops. *Trends in Plant Science*, *11*(10), 499–507. DOI: 10.1016/j.tplants.2006.08.006 PMID: 16949856

Kumar, G. P., & Khanum, F. (2012). Neuroprotective potential of phytochemicals. *. *Pharmacognosy Reviews*, *6*(12), 81. DOI: 10.4103/0973-7847.99898 PMID: 23055633

Kumar, R., Aadil, K. R., Mondal, K., Mishra, Y. K., Oupicky, D., Ramakrishna, S., et al. (2022). Neurodegenerative disorders management: State-of-art and prospects of nano-biotechnology. *Critical Reviews in Biotechnology, 42*(8), 1180–1212. https://doi.org/DOI: 10.1080/07388551.2022.2127602

Kumar, S., Korra, T., Thakur, R., Arutselvan, R., Kashyap, A. S., & Nehela, Y.. (2023). Role of plant secondary metabolites in defence and transcriptional regulation in response to biotic stress. *Plant Stress*, *8*, 100154. DOI: 10.1016/j.stress.2023.100154

Kunle, O. F., Egharevba, H. O., & Ahmadu, P. O. (2012). Standardization of herbal medicines—A review. *International Journal of Biodiversity and Conservation, 4*(3), 101-112. https://doi.org/DOI: 10.5897/IJBC11.028

Laadraoui, J., Aboufatima, R., El Gabbas, Z., Ferehan, H., Bezza, K., & Laaradia, M. A.. (2018). Effect of *Artemisia herba-alba* consumption during pregnancy on fertility, morphological and behaviors of mice offspring. *Journal of Ethnopharmacology, 226*, 105–110. DOI: 10.1016/j.jep.2018.08.017 PMID: 30118834

Leonoudakis, D., Rane, A., Angeli, S., Lithgow, G. J., Andersen, J. K., & Chinta, S. J. (2017). Anti-inflammatory and neuroprotective role of natural product securinine in activated glial cells: Implications for Parkinson's disease. *Mediators of Inflammation, 2017*, 1–11. DOI: 10.1155/2017/8302636 PMID: 28473732

Li, N., Lu, W., Ren, H., & Chen, Z. (2024). Chemistry, bioactivities, structure–activity relationship, biosynthesis and metabolism of prenylated flavonoids in *Moraceae* plants. *Food & Function, 15*(19), 9598–9631. DOI: 10.1039/D4FO02688H PMID: 39238316

Li, Q., Zhao, H. F., Zhang, Z. F., Liu, Z. G., Pei, X. R., Wang, J. B., et al. (2009). Long-term green tea catechin administration prevents spatial learning and memory impairment in senescence-accelerated mouse prone-8 mice by decreasing Aβ1-42 oligomers and upregulating synaptic plasticity–related proteins in the hippocampus. *Neuroscience, 163*(3), 741-749. DOI: 10.1016/j.neuroscience.2009.06.015

Li, Y., Xia, Y., Yin, S., Wan, F., Hu, J., Kou, L., & Liu, L. (2021). Targeting microglial α-synuclein/TLRs/NF-kappaB/NLRP3 inflammasome axis in Parkinson's disease. *Frontiers in Immunology, 12*, 719807. DOI: 10.3389/fimmu.2021.719807 PMID: 34691027

Lim, Y. J., Jeong, H. Y., Gil, C. S., Kwon, S. J., Na, J. K., Lee, C., & Eom, S. H. (2020). Isoflavone accumulation and the metabolic gene expression in response to persistent UV-B irradiation in soybean sprouts. *Food Chemistry, 303*, 125376. DOI: 10.1016/j.foodchem.2019.125376 PMID: 31442900

Lima, E., & Medeiros, J. (2024). Terpenes as potential anti-Alzheimer's disease agents. *Applied Sciences (Basel, Switzerland), 14*(9), 3898. DOI: 10.3390/app14093898

Lo Van, A., Sakayori, N., Hachem, M., Belkouch, M., Picq, M., Fourmaux, B., & Charriaut-Marlangue, C. (2019). Targeting the brain with a neuroprotective omega-3 fatty acid to enhance neurogenesis in hypoxic condition in culture. *Molecular Neurobiology, 56*(2), 986–999. DOI: 10.1007/s12035-018-1139-0 PMID: 29858775

Long, J. M., & Holtzman, D. M. (2019). Alzheimer disease: An update on pathobiology and treatment strategies. *Cell, 179*(2), 312–339. DOI: 10.1016/j.cell.2019.09.001 PMID: 31564456

López de Dicastillo, C., Piña, C., Garrido, L., Arancibia, C., & Galotto, M. J. (2019). Enhancing thermal stability and bioaccessibility of açaí fruit polyphenols through electrohydrodynamic encapsulation into zein electrosprayed particles. *Antioxidants, 8*(10), 464. DOI: 10.3390/antiox8100464 PMID: 31600875

Loy, C., & Schneider, L. (2006). Galantamine for Alzheimer's disease and mild cognitive impairment. *Cochrane Database of Systematic Reviews, 2006*(1). DOI: 10.1002/14651858.CD001747.pub3

Luca, S. V., Macovei, I., Bujor, A., Miron, A., Skalicka-Woźniak, K., Aprotosoaie, A. C., & Trifan, A. (2020). Bioactivity of dietary polyphenols: The role of metabolites. *Critical Reviews in Food Science and Nutrition, 60*(4), 626–659. DOI: 10.1080/10408398.2018.1546669 PMID: 30614249

Luckner, M. (2013). *Secondary metabolism in microorganisms, plants and animals*. Springer Science & Business Media.

Luo, C. F., Yuan, M., Chen, M. S., Liu, S. M., Zhu, L., Huang, B. Y., Liu, X.-W., & Xiong, W. (2011). Pharmacokinetics, tissue distribution, and relative bioavailability of puerarin solid lipid nanoparticles following oral administration. *International Journal of Pharmaceutics, 410*(1-2), 138–144. DOI: 10.1016/j.ijpharm.2011.02.064 PMID: 21392565

Mahad, D. H., Trapp, B. D., & Lassmann, H. (2015). Pathological mechanisms in progressive multiple sclerosis. *Lancet Neurology, 14*(2), 183–193. DOI: 10.1016/S1474-4422(14)70256-X PMID: 25772897

Malik, J. A., Bhadauria, M., Lone, R., & Hajam, Y. A. (2020). Exploitation of plant phenolics in animal farming. In Lone, R., Shuab, R., & Kamili, A. N. (Eds.), *Plant phenolics in sustainable agriculture* (pp. 69–89). Springer Singapore., DOI: 10.1007/978-981-15-4890-1_3

Mandel, S. A., Avramovich-Tirosh, Y., Reznichenko, L., Zheng, H., Weinreb, O., Amit, T., & Youdim, M. B. H. (2005). Multifunctional activities of green tea catechins in neuroprotection. *Neuro-Signals, 14*(1–2), 46–60. DOI: 10.1159/000085385 PMID: 15956814

Manochkumar, J., Doss, C. G. P., El-Seedi, H. R., Efferth, T., & Ramamoorthy, S. (2021). The neuroprotective potential of carotenoids in vitro and in vivo. *Phytomedicine, 91*, 153676. DOI: 10.1016/j.phymed.2021.153676

Mansour, M., Salah, M., & Xu, X. (2020). Effect of microencapsulation using soy protein isolate and gum arabic as wall material on red raspberry anthocyanin stability, characterization, and simulated gastrointestinal conditions. *Ultrasonics Sonochemistry*, *63*, 104927. DOI: 10.1016/j.ultsonch.2019.104927 PMID: 31952001

Marino, P. (2023). *Isolation, characterization and biological evaluation of onco-nutraceuticals compounds in the Mediterranean area: New tools for the treatment of oncological diseases*. https://iris.unibas.it/handle/11563/172735

Martin, L. J. (2010). Mitochondrial and cell death mechanisms in neurodegenerative diseases. *Pharmaceuticals (Basel, Switzerland)*, *3*(4), 839–915. DOI: 10.3390/ph3040839 PMID: 21258649

Martin, L. J., Al-Abdulla, N. A., Brambrink, A. M., Kirsch, J. R., Sieber, F. E., & Portera-Cailliau, C. (1998). Neurodegeneration in excitotoxicity, global cerebral ischemia, and target deprivation: A perspective on the contributions of apoptosis and necrosis. *Brain Research Bulletin*, *46*(4), 281–309. DOI: 10.1016/S0361-9230(98)00024-0 PMID: 9671259

Merecz-Sadowska, A., Sitarek, P., Kowalczyk, T., Palusiak, M., Hoelm, M., Zajdel, K., & Zajdel, R. (2023). In vitro evaluation and in silico calculations of the antioxidant and anti-inflammatory properties of secondary metabolites from *Leonurus sibiricus* L. root extracts. *Molecules (Basel, Switzerland)*, *28*(18), 6550. DOI: 10.3390/molecules28186550 PMID: 37764326

Mérillon, J. M., & Ramawat, K. G. (Eds.). (2020). *Co-evolution of secondary metabolites* (Reference Series in Phytochemistry). Springer. DOI: 10.1007/978-3-319-96397-6

Miguel, C. A., Noya-Riobó, M. V., Mazzone, G. L., Villar, M. J., & Coronel, M. F. (2021). Antioxidant, anti-inflammatory and neuroprotective actions of resveratrol after experimental nervous system insults. Special focus on the molecular mechanisms involved. *Neurochemistry International*, *150*, 105188. DOI: 10.1016/j.neuint.2021.105188 PMID: 34536545

Miller, A. P., Coronel, J., & Amengual, J. (2020). The role of β-carotene and vitamin A in atherogenesis: Evidences from preclinical and clinical studies. *Biochimica et Biophysica Acta (BBA)—Molecular and Cell Biology of Lipids, 1865*(11), 158635. DOI: 10.1016/j.bbalip.2020.158635

Miller, N. J., Sampson, J., Candeias, L. P., Bramley, P. M., & Rice-Evans, C. A. (1996). Antioxidant activities of carotenes and xanthophylls. *FEBS Letters*, *384*(3), 240–242. DOI: 10.1016/0014-5793(96)00323-7 PMID: 8617362

Mitra, I., Saha, A., & Roy, K. (2010). Exploring quantitative structure–activity relationship studies of antioxidant phenolic compounds obtained from traditional Chinese medicinal plants. *Molecular Simulation, 36*(13), 1067–1079. DOI: 10.1080/08927022.2010.503326

Mittal, K. R., Pharasi, N., Sarna, B., & Singh, M., Rachana, Haider, S., ... & Jha, N. K. (2022). Nanotechnology-based drug delivery for the treatment of CNS disorders. *Translational Neuroscience, 13*(1), 527–546.

Mogi, M., Harada, M., Kondo, T., Riederer, P., Inagaki, H., Minami, M., & Nagatsu, T. (1994). Interleukin-1β, interleukin-6, epidermal growth factor and transforming growth factor-α are elevated in the brain from parkinsonian patients. *Neuroscience Letters, 180*(2), 147–150. DOI: 10.1016/0304-3940(94)90508-8 PMID: 7700568

Mondal, A., Gandhi, A., Fimognari, C., Atanasov, A. G., & Bishayee, A. (2019). Alkaloids for cancer prevention and therapy: Current progress and future perspectives. *European Journal of Pharmacology, 858*, 172472. DOI: 10.1016/j.ejphar.2019.172472 PMID: 31228447

Mortada, I., Farah, R., Nabha, S., Ojcius, D. M., Fares, Y., Almawi, W. Y., et al. (2021). Immunotherapies for neurodegenerative diseases. *Frontiers in Neurology, 12*, 654739. DOI: 10.3389/fneur.2021.654739

Mouton-Liger, F., Rosazza, T., Sepulveda-Diaz, J., Ieang, A., Hassoun, S. M., Claire, E., & Corvol, J. C. (2018). Parkin deficiency modulates NLRP3 inflammasome activation by attenuating an A20-dependent negative feedback loop. *Glia, 66*(8), 1736–1751. DOI: 10.1002/glia.23337 PMID: 29665074

Muscolo, A., Mariateresa, O., Giulio, T., & Mariateresa, R. (2024). Oxidative stress: The role of antioxidant phytochemicals in the prevention and treatment of diseases. *International Journal of Molecular Sciences, 25*(6), 3264. DOI: 10.3390/ijms25063264

Mushtaq, Z., Sadeer, N. B., Hussain, M., Mahwish, , Alsagaby, S. A., Imran, M., Mumtaz, T., Umar, M., Tauseef, A., Al Abdulmonem, W., Tufail, T., Al Jbawi, E., & Mahomoodally, M. F. (2023). Therapeutical properties of apigenin: A review on the experimental evidence and basic mechanisms. *International Journal of Food Properties, 26*(1), 1914–1939. DOI: 10.1080/10942912.2023.2236329

Muthukrishnan, S. D., & Annapoorani Subramaniyan, A. S. (2012). Phytochemical constituents of *Gloriosa superba* seed, tuber and leaves. *CAB Direct*. https://www.cabidigitallibrary.org/doi/full/10.5555/20123285124

Naija, D. S., Gueddes, S. B. M., Flamini, G., Khiareddine, H. J., Remadi, M. D., & Mariem, F. B.. (2021). Assessment of antioxidant and antimicrobial compounds of volatiles from leaves, stems and flowers of olives. *Polish Journal of Environmental Studies*, *30*(2), 1325–1338. DOI: 10.15244/pjoes/121514

Najmi, A., Javed, S. A., Al Bratty, M., & Alhazmi, H. A. (2022). Modern approaches in the discovery and development of plant-based natural products and their analogues as potential therapeutic agents. *Molecules (Basel, Switzerland)*, *27*(2), 349. DOI: 10.3390/molecules27020349 PMID: 35056662

Niedzielska, E., Smaga, I., Gawlik, M., Moniczewski, A., Stankowicz, P., Pera, J., et al. (2016). Oxidative stress in neurodegenerative diseases. *Molecular Neurobiology, 53*(6), 4094–4125. https://doi.org/DOI: 10.1007/s12035-016-9820-z

Nobre, M. E. P., Correia, A. O., Mendonça, F. N. M., Uchoa, L. R. A., Vasconcelos, J. T. N., De Araújo, C. N. A., & de Lima, M. A. (2016). Omega-3 fatty acids: Possible neuroprotective mechanisms in the model of global ischemia in rats. *Journal of Nutrition and Metabolism*, *2016*, 1–13. DOI: 10.1155/2016/6462120 PMID: 27313881

Nolaou, K. C., Chen, J. S., & Corey, E. J. (2011). *Classics in total synthesis III: Further targets, strategies, methods*. Wiley.

Olney, J. W. (1969). Glutamate-induced retinal degeneration in neonatal mice: Electron microscopy of the acutely evolving lesion. *Journal of Neuropathology and Experimental Neurology*, *28*(3), 455–474. DOI: 10.1097/00005072-196907000-00007 PMID: 5788942

Orlando, F. A., & Mainous, A. G.III. (2024). Editorial: Inflammation and chronic disease. *Frontiers in Medicine*, *11*, 1434533. https://www.frontiersin.org/articles/10.3389/fmed.2024.1434533/full. DOI: 10.3389/fmed.2024.1434533 PMID: 39015780

Oufquir, S., Kabdy, H., Laaradia, M. A., Tazart, Z., Raoui, K., & Aboufatima, R.. (2024). Phytochemical characterization and evaluation of therapeutic benefit of *Annona muricata* L. leaves against tumor growth in the P815 murine tumor model. *South African Journal of Botany*, *172*, 407–414. DOI: 10.1016/j.sajb.2024.07.044

Pannucci, E., Spagnuolo, L., De Gara, L., Santi, L., & Dugo, L. (2023). Phenolic compounds as preventive and therapeutic agents in diabetes-related oxidative stress, inflammation, advanced glycation end-products production and insulin sensitivity. *Discovery Medicine*, *35*(178), 715. https://www.iris.unicampus.it/handle/20.500.12610/83723. DOI: 10.24976/Discov.Med.202335178.68 PMID: 37811611

Piguet, F., Alves, S., & Cartier, N. (2017). Clinical gene therapy for neurodegenerative diseases: Past, present, and future. *Human Gene Therapy, 28*(11), 988–1003. DOI: 10.1089/hum.2017.157

Pilipović, K., Jurišić Grubešić, R., Dolenec, P., Kučić, N., Juretić, L., & Mršić-Pelčić, J. (2023). Plant-based antioxidants for prevention and treatment of neurodegenerative diseases: Phytotherapeutic potential of *Laurus nobilis, Aronia melanocarpa*, and celastrol. *Antioxidants*, *12*(3), 746. DOI: 10.3390/antiox12030746 PMID: 36978994

Poewe, W., Seppi, K., Tanner, C. M., Halliday, G. M., Brundin, P., Volkmann, J., Schrag, A.-E., & Lang, A. E. (2017). Parkinson disease. *Nature Reviews. Disease Primers*, *3*(1), 17013. DOI: 10.1038/nrdp.2017.13 PMID: 28332488

Poovaiah, N., Davoudi, Z., Peng, H., Schlichtmann, B., Mallapragada, S., Narasimhan, B., et al. (2018). Treatment of neurodegenerative disorders through the blood–brain barrier using nanocarriers. *Nanoscale, 10*(36), 16962–16983. https://doi.org/DOI: 10.1039/C8NR04256H

Potì, F., Santi, D., Spaggiari, G., Zimetti, F., & Zanotti, I. (2019). Polyphenol health effects on cardiovascular and neurodegenerative disorders: A review and meta-analysis. *International Journal of Molecular Sciences, 20*(2), 351. DOI: 10.3390/ijms20020351

Prakash, A., & Kumar, A. (2014). Implicating the role of lycopene in restoration of mitochondrial enzymes and BDNF levels in β-amyloid induced Alzheimer's disease. *European Journal of Pharmacology*, *741*, 104–111. DOI: 10.1016/j.ejphar.2014.07.036 PMID: 25066110

Przedborski, S. (2017). The two-century journey of Parkinson disease research. *Nature Reviews. Neuroscience*, *18*(4), 251–259. DOI: 10.1038/nrn.2017.25 PMID: 28303016

Rabie, O., El-Nashar, H. A. S., George, M. Y., Majrashi, T. A., Al-Warhi, T., Hassan, F. E., Eldehna, W. M., & Mostafa, N. M. (2023). Phytochemical profiling and neuroprotective activity of *Callistemon subulatus* leaves against cyclophosphamide-induced chemobrain. *Biomedicine and Pharmacotherapy*, *167*, 115596. DOI: 10.1016/j.biopha.2023.115596 PMID: 37797461

Rahman, M. H., Bajgai, J., Fadriquela, A., Sharma, S., Trinh, T. T., Akter, R., et al. (2021). Therapeutic potential of natural products in treating neurodegenerative disorders and their future prospects and challenges. *Molecules, 26*(17), 5327. DOI: 10.3390/molecules26175327

Rakotoarisoa, M., & Angelova, A. (2019). Amphiphilic nanocarrier systems for curcumin delivery in neurodegenerative disorders. In *The Road from Nanomedicine to Precision Medicine* (pp. 1027–1065). Springer., DOI: 10.1201/9780429295010-33

Rao, S. R., & Ravishankar, G. A. (2002). Plant cell cultures: Chemical factories of secondary metabolites. *Biotechnology Advances*, *20*(2), 101–153. DOI: 10.1016/S0734-9750(02)00007-1 PMID: 14538059

Rashidinejad, A., Birch, E. J., Sun-Waterhouse, D., & Everett, D. W. (2016). Effect of liposomal encapsulation on the recovery and antioxidant properties of green tea catechins incorporated into a hard low-fat cheese following in vitro simulated gastrointestinal digestion. *Food and Bioproducts Processing*, *100*, 238–245. DOI: 10.1016/j.fbp.2016.07.005

Rasmus, P., & Kozłowska, E. (2023). Antioxidant and anti-inflammatory effects of carotenoids in mood disorders: An overview. *Antioxidants, 12*(3), 676. DOI: 10.3390/antiox12030676

Renaud, J., & Martinoli, M. G. (2019). Considerations for the use of polyphenols as therapies in neurodegenerative diseases. *International Journal of Molecular Sciences*, *20*(8), 1883. DOI: 10.3390/ijms20081883 PMID: 30995776

Rex, J. R. S., Muthukumar, N., & Selvakumar, P. M. (2018). Phytochemicals as a potential source for antimicrobial, antioxidant and wound healing: A review. *MOJ Bioorganic & Organic Chemistry*, *2*(2), 61–70. DOI: 10.15406/mojbo.2018.02.00052

Rezai-Zadeh, K., Arendash, G. W., Hou, H., Fernandez, F., Jensen, M., Runfeldt, M., Shytle, R. D., & Tan, J. (2008). Green tea epigallocatechin-3-gallate (EGCG) reduces β-amyloid-mediated cognitive impairment and modulates tau pathology in Alzheimer transgenic mice. *Brain Research*, *1214*, 177–187. DOI: 10.1016/j.brainres.2008.02.107 PMID: 18457818

Riccardi, C., Napolitano, F., Montesarchio, D., Sampaolo, S., & Melone, M. A. B. (2021). Nanoparticle-guided brain drug delivery: Expanding the therapeutic approach to neurodegenerative diseases. *Pharmaceutics, 13*(11), 1897. DOI: 10.3390/pharmaceutics13111897

Rodrigues, F., Reis, M., Ferreira, L., Grosso, C., Ferraz, R., Vieira, M., Vasconcelos, V., & Martins, R. (2024). The neuroprotective role of cyanobacteria with focus on the anti-inflammatory and antioxidant potential: Current status and perspectives. *Molecules (Basel, Switzerland)*, *29*(20), 4799. DOI: 10.3390/molecules29204799 PMID: 39459167

Rushendran, R., Begum, R. F., Singh, A., Narayanan, P. L., Vellapandian, C., & Prajapati, B. G.. (2024). Navigating neurological disorders: Harnessing the power of natural compounds for innovative therapeutic breakthroughs. *EXCLI Journal*, *23*, 534. PMID: 38741726

Sala Frigerio, C., & De Strooper, B. (2016). Alzheimer's disease mechanisms and emerging roads to novel therapeutics. *Annual Review of Neuroscience*, *39*(1), 57–79. DOI: 10.1146/annurev-neuro-070815-014015 PMID: 27050320

Salińska, E., Danysz, W., & Łazarewicz, J. W. (2005). The role of excitotoxicity in neurodegeneration. *Folia Neuropathologica*, *43*(4), 322–339. PMID: 16416396

Samanta, S., Banerjee, J., Ahmed, R., & Dash, S. K. (2023). Potential benefits of bioactive functional components of citrus fruits for health promotion and disease prevention. In Singh Purewal, S., Punia Bangar, S., & Kaur, P. (Eds.), *Recent advances in citrus fruits* (pp. 451–499). Springer., https://link.springer.com/10.1007/978-3-031-37534-7_15 DOI: 10.1007/978-3-031-37534-7_15

Sarlus, H., & Heneka, M. T. (2017). Microglia in Alzheimer's disease. *The Journal of Clinical Investigation*, *127*(9), 3240–3249. DOI: 10.1172/JCI90606 PMID: 28862638

Scheffer, I. E., Bhatia, K. P., Lopes-Cendes, I., Fish, D. R., Marsden, C. D., Andermann, E., Andermann, F., Desbiens, R., Keene, D., Cendes, F., Manson, J. I., Constantinou, J. E. C., McIntosh, A., & Berkovic, S. F. (1995). Autosomal dominant nocturnal frontal lobe epilepsy: A distinctive clinical disorder. *Brain*, *118*(1), 61–73. DOI: 10.1093/brain/118.1.61 PMID: 7895015

Schmatz, R., Mazzanti, C. M., Spanevello, R., Stefanello, N., Gutierres, J., Corrêa, M., et al. (2009). Resveratrol prevents memory deficits and the increase in acetylcholinesterase activity in streptozotocin-induced diabetic rats. *European Journal of Pharmacology, 610*(1), 42-48. DOI: 10.1016/j.ejphar.2009.04.019

Schöll, M., Maass, A., Mattsson, N., Ashton, N. J., Blennow, K., Zetterberg, H., & Hansson, O. (2019). Biomarkers for tau pathology. *Molecular and Cellular Neurosciences*, *97*, 18–33. DOI: 10.1016/j.mcn.2018.12.001 PMID: 30529601

Setyorini, D., & Antarlina, S. S. (2022). Secondary metabolites in sorghum and its characteristics. *Food Science and Technology (Campinas)*, *42*, e49822. DOI: 10.1590/fst.49822

Shankar, E., Goel, A., Gupta, K., & Gupta, S. (2017). Plant flavone apigenin: An emerging anticancer agent. *Current Pharmacology Reports*, *3*(6), 423–446. DOI: 10.1007/s40495-017-0113-2 PMID: 29399439

Sharma, S., & Dang, S. (2023). Nanocarrier-based drug delivery to the brain: Interventions of surface modification. *CN, 21*(3), 517–535. DOI: 10.1016/j.jnn.2023.03.004

Shaygannejad, V., Janghorbani, M., Ashtari, F., Zanjani, H. A., & Zakizade, N. (2008). Effects of rivastigmine on memory and cognition in multiple sclerosis. *The Canadian Journal of Neurological Sciences*, *35*(4), 476–481. DOI: 10.1017/S0317167100009148 PMID: 18973065

Shi, Y., & Holtzman, D. M. (2018). Interplay between innate immunity and Alzheimer disease: APOE and TREM2 in the spotlight. *Nature Reviews. Immunology*, *18*(12), 759–772. DOI: 10.1038/s41577-018-0051-1 PMID: 30140051

Shoji, Y., & Nakashima, H. (2004). Nutraceutics and delivery systems. *Journal of Drug Targeting*, *12*(6), 385–391. DOI: 10.1080/10611860400003817 PMID: 15545088

Singh, B., & Sharma, R. A. (2015). Plant terpenes: Defense responses, phylogenetic analysis, regulation and clinical applications. *3 Biotech, 5*(2), 129–151. https://doi.org/DOI: 10.1007/s13205-015-0279-6

Singh, P. K., Nath, R., Naraian, R., & Gupta, M. K. (2020). Structural and functional aspects of muscarinic receptors in correlation with anticholinergic drugs. In Singh, D. B., & Tripathi, T. (Eds.), *Frontiers in protein structure, function, and dynamics* (pp. 317–338). Springer., DOI: 10.1007/978-981-15-5530-5_13

Somova, L. I., Shode, F. O., Ramnanan, P., & Nadar, A. (2003). Antihypertensive, antiatherosclerotic and antioxidant activity of triterpenoids isolated from *Olea europaea* subspecies *africana* leaves. *Journal of Ethnopharmacology*, *84*(2–3), 299–305. DOI: 10.1016/S0378-8741(02)00332-X PMID: 12648829

Souza, A. C. P., Gurak, P. D., & Marczak, L. D. F. (2017). Maltodextrin, pectin, and soy protein isolate as carrier agents in the encapsulation of anthocyanins-rich extract from jaboticaba pomace. *Food and Bioproducts Processing*, *102*, 186–194. DOI: 10.1016/j.fbp.2016.12.012

Subhan, S., Zeeshan, M., Rahman, A. U., & Yaseen, M. (2024). Fundamentals of polyphenols: Nomenclature, classification and properties. In Verma, C. (Ed.), *Science and engineering of polyphenols* (1st ed., pp. 1–36). Wiley., DOI: 10.1002/9781394203932.ch1

Sun, M., Su, X., Ding, B., He, X., Liu, X., Yu, A., et al. (2012). Advances in nanotechnology-based delivery systems for curcumin. *Nanomedicine, 7*(7), 1085-1100. DOI: 10.2217/nnm.12.48

Sung, B., Chung, H. Y., & Kim, N. D. (2016). Role of apigenin in cancer prevention via the induction of apoptosis and autophagy. *Journal of Cancer Prevention*, *21*(4), 216–226. DOI: 10.15430/JCP.2016.21.4.216 PMID: 28053955

Suri, S., Singh, A., & Nema, P. K. (2023). Bioactive compounds in citrus fruits: Extraction and identification. In Singh Purewal, S., Punia Bangar, S., & Kaur, P. (Eds.), *Recent advances in citrus fruits* (pp. 427–450). Springer., https://link.springer.com/10.1007/978-3-031-37534-7_14 DOI: 10.1007/978-3-031-37534-7_14

Sutherland, B. A., Rahman, R. M., & Appleton, I. (2006). Mechanisms of action of green tea catechins, with a focus on ischemia-induced neurodegeneration. *The Journal of Nutritional Biochemistry*, *17*(5), 291–306. DOI: 10.1016/j.jnutbio.2005.10.005 PMID: 16443357

Szeja, W., Grynkiewicz, G., & Rusin, A.Synthesis and Biological Activity. (2017). Isoflavones, their glycosides and glycoconjugates: Synthesis and biological activity. *Current Organic Chemistry*, *21*(3), 218–235. DOI: 10.2174/1385272820666160928120822 PMID: 28553156

Tanzi, R. E. (2012). The genetics of Alzheimer disease. *Cold Spring Harbor Perspectives in Medicine*, *2*(10), a006296. DOI: 10.1101/cshperspect.a006296 PMID: 23028126

Tchekalarova, J., & Tzoneva, R. (2023). Oxidative stress and aging as risk factors for Alzheimer's disease and Parkinson's disease: The role of the antioxidant melatonin. *International Journal of Molecular Sciences*, *24*(3), 3022. DOI: 10.3390/ijms24033022 PMID: 36769340

Tunon, M. J., Garcia-Mediavilla, M. V., Sanchez-Campos, S., & González-Gallego, J. (2009). Potential of flavonoids as anti-inflammatory agents: Modulation of pro-inflammatory gene expression and signal transduction pathways. *Current Drug Metabolism*, *10*(3), 256–271. DOI: 10.2174/138920009787846369 PMID: 19442088

Tzeng, N. S., Chung, C. H., Lin, F. H., Chiang, C. P., Yeh, C. B., Huang, S. Y., Lu, R.-B., Chang, H.-A., Kao, Y.-C., Yeh, H.-W., Chiang, W.-S., Chou, Y.-C., Tsao, C.-H., Wu, Y.-F., & Chien, W. C. (2018). Anti-herpetic medications and reduced risk of dementia in patients with herpes simplex virus infections—A nationwide, population-based cohort study in Taiwan. *Neurotherapeutics; the Journal of the American Society for Experimental NeuroTherapeutics*, *15*(2), 417–429. DOI: 10.1007/s13311-018-0611-x PMID: 29488144

Van Den Bosch, L., Van Damme, P., Bogaert, E., & Robberecht, W. (2006). The role of excitotoxicity in the pathogenesis of amyotrophic lateral sclerosis. *Biochimica et Biophysica Acta (BBA) -. Biochimica et Biophysica Acta. Molecular Basis of Disease*, *1762*(11–12), 1068–1082. DOI: 10.1016/j.bbadis.2006.05.002 PMID: 16806844

Velderrain-Rodríguez, G. R., Palafox-Carlos, H., Wall-Medrano, A., Ayala-Zavala, J. F., Chen, C. O., Robles-Sánchez, M., Astiazaran-García, H., Alvarez-Parrilla, E., & González-Aguilar, G. A. (2014). Phenolic compounds: Their journey after intake. *Food & Function*, *5*(2), 189–197. DOI: 10.1039/C3FO60361J PMID: 24336740

Venegas, C., & Heneka, M. T. (2017). Danger-associated molecular patterns in Alzheimer's disease. *Journal of Leukocyte Biology*, *101*(1), 87–98. DOI: 10.1189/jlb.3MR0416-204R PMID: 28049142

Voet, S., Srinivasan, S., Lamkanfi, M., & Van Loo, G. (2019, April 23). Inflammasomes in neuroinflammatory and neurodegenerative diseases. *EMBO Molecular Medicine*, *11*(6), e10248. Advance online publication. DOI: 10.15252/emmm.201810248 PMID: 31015277

Voet, S., Srinivasan, S., Lamkanfi, M., & Van Loo, G. (2019). Inflammasomes in neuroinflammatory and neurodegenerative diseases. *EMBO Molecular Medicine*, *11*(6), e10248. DOI: 10.15252/emmm.201810248 PMID: 31015277

Wagner, K. H., & Elmadfa, I. (2003). Biological relevance of terpenoids: Overview focusing on mono-, di- and tetraterpenes. *Annals of Nutrition and Metabolism, 47*(3–4), 95–106. DOI: 10.1159/000073377

Wang, B., Wang, Q., Yuan, R., Yang, S., Lu, M., Yuan, F., Dong, Z., Mo, M., Pan, Q., & Gao, H. (2023). Prenylated chromones and flavonoids isolated from the roots of *Flemingia macrophylla* and their anti-lung cancer activity. *Chinese Medicine*, *18*(1), 153. DOI: 10.1186/s13020-023-00860-3 PMID: 37996917

Wang, Y., Huang, M., Zhou, X., Li, H., Ma, X., & Sun, C. (2024). Potential of natural flavonoids to target breast cancer angiogenesis [Review]. *British Journal of Pharmacology*. Advance online publication. DOI: 10.1111/bph.16275 PMID: 37940117

Wang, Y., Wang, W., Li, Z., Hao, S., & Wang, B. (2016). A novel perspective on neuron study: Damaging and promoting effects in different neurons induced by mechanical stress. *Biomechanics and Modeling in Mechanobiology*, *15*(5), 1019–1027. DOI: 10.1007/s10237-015-0743-4 PMID: 26591000

White, H. S. (1999). Comparative anticonvulsant and mechanistic profile of the established and newer antiepileptic drugs. *Epilepsia*, *40*(s5). Advance online publication. DOI: 10.1111/j.1528-1157.1999.tb00913.x PMID: 10530688

Whone, A. L. (2022). Monoclonal antibody therapy in Parkinson's disease—The End? *New England Journal of Medicine, 387*(5), 466–467. https://doi.org/DOI: 10.1056/NEJMp2203904

Wilson, D. M.III, Cookson, M. R., Van Den Bosch, L., Zetterberg, H., Holtzman, D. M., & Dewachter, I. (2023). Hallmarks of neurodegenerative diseases. *Cell*, *186*(4), 693–714. DOI: 10.1016/j.cell.2022.12.032 PMID: 36803602

Wu, X., Xie, J., Qiu, L., Zou, L., Huang, Y., Xie, Y., Xu, H., He, S., & Zhang, Q. (2021). The anti-inflammatory and analgesic activities of the ethyl acetate extract of *Viburnum taitoense* Hayata. *Journal of Ethnopharmacology*, *269*, 113742. DOI: 10.1016/j.jep.2020.113742 PMID: 33359186

Xie, L., Roto, A. V., & Bolling, B. W. (2012). Characterization of ellagitannins, gallotannins, and bound proanthocyanidins from California almond (Prunus dulcis) varieties. *Journal of Agricultural and Food Chemistry*, *60*(49), 12151–12156. DOI: 10.1021/jf303673r PMID: 23167850

Xing, S. H., Zhu, C. X., Zhang, R., & An, L. (2014). Huperzine A in the treatment of Alzheimer's disease and vascular dementia: A meta-analysis. *Evidence-Based Complementary and Alternative Medicine : eCAM*, *2014*(1), 363985. DOI: 10.1155/2014/363985 PMID: 24639880

Xu, B., Watkins, R., Wu, L., Zhang, C., & Davis, R. (2015). Natural product-based nanomedicine: Recent advances and issues. *International Journal of Nanomedicine, 10*, 6055-6070. https://doi.org/DOI: 10.2147/IJN.S90773

Xu, Z., Chen, S., Li, X., Luo, G., Li, L., & Le, W. (2006). Neuroprotective effects of (-)-epigallocatechin-3-gallate in a transgenic mouse model of amyotrophic lateral sclerosis. *Neurochemical Research*, *31*(10), 1263–1269. DOI: 10.1007/s11064-006-9166-z PMID: 17021948

Yahfoufi, N., Alsadi, N., Jambi, M., & Matar, C. (2018). The immunomodulatory and anti-inflammatory role of polyphenols. *Nutrients*, *10*(11), 1618. DOI: 10.3390/nu10111618 PMID: 30400131

Yan, Y., Jiang, W., Liu, L., Wang, X., Ding, C., Tian, Z., & Sun, B. (2015). Dopamine controls systemic inflammation through inhibition of NLRP3 inflammasome. *Cell*, *160*(1–2), 62–73. DOI: 10.1016/j.cell.2014.11.047 PMID: 25594175

Yang, L., Mao, K., Yu, H., & Chen, J. (2020). Neuroinflammatory responses and Parkinson's disease: Pathogenic mechanisms and therapeutic targets. *Journal of Neuroimmune Pharmacology*, *15*(4), 830–837. DOI: 10.1007/s11481-020-09926-7 PMID: 32529463

Yang, L. Y., Lei, S. Z., Xu, W. J., Lai, Y., Zhang, Y., Wang, Y., & Wang, Z.-L. (2025). Rising above: Exploring the therapeutic potential of natural product-based compounds in human cancer treatment. *Traditional Medicine Research, 10*(3), 18. DOI: 10.53388/TMR20240618001

Yang, X. B., & Huang, Y. (2020). Protective effects of apigenin, apigenin-8-sulfonate, and apigenin-3′,8-disulfonate on D-galactosamine-induced acute liver damage in mice. *Medicinal Chemistry Research, 29*(10), 1867–1873. DOI: 10.1007/s00044-020-02608-2

Ying, J. Y., Zhang, M. M., Qiu, X. Y., & Lu, Y. (2018). The potential of herb medicines in the treatment of esophageal cancer. *Retrieved March 2, 2025*.

Zeng, T., Song, Y., Qi, S., Zhang, R., Xu, L., & Xiao, P. (2023). A comprehensive review of vine tea: Origin, research on materia medica, phytochemistry and pharmacology. *Journal of Ethnopharmacology, 317*, 116788. DOI: 10.1016/j.jep.2023.116788 PMID: 37343650

Zhang, B., Safa, R., Rusciano, D., & Osborne, N. N. (2007). Epigallocatechin gallate, an active ingredient from green tea, attenuates damaging influences to the retina caused by ischemia/reperfusion. *Brain Research, 1159*, 40–53. DOI: 10.1016/j.brainres.2007.05.029 PMID: 17573045

Zhang, W., Xiao, D., Mao, Q., & Xia, H. (2023). Role of neuroinflammation in neurodegeneration development. *Signal Transduction and Targeted Therapy, 8*(1), 267. DOI: 10.1038/s41392-023-01486-5 PMID: 37433768

Zhao, L., Hou, L., Sun, H., Yan, X., Sun, X., Li, J., Bian, Y., Chu, Y., & Liu, Z. (2011). Apigenin isolated from the medicinal plant *Elsholtzia rugulosa* prevents β-amyloid 25-35-induced toxicity in rat cerebral microvascular endothelial cells. *Molecules (Basel, Switzerland), 16*(5), 4005–4019. DOI: 10.3390/molecules16054005

Zhao, L., Wang, J. L., Liu, R., Li, X. X., Li, J. F., & Zhang, L. (2013). Neuroprotective, anti-amyloidogenic and neurotrophic effects of apigenin in an Alzheimer's disease mouse model. *Molecules (Basel, Switzerland), 18*(8), 9949–9965. DOI: 10.3390/molecules18089949 PMID: 23966081

Zhou, Y., Lu, M., Du, R. H., Qiao, C., Jiang, C. Y., Zhang, K. Z., Ding, J.-H., & Hu, W. (2016). MicroRNA-7 targets Nod-like receptor protein 3 inflammasome to modulate neuroinflammation in the pathogenesis of Parkinson's disease. *Molecular Neurodegeneration, 11*(1), 28. DOI: 10.1186/s13024-016-0094-3 PMID: 27084336

Zia-Ul-Haq, M. (2021). Historical and introductory aspects of carotenoids. In Zia-Ul-Haq, M., Dewanjee, S., & Riaz, M. (Eds.), *Carotenoids: Structure and function in the human body* (pp. 1–42). Springer International Publishing., DOI: 10.1007/978-3-030-46459-2_1

Chapter 6
Unveiling the Anti-Inflammatory and Immunomodulatory Effects of Secondary Metabolites

Chitralekha Kataki
https://orcid.org/0000-0001-5375-164X
Assam Down Town University, India

ABSTRACT

Inflammation and immune modulation are critical for the body's defense against infection, injury, and stress, but chronic inflammation underlies many diseases, including autoimmune disorders, metabolic diseases, and neurodegenerative conditions. Secondary metabolites—bioactive compounds from plants and organisms—offer promising anti-inflammatory and immunomodulatory effects. These include alkaloids, flavonoids, terpenoids, and polyphenols, which can inhibit pro-inflammatory cytokines, reduce oxidative stress, and modulate immune cell function. For example, compounds like curcumin, quercetin, and resveratrol target inflammatory pathways such as NF-κB and COX-2. These natural agents often have fewer side effects compared to conventional drugs, making them appealing for treating inflammation-driven diseases. The growing evidence suggests secondary metabolites could provide safer, effective alternatives to traditional anti-inflammatory treatments, offering hope for more natural therapies with broad applications.

DOI: 10.4018/979-8-3693-9112-9.ch006

INTRODUCTION

Metabolism is defined as the sum of all biochemical reactions occurring within an organism. Metabolites, which are intermediates and products of metabolism, are generally small molecules. In 1891, A. Kossel introduced the term "secondary" to distinguish secondary metabolites from primary ones. Unlike primary metabolites—found in every actively dividing cell and essential for basic cellular function—secondary metabolites are present only incidentally and are not crucial for the immediate survival of an organism. Although secondary metabolites are derived from primary metabolic pathways, they do not constitute the fundamental molecular structure of the organism. Their absence does not directly threaten life, unlike primary metabolites, yet their presence significantly enhances survival, especially in ecologically disadvantaged species within a phylogenetic group (Tiwari and Rana, 2015). Secondary metabolites, or natural products, are a diverse group of metabolic compounds that, while not essential for the vegetative growth of the organisms that produce them, play key roles in adaptation. Secondary metabolites represent a remarkably diverse range of natural compounds produced by plants, fungi, bacteria, algae, and animals. These metabolites, which include terpenes, phenolic compounds, and alkaloids, are typically classified according to their biosynthetic pathways. Often, specific classes of these compounds are found only within certain phylogenetic groups, reflecting their unique evolutionary roles (Roze, Chanda, and Linz, 2011). They function as differentiation compounds, supporting ecological interactions by acting as defence agents, signalling molecules, and mediators in processes like symbiosis, metal transport, and competition. Humankind harnesses the vast array of secondary metabolites to enhance health (such as antibiotics, enzyme inhibitors, immunomodulators, antitumor agents, and growth promoters for animals and plants), expand nutritional benefits (through pigments and nutraceuticals), and boost agricultural productivity (including pesticides, insecticides, ecological competitors, symbiotic effectors, and pheromones). These applications have a positive economic impact on society by supporting health, nutrition, and agricultural industries (Demain and Fang, 2000).

Inflammation is a complex physiological response driven by signalling molecules released by immune cells such as leukocytes, macrophages, and mast cells. This response, along with complement factor activation, leads to fluid and protein leakage (edema) and the accumulation of leukocytes at the site of inflammation. The inflammatory response generally serves a protective role, helping to eliminate both the cause of tissue injury and its resulting effects, thus supporting the body's defence mechanisms (White, 1999 and Charles and Catherine, 2011). Anti-inflammatory drugs are generally divided into two main types: steroidal and non-steroidal anti-inflammatory drugs (NSAIDs). Steroidal drugs work by targeting inflammatory cells and mediators, while NSAIDs reduce inflammation by inhibiting the enzymes Cyclooxygenase 1 and 2 (COX-1 and COX-2). Secondary metabolites from plants have been a key source of medicines since ancient times, with about half of today's active drugs derived from natural sources. Many of these herbal compounds are widely used to treat inflammatory conditions (Mona et al.,2014).

With a growing understanding of immune cell communication, researchers have developed ways to influence these signalling pathways, allowing for targeted adjustments in immune responses. By focusing on specific immune cell types—such as neutrophils, macrophages, natural killer (NK) cells, or lymphocytes—and modulating cytokine production, it is possible to regulate immune activity. This process, known as immunomodulation, can generally be categorized into immunosuppressive or immunostimulatory approaches (Eduardo et al., 2022). Immunomodulatory drugs adjust the immune system's activity by either boosting (immunostimulators) or reducing (immunosuppressives) the production of antibodies. Immunostimulators are used to strengthen the immune response in cases of infections, tumours, immune deficiencies, and antibody transfer issues. Conversely, immunosuppressive drugs help lower immune activity to prevent organ transplant rejection and manage autoimmune conditions like pemphigus, lupus, and allergies (Bascones et al., 2014).

Inflammation and immune malfunctioning are key contributors to the pathophysiology of innumerable chronic diseases. Although conventional drugs provide some relief, they are often accompanied by side effects and limited efficacy. As a result, there has been growing attention in exploring natural alternatives. In this context, secondary metabolites from plants and other organisms increasingly being recognized as valuable therapeutic agents due to their multifaceted biological activities. This chapter explores the miscellaneous array of such metabolites, focusing on their anti-inflammatory and immunomodulatory potential along with the underlying molecular mechanisms involved.

UNDERSTANDING INFLAMMATION AND IMMUNE RESPONSE

Inflammation:

Inflammation arises from the coordinated involvement of numerous vasoactive, chemotactic, and proliferative factors at various stages, providing multiple targets for anti-inflammatory intervention. A key component of the inflammatory process is the arachidonic acid (AA) pathway. Arachidonic acid is quickly released from damaged cellular membranes by the enzyme phospholipase A2 (PLA2). Once released, arachidonic acid is acted upon by cyclooxygenases (COX-1 and COX-2), producing prostaglandin G2 (PGG2). Through a subsequent peroxidase reaction,

PGG2 is reduced to PGH2, which can then be converted by various enzymes into several active compounds, including prostaglandins (PGD2, PGE2, PGF2α), prostacyclin (PGI2), and thromboxane (THA2). These prostaglandins are central to inflammation, as they not only drive the inflammatory response necessary for healing but also contribute to pain and fever. Additionally, they aid in blood clotting and protect the stomach lining from acid damage. The lipoxygenase (LOX) pathway is another powerful mediator of inflammation. Lipoxygenase enzymes (LOX) catalyse the incorporation of molecular oxygen into specific positions on arachidonic acid—namely, the 5-, 12-, or 15-carbon positions—resulting in the formation of 5-LOX, 12-LOX, and 15-LOX, respectively. The main products of this pathway are 5S-, 12S-, or 15S-hydroperoxyeicosatetraenoic acid (5-, 12-, or 15-HPETE), which can then be further reduced by glutathione peroxidase to their hydroxy derivatives: 5-, 8-, 12-, and 15-HETE, respectively (Pushpangadan, Ijinu and George, 2015). NF-κB is located in the cell cytoplasm, where it is bound to inhibitory IκB proteins that prevent its movement into the nucleus by blocking its nuclear localization signal. When exposed to certain stimuli, IκB proteins are degraded, allowing NF-κB to enter the nucleus and activate the expression of genes that promote inflammation (Gupta et al., 2001, Wang et al., 2004 and Maroon, Bost and Maroon, 2010). This activation includes the transcription of pro-inflammatory cytokines (e.g., IL-1, IL-2, IL-6, TNF-α), chemokines (e.g., IL-8, MIP-1α, MCP-1, RANTES, eotaxin), adhesion molecules (e.g., ICAM, VCAM, E-selectin), inducible enzymes (e.g., COX-2, iNOS), growth factors, acute phase proteins, and immune receptors. Together, these factors play essential roles in regulating inflammatory processes (Barnes and Karin, 1997 and Ghosh and Karin, 2002). Proinflammatory molecules, together with chemokines and various co-stimulatory molecules, aid in recruiting effector cells like monocytes and neutrophils to sites of disturbance. Neutrophils then generate a cytotoxic environment by releasing harmful substances from cytoplasmic granules, a process called degranulation. This rapid release demands both glucose and oxygen, initiating a respiratory burst. The toxic chemicals released, including reactive oxygen species (ROS), reactive nitrogen species (RNS), and a variety of proteinases, are highly destructive to both pathogens and host tissues. This action ultimately liquefies surrounding tissue, helping to prevent microbial spread. These interactions collectively result in the classic cardinal signs of local inflammation: heat, swelling, redness, pain, and loss of function (Nathan, 2002 and Ashley, Weil and Nelson, 2012).

IMMUNOMODULATION:

Immunomodulation refers to any alteration in the immune response, which may involve inducing, expressing, amplifying, or inhibiting various components or phases of immunity. An immunomodulatory substance is used specifically for its effects on the immune system. Immunomodulators are generally classified into two types based on their effects: immunostimulators and immunosuppressants. Specific immunomodulators, called immunological adjuvants, are often administered with antigens to enhance the immune response to vaccine components. Immunostimulators are inherently nonspecific, designed to enhance the body's resistance to infections. They can function through both innate and adaptive immune responses. In healthy individuals, immunostimulants are intended to act as prophylactic and promoter agents, serving as immunopotentiators by boosting the baseline immune response. In individuals with impaired immune responses, they function as immunotherapeutic agents. Immunosuppressants form a structurally and functionally diverse group, often administered in combination regimens to manage organ transplant rejection and treat various autoimmune diseases. Immunoadjuvants are used to enhance vaccine efficacy and can therefore be considered specific immune stimulants, with Freund's adjuvant being a notable example. Immunoadjuvants hold significant potential as true modulators of immune response. They are proposed for use in guiding the immune system towards specific pathways, such as cellular versus humoral immunity, Th1 versus Th2 responses, or immunoprotective versus immunodestructive effects. Additionally, they may help direct the immune response toward IgE or IgG production—a challenge for vaccine developers (Singune, Vaghela and Sisodia, 2018).

ANTI-INFLAMMATORY AND IMMUNOMODULATORY DRUG

The most commonly used drug for management of inflammatory conditions are steroidal and non-steroidal anti-inflammatory drugs (NSAIDs). Both steroidal and non-steroidal anti-inflammatory drugs (NSAIDs) appear to inhibit the production of pro-inflammatory prostaglandins (PGs) across various biological systems, including cultured cells and isolated tissues under appropriate incubation conditions. Glucocorticoids seem to suppress PG production or release by inhibiting phospholipase A2 activity or potentially through other unknown mechanisms. NSAIDs, such as indomethacin, inhibit PG synthesis by blocking cyclooxygenase 1 and 2 (COX- 1 and COX-2). However, it remains unclear whether the reduction in PG production or release at the site of inflammation occurs in parallel with the inhibition of vascular permeability (Tsurufuji et al., 1980). Secondary metabolites have been a crucial source of medicinal compounds since ancient times, with nearly half of today's widely used drugs derived from natural sources. Many of these herbal constituents are commonly prescribed for treating inflammatory conditions (Mona et al., 2014). Immunomodulatory drugs are designed to modulate the immune system, either by boosting (immunostimulators) or suppressing (immunosuppressives) its response, affecting serum antibody production. Immunostimulators are typically prescribed to strengthen the immune response against infections, tumours, immunodeficiencies, and impaired antibody transfer. In contrast, immunosuppressive agents help diminish the immune response in conditions like organ transplantation and autoimmune diseases (e.g., pemphigus, lupus, and allergies) (Bascones, et al., 2014).

USES OF SECONDARY METABOLITES AS ANTI-INFLAMMATORY AND IMMUNOMODULATORY DRUG

Plant-derived compounds have long been utilized as anti- inflammatory and immunomodulatory drug, either in their natural or semi-synthetic forms. These plant secondary metabolites act as precursors, prototypes, or pharmacological tools for drug development. Despite advancements in drug discovery using molecular modelling, combinatorial chemistry, and synthetic methods, plant-based compounds continue to be an invaluable source of therapeutic agents. Numerous studies confirm that bioactive plant compounds offer protective effects against both acute and chronic inflammatory diseases. Traditionally, many plants have been used to treat inflammation, and isolated natural compounds from these plants often exhibit strong anti-inflammatory properties in both in vitro and in vivo animal studies. These compounds inhibit inflammatory pathways in mechanisms similar to those of NSAIDs. The anti-inflammatory effects of phytochemicals include (i) antioxidative properties and radical-scavenging activity, (ii) regulation of cellular functions in inflammation-related cells such as mast cells, macrophages, lymphocytes, and neutrophils, (iii) inhibition of proinflammatory enzyme activities, including PLA2, COX, LOX, and the NO-producing enzyme NOS, (iv) reduction of other proinflammatory molecule production, and (v) influence on the expression of proinflammatory genes (Pushpangadan, Ijinu and George, 2015). The immunosuppressive effects of plant secondary metabolites arise from their ability to interact with various molecular targets, enabling them to modulate the complex immune system through diverse mechanisms of action. A wide range of phytochemicals show potent immunomodulatory activity (Yuandani, et al., 2014). Outlined below are some powerful plant-derived bioactive compounds identified in recent years, along with the mechanisms underlying their anti-inflammatory and immunomodulatory effects.

Phenolic Compounds

Phenolic compounds hold significant pharmacological value, with some demonstrating anti-inflammatory effects. Various types, including flavonoids, condensed tannins, and gallotannins, are known to inhibit molecular targets involved in the production of pro-inflammatory mediators during inflammatory responses (Fawole, et al., 2009).

Flavonoids:

Flavonoids are a class of polyphenolic compounds widely found in plant-based foods. With over 4,000 identified varieties, flavonoids are classified into several groups, including flavonols, flavones, catechins, flavanones, anthocyanidins, and isoflavonoids. Flavonoids exhibit a wide range of biological effects across various mammalian cell systems, both in vitro and in vivo. Research has demonstrated their capabilities in antimicrobial, antiviral, and antiulcerogenic activities, as well as cytotoxic and antineoplastic effects. Additionally, they possess mutagenic, anti-inflammatory, antioxidant, antihepatotoxic, antihypertensive, hypolipidemic, and antiplatelet properties (Rodrigo et al., (2010). Flavonoids are recognized for their ability to modulate the inflammatory response through various pathways. They inhibit key molecules involved in inflammation, such as cyclooxygenase (COX), insulin, cytokines, nuclear factor-kappa B (NF-κB), and matrix metalloproteinases (Fawole, et al., 2009). A study in rats demonstrated that flavonoids exhibit significant activity in both the proliferative and exudative phases of inflammation. These compounds showed anti-inflammatory effects by inhibiting granuloma formation, especially when a catechol or guaiacol-like B ring was present in their structure. For instance, quercetin blocked both cyclooxygenase and lipoxygenase pathways at higher concentrations, while at lower concentrations, it primarily targeted the lipoxygenase pathway for its anti-inflammatory action. A micronized flavonoid complex containing 90% diosmin and 10% hesperidin (Daflon 500 mg) effectively protected against perivascular edema, with its therapeutic potential linked to its inhibition of inflammatory processes. Additionally, subcutaneous administration of hesperidin (hesperetin-7-rutinoside) significantly reduced rat paw edema induced by carrageenan and dextran, as well as carrageenan-induced pleurisy, without causing the side effects associated with other anti-inflammatory drugs. Furthermore, studies have shown that flavonoids like rutin (quercetin-3-rutinoside) and quercetin also exhibit antioxidant properties (Fawole, et al., 2009). Dioclein, a flavonoid from the flavanone family, is derived from the roots of *Dioclea grandiflora* Mart. ex Benth. It has been shown to significantly inhibit the production of key pro-inflammatory mediators, including IL-6, TNF-α, CXCL1/KC, CCL2/JE, and nitric oxide (NO), in LPS-stimulated macrophages in vitro. Dioclein also demonstrates notable reactive oxygen species (ROS) scavenging activity in both macrophages and cell-free systems, with its anti-inflammatory effects partly attributed to reduced ROS levels in the medium. This unique combination of actions makes dioclein a distinct anti-inflammatory agent among flavonoids (Chen et al., 2011). The anti-inflammatory effects of 30 flavonoids isolated from various plants of the Compositae (Asteraceae) family were assessed using carrageenan-induced paw edema in mice and cotton pellet-induced granuloma in rats. The results indicated that flavonoids, particularly those with a catechol or guaiacol-like B ring, effectively inhibited granuloma formation, with jaceosidin emerging as the most active compound among those tested (Jeon et al., 2010). Among the compounds isolated from the roots of *Sophora flavescens*, prenylated flavonoids such as sophoraflavanone G, kuraridin, and kurarinone have been shown to inhibit eicosanoid-producing enzymes, including COX-1, COX-2, 5-lipoxygenase (5-LOX), and 12-LOX. Sophoraflavanone G demonstrated in vivo anti-inflammatory effects in various animal models through both oral and topical applications. Additionally, kurarinone was found to inhibit chemotaxis induced by monocyte chemoattractant protein-1. These findings collectively suggest that the prenylated flavonoid-enriched fraction from *Sophora flavescens* possesses significant anti-inflammatory potential (Li et al., 2011).

Flavonoids also have the potential to impact immune responses and may act as immunomodulators. A study on treatment of quercetin on dendritic cells (DCs) obtained from mouse bone marrow showed that this flavonoid can effectively reduce the production of pro-inflammatory cytokines and chemokines, as well as the expression of MHC class II and co-stimulatory molecules, thereby inhibiting lipopolysaccharide (LPS) induced activation of dendritic cells (DCs). Additionally, quercetin treatment has been shown to decrease both the endocytosis of DCs and their LPS-induced migration (Sun et al., 2015). In a study investigating airway allergic inflammation, the effects of quercetin-loaded micro-emulsion (QU-ME) were assessed in mice given daily oral doses of QU-ME (3 or 10 mg/kg) for 22 days. Compared to the control group, QU-ME treatment reduced inflammatory markers IL-5 and IL-4, though CCL11, IFN-gamma, and LTB levels remained unchanged. Additionally, oral QU-ME inhibited nuclear transcription factor kappa B (NF-kappa B) activation, reduced P-selectin expression, and suppressed mucus production in the lungs (Rogerio et al., 2010). In a study on peripheral blood mononuclear cells (PBMC) from multiple sclerosis (MS) patients and healthy subjects, Sternberg et al. demonstrated that quercetin reduced PBMC proliferation and modulated IL-1β and TNF-α levels in a dose-dependent manner. Additionally, the modulation of TNF-α was enhanced when quercetin was combined with human interferon-beta (IFN-β) (Sternberg et al., 2008). In a mouse model of asthma, Gupta et al. investigated quercetin's potential to alleviate asthma symptoms, revealing its promising anti-asthmatic effects. Quercetin treatment significantly reduced specific immunoglobulin E (sIgE) levels and signs of anaphylaxis. Additionally, quercetin modulated Th2 cytokines, including IL-4 and IL-5, which are involved in IgE class switching and the suppression of various chemical mediators (PGD2, mMCPT-1, Cys-L, and TSLP) released from activated mast cells (Gupta et al., 2016).

Luteolin (3′,4′,5,7-tetrahydroxyflavone) and its glycosylated form luteolin-7-glucoside (L7G) belong to the flavone subclass of flavonoids have beneficial effects on the modulation of immune responses though the mechanisms of this action are not clearly known. Apigenin, scientifically known as 4′,5,7-trihydroxyflavone, is a widely occurring dietary flavonoid found in various fruits, vegetables, and herbs, including oranges, grapefruits, onions, wheat sprouts, parsley, celery, and chamomile tea (Hosseinzade et al., 2019). In an experimental study, Cardenas et al. demonstrated that Apigenin notably influenced NF-kB activity within lung tissue, highlighting its potential for organ-specific immune regulation (Cardenas et al., 2016). In a separate study using rat models of colitis, treatment with apigenin K, a soluble form of Apigenin, led to decreased inflammation, reduced colonic damage scores, and a lower colonic weight-to-length ratio (Wang et al., 2017). In an experimental study on asthma in mice, Li et al. found that administering Apigenin (at doses of 5 mg/kg and 10 mg/kg) suppressed OVA-induced increases in eosinophil count and Th17 cell levels. These results suggest that Apigenin could potentially slow asthma progression. Overall, Apigenin shows potential as a modulator of the immune system (Li and Zhang, 2013).

Research on Fisetin (3, 3′, 4′, 7-tetrahydroxy flavone), a type of flavonoid, and its impact on the immune system is limited, but Song et al. investigated its immunosuppressive effects on T-cell activation both in vitro and in vivo. Their findings revealed that Fisetin significantly reduced Th1 and Th2 cytokine production, cell cycle progression, and the CD4+/CD8+ T-cell ratio in vitro. Additionally, Fisetin inhibited mouse T lymphocytes by downregulating nuclear factor kappa B and nuclear factor of activated T cells signalling in a dose-dependent manner. In vivo, Fisetin was also found to reduce delayed-type hypersensitivity reactions in mice (Song et al., 2013). In an experimental study using a mouse model of atopic dermatitis (AD), Kim et al., in 2014 examined the effects of Fisetin on AD-like symptoms. Their results showed that Fisetin administration reduced the infiltration of inflammatory cells, including eosinophils, mast cells, and CD4+ and CD8+ T cells. Additionally, Fisetin suppressed cytokines and chemokines linked to skin inflammation in AD-like lesions. In a dose-dependent manner, Fisetin decreased CD4+ T cell-induced production of interferon-gamma and interleukin-4 while increasing the anti-inflammatory cytokine interleukin-10 (Pathak et al., 2016). A study investigating Fisetin's effects on human mast cells (HMC-1) found that Fisetin could reduce mast cell activation (Park et al., 2009). Based on these findings,

Fisetin has a notable impact on immune system responses. Genistein and daidzein are the key bioactive isoflavones, predominantly found in soybeans and soy-based products. Genistein was found to inhibit the activation of STAT-1 and NF-κB. It also reduced the production of NO and PGE2 by suppressing the expression of iNOS and COX-2 (Kyong et al., 2009). Additionally, genistein significantly diminished the release and expression of inflammatory cytokines, such as IL-1β and TNF-α, which were elevated by LPS stimulation. Genistein and daidzein were found to lower serum concentrations of TNF-α, IL-6, adiponectin, and leptin, leading to significant improvement in rheumatoid arthritis symptoms. Additionally, pre-treatment with daidzein notably reduced TNF-α-induced lung inflammation and inhibited CxCl2 expression in lung tissues, as well as in MLE-12 cells in vitro. The study demonstrated that daidzein significantly inhibited both the production of NO and IL-6, as well as their mRNA expression, in LPS-treated RAW264.7 cells (Pushpangadan, Ijinu and George, 2015).

Condensed tannins:

Condensed tannins, or proanthocyanidins, are primarily composed of derivatives of gallocatechin, epicatechin, catechin, and epigallocatechin. Proanthocyanidins are linked to various biological activities, including anti-inflammatory, anti-asthmatic, anticancer, antimicrobial, anti-allergic, antihypertensive, and cardioprotective effects. Their positive impact on human health is largely due to their potent free radical-scavenging and antioxidant properties. Additionally, these compounds act as antagonists to specific hormone receptors and inhibit certain enzymes, such as COX enzymes (Mona, et al., 2014). Supplementing the diet with 1.5% condensed tannins from a mixture of *F. infectoria* and *P. guajava* leaves significantly enhanced both humoral and cell-mediated immune responses while reducing fecal egg counts (FECs) in sheep infected with *H. contortus* (Pathak et al., 2016). Recent studies have shown that plant tannins exert anti-inflammatory effects by inhibiting nitric oxide (NO) and prostaglandin E2 (PGE2) production. Tannins extracted from various plants generally exhibit anti-inflammatory properties. For instance, an in vitro study using obese Zucker rats demonstrated that grape seed procyanidin extract can reduce obesity-induced inflammation by regulating cytokine expression. Additionally, the tannin fraction from black raspberry seed extract has been shown to reduce LPS-induced nitric oxide (NO) production in RAW 264.7 cells, highlighting its anti-inflammatory potential. This anti-inflammatory activity has also been confirmed in a croton oil-induced ear edema mouse model. It is believed that the anti-inflammatory effects of tannins from various sources may arise from their ability to regulate cytokine expression, decrease the production of inflammatory mediators, and enhance their interaction with other molecules (Zhenkai et al., 2022).

Gallotannins:

Gallotannins exhibit a range of biological effects, including anti-inflammatory, anticancer, and antiviral properties. Their anti-inflammatory mechanisms involve scavenging free radicals and inhibiting the expression of inflammatory mediators, such as certain cytokines, inducible nitric oxide synthase (iNOS), and COX-2. Notably, a high concentration of gallotannins has been found in the leaves of Protea simplex (Fawole et al., 2009).

Ellagic acid:

Ellagic acid, phenolic acid is considered a promising therapeutic agent for inflammation associated with acute lung injury by reducing COX-2-induced exacerbation. It also inhibits several cell-signalling pathways critical to tumour growth, including inflammatory pathways such as TNF-α-induced COX-2 protein expression and NOS inhibition. Ellagic acid-rich pomegranate juice (*Punica granatum*) significantly reduced TNF-α-induced COX-2 protein expression in human colon cancer cells. Additionally, ellagitannins and punicalagin from *P. granatum* have been shown to inhibit cancer cell proliferation and promote apoptosis by modulating the NF-κB signalling pathway and suppressing NF-κB-regulated gene expression (Adams et al., 2006 and Chiang, et al., 2003).

Epigallocatechin-3-gallate:

The compound (-)-epigallocatechin-3-gallate (EGCG), a predominant catechin found in *Camellia sinensis*, has demonstrated significant anti-inflammatory and cancer chemo preventive properties across various models, including animal tumor bioassays, cell culture systems, and epidemiological studies (Ahmad, Gupta and Mukhtar, 2000 and Le, 2002). The anti-inflammatory effects of EGCG are mediated through the activation of AMPK, which has been shown to suppress the production of several key proinflammatory mediators, including TNF-α, IL-1β, IL-6, MCP-1, iNOS, and COX-2 in response to LPS stimulation. Additional research indicates that EGCG inhibits IL-1β-induced NO production in human chondrocytes by uniquely interfering with NF-κB activation. Furthermore, EGCG has been found to inhibit metalloproteinase, COX-2, PGE2, MAPKs, and AP-1 in IL-1β-stimulated human osteoarthritic chondrocytes (Pushpangadan, Ijinu and George, 2015).

Tannic Acid:

Tannic acid, the simplest hydrolysable tannin is composed of a core glucose molecule connected to 10 galloyls by aliphatic ester bonds. The anti-inflammatory effects of tannic acid have been investigated using a formalin-induced paw edema model. The results showed that tannic acid inhibits edema, likely by reducing myeloperoxidase (MPO) enzyme activity; however, the exact molecular mechanism behind this action remains unclear. Additionally, numerous epidemiological studies indicate that tannic acid is effective in the external treatment of skin inflammation and injuries, and that its intake may help prevent the development of chronic diseases. Further studies have shown that tannic acid exerts a protective effect on retinal pigment epithelium cells against UVB radiation by modulating the inflammatory response. This protection is mediated through the IL-6/STAT3/CFB signalling pathway (Wang et al., 2022).

Coumarins

Coumarins are a large family of naturally occurring compounds found in plants. Research has shown that several coumarin derivatives exhibit significant anti-inflammatory and antioxidant activities, making them potentially effective for treating high-protein edema. Some coumarins have been identified for their ability to scavenge superoxide anion radicals, while others can inhibit both the lipoxygenase and cyclooxygenase pathways involved in arachidonic acid metabolism (Kyong et al., 2009). Stefanova TH et al. studied the immunomodulatory effect of coumarins against sarcoma 180 in mice and found that The immunomodulatory activity of coumarins enhances their direct cytostatic effects, highlighting their potential to act as immunostimulators when combined with other antitumor agents (Stefanova et al., 2007).

Alkaloids

Certain alkaloids, including isoquinoline, indole, and diterpene, are recognized for their strong anti-inflammatory properties. Bisbenzylisoquinoline, a type of alkaloids possesses anti-inflammatory, immunomodulatory and antimalarial activities. Recently, there has been growing interest in bisbenzylisoquinoline alkaloids as potential anti-inflammatory agents due to their ability to inhibit the synthesis or action of certain pro-inflammatory cytokines. Among these, tetrandrine, along with its analogues berbamine and fangchinoline, has been the focus of extensive research (Mona, et al., 2014). Bisbenzylisoquinoline alkaloids such as cepharanthine, cycleanine, and isotetrandrine, derived from *Stephania cephararantha*, demonstrated significant suppression of in vitro histamine release and nitric oxide production. Notably, cepharanthine was found to be a highly effective inhibitor of HIV replication in a chronically infected monocytic cell line and also reduced the production of inflammatory cytokines and neural cell death (Dongdong et al., 2011). Other alkaloids, including imperialine and chuanbeinone from *Bulbus Fritillariae Cirrhosae*, as well as imperialine, imperialine-β-N-oxide, isoverticine, and isoverticine-β-N-oxide from bulbus of *Fritillaria wabuensis*, along with berberine and 8-hydroxydihydrosanguinarine from *Chelidonium majus*, have demonstrated significant anti-inflammatory activity (Mona, et al., 2014). Berberine, isolated from *Berberis aristata*, has been shown to inhibit NF-κB activation induced by various inflammatory agents and carcinogens, as well as suppress constitutive NF-κB activation observed in certain tumor cells. This suppression occurs through the inhibition of IκB-α phosphorylation and degradation, mediated by the blockade of IκB kinase activation. As a result, berberine prevents the phosphorylation and nuclear translocation of p65, ultimately inhibiting NF-κB reporter activity. The inhibition of IκB kinase by berberine is direct and can be reversed by reducing agents. Furthermore, berberine reduces the expression of NF-κB-regulated genes involved in antiapoptosis, cell proliferation, inflammation, and invasion. Notably, the suppression of antiapoptotic gene products enhances apoptosis induced by TNF and chemotherapy agents and inhibits TNF-induced cellular invasion (Pandey, 2008). Amide alkaloids such as riparin I (N-benzoyl tyramine) and riparin II (N-(2-hydroxybenzoyl) tyramine), isolated from the unripe fruit of *Aniba riparia*, have been shown to reduce carrageenan-induced paw edema at 4 hours and 2 hours, respectively, compared to a control group (Ahmad, Gupta and Mukhtar, 2000 and Le, 2002). These findings suggest that the presence of a hydroxyl group on the benzoyl moiety enhances the anti-inflammatory activity of the compounds. A bisindolic alkaloid called caulerpin, isolated from the lipid extract of the algae *Caulerpa racemosa*, demonstrated anti-inflammatory activity in mice when administered orally at a dose of 100 μmol/kg (Souto et al., 2011).

Curcumin:

Curcuma longa has a long-standing history of use in Ayurvedic medicine for treating inflammatory conditions. The anti-inflammatory effects of curcumin, a highly versatile compound derived from this plant, are primarily mediated by its ability to inhibit COX-2, LOX, and iNOS. Dysregulated expression of COX-2 and/or iNOS has been linked to the pathophysiology of certain cancers and inflammatory disorders. Curcumin also downregulates the expression of various pro-inflammatory cytokines, including TNF-α, interleukins (IL-1, IL-2, IL-6, IL-8, IL-12), and chemokines, likely through the inactivation of NF-κB. In animal models, curcumin has been shown to inhibit arachidonic acid metabolism and inflammation in mouse skin epidermis by downregulating the COX and LOX pathways. However, a significant challenge in using curcumin therapeutically is its limited systemic bioavailability (Pushpangadan, Ijinu and George, 2015). Yadav et al., (2005) explored the effects of curcumin on T-cell proliferation stimulated by mitogen (phytohaemagglutinin; PHA), natural killer (NK) cell cytotoxicity, cytokine production by human peripheral blood mononuclear cells (PBMCs), and nitric oxide (NO) production in mouse macrophage cells (RAW-264.7). The study revealed that curcumin suppresses PHA-induced T-cell proliferation, interleukin-2 production, nitric oxide generation, and the activation of nuclear factor-kappaB (NF-κB) triggered by lipopolysaccharide, while also enhancing the cytotoxicity of NK cells. These findings indicate that curcumin may inhibit cell proliferation and cytokine production by targeting NF-κB-related genes that regulate these immune functions.

Saponins

Saponins, which are steroid or triterpene glycosides, are widely distributed in the plant kingdom and encompass a variety of biologically active compounds. Research has shown that saponins isolated from around 50 different plants exhibit anti-inflammatory activity in various experimental models involving mice and rats. The mechanisms of action include both indirect effects (as seen with many saikosaponins) and direct effects (such as those from saikosaponin D and ginsenosides), which can mimic corticoid activity, inhibit glucocorticoid degradation (e.g., glycyrrhizin), and block the enzymatic formation and release of inflammatory mediators (e.g., ginsenosides Rb2, Re, R, and saikosaponins A, C, D). Recently, two triterpene saponins from *Quercus imbricaria* and a bidesmosidic echinocystic acid glycoside from *Pithecellobium dulce* have also been identified for their anti-inflammatory properties. Additionally, a new steroid saponin, dracoside, was isolated during the search for anti-rheumatic compounds in the roots of *Helleborus purpurascens*, and its anti-inflammatory effect has been attributed to a counter-irritation mechanism (Wang et al., 2008). Three triterpenoid saponins (saponins 1, 4, and 5) with notable anti-inflammatory activity were isolated from *Polygala japonica*. Numerous reports highlight the anti-inflammatory properties of saponins. For example, fruticesaponin B, a bidesmosidic saponin with an unbranched saccharide moiety from *Bupleurum fruticescens* (Apiaceae), demonstrated the highest anti-inflammatory activity among all tested saponins in mouse edema assays. In vivo studies of saponins from *Bupleurum rotundifolium* (Apiaceae) also revealed anti-inflammatory effects against 12-O-tetradecanoylphorbol-13-acetate (TPA)-induced ear edema and chronic skin inflammation. Out of seven saponins evaluated, five effectively reduced TPA-induced ear edema in a dose-dependent manner. However, only two saponins were effective in alleviating chronic skin inflammation and were associated with a reduction in neutrophil infiltration. Aescin, a mixture of triterpenoid saponins and the primary active component of *Aesculus hippocastanum* L. (Hippocastanaceae), has demonstrated anti-inflammatory, anti-edematous, and venotonic properties. A novel steroidal saponin isolated from the leaves of *Agave attenuata* Salm-Dyck (Agavaceae) was assessed for its anti-inflammatory activity. This steroidal saponin effectively inhibited the increase in vascular permeability induced by acetic acid, a common model for the initial stage of inflammation. Importantly, this activity was not associated with any undesirable hemolytic effects, suggesting its potential as an anti-inflammatory drug that merits further investigation. Additionally, the triterpenoid saponin loniceroside C, extracted from the aerial parts of *Lonicera japonica* Thunb. (Caprifoliaceae), exhibited anti-inflammatory activity in vivo (Mona et al., 2014). The potential immunomodulatory effects of saponins have garnered significant interest since their discovery in 1925 as enhancers of the immune response to diphtheria and tetanus. Since 1964, the saponin extracted from the bark of a South American tree *Quillaja saponaria*, has been a primary focus of research investigating its immunoregulatory activity. *Panax notoginseng* and *Astragalus membranaceus* have demonstrated significant immunomodulatory activity. These saponins can stimulate the mammalian immune system by activating the innate immune response and enhancing the production of cytotoxic T lymphocytes (CTLs) that target exogenous antigens, among other effects (Shen et al., 2023). Steroidal saponins offer promising therapeutic potential for treating inflammatory diseases due to their ability to directly target pro-inflammatory cytokines like tumor necrosis factor alpha (TNF-α) and interleukin-6 (IL-6). Additionally, they can inhibit macrophage activity and modulate the arachidonic acid (AA) pathway, leading to reduced cyclooxygenase-2 (COX-2) and prostaglandin E2 (PGE2) activity. Steroidal saponins are found in abundance in plants with reduced side effects and therefore can be new therapeutic options (Fabiolla et al., 2022).

Sterols

Phytosterols and their derivatives are vital components of plant bio membranes and serve as biogenetic precursors for various metabolites, including plant steroid hormones. Research has explored the use of plant sterols as an alternative for lowering plasma cholesterol levels, with several studies indicating that they can significantly reduce total and LDL cholesterol. The anti-atherosclerotic effects of plant sterols are well-documented, attributed not only to their cholesterol-lowering properties but also to other beneficial effects on the coagulation system, antioxidant activity, and the functions of hepatic and lipoprotein lipase. Additionally, plant sterols have been associated with other metabolic benefits; for instance, numerous epidemiological and animal studies suggest that phytosterols may help suppress the growth of colon tumors. *Lepidium sativum* contains the highest concentration of sterols, with γ-sitosterol (12.2%) and ergost-5-en-3-ol (3β) (4.5%) identified as the major constituents. Additionally, three unique compounds—stigmasta-5,23-dien-3β-ol, stigmasta-5,24(28)-dien-3-ol (3β,22E), and 9,19-cyclolanost-24-en-3-ol (3γ)—were found exclusively in this plant. Strong anti-inflammatory activity has been observed in the leaves of *Picris hieracioides*, *Foeniculum vulgare*, *Cichorium intybus*, and *Cynara cardunculus*. Notably, *P. hieracioides* contained only γ-sitosterol. Both γ-sitosterol and stigmasterol were predominant sterols, widely distributed across various plants. The former was present in every plant examined, except for *Foeniculum vulgare*, and was primarily concentrated in *Lepidium sativum*, *Cichorium intybus* leaves, and *Sonchus oleraceus* (12.2%, 9.5%, and 6.5%, respectively). Stigmasterol was also identified in the extracts, with particularly high levels found in *Cichorium intybus* extracts (4.3% in root extract and 3.6% in leaves). Ergost-5-en-3-ol (3β) and campesterol were less widely distributed among the plants (Haiyin et al., 1995). Marine invertebrates have demonstrated a remarkable ability to produce novel sterols, although relatively few secosterols have been isolated to date. Among the known secosterols, most have only been reported for their in vitro cytotoxicity. Specifically, secosterols 1-3, 6, and 7, isolated from the Gorgonian *Pseudopterogorgia* sp., exhibited moderate inhibitory activity against protein kinase C. Notably, secosterol 6 displayed potent antiproliferative and anti-inflammatory effects (Mendesa et al., 2010).

Terpenoids and Essential Oils

Essential oils are volatile, natural, and complex compounds characterized by their strong aromas, produced by aromatic plants as secondary metabolites. These oils are rich in compounds with an isoprene structure, known as terpenes, which have a general chemical formula of $C10H16$. They can be categorized into various types, including diterpenes (C20), triterpenes (C30), tetraterpenes (C40), hemiterpenes (C5), and sesquiterpenes (C15). When these compounds contain additional elements, typically oxygen, they are referred to as terpenoids. Common examples of terpenoids include menthol and camphor (monoterpenes) and farnesol and artemisinin (sesquiterpenoids). Artemisinin and its derivative, α-arteether (also known as qinghaosu), are widely used as antimalarial agents. The compounds mentioned possess notable antiseptic properties, exhibiting bactericidal, virucidal, and fungicidal effects. Additionally, they are employed in embalming, food preservation, and as remedies with antimicrobial, analgesic, sedative, anti-inflammatory, spasmolytic, and local anesthetic effects (Sharif et al., 2010). Parthenolide is a sesquiterpene lactone derived from the medicinal herb *Tanacetum parthenium*. It has been shown to inhibit pro-inflammatory enzymes, including 5-lipoxygenase (5-LOX), phosphodiesterase-3, and phosphodiesterase-4. Additionally, parthenolide suppresses the release of key pro-inflammatory mediators such as nitric oxide (NO), prostaglandin E2 (PGE2), and tumor necrosis factor-alpha (TNF-α) from macrophages, as well as TNF-α, interleukin-2 (IL-2), interferon-gamma (IFN-γ), and IL-4 from human peripheral blood mononuclear cells. Research exploring its molecular mechanisms suggests that parthenolide could be beneficial in treating periodontitis. Its therapeutic effects are primarily attributed to the inhibition of NF-κB signaling, but beyond this, it is also demonstrated that parthenolide is a potent inhibitor of the NLRP3 inflammasome (Pushpangadan, Ijinu and George, 2015). Cucurbitacin E, is a triterpenoid compound, isolated from *Cucurbitaceae* plants, exhibits a broad spectrum of biological activities, including notable anti-inflammatory effects. Its anti-inflammatory action is mediated by the inhibition of NF-κB nuclear translocation, which in turn reduces the expression of TNF-α and IL-1β in LPS-stimulated RAW 264.7 cells and inhibition of COX-2 (Qiao et al., 2013). Dihydrocucurbitacin B is a triterpene compound isolated from the roots of *Cayaponia tayuya*, a plant known for its medicinal properties. Studies have demonstrated that dihydrocucurbitacin B significantly modulates the progression of clinical symptoms associated with inflammation and tissue damage. It effectively reduces swelling in both bone and surrounding tissues while limiting the overall development of the disease. This compound also alters the infiltration of immune cells at the site of inflammation and regulates the expression of key inflammatory enzymes, including nitric oxide synthase (NOS) and cyclooxygenase-2 (COX-2), which play critical roles in the inflammatory response. Furthermore, dihydrocucurbitacin B has been shown to decrease the production of pro-inflammatory cytokines, such as TNF-α and IL-1β, in lymphocytes, suggesting its potential as a therapeutic agent in conditions characterized by excessive inflammation (Escandell et al., 2006). Furthermore, a detailed analysis of inflamed tissues revealed that dihydrocucurbitacin B significantly reduced the levels of several key cytokines that play critical roles in the inflammatory processes. Among the cytokines decreased were IL-1β, IL-4, and TNF-α, which are known to be highly involved in mediating inflammation and immune responses. In addition to its effects on cytokine production, dihydrocucurbitacin B was found to inhibit the proliferation of phytohemagglutinin-stimulated human T lymphocytes, effectively halting the cell cycle at the G_0 phase. This interruption in the cell cycle prevents the expansion of T cells, which are crucial to immune responses. Furthermore, dihydrocucurbitacin B was shown to exert a selective inhibitory effect on the nuclear factor of activated T cells (NFAT) in human lymphocytes. By inhibiting NFAT, a key transcription factor involved in T cell activation and differentiation, dihydrocucurbitacin B effectively dampens delayed-type hypersensitivity (DTH) reactions. This action suppresses the proliferation of T cells, which are central to the development and progression of DTH responses, thus reducing the severity of these immune-mediated inflammatory reactions (Escandell et al., 2007). Comparing results from different studies can be challenging due to the significant variability in essential oil compositions. Factors such as geographical region, plant variety, age, drying methods, and oil extraction techniques can all influence these compositions. In recent years, researchers have identified mono- and sesquiterpene hydrocarbons, along with their oxygenated derivatives, as the primary components of essential oils derived from plants, which are known to exhibit potent anti-inflammatory effects (Jeane et al., 2003). The analgesic and anti-inflammatory properties of essential oils from various species have been established, including those from the genus *Eucalyptus* (Myrtaceae), *Cordia verbenacea* (Boraginaceae), *Lippia sidoides* (Verbenaceae), *Lippia gracilis* (Verbenaceae), and the seeds of *Zizyphus jujube* (Mona et al., 2014). Madecassoside, a triterpenoid compound isolated from *Centella asiatica*, has been shown to effectively reduce the inflammatory response in collagen-induced arthritis. Its anti-inflammatory effects are attributed to the inhibition of proinflammatory mediators, including the expression of COX-2, production of PGE2, and elevated levels of TNF-α and IL-6. Additionally, madecassoside promotes the upregulation of the anti-inflammatory molecule IL-10, further contributing to its anti-inflammatory action (Li et al., 2009). In a separate study, Won et al. (2020) found that the anti-inflammatory effects of madecassic acid result from the inhibition of iNOS, COX-2, TNF-α, IL-1β, and IL-6, which occurs through the downregulation of NF-κB activation in RAW 264.7 macrophage cells. Triptolide is a diterpenoid triepoxide extracted from the Chinese herb *Tripterygium wilfordii*. It inhibits both Ca2+-dependent and Ca2+-independent pathways, affecting T-cell activation by suppressing IL-2 transcription at a site distinct from the target of cyclosporin A. Additionally, triptolide exerts inhibitory effects on a range of proinflammatory cytokines, mediators, and the expression of adhesion molecules in endothelial cells (Chen, 2001). It inhibits the transcriptional activation of the IL-2 gene by blocking the purine-box regulator that controls the NFAT target DNA sequence in the IL-2 enhancer, as well as by preventing NF-κB activation (Qiu, 1999). Wen et al. (2013) found that triptolide treatment significantly reduces cardiac inflammation and fibrosis by inhibiting the activity and expression of NF-κB, leading to improved left ventricular function in a model of experimental diabetic cardiomyopathy.

Acetylsalicylic Acid or Aspirin

This drug is one of the most widely used medications globally and is often considered the first-line treatment for inflammation and related disorders. It was originally derived from salicylic acid, a compound found in the bark of *Spiraea ulmaria* (meadowsweet), a plant that has long been used in traditional medicine for its ability to alleviate fever and reduce inflammation (Recio, Andújar and Ríos,

2012). The therapeutic effects of this drug, particularly its anti-inflammatory and antithrombotic properties, stem from its ability to acetylate the enzymes COX-1 and COX-2. By acetylating these cyclooxygenases, the drug permanently inhibits their function, preventing the conversion of arachidonic acid into a variety of important bioactive lipids known as prostanoids. These include prostaglandins, thromboxanes, and prostacyclins, all of which are essential mediators in processes such as inflammation, pain, fever, and blood clotting. Through this inhibition, the drug effectively reduces the production of these key signalling molecules, helping to control the inflammatory response and blood clot formation, making it a cornerstone treatment for conditions associated with these processes (Amann and Peskar, 2002; Vane and Botting, 2003 and Bala et al., 2008). Recently, Alfonso et al., (2014) proposed the intriguing idea that aspirin may interact with and acetylate cellular molecules like RNA, as well as metabolites such as CoA, potentially altering their function. Further research in this area could offer deeper insights into the drug's mechanisms of action.

Pinitol

Pinitol, a bioactive compound derived from *Abies pindrow* (Himalayan fir), has been shown to play a significant role in modulating the inflammatory and carcinogenic pathways, particularly through its ability to inhibit NF-κB activation. This includes the activation of NF-κB in response to both inflammatory stimuli and carcinogens, as well as the constitutive NF-κB activation frequently observed in various tumour cells. The underlying mechanism by which pinitol exerts its effects involves the inhibition of IκBα kinase (IKK) activation, which is crucial for the regulation of NF-κB signalling. By preventing IKK activation, pinitol stops the phosphorylation and subsequent degradation of IκBα, an inhibitory protein that normally prevents NF-κB from translocating to the nucleus. As a result, the phosphorylation and nuclear translocation of the p65 subunit of NF-κB are hindered, leading to a significant reduction in NF-κB-dependent gene expression. This disruption of NF-κB signalling has profound consequences on a range of cellular processes. Pinitol downregulates the expression of several genes involved in inflammation, such as COX-2, which plays a pivotal role in the inflammatory response. It also suppresses genes associated with cell proliferation, including cyclin D1 and c-Myc, both of which are critical for cell cycle regulation and tumour growth. Furthermore, pinitol inhibits genes involved in cell invasion (e.g., MMP-9), angiogenesis (e.g., VEGF), and cell survival (e.g., cIAP1, cIAP2, XIAP, Bcl-2, and Bcl-xL), all of which contribute to cancer progression and metastasis. By modulating these pathways, pinitol not only dampens the inflammatory response but also enhances apoptosis (programmed cell death) induced by TNF (tumour necrosis factor) and chemotherapy agents. Additionally, pinitol has been shown to inhibit TNF-induced cellular invasion, further highlighting its potential as a therapeutic agent in cancer treatment and inflammation-related diseases. This combination of effects underscores the therapeutic promise of pinitol in controlling both inflammation and tumorigenesis, making it a compound of interest in cancer therapy and inflammatory disease management (Sethi et al., 2008 and Aggarwal et al., (2011).

Resveratrol

Resveratrol, a naturally occurring stilbene compound, is widely recognized for its diverse array of beneficial biological effects. These include anticancer, antiatherogenic, ant oxidative, anti-inflammatory, antimicrobial, and estrogenic properties, making it a highly studied phytochemical with considerable therapeutic potential (Piotrowska, Kucinska and Murias, 2012). When it comes to its anti-inflammatory effects, resveratrol works through multiple mechanisms that target various pathways involved in inflammation. One of the key mechanisms is the inhibition of cyclooxygenase (COX) activity, which prevents the conversion of arachidonic acid into pro-inflammatory prostaglandins. In addition to this, resveratrol has been shown to suppress the activation of immune cells, which are typically involved in propagating inflammatory responses. By curbing the activity of these immune cells, resveratrol limits the production of several pro-inflammatory mediators that contribute to chronic inflammation. It also plays a significant role in the inhibition of key transcription factors, such as NF-κB (Nuclear Factor kappa-light-chain-enhancer of activated B cells) and AP-1 (Activator Protein-1), which are crucial in regulating the expression of genes responsible for inflammation, cell survival, and immune responses. Furthermore, resveratrol exerts additional anti-inflammatory effects through the inhibition of IκB kinase, an enzyme involved in the activation of NF-κB. This reduces the nuclear translocation of NF-κB, thus preventing the activation of inflammatory gene expression. Additionally, resveratrol has been shown to decrease the production of prostaglandin E2 (PGE2), a potent mediator of inflammation, and to lower the levels of reactive oxygen species (ROS), which are highly reactive molecules that contribute to oxidative stress and inflammation. These effects have been particularly noted in LPS-activated microglial cells, which are immune cells in the brain that play a significant role in neuroinflammatory responses. In summary, resveratrol's anti-inflammatory actions are multifaceted, involving the suppression of COX enzymes, immune cell activation, inflammatory mediators, and key transcription factors. Its ability to regulate NF-κB and reduce oxidative stress further enhances its potential as a therapeutic agent in managing inflammatory diseases and conditions associated with oxidative damage (Pushpangadan, Ijinu and George, 2015).

Shikonin

Shikonin, a naturally occurring pigment belonging to the naphthoquinone class, is predominantly isolated from the roots of *Lithospermum erythrorhizon*, a medicinal plant known for its therapeutic properties. Several scientific evidences have demonstrated that shikonin possesses notable anti-inflammatory activity. In particular, research has shown that shikonin can effectively diminish inflammation in cases of acute lung injury (ALI) which are brought about by exposure to lipopolysaccharide (LPS), a component of the outer membrane of Gram-negative bacteria. The elemental mechanism responsible for this protective effect appears to be closely linked to the suppression of the nuclear factor kappa-light-chain-enhancer of activated B cells (NF-κB) signaling pathway, which plays a critical role in the regulation of immune and inflammatory responses. (Liang et al., 2013). Shikonin has been found to exert significant anti-inflammatory effects by interfering with macrophage polarization, specifically by inhibiting the conversion of pro-inflammatory M1 macrophages to the anti-inflammatory M2 phenotype within the joint tissues of mice suffering from collagen-induced arthritis (CIA). This regulatory action plays a crucial role in diminishing the overall inflammatory response localized in the affected joint regions. In parallel, earlier studies have reported that Nano gels engineered to self-assemble and incorporate comfreyin as an active component display potent anti-inflammatory properties. These therapeutic effects are achieved through the modulation of the innate immune system's inflammatory response. Moreover, the Nano gels contribute to the activation of the NOD-like receptor protein 3 (NLRP3) inflammasomes, a key molecular complex involved in initiating and regulating inflammation, thereby enhancing their immunomodulatory potential. (Song et al., 2023).

CONCLUSION

This chapter highlights the vast potential of secondary metabolites as effective anti-inflammatory and immunomodulatory agents, underscoring their capacity to act as natural therapeutic alternatives to synthetic drugs. The wide range of secondary metabolites—including flavonoids, alkaloids, terpenoids, and polyphenols—demonstrates versatile mechanisms in modulating immune responses and reducing inflammation, driven by their biochemical interactions with critical molecular targets. For example, flavonoids such as quercetin, dioclein etc. have been shown to inhibit key pro-inflammatory cytokines, including TNF-α, IL-1β, and IL-6, through modulation of NF-κB and MAPK signaling pathways. Similarly, alkaloids like berberine and curcumin have demonstrated efficacy in suppressing inflammatory pathways, such as COX-2 and iNOS, both crucial mediators of inflammation in chronic conditions like arthritis, cardiovascular disease, and neurodegenerative disorders. A pivotal benefit of secondary metabolites is their ability to mitigate oxidative stress, a key factor in inflammatory processes and immune dysregulation. This dual action on oxidative stress and immune modulation is particularly valuable, as it targets the root cause of many chronic inflammatory conditions, thereby offering a comprehensive approach to disease management. Additionally, polyphenols such as resveratrol and epigallocatechin gallate (EGCG) have shown immunomodulatory effects by regulating T-cell responses, thereby balancing immune function and preventing autoimmune responses. These mechanistic insights emphasize the potential of secondary metabolites to be incorporated into therapeutic strategies for inflammatory and autoimmune disorders. Emerging studies also suggest the synergistic potential of combining multiple secondary metabolites to enhance their bioactivity. For instance, the co-administration of curcumin and resveratrol has shown enhanced anti-inflammatory effects through concurrent modulation of the NF-κB and Nrf2 pathways. Such combinations may offer more robust therapeutic outcomes by targeting multiple inflammatory and immune pathways simultaneously, potentially delaying disease progression and reducing the need for high drug dosages. In conclusion, secondary metabolites as anti-inflammatory and immunomodulatory agents offer a promising frontier in both preventive and therapeutic medicine. Their ability to act on multiple molecular targets and their potential for low toxicity make them attractive candidates for addressing complex, multifactorial diseases.

Although the secondary metabolites reveal remarkable anti-inflammatory and immunomodulatory potential; however, their clinical utility is often retarded by poor bioavailability. This constraint arises from factors such as low aqueous solubility, chemical instability in the gastrointestinal tract, rapid metabolic degradation in the liver and poor membrane permeability. As a result, only a small fraction of the administered dose reaches systemic circulation in an active form, reducing the compound's pharmacological effectiveness. Overcoming these challenges is critical for successful drug development, and current strategies include the use of nano formulations, prodrugs, encapsulation techniques, and co-administration with absorption enhancers. Enhancing the bioavailability of these compounds can significantly improve their therapeutic outcomes and broaden their clinical applications. With continued research into their mechanisms of action, enhanced delivery systems, and synergistic formulations, secondary metabolites could be pivotal in advancing novel, natural-based therapies, contributing significantly to the future landscape of medicine focused on safety, efficacy, and holistic health.

REFERENCES

Adams, L. S., Seeram, N. P., Aggarwal, B. B., Takada, Y., Sand, D., & Heber, D. (2006). Pomegranate juice, total pomegranate ellagitannins, and punicalagin suppress inflammatory cell signalling in colon cancer cells. *Journal of Agricultural and Food Chemistry*, *54*(3), 980–985. DOI: 10.1021/jf052005r PMID: 16448212

Aggarwal, B. B.. (2011). Identification of novel anti-inflammatory agents from Ayurvedic medicine for prevention of chronic diseases: Reverse pharmacology and bedside to bench approach. *Current Drug Targets*, *12*(11), 1595–1653. DOI: 10.2174/138945011798109464 PMID: 21561421

Ahmad, N., Gupta, S., & Mukhtar, H. (2000). Green tea polyphenol epigallocatechin-3-gallate differentially modulates nuclear factor kB in cancer cells versus normal cells. *Archives of Biochemistry and Biophysics*, *376*(2), 338–346. DOI: 10.1006/abbi.2000.1742 PMID: 10775421

Alfonso, L., Ai, G., Spitale, R. C., & Bhat, G. J. (2014). Molecular targets of aspirin and cancer prevention. *British Journal of Cancer*, *111*(1), 61–67. DOI: 10.1038/bjc.2014.271 PMID: 24874482

Amann, R., & Peskar, B. A. (2002). Anti-inflammatory effects of aspirin and sodium salicylate. *European Journal of Pharmacology*, *447*(1), 1–9. DOI: 10.1016/S0014-2999(02)01828-9 PMID: 12106797

Ashley, N. T., Weil, Z. M., & Nelson, R. J. (2012). Inflammation: Mechanisms, costs, and natural variation. *Annual Review of Ecology, Evolution, and Systematics*, *43*(1), 385–406. DOI: 10.1146/annurev-ecolsys-040212-092530

Bala, M., Chin, C. N., Logan, A. T., Amin, T., Marnett, L. J., Boutaud, O., & Oates, J. A. (2008). Acetylation of prostaglandin H2 synthases by aspirin is inhibited by redox cycling of the peroxidase. *Biochemical Pharmacology*, *75*(7), 1472–1481. DOI: 10.1016/j.bcp.2007.12.005 PMID: 18242581

Barnes, P. J., & Karin, M. (1997). Nuclear factor-κB-a pivotal transcription factor in chronic inflammatory diseases. *The New England Journal of Medicine*, *336*(15), 1066–1071. DOI: 10.1056/NEJM199704103361506 PMID: 9091804

Bascones, M. A. et al., (2014) Immunomodulatory drugs: oral and systemic adverse effects. *Med Oral Patol Oral Cir Bucal*, 1;19(1):e24-31. .DOI: 10.4317/medoral.19087

Cardenas, H., Arango, D., Nicholas, C., Duarte, S., Nuovo, G., He, W., Voss, O., Gonzalez-Mejia, M., Guttridge, D., Grotewold, E., & Doseff, A. (2016). Dietary apigenin exerts immune-regulatory activity in vivo by reducing NF- kB activity, halting leukocyte infiltration and restoring normal metabolic function. *International Journal of Molecular Sciences*, *17*(3), 323. DOI: 10.3390/ijms17030323 PMID: 26938530

Charles, N. S. and Catherine, G. (2011) Endogenous Anti-inflammatory and Proresolving Lipid Mediators in Renal Disease. *Regenerative Nephrology*;69-92.

Chen, B. J. (2001). Triptolide, a novel immunosuppressive and anti-inflammatory agent purified from a Chinese herb *Tripterygium wilfordii* Hook F. *Leukemia & Lymphoma*, *42*(3), 253–265. DOI: 10.3109/10428190109064582 PMID: 11699390

Chen, H. J., Chung, C.-P., Chiang, W., & Lin, Y.-L. (2011). nti-inflammatory effects and chemical study of a flavonoid-enriched fraction from adlay bran. *Food Chemistry*, *126*(4), 1741–1748. DOI: 10.1016/j.foodchem.2010.12.074 PMID: 25213953

Chiang, L. C.. (2003). Immunomodulatory activities of flavonoids, monoterpenoids, triterpenoids, iridoid glycosides and phenolic compounds of *Plantago* species. *Planta Medica*, *69*(7), 600–604. DOI: 10.1055/s-2003-41113 PMID: 12898413

Demain, A. L., & Fang, A. (2000). The natural functions of secondary metabolites. *Advances in Biochemical Engineering/Biotechnology*, *69*, 1–39. DOI: 10.1007/3-540-44964-7_1 PMID: 11036689

Dongdong, W.. (2011). Antitussive, expectorant and anti-inflammatory alkaloids from *Bulbus fritillariae* Cirrhosae. *Fitoterapia*, *82*(8), 1290–1294. DOI: 10.1016/j.fitote.2011.09.006 PMID: 21958967

Eduardo, C., ... (2022) Chapter 12 - Biological macromolecules as immunomodulators, Editor(s): Amit, K. N.; Amal, K. D.; Dilip, K. P. *Biological Macromolecules, Academic Press*; 273-287

Escandell, J. M., Recio, M. C., Máñez, S., Giner, R. M., Cerdá-Nicolás, M., Gil-Benso, R., & Ríos, J.-L. (2007). Dihydrocucurbitacin B inhibits delayed type hypersensitivity reactions by suppressing lymphocyte proliferation. *The Journal of Pharmacology and Experimental Therapeutics*, *322*(3), 1261–1268. DOI: 10.1124/jpet.107.122671 PMID: 17562851

Escandell, J. M., Recio, M.-C., Máñez, S., Giner, R.-M., Cerdá-Nicolás, M., & Ríos, J.-L. (2006). Dihydrocucurbitacin B, isolated from *Cayaponia tayuya*, reduces damage in adjuvant-induced arthritis. *European Journal of Pharmacology*, *532*(1-2), 145–154. DOI: 10.1016/j.ejphar.2005.12.028 PMID: 16443215

Fabiolla, R. S. P.. (2022). Anti-inflammatory and modulatory effects of steroidal saponins and sapogenins on cytokines: A review of pre-clinical research. *Phytomedicine, 96*, 153842. DOI: 10.1016/j.phymed.2021.153842 PMID: 34952766

Fawole, O. A., Ndhlala, A. R., Amoo, S. O., Finnie, J. F., & Van Staden, J. (2009). Anti-inflammatory and phytochemical properties of twelve medicinal plants used for treating gastro-intestinal ailments in South Africa. *Journal of Ethnopharmacology*, *123*(2), 237–243. DOI: 10.1016/j.jep.2009.03.012 PMID: 19429367

Ghosh, S., & Karin, M. (2002). Missing pieces in the NF-kB puzzle. *Cell*, *109*(2), 81–96. DOI: 10.1016/S0092-8674(02)00703-1

Gupta, I., Parihar, A., Malhotra, P., Gupta, S., Lüdtke, R., Safayhi, H., & Ammon, H. P. T. (2001). Effects of gum resin of *Boswellia serrata* in patients with chronic colitis. *Planta Medica*, *67*(5), 391–395. DOI: 10.1055/s-2001-15802 PMID: 11488449

Gupta, K., Kumar, S., Gupta, R. K., Sharma, A., Verma, A. K., Stalin, K., Chaudhari, B. P., Das, M., Singh, S. P., & Dwivedi, P. D. (2016). Reversion of asthmatic complications and mast cell signalling pathways in BALB/c mice model using quercetin nanocrystals. *Journal of Biomedical Nanotechnology*, *12*(4), 717–731. DOI: 10.1166/jbn.2016.2197 PMID: 27301198

Haiyin, H.. (1995). New antiproliferative and anti-inflammatory 9,11-secosterols from the *Gorgonian pseudopterogorgia* sp. *Tetrahedron*, *51*(1), 51–58. DOI: 10.1016/0040-4020(94)00962-T

Hosseinzade, A., Sadeghi, O., Naghdipour Biregani, A., Soukhtehzari, S., Brandt, G. S., & Esmaillzadeh, A. (2019). Immunomodulatory Effects of Flavonoids: Possible Induction of TCD4+ Regulatory Cells Through Suppression of mTOR Pathway Signaling Activity. *Frontiers in Immunology*, *10*, 51. DOI: 10.3389/fimmu.2019.00051 PMID: 30766532

Jeane, S.. (2003). Analgesic and anti-inflammatory effects of essential oils of Eucalyptus. *Journal of Ethnopharmacology*, *89*(2-3), 277–283. DOI: 10.1016/j.jep.2003.09.007 PMID: 14611892

Jeon, H. J.. (2010). Anti-inflammatory and anti-arthritic activity of total flavonoids of the roots of *Sophora flavescens*. *Journal of Ethnopharmacology*, *127*(3), 589–595. DOI: 10.1016/j.jep.2009.12.020 PMID: 20034551

Kim, G. D., Lee, S. E., Park, Y. S., Shin, D.-H., Park, G. G., & Park, C.-S. (2014). Immunosuppressive effects of fisetin against dinitrofluorobenzene-induced atopic dermatitis-like symptoms in NC/Nga mice. *Food and Chemical Toxicology*, *66*, 341–349. DOI: 10.1016/j.fct.2014.01.057 PMID: 24525099

Kyong, H. K.. (2009). Anti-inflammatory effect of coumarins isolated from *Corydalis heterocarpa* in HT-29 human colon carcinoma cells. *Food and Chemical Toxicology*, *47*(8), 2129–2134. DOI: 10.1016/j.fct.2009.05.036 PMID: 19500635

Le, M. L. (2002). Cancer preventive effects of flavonoids-a review. *Biomedicine and Pharmacotherapy*, *56*(6), 296–301. DOI: 10.1016/S0753-3322(02)00186-5 PMID: 12224601

Li, H., Gong, X., Zhang, L., Zhang, Z., Luo, F., Zhou, Q., Chen, J., & Wan, J. (2009). Madecassoside attenuates inflammatory response on collagen-induced arthritis in DBA/1 mice. *Phytomedicine*, *16*(6-7), 538–546. DOI: 10.1016/j.phymed.2008.11.002 PMID: 19135346

Li, J., & Zhang, B. (2013). Apigenin protects ovalbumin-induced asthma through the regulation of Th17 cells. *Fitoterapia*, *91*, 298–304. DOI: 10.1016/j.fitote.2013.09.009 PMID: 24060907

Li, Z. P., Hu, J.-F., Sun, M.-N., Ji, H.-J., Zhao, M., Wu, D.-H., Li, G.-Y., Liu, G., & Chen, N.-H. (2011). Effect of compound IMMLG5521, a novel coumarin derivative, on carrageenan-induced pleurisy in rats. *European Journal of Pharmacology*, *661*(1-3), 118–123. DOI: 10.1016/j.ejphar.2011.04.024 PMID: 21549112

Liang, D., Sun, Y., Shen, Y., Li, F., Song, X., Zhou, E., Zhao, F., Liu, Z., Fu, Y., Guo, M., Zhang, N., Yang, Z., & Cao, Y. (2013). Shikonin exerts anti-inflammatory effects in a murine model of lipopolysaccharide-induced acute lung injury by inhibiting the nuclear factor-kappaB signalling pathway. *International Immunopharmacology*, *16*(4), 475–480. DOI: 10.1016/j.intimp.2013.04.020 PMID: 23651796

Maroon, J. C., Bost, J. W., & Maroon, A. (2010). Natural anti-inflammatory agents for pain relief. *Surgical Neurology International*, *1*(1), 80. DOI: 10.4103/2152-7806.73804 PMID: 21206541

Mendesa, S. S.. (2010). Evaluation of the analgesic and anti-inflammatory effects of the essential oil of *Lippia gracilis* leaves. *Journal of Ethnopharmacology*, *129*(3), 391–397. DOI: 10.1016/j.jep.2010.04.005 PMID: 20420889

Mona, S. M.. (2014). Secondary metabolites as anti-inflammatory agents. *The Journal of Phytopharmacology*, *3*(4), 275–285. DOI: 10.31254/phyto.2014.3409

Nathan, C. (2002). Points of control in inflammation. *Nature*, *420*(6917), 846–852. DOI: 10.1038/nature01320 PMID: 12490957

Pandey, M. K., Sung, B., Kunnumakkara, A. B., Sethi, G., Chaturvedi, M. M., & Aggarwal, B. B. (2008). Berberine modifies cysteine 179 of IκB alpha kinase, suppresses nuclear factor-kappaB-regulated antiapoptotic gene products, and potentiates apoptosis. *Cancer Research*, *68*(13), 5370–5379. DOI: 10.1158/0008-5472.CAN-08-0511 PMID: 18593939

Park, H. H., Lee, S., Oh, J.-M., Lee, M.-S., Yoon, K.-H., Park, B. H., Kim, J. W., Song, H., & Kim, S.-H. (2009). Antiinflammatory activity of fisetin in human mast cells (HMC-1). *Pharmaceutical Research*, *55*(1), 31–37. DOI: 10.1016/j.phrs.2006.10.002 PMID: 17079162

Pathak, A. K., Dutta, N., Banerjee, P. S., Goswami, T. K., & Sharma, K. (2016). Effect of condensed tannins supplementation through leaf meal mixture on voluntary feed intake, immune response and worm burden in Haemonchus contortus infected sheep. *Journal of Parasitic Diseases : Official Organ of the Indian Society for Parasitology*, *40*(1), 100–105. DOI: 10.1007/s12639-014-0455-1 PMID: 27065606

Piotrowska, H., Kucinska, M., & Murias, M. (2012). Biological activity of piceatannol: Leaving the shadow of resveratrol. *Mutation Research*, *750*(1), 60–82. DOI: 10.1016/j.mrrev.2011.11.001 PMID: 22108298

Pushpangadan, P., Ijinu, T. P., & George, V. (2015). Plant based anti-inflammatory secondary metabolites. *Annals of Phytomedicine*, *4*(1), 17–36.

Qiao, J., Xu, L., He, J., Ouyang, D., & He, X. (2013). Cucurbitacin E exhibits anti-inflammatory effect in RAW 264.7 cells via suppression of NF-κB nuclear translocation. *Inflammation Research*, *62*(5), 461–469. DOI: 10.1007/s00011-013-0598-z PMID: 23360962

Qiu, D., Zhao, G., Aoki, Y., Shi, L., Uyei, A., Nazarian, S., Ng, J. C.-H., & Kao, P. N. (1999). Immunosuppressant PG490 (Triptolide) inhibits T-cell interleukin-2 expression at the level of purine-box/nuclear factor of activated T-cells and NF-κB transcriptional activation. *The Journal of Biological Chemistry*, *274*(19), 13443–13450. DOI: 10.1074/jbc.274.19.13443 PMID: 10224109

Recio, M. C., Andújar, I., & Ríos, J. L. (2012). Anti-Inflammatory agents from plants: Progress and potential. *Current Medicinal Chemistry*, *19*, 2088–2103. DOI: 10.2174/092986712800229069 PMID: 22414101

Rodrigo, G.. (2010). The flavonoid dioclein reduces the production of pro-inflammatory mediators in vitro by inhibiting PDE4 activity and scavenging reactive oxygen species. *European Journal of Pharmacology*, *633*(1-3), 85–92. DOI: 10.1016/j.ejphar.2010.01.021 PMID: 20152831

Rogerio, A. P., Dora, C. L., Andrade, E. L., Chaves, J. S., Silva, L. F. C., Lemos-Senna, E., & Calixto, J. B. (2010). Anti-inflammatory effect of quercetin-loaded micro emulsion in the airways allergic inflammatory model in mice. *Pharmacological Research*, *61*(4), 288–297. DOI: 10.1016/j.phrs.2009.10.005 PMID: 19892018

Roze, L. V., Chanda, A., & Linz, J. E. (2011). Compartmentalization and molecular traffic in secondary metabolism: A new understanding of established cellular processes. *Fungal Genetics and Biology*, *48*(1), 35–48. DOI: 10.1016/j.fgb.2010.05.006 PMID: 20519149

Sethi, G., Ahn, K. S., Sung, B., & Aggarwal, B. B. (2008). Pinitol targets nuclear factor-kappaB activation pathway leading to inhibition of gene products associated with proliferation, apoptosis, invasion, and angiogenesis. *Molecular Cancer Therapeutics*, *7*(6), 1604–1614. DOI: 10.1158/1535-7163.MCT-07-2424 PMID: 18566231

Sharif, M. A. R.. (2010). Anti-inflammatory activity of seed essential oil from *Zizyphus jujuba.Food and Chemical Toxicology*, *48*(2), 639–643. DOI: 10.1016/j.fct.2009.11.045 PMID: 19944733

Shen, L. et alo., (2023) Potential Immunoregulatory Mechanism of Plant Saponins: A Review. *Molecules*; 23;29(1):113. DOI: 10.3390/molecules29010113

Singune, S.; Vaghela, J.S. Sisodia S.S. (2018) Review on Immunomodulation and Immunomodulatory Activity of Some Medicinal Plants. *European Journal of Biomedical and Pharmaceutical sciences*; 5(8): 163-174

Song, B., Guan, S., Lu, J., Chen, Z., Huang, G., Li, G., Xiong, Y., Zhang, S., Yue, Z., & Deng, X. (2013). Suppressive effects of fisetin on mice T lymphocytes in vitro and in vivo. *The Journal of Surgical Research*, *185*(1), 399–409. DOI: 10.1016/j.jss.2013.05.093 PMID: 23993202

Song, Y., Ding, Q., Hao, Y., Cui, B., Ding, C., & Gao, F. (2023). Pharmacological Effects of Shikonin and Its Potential in Skin Repair: A Review. *Molecules (Basel, Switzerland)*, *28*(24), 7950. DOI: 10.3390/molecules28247950 PMID: 38138440

Souto, A. L., Tavares, J. F., Da Silva, M. S., Diniz, M. F. F. M., De Athayde-Filho, P. F., & Barbosa Filho, J. M. (2011). Anti-inflammatory activity of alkaloids: An update from 2000 to 2010. *Molecules (Basel, Switzerland)*, *16*(10), 8515–8534. DOI: 10.3390/molecules16108515 PMID: 21989312

Stefanova, T. H.. (2007). Antitumor and immunomodulatory effect of coumarin and 7-hydroxycoumarin against Sarcoma 180 in mice. *Journal of Experimental Therapeutics & Oncology*, *6*(2), 107–115. PMID: 17407969

Sternberg, Z., Chadha, K., Lieberman, A., Hojnacki, D., Drake, A., Zamboni, P., Rocco, P., Grazioli, E., Weinstock-Guttman, B., & Munschauer, F. (2008). Quercetin and interferon-β modulate immune response (s) in peripheral blood mononuclear cells isolated from multiple sclerosis patients. *Journal of Neuroimmunology*, *205*(1-2), 142–147. DOI: 10.1016/j.jneuroim.2008.09.008 PMID: 18926575

Sun, X., Yamasaki, M., Katsube, T., & Shiwaku, K. (2015). Effects of quercetin derivatives from mulberry leaves: Improved gene expression related hepatic lipid and glucose metabolism in short-term high-fat fed mice. *Nutrition Research and Practice*, *9*(2), 137–143. DOI: 10.4162/nrp.2015.9.2.137 PMID: 25861419

Tiwari, R., & Rana, C. S. (2015). Plant secondary metabolites: A review. *International Journal of Engineering Research and General Science*, *3*(5), 661–670.

Tsurufuji, S.. (1980). A review of mechanism of action of steroid and non-steroid anti-inflammatory drugs. In Willoughby, D. A., & Giroud, J. P. (Eds.), *Inflammation: Mechanisms and Treatment. Inflammation: Mechanisms and Treatment* (Vol. 4). Springer., DOI: 10.1007/978-94-010-9423-8_7

Vane, J. R., & Botting, R. M. (2003). The mechanism of action of aspirin. *Thrombosis Research*, *110*(5-6), 255–258. DOI: 10.1016/S0049-3848(03)00379-7 PMID: 14592543

Wang, C.. (2004). Effects of omega-3 fatty acids on cardiovascular disease (Summary). *Evid. Rep. Technol. Assess.*, *94*, 1–8.

Wang, H. et al., (2008) Anti-inflammatory activities of triterpenoid saponins from *Polygala japonica. Phytomedicine*; 1 15: 321–326

Wang, J.. (2022). Pharmacological effects and mechanisms of tannic acid. *Biomedicine and Pharmacotherapy*, *154*, 113561. DOI: 10.1016/j.biopha.2022.113561 PMID: 36029537

Wang, J., Li, T. M., Zang, L., Pan, X., Wang, S., Wu, Y., & Wang, G. (2017). Apigenin inhibits human SW620 cell growth by targeting polyamine catabolism. *Evidence-Based Complementary and Alternative Medicine : eCAM*, *3684581*(1), 3684581. Advance online publication. DOI: 10.1155/2017/3684581 PMID: 28572828

Wen, H. L., Liang, Z.-S., Zhang, R., & Yang, K. (2013). Antiinflammatory effects of triptolide improve left ventricular function in a rat model of diabetic cardiomyopathy. *Cardiovascular Diabetology*, *12*(1), 50. DOI: 10.1186/1475-2840-12-50 PMID: 23530831

White, M. (1999). Mediators of inflammation and inflammatory process. *The Journal of Allergy and Clinical Immunology*, *103*(3), 378–381. DOI: 10.1016/S0091-6749(99)70215-0 PMID: 10069896

Won, J. H., Shin, J.-S., Park, H.-J., Jung, H.-J., Koh, D.-J., Jo, B.-G., Lee, J.-Y., Yun, K., & Lee, K.-T. (2020). Anti-inflammatory effects of madecassic acid *via* the suppression of NF-kappaB pathway in LPS-induced RAW 264.7 macrophage cells. *Planta Medica*, *76*(3), 251–257. DOI: 10.1055/s-0029-1186142 PMID: 19774506

Yadav, V. S., Mishra, K. P., Singh, D. P., Mehrotra, S., & Singh, V. K. (2005). Immunomodulatory effects of curcumin. *Immunopharmacology and Immunotoxicology*, *27*(3), 485–497. DOI: 10.1080/08923970500242244 PMID: 16237958

Yuandani, J. I., Jantan, I., Salim, E., Septama, A. W., Rullah, K., Nainu, F., Fasihi Mohd Aluwi, M. F., Emran, T. B., Roney, M., Khairunnisa, N. A., Nasution, H. R., Fadhil As'ad, M., Shamsudin, N. F., Abdullah, M. A., Marwa Rani, H. L., Al Chaira, D. M., & Aulia, N. (2014). Mechanistic insights into anti-inflammatory and immunosuppressive effects of plant secondary metabolites and their therapeutic potential for rheumatoid arthritis. *Phytotherapy Research*, *38*(6), 2931–2961. DOI: 10.1002/ptr.8147 PMID: 38600726

Zhenkai, T.. (2022). Biological Function of Plant Tannin and Its Application in Animal Health. *Frontiers in Veterinary Science*, *8*, 803657. Advance online publication. DOI: 10.3389/fvets.2021.803657 PMID: 35083309

Chapter 7
Medicinal Plants and Secondary Metabolite for the Treatments of Hypertension

Bui Thanh Tung
https://orcid.org/0000-0002-7308-5039
VNU University of Medicine and Pharmacy, Vietnam

Dinh Van Anh
VNU University of Medicine and Pharmacy, Vietnam

Nguyen Thi Van Anh
VNU University of Medicine and Pharmacy, Vietnam

Nguyen Thi Anh Hong
VNU University of Medicine and Pharmacy, Vietnam

ABSTRACT

Traditional medicine encompasses a range of ancient, culturally-rooted health practices that were developed long before modern scientific approaches were applied to healthcare. Used for centuries, these practices often involve medicinal plants, which play a role in treating cardiovascular conditions such as heart disease, cerebrovascular disorders, hypertension, and heart failure. Hypertension complicates heart function and contributes to atherosclerosis, thereby increasing the risk of heart attacks and strokes. Although numerous drugs are available to manage these conditions, many commonly used anti- hypertensive medications carry significant side effects. Medicinal herbs contain active compounds with both therapeutic and

DOI: 10.4018/979-8-3693-9112-9.ch007

preventive properties, offering potential for the treatment of hypertension. This review provides an overview of several medicinal plants and secondary metabolites that have demonstrated hypertensive or anti-hypertensive effects.

INTRODUCE

Cardiovascular diseases (CVDs) are a leading cause of morbidity and premature mortality worldwide, posing a significant public health challenge. Hypertension, often referred to as the "silent killer," arises from a complex interplay between genetic predisposition and environmental factors, leading to dysregulation of blood pressure control mechanisms (Kamyab et al., 2021). Hypertension (HTN) is the most prevalent risk factor for acute myocardial infarction and is responsible for approximately 16.5% of deaths worldwide each year. It also represents the leading cause of morbidity and mortality associated with cardiovascular diseases (CVDs) (Kamyab et al., 2021). Hypertension is broadly classified into two main types: primary (essential) and secondary. Primary hypertension, accounting for approximately 90–95% of cases, refers to elevated blood pressure without an identifiable medical cause. In contrast, secondary hypertension, comprising 5–10% of cases, results from underlying conditions affecting the kidneys, arteries, heart, or endocrine system. (Tabassum & Ahmad, 2011).

Essential hypertension is characterized by elevated blood pressure of unknown etiology and significantly increases the risk of cerebrovascular, cardiac, and renal events. In industrialized countries, the lifetime risk of developing hypertension (defined as blood pressure >140/90 mmHg) exceeds 90%. Essential hypertension often coexists with other cardiovascular risk factors, including aging, obesity, insulin resistance, diabetes mellitus, and hyperlipidemia. Subclinical target-organ damage—such as left ventricular hypertrophy, microalbuminuria, and cognitive impairment—can occur early in the disease course, whereas major adverse events, including stroke, myocardial infarction, renal failure, and dementia, typically arise after prolonged periods of uncontrolled hypertension. (Messerli et al., 2007).

Secondary hypertension refers to elevated blood pressure resulting from an identifiable and often reversible underlying cause. Recognizing secondary hypertension is crucial for effective management, as it enables targeted treatment by addressing the root cause. Several conditions are known to induce secondary hypertension, including endocrine disorders such as Cushing's syndrome (characterized by excess cortisol production), hyperthyroidism, hypothyroidism, and adrenal gland tumors. Other common contributors include chronic kidney disease, obesity and metabolic disorders, pre-eclampsia during pregnancy, congenital abnormalities like coarctation of the aorta, and the use of certain prescription or illicit drugs. (Tabassum & Ahmad, 2011).

Pathophysiology of Hypertension: Although the pathophysiology of hypertension remains incompletely understood, it is recognized that 2–5% of patients have an identifiable secondary cause, such as renal or adrenal disease. In the majority of cases, however, no single underlying cause can be determined, and the condition is classified as "essential hypertension." The regulation of normal blood pressure involves multiple physiological mechanisms, including renal, neural, hormonal, and vascular factors. Dysregulation within these systems is thought to contribute to the development and progression of essential hypertension (Beevers et al., 2001). It is likely that multiple interrelated factors contribute to elevated blood pressure in hypertensive patients, with the relative impact of each factor varying between individuals. Key contributors that have been extensively studied include high salt intake, obesity and insulin resistance, dysregulation of the renin-angiotensin system, and overactivity of the sympathetic nervous system. More recently, additional factors such as genetic predisposition, endothelial dysfunction (reflected by alterations in endothelin and nitric oxide levels), low birth weight and intrauterine nutritional status, as well as neurovascular anomalies, have also been implicated in the pathogenesis of hypertension (Beevers et al., 2001). Moreover different physiological effectors like potassium channels, nitric oxide (NO), renin angiotensin system, reactive oxygen species and calciumions modulate the vascular tone and any imbalance in these factors may lead to hypertension (Nelson & Quayle, 1995).

Despite clinical interventions, hypertension remains a major risk factor for cardiovascular diseases, including heart failure, widespread atherosclerosis, cognitive impairment, and dementia. Although synthetic antihypertensive drugs are commonly used in clinical practice, their overall efficacy is limited and they are frequently associated with adverse effects such as dry mouth, dizziness, emotional disturbances, gastrointestinal discomfort, and visual disorders. These side effects can significantly impair health-related quality of life. Consequently, there is a growing need to explore natural, cost-effective, and non-toxic alternatives. Plants, extensively utilized in traditional medicine systems, offer promising potential for the treatment and management of hypertension and related disorders (Sultana & Asif, 2017). Plants are a rich source of secondary metabolites, many of which have demonstrated antihypertensive properties in vivo. The present study focuses on reviewing the antihypertensive activities of medicinal plants and their associated metabolites. A comprehensive search was conducted using the keywords "plants," "medicinal plants," and "plant extracts," cross-referenced with "hypertension" and "antihypertensive activity." The use of natural plant-derived compounds as cardioprotective and antihypertensive agents presents a promising strategy for the discovery of novel bioactive products. Plants are particularly abundant in secondary metabolites such as flavonoids, alkaloids, tannins, and terpenoids, which have shown significant antihypertensive effects in experimental models. This review thus provides a strong foundation for the identification and selection of specific molecules within these categories that may serve as effective therapeutic agents in the future (Sultana & Asif, 2017).

MEDICINAL PLANTS USING FOR TREATMENT OF HYPERTENSION

Allium Sativum (Garlic)

Garlic (Allium sativum), a member of the Amaryllidaceae family, has been widely utilized by humans not only as a culinary spice and vegetable but also for its medicinal properties. Since ancient times, it has been employed in traditional medicine across the world for the prevention and treatment of various diseases, continuing its relevance into modern healthcare practices (Ryu & Kang, 2017). Garlic has been traditionally utilized for the management of various cardiovascular conditions, particularly hyperlipidemia. In addition, it has been reported to exhibit antihypertensive effects, primarily through the enhancement of nitric oxide production, leading to smooth muscle relaxation and vasodilation. One of the key bioactive compounds responsible for garlic's characteristic odor and numerous therapeutic properties is allicin (Tabassum & Ahmad, 2011). Since it has been reported to exert angiotensin II-inhibiting and vasodilating effects (Matsutomo, 2020). Allicin has also been shown to suppress cholesterol biosynthesis by inhibiting squalene monooxygenase and acetyl-CoA synthetase (Ali et al., 2023). Therefore, it help lower blood pressure. In summary, garlic has a significant effect in the treatment and prevention of high blood pressure.

Camellia Sinensis (Tea)

Tea (*Camellia sinensis*), a plant species in the Theaceae family, primarily thrives in tropical and subtropical climates (Sanchez et al., 2020). Tea has a long-standing history, originating in China and subsequently spreading worldwide through both direct and indirect routes. (Zhao et al., 2022). There is considerable research interest in the effects of tea on cardiovascular diseases (Tabassum & Ahmad, 2011). Tea, characterized by its unique flavonoid compositions, has been studied for its effects on nitric oxide (NO) production and related protein expression in the aorta of spontaneously hypertensive rats (SHRs) fed a high-salt diet. Results showed that the reduction in urinary NO metabolites (NOx), which reflect whole-body NO production, induced by the high-salt diet was significantly prevented by all three tea infusions. Notably, the improvement in NOx levels observed in the tea-treated groups was unlikely to be attributed to changes in oxidative damage (Nomura et al., 2017). In addition to their cardiovascular benefits, tea polyphenols exert four major effects: vasorclaxant activity, protection against endothelial dysfunction, antioxidant properties, and hypolipidemic effects (San Cheang et al., 2015). Moreover, black tea has been shown to protect against endothelial dysfunction in angiotensin II-induced hypertensive rats by inhibiting endoplasmic reticulum stress and oxidative stress within the vascular wall (San Cheang et al., 2015). Conclusion, tea brings about many benefits in treatment hypertension.

Daucus Carota L (Carrot)

Carrot (*Daucus carota* L.), a member of the Apiaceae family, is one of the most significant plant species in the field of molecular farming. It is particularly notable for being the first plant species approved for the production of biopharmaceuticals intended for human use (Rosales-Mendoza & Tello-Olea, 2015). Daucus carota has been traditionally used to treat hypertension. Activity-guided fractionation of the aerial parts of D. carota led to the isolation of two coumarin glycosides, designated as DC-2 (Daucus carota-2) and DC-3 (Daucus carota-3). These compounds are believed to exert their blood pressure-lowering effects by blocking calcium channels, as demonstrated in in vivo studies.(Gilani et al., 2000). Furthermore, antioxidant compounds in carrots, including carotenoids and polyphenols, possess the ability to scavenge reactive oxygen species (ROS) and enhance endogenous defense systems, thereby reducing oxidative stress and ultimately lowering the risk of cardiovascular diseases (Soleti et al., 2021). In summary, carrot offers substantial benefits in the prevention and management of vascular and metabolic diseases.

Lycopersicon Esculentum L. (Tomato)

The tomato (*Solanum lycopersicum* L., also known as *Lycopersicum esculentum* L.), is the fruit of a herbaceous plant belonging to the Solanaceae family (Marcolongo et al., 2020) and one of the most widely consumed vegetables. This widely consumed vegetable is rich in antioxidants and various bioactive compounds, including vitamins E and C, flavonoids (such as rutin), phenolic compounds (such as chlorogenic acid), carotenoids (β-carotene and lycopene), and glycoalkaloids (such as tomatine) (Marcolongo et al., 2020). All these components of tomato have demonstrated potent protective effects against cancer and cardiovascular diseases, ischemia/reperfusion injury, and also exhibit strong antioxidant properties (Marcolongo et al., 2020), which is one of the mechanisms for the cardiovascular protective effect (Wolak et al., 2019). Beside the beneficial properties of tomato have been well-documented, and tomato extracts have demonstrated inhibitory effects on angiotensin-converting enzyme (ACE) activity and platelet aggregation (Marcolongo et al., 2020). Moreover tomato extract, when administered to patients receiving low doses of angiotensin-converting enzyme (ACE) inhibitors, calcium channel blockers, or their combination with low-dose diuretics, has shown additional beneficial effects (Paran et al., 2009). In short, the use of standardized tomato extract significant in arterial hypertension patients with high total cardiovascular risk; it is associated with better blood pressure control and improvements in the daily blood pressure profile (Osinska et al., 2017).

Glycine Max L. (Soybean)

Soybean (Glycine max L.) is a member of the Fabaceae family and originates from East Asia, particularly regions in North and Central Asia (Ramlal et al., 2022). It is rich in various nutrients such as proteins (approximately 40–42%) and fats (15–20%). The lipid fraction primarily consists of polyunsaturated fatty acids (PUFAs), such as alpha-linolenic acid, alongside essential micronutrients like vitamins and minerals (Ramlal et al., 2022). Soy peptides play a role in combating high blood pressure. They offer protective effects against complications related to hypertension, including cognitive decline and renal impairment (Li et al., 2022). In addition, a relatively understudied aspect of soy isoflavone research involves their impact on vascular function and the regulation of blood pressure. Evidence suggests that soy isoflavones, particularly genistein, may influence blood pressure control mechanisms. Genistein functions as an estrogen receptor agonist, and estrogen is known to support cardiovascular health by regulating blood lipid profiles and acting directly on blood vessels and the nervous system (Martin et al., 2001). Other study is suggested that the antihypertensive effects of black soybean-derived peptides may stem from their ability to reduce oxidative stress, stimulate nitric oxide (NO) production, and inhibit angiotensin-converting enzyme (ACE) activity (Kwak et al., 2013). In summary, soybean offers numerous benefits in the treatment and management of hypertension.

Sesamum Indicum (Sesamin)

Sesame seeds have been recognized as a traditional health food in East Asia for centuries, and their oil has been a key component in natural remedies in India and traditional Chinese medicine, known for its ability to enhance energy and prevent aging (Miyawaki et al., 2009). Sesame seeds have been a staple in traditional health foods across East Asia for centuries, and their oil has been an essential element in natural remedies in India and Chinese medicine, known for boosting energy and combating aging (Dalibalta et al., 2020). It is recognized for its antioxidant and anti-inflammatory effects, which are crucial in the management of various cardiovascular diseases (CVDs) (Dalibalta et al., 2020). Moreover by reducing ROS production, sesamin boosts the bioactivity of NO in blood vessels, thereby improving endothelial function, alleviating hypertension, and reducing vascular inflammation (Dalibalta et al., 2020). In addition, a significant association was observed between systolic blood pressure and elevated aortic $O2-$ levels. These results indicate that sesamin intake suppresses the increased vascular $O2-$ generation in deoxycorticosterone acetate (DOCA)-salt-induced hypertensive rats, suggesting that its antioxidant capacity may underlie its blood pressure-lowering effects (Nakano et al., 2002). In summary, the blood pressure-lowering effect of sesamin may play a significant role in the prevention of cardiovascular diseases (Miyawaki et al., 2009).

Zingiber Officinale Roscoe (Ginger)

Ginger (*Zingiber officinale Roscoe*, Zingiberaceae), a medicinal herb from the Zingiberaceae family, is characterized by its perennial rhizome. It is naturally cultivated in Southern Asia and thrives in both tropical and subtropical climates (Salaramoli et al., 2022). Additionally, ginger is among the most widely used dietary spices globally (Bode & Dong, 2011). Traditionally, it has been employed to treat a broad spectrum of ailments, including hypertension (Ghayur & Gilani, 2005). The primary non-volatile compound in ginger, 6-gingerol, has been shown to improve hypertension-related biomarkers and reduce lipid accumulation. This is achieved by enhancing the expression of phosphorylated endothelial nitric oxide synthase (eNOS), vascular cell adhesion molecule 1 (VCAM1), TNFα, and epithelial sodium channel (ENaC) protein via activation of PPARδ in mouse preadipocytes (3T3-L1 cells), human embryonic kidney cells (HEK293 cells), and human umbilical vein endothelial cells (HUVECs) (Salaramoli et al., 2022). Moreover the suppression of arginase activity, along with elevated levels of nitric oxide (NO) and testosterone induced by both ginger and turmeric rhizomes, may represent a potential mechanism underlying their protective effects against male infertility associated with hypertension (Akinyemi et al., 2015). Conclusion, the daily inclusion of ginger in the diet as a choice for managing hypertension along with its potential to lower the risk of hypertension-related complications.

Panax Ginseng

Panax ginseng is a slow-growing perennial plant that belongs to the genus Panax in the Araliaceae family (Zhou et al., 2019). Panax ginseng holds a significant position in traditional herbal medicine due to its wide-ranging therapeutic properties, including anti-inflammatory, antiallergic, antidiabetic, cardioprotective, and anticancer effects. Its beneficial and restorative actions are primarily attributed to bioactive compounds such as ginsenosides, polysaccharides, peptides, alkaloids, polyacetylenes, and phenolic substances, which are regarded as the key pharmacologically active constituents across various P. ginseng species (Irfan et al., 2020). Notably, ginsenosides are capable of suppressing reactive oxygen species (ROS) production, enhancing nitric oxide (NO) synthesis, improving blood circulation, regulating vasomotor tone, and modulating lipid metabolism. Furthermore, they exert diverse biological effects under both normal and pathological conditions related to cardiovascular diseases (CVD) (Kim, 2012). Moreover, P. ginseng exhibits antihypertensive properties primarily through its vasorelaxant effects. Paradoxically, it has also been reported to elevate blood pressure via vasoconstrictive mechanisms, suggesting a dual role in supporting cardiovascular homeostasis (Irfan et al., 2020). In short, ginseng exhibits various effects in both the prevention and treatment of hypertension.

Curcuma Longa (Turmeric)

Turmeric is prepared by grinding of dried rhizomes mainly from *Curcuma longa* L. of the Zingiberaceae family (Basnet & Skalko-Basnet, 2011). Turmeric *(Curcuma longa),* along with curcumin, its primary bioactive compound derived from the plant's rhizome (Vafaeipour et al., 2022). Curcumin has been shown to prevent and treat cardiovascular diseases (CVDs) through the modulation of multiple signaling pathways involved in cellular proliferation, growth, survival, oxidative stress, and inflammation. It prevents cardiovascular dysfunction and its key risk factors, including atherosclerosis, aortic aneurysm, myocardial infarction, and stroke, by activating endogenous antioxidant, anti-inflammatory, and anti-apoptotic pathways, thereby improving cardiovascular health, alleviating heart failure, and reducing cardiotoxicity (Nurcahyanti et al., 2022). Besides the other mechanisms of action of curcumin in cardiovascular diseases is anti- oxidant, inhibits sarcoplasmic Ca^{2+}- ATPase, membrane stabilizing effect, prevents Adriamycin- induced cardiomyopathy and decreases serum cholesterol levels (Sundar Dhilip Kumar et al., 2018). To sum up curcumin is a well-known plant-derived compound that exhibits a wide range of biological and pharmacological effects in modern medicine (Sundar Dhilip Kumar et al., 2018).

Cynara Scolymus L (Artichoke)

Artichoke or globe artichoke (*Cynara cardunculus* var. *scolymus* L.) belongs to the *Asteraceae* family (Colombo et al., 2024). It is cultivated as a food primarily in the Mediterranean, Canary Islands, and Egypt, as well as in Asia and South

America (Olas, 2024). It is one of the therapeutic plants with a beneficial impact on HTN (Amini et al., 2022). The leaves of the artichoke are the primary part known to influence blood pressure elevation. It contains polyphenolic compounds, prebiotics (such as inulin), minerals, ascorbic acid, and folate. The leaf extract is rich in dietary fibers and antioxidant components, suggesting its potential benefits in managing hypertension (HTN). Furthermore, artichoke leaf extract has been shown to increase endothelial nitric oxide synthase (eNOS) gene expression and nitric oxide (NO) production in cultured human vascular endothelial cells, as well as enhance endothelium-dependent vasodilation in the aorta of mice (Amini et al., 2022). Moreover, artichoke extracts have also been shown to have beneficial effects on dyslipidemia, a key risk factor for cardiovascular diseases (CVDs) (Olas, 2024). It has been shown to decrease LDL concentration, total cholesterol, and triglyceride levels. Luteolin and chlorogenic acid, two key components of this extract, are believed to play a significant role in cardioprotection. Additionally, the beneficial effects of cooked artichoke hearts are primarily attributed to their fiber content, particularly inulin (Olas, 2024). Overall artichoke supplementation may potentially lead to blood pressure reduction in hypertensive patients (Moradi et al., 2021).

Apium Graveolens (Celery)

Celery (Apium graveolens), a biennial herb native to the Mediterranean region, has been cultivated for centuries. It is rich in vitamins, minerals, phthalides, and flavonoids such as apigenin and luteolin, which are known for their potent anti-inflammatory and anti-tumor properties (Alobaidi & Saleh, 2024). Apigenin exhibited an endothelium-dependent vasorelaxant effect in aortic rings, which was mediated by the influx and release of Ca2+, cGMP, and nitric oxide (Sohrabi et al., 2021). Luteolin also demonstrated endothelium-dependent vasorelaxation in the aorta (Sohrabi et al., 2021). It was shown that luteolin induces relaxation in the thoracic aorta of rats through an endothelium-independent mechanism (Sohrabi et al., 2021). Moreover, active components of celery, such as 3-n-butylphthalide (NBP) and apigenin, help lower blood pressure by acting as diuretics and vasodilators. Their effectiveness is comparable to that of calcium channel blocker drugs They can also reduce cholesterol levels and prevent arterial plaque formation, further contributing to the reduction of blood pressure. Additionally, hexane, methanol, and aqueous ethanol extracts of A. graveolens seeds have been reported to reduce blood pressure in deoxycorticosterone acetate-induced hypertensive rats (Nugraha et al., 2022). Therefore, hypertension can be managed both pharmaceutically and non-pharmaceutically through the use of herbal plants such as celery (Alobaidi & Saleh, 2024).

Olea Europaea L. (Olive)

Olea europaea L., a fruit tree native to Asia Minor and Syria, is now cultivated throughout the entire Mediterranean region (Romani et al., 2019). It contains high levels of fatty acids (98–99% of the total weight of extra-virgin olive oil, EVOO) and small amounts (1–2%) of phenolics, phytosterols, tocopherols, and squalene (Romani et al., 2019). The cardio-protective effects of olive oil are now believed to stem from its phenolic compounds, which are derived from the water-soluble fraction. These include primarily the low-molecular weight molecule hydroxytyrosol, as well as oleuropein, both of which are potent antioxidants, free radical scavengers, and enzyme modulators (Widmer et al., 2015). Additionally, the leaves of the olive tree have been used to treat high blood pressure, atherosclerosis, diabetes, and other medicinal conditions. The anti-hypertensive effects of active compounds in the olive tree leaves, such as oleuropein and oleacein, may be linked to the inhibition of angiotensin-converting enzyme. Chronic treatment with oleuropein in rats with concurrent type 2 diabetes and renal hypertension demonstrated anti-hypertensive effects, which appear to be partially mediated by enhanced nitric oxide (NO) release, as well as antioxidant and sympatholytic activities (Romero et al., 2016). In summary, olive polyphenols induce a marked reduction in blood pressure in hypertensive subjects (Saibandith et al., 2017).

Crataegus spp (Hawthorns)

Hawthorn is a member of the *Crataegus* species and *Rosacea* family (Dehghani et al., 2019). Hawthorn extract has been utilized for the treatment of cardiovascular diseases for centuries. Recent studies have shown its effectiveness in managing heart failure, and the outcomes of several small trials indicate that it may help reduce blood pressure (Asher et al., 2012). In addition, research has indicated that extracts derived from the fruits, leaves, and flowers of *C. pinnatifida* may have the potential to prevent heart failure and hypertension (Dehghani et al., 2019). In which the total flavonoids, proanthocyanidins, triterpenoid acid extracts, and polysaccharide active components isolated from hawthorn leaves have exhibited anti-hypertensive effects (Guo et al., 2023). Potential mechanisms of Crataegus tincture (TCR) include inhibiting the rise in lipid peroxidation and the activity of marker enzymes, preventing the isoproterenol-induced reduction in antioxidant enzymes in the heart, and enhancing the rate of ADP-stimulated oxygen consumption and respiratory coupling ratio in isoproterenol-treated rats (Wang et al., 2013). Another mechanism for hawthorn's blood pressure-lowering effect is its association with nitric oxide-mediated vasodilation (Asher et al., 2012). In conclusion, hawthorn offers significant therapeutic potential in both the treatment and prevention of hypertension, thanks to its cardiovascular benefits, including blood pressure-lowering effects and improvements in vascular function.

Punica Granatum L (Pomegranate)

Pomegranate (*Punica granatum* L.), a fruit from the *Punica* genus and *Punicaceae* family, is an ancient species originally from Central Asia. Its cultivation extends from Iran and Turkmenistan to northern India, as well as across the Mediterranean and the Middle East (Wang et al., 2018). It is a popular edible fruit with wide applications in traditional medicine (Asgary et al., 2013). The pomegranate is characterized by considerable amounts of biologically active phytochemicals including flavonoids (e.g. anthocyanins, catechins, quercetin, and rutin), other types of polyphenols, ellagitannins, and antioxidant vitamins. Many of these phytochemicals have been shown to possess antioxidant and anti-inflammatory properties plus additional biological activities such as inhibition of angiotensin converting enzyme (Asgary et al., 2013). Pomegranate extract alleviates symptoms of hypertension by reducing oxidative stress, improving mitochondrial function, and decreasing chronic activation of the sympathetic nervous system in the para-ventricular nucleus, and have identified the AMPK-Nrf2 pathway as a mechanistic link between pomegranate extract-induced reduction of oxidative stress (Sun et al., 2016). To sum up, all these activities of the pomegranate are potentially beneficial for the treatment of hypertension and improvement of endothelial function (Asgary et al., 2013).

BIOACTIVE COMPOUNDS USING FOR TREATMENT OF HYPERTENSION

Flavonoids

Flavonoids are important natural compounds with diverse biological activities (Alam et al., 2014) and common compounds found in fruits and vegetables as secondary metabolites (Maaliki et al., 2019). By blocking the production and release of inflammatory mediators, flavonoids help prevent endothelial damage and myocardial inflammation, stimulate the production and secretion of vasoactive substances like NO and eNOS, promote autophagic processes, and reduce platelet aggregation and thrombosis. These compounds offer therapeutic benefits for inflammatory damage associated with hypertension, coronary atherosclerotic heart disease, myocarditis, and other conditions. Furthermore, flavonoids participate in the modulation of ion channels, preserving the balance of sodium and calcium ion concentrations in the myocardium. Through their regulation of ions and associated myofilaments, flavonoids influence myocardial contractility, contributing to the improvement of restrictive heart diseases (Liu et al., 2024).Moreover, some flavonoids, such as quercetin, catechin, puerarin, and hesperidin, also have therapeutic effects on hypertension. Quercetin and catechin, which are plentiful in tea, provide benefits for individuals with coronary artery disease, while puerarin helps mitigate pathological cardiac remodeling. Hesperidin, found in citrus fruits, and flavonoid luteolin, a widely researched and common compound, exhibit blood pressure-lowering properties (Liu et al., 2024). For example, luteolin notably reduced blood pressure in spontaneous hypertensive rats (SHRs) and enhanced vascular relaxation in aortic rings. The relaxation of vascular smooth muscle cells (VSMCs) induced by luteolin takes place through both endothelium-NO dependent and endothelium-NO-independent pathways, the latter being driven by Ca2+ and K+ channels (Maaliki et al., 2019). Overall, the solubility and multifaceted cardiovascular benefits of flavonoids make them promising candidates for hypertension management (Chen & Zhang, 2021).

Alkaloid

Alkaloids have gained greater focus in the quest for novel vasodilatory compounds (Amssayef & Eddouks, 2023). The majority of these alkaloids promote vasodilation via both endothelium-dependent and endothelium-independent pathways, primarily facilitated by the activation of the eNOS/NO/sGC/cGMP cascade, the opening of multiple potassium (K+) channels, or the modulation of calcium (Ca2+) channels (Amssayef & Eddouks, 2023). Additionally, various alkaloids have shown the capacity to safeguard endothelial function by mitigating oxidative stress, endoplasmic reticulum stress, and inflammation (Amssayef & Eddouks, 2023). For instance, tetrandrine is a key constituent of alkaloids derived from the Radix S. tetrandra S. Moore. It is widely recognized as a non-selective Ca2+ channel antagonist. Numerous studies, both in vivo and in vitro, suggest that tetrandrine's antihypertensive effect is due to its suppression of L-type calcium channels (Huang et al., 2016). Furthermore, reserpine, the isolated alkaloid from Rauwolfia serpentina, was the first powerful medication extensively employed in the long-term management of hypertension. Moreover, selective inhibitors can be developed from phytopharmaceuticals, like alkaloids, owing to their extensive therapeutic history and varied clinical uses. Research on alkaloids has yielded remarkable results, leading to continued investigation into these and other alkaloids to discover new, potent, and targeted ACE inhibitors(Islam et al., 2023). In conclusion, alkaloids present considerable promise for managing and preventing hypertension, owing to their vessel-relaxing, anti-inflammatory, and free-radical scavenging characteristics

Polysaccharide

In recent years, there has been an significant interest in the bioactivities of polysaccharides from natural sources (Xie et al., 2021). Natural polysaccharides show fewer adverse effects than synthetic medicines, but their inherent physicochemical features can complicate comparisons. For example, the mean arterial blood pressure in both normotensive and hypertensive rats was significantly reduced by polysaccharides derived from white mulberry fruit. This action is probably linked to the increased production of nitric oxide (NO) in vascular endothelial cells (Dong et al., 2021). The generation of NO could be linked to the initiation of intracellular calcium signaling and the PI3K/AKT signaling cascade. Furthermore, treatment with Astragalus polysaccharides also lowered the average pulmonary artery pressure in rats with monocrotaline-induced pulmonary hypertension through the activation of the eNOS/NO signaling pathway (Dong et al., 2021). Moreover, plant-derived polysaccharides have the potential to lower elevated blood pressure by blocking the activity of angiotensin-converting enzyme (ACE) (Dong et al., 2021). Some examples include Astragalus polysaccharide extract (APS), which notably lowered blood pressure in mice treated with DOCA-salt and Ang II, alleviated inflammation and renal scarring, thus enhancing kidney function (Zheng et al., 2021). Similary, *Angelica sinensis* polysaccharide (ASP) prevents hypertensive heart disease by improving cardiac function, inhibiting cardiac fibrosis, suppressing cardiomyocyte apoptosis, and alleviating oxidative stress (Song et al., 2021). To sum up, polysaccharides are promising compound in the prevention and treatment of hypertension.

Terpenoids

Terpenes are a class of secondary metabolites that can be found in a variety of animal and plants species (Silva et al., 2019). They are widely recognized for their diverse biological activities, including their ability to regulate metabolic processes and provide therapeutic effects in various diseases. Terpenes have shown efficacy in the treatment of chronic disorders such as obesity, diabetes, hypertension and vascular conditions (Oliveira et al., 2021). Some of the terpenoids commonly studied for cardiovascular diseases (CVD) include platycodin D, rubiarbonol C, rubiarbononeC, 3,4-*seco*-Olean-18-ene- 3,2,8-dioic acid, β-Sitosterol glycoside, ursolic acid, triterpenic acid, asiatic acid, astragaloside IV, betulinic acid, 6β-OH-Betulinic acid, boswellic acid, and celastrol (Bachheti et al., 2022). These compounds are notable for their vasorelaxant properties, which are critical for managing high blood pressure. A number of terpenoids were reported exhibiting vasorelaxant activities and have shown significant therapeutic potential in the medical field. For example, the terpenoid extracted from liverwort has anti-hypertensive effects(Qiao et al., 2018). Moreover the diterpene Sclareol showed in vivo hypertensive and in-vitro vasodilator effects (Campos et al., 2017). Terpenoids also exert their anti-hypertensive effects through multiple mechanisms, such as modulating calcium ion channels, enhancing nitric oxide (NO) release, and reducing oxidative stress. These mechanisms not only contribute to blood pressure regulation but also help improve vascular endothelial function, which is essential for overall cardiovascular health. In conclusion, terpenoids offer significant potential in the prevention and treatment of hypertension due to their vasorelaxant and antihypertensive properties.

Tannic Acid

Tannic acid is a water-soluble polyphenol that is present in tea, green tea, coffee, red wine, nuts, fruits and many plant foods. Tannic acid is widely recognized for its versatile biological activities and its role in modulating oxidative and inflammatory processes in the body. It is known to act as either an antioxidant or a pro-oxidant, depending on the type of cells and its concentration.. Studies have highlighted the impact of tannic acid in lowering blood pressure in hypertensive rats (Turgut Cosan et al., 2015). It has also been observed to significantly suppress cardiac enlargement caused by Abdominal Aortic Banding (AAB) in rats, making it a potential therapeutic agent for cardiovascular diseases. The heart-protective properties of tannic acid (TA) are likely due to its ability to act on multiple pathways, such as reducing oxidative stress, inflammation, fibrosis, and cell death, while also enhancing nitric oxide (NO) levels, lowering endothelin-1 (ET-1) concentrations, and suppressing angiotensin receptor expression along with ERK1/2 phosphorylation (Chu et al., 2017). Moreover, certain tannins extracted from medicinal plants have been shown to non-selectively inhibit angiotensin-converting enzyme (ACE) activity. The blood pressure-lowering effects of these tannins may be attributed to their ability to inhibit angiotensin-converting enzyme (ACE) activity (Liu et al., 2003). This ACE inhibitory action may provide a mechanistic basis for tannins' hypotensive effects. Additionally, tannic acid's role as an antioxidant contributes to its ability to mitigate endothelial dysfunction and improve vascular health. Its anti-inflammatory properties further enhance its therapeutic value by reducing systemic inflammation, which is often linked to hypertension and other cardiovascular disorders. In conclusion, tannic acid and related tannins show great promise in the prevention and treatment of hypertension.

Carotenoids

Carotenoids are plant-based compounds recognized for their biological properties. They are present in nature in various sources, include vegetation, seaweeds, mushrooms, and microbial organisms (Bhatt & Patel, 2020). Due to their significant medicinal properties and safety, they have been identified as distinctive treatment options for a wide array of ailments. Carotenoids regulate blood pressure by reducing the production of reactive oxygen species (ROS), blocking angiotensin-II, endothelin-1, and oxidized low-density lipoprotein; while also promoting the synthesis of nitric oxide (NO). These mechanisms contribute to their ability to lower blood pressure. Some carotenoids such as astaxanthin, β-carotene, bixin, capsanthin, lutein, crocin, and lycopene, exhibit blood pressure-lowering effects (Abbasian et al., 2023). These effects are partly due to their role in reducing oxidized LDL and improving the balance between LDL and high-density lipoprotein (HDL) (Bhatt & Patel, 2020). Another mechanism of high blood pressure reduction by carotenoids is their interaction with angiotensin II (Abbasian et al., 2023). Besides, carotenoids reduce inflammation and oxidative stress by facilitating normal cellular mechanisms. They work directly by evacuating superoxide anions ($O2-$) and reducing the production of reactive oxygen species (ROS). Carotenoids have also been shown to restore the bioavailability of nitric oxide (NO) in endothelial cells. As a result, carotenoids may be considered a promising source of oxidant modulators that influence endothelial reactions to pro-oxidant/inflammatory stimuli (Bhatt & Patel, 2020). In conclusion, additional properties of carotenoids that may contribute to a potential reduction in cardiovascular risk include the lowering of blood pressure, reduction of pro-inflammatory cytokines and inflammation markers, as well as enhancement of insulin sensitivity in muscle, liver, and adipose tissues (Gammone et al., 2015).

CONCLUSION

Currently, herbal treatments and the use of secondary metabolites in managing hypertension are gaining significant attention and are becoming a preferred option for many patients. Compared to conventional therapies, herbal medicine offers numerous advantages: natural origin, minimal side effects, high safety—especially for individuals with sensitive conditions—and greater affordability. Beyond merely alleviating symptoms, herbal remedies contribute to improving overall health, strengthening the immune system, and addressing the root causes of hypertension, thereby reducing the likelihood of recurrence. What sets medicinal plants apart lies in their rich content of bioactive secondary metabolites, such as flavonoids, alkaloids, terpenoids, polysaccharides, tannins, and carotenoids. These compounds exert antihypertensive effects through various mechanisms, including vasodilation, antioxidative stress reduction, anti-inflammatory activity, and modulation of enzymes and signaling pathways involved in blood pressure regulation. As such, secondary metabolites not only complement modern medicine but also represent a valuable resource for the development of natural, multi-targeted therapeutic strategies. Their role as key agents in combating hypertension opens new directions for research and clinical application, emphasizing the need for continued exploration into their mechanisms and potential.

REFERENCES

Abbasian, F., Alavi, M. S., & Roohbakhsh, A. (2023). Dietary carotenoids to improve hypertension. *Heliyon*, *9*(9), e19399. DOI: 10.1016/j.heliyon.2023.e19399 PMID: 37662767

Akinyemi, A. J., Adedara, I. A., Thome, G. R., Morsch, V. M., Rovani, M. T., Mujica, L. K. S., Duarte, T., Duarte, M., Oboh, G., & Schetinger, M. R. C. (2015). Dietary supplementation of ginger and turmeric improves reproductive function in hypertensive male rats. *Toxicology Reports*, *2*, 1357–1366. DOI: 10.1016/j.toxrep.2015.10.001 PMID: 28962478

Alam, M. A., Subhan, N., Rahman, M. M., Uddin, S. J., Reza, H. M., & Sarker, S. D. (2014). Effect of citrus flavonoids, naringin and naringenin, on metabolic syndrome and their mechanisms of action. *Advances in Nutrition*, *5*(4), 404–417. DOI: 10.3945/an.113.005603 PMID: 25022990

Ali, U., Wabitsch, M., Tews, D., & Colitti, M. (2023). Effects of allicin on human Simpson-Golabi-Behmel syndrome cells in mediating browning phenotype. *Frontiers in Endocrinology (Lausanne)*, *14*, 1141303. DOI: 10.3389/fendo.2023.1141303 PMID: 36936145

Alobaidi, S., & Saleh, E. (2024). Antihypertensive Property of Celery: A Narrative Review on Current Knowledge. *International Journal of Food Sciences*, *9792556*, 1–8. Advance online publication. DOI: 10.1155/2024/9792556 PMID: 38505582

Amini, M. R., Sheikhhossein, F., Alvani, M., Shoura, S. M. S., Sohrabnavi, A., Heidarian, E., & Hekmatdoost, A. (2022). Anti-hypertensive Effects of Artichoke Supplementation in Adults: A Systematic Review and Dose-response Meta-analysis of Randomized Controlled Trials. *Clinical Nutrition Research*, *11*(3), 214–227. DOI: 10.7762/cnr.2022.11.3.214 PMID: 35949557

Amssayef, A., & Eddouks, M. (2023). Alkaloids as Vasodilator Agents: A Review. *Current Pharmaceutical Design*, *29*(24), 1886–1895. DOI: 10.2174/1381612829666230809094313 PMID: 37559238

Asgary, S., Keshvari, M., Sahebkar, A., Hashemi, M., & Rafieian-Kopaei, M. (2013). Clinical investigation of the acute effects of pomegranate juice on blood pressure and endothelial function in hypertensive individuals. *ARYA Atherosclerosis*, *9*(6), 326–331. https://www.ncbi.nlm.nih.gov/pubmed/24575134 PMID: 24575134

Asher, G. N., Viera, A. J., Weaver, M. A., Dominik, R., Caughey, M., & Hinderliter, A. L. (2012). Effect of hawthorn standardized extract on flow mediated dilation in prehypertensive and mildly hypertensive adults: A randomized, controlled cross-over trial. *BMC Complementary and Alternative Medicine*, *12*(1), 26. DOI: 10.1186/1472-6882-12-26 PMID: 22458601

Bachheti, R. K., Worku, L. A., Gonfa, Y. H., Zebeaman, M., Deepti, , Pandey, D. P., & Bachheti, A. (2022). Deepti, Pandey, D. P., & Bachheti, A. (2022). Prevention and Treatment of Cardiovascular Diseases with Plant Phytochemicals: A Review. *Evidence-Based Complementary and Alternative Medicine : eCAM*, *5741198*, 1–21. Advance online publication. DOI: 10.1155/2022/5741198 PMID: 35832515

Basnet, P., & Skalko-Basnet, N. (2011). Curcumin: An anti-inflammatory molecule from a curry spice on the path to cancer treatment. *Molecules (Basel, Switzerland)*, *16*(6), 4567–4598. DOI: 10.3390/molecules16064567 PMID: 21642934

Beevers, G., Lip, G. Y., & O'Brien, E. (2001). ABC of hypertension: The pathophysiology of hypertension. *BMJ (Clinical Research Ed.)*, *322*(7291), 912–916. DOI: 10.1136/bmj.322.7291.912 PMID: 11302910

Bhatt, T., & Patel, K. (2020). Carotenoids: Potent to Prevent Diseases Review. *Natural Products and Bioprospecting*, *10*(3), 109–117. DOI: 10.1007/s13659-020-00244-2 PMID: 32405969

Bode, A. M., & Dong, Z. (2011). The Amazing and Mighty Ginger. In Benzie, I. F. F., & Wachtel-Galor, S. (Eds.), *Herbal Medicine: Biomolecular and Clinical Aspects* (2nd ed.)., https://www.ncbi.nlm.nih.gov/pubmed/22593941 DOI: 10.1201/b10787-8

Campos, D. R., Celotto, A. C., Albuquerque, A. A. S., Ferreira, L. G., Monteiro, A., Coelho, E. B., & Evora, P. R. B. (2017). The Diterpene Sclareol Vascular Effect in Normotensive and Hypertensive Rats. *Arq Bras Cardiol*, *109*(2), 0. DOI: 10.5935/abc.20170086

Chen, Z., & Zhang, S. L. (2021). The role of flavonoids in the prevention and management of cardiovascular complications: A narrative review. *Annals of Palliative Medicine*, *10*(7), 8254–8263. DOI: 10.21037/apm-21-1343 PMID: 34353106

Chu, L., Li, P., Song, T., Han, X., Zhang, X., Song, Q., Liu, T., Zhang, Y., & Zhang, J. (2017). Protective effects of tannic acid on pressure overload-induced cardiac hypertrophy and underlying mechanisms in rats. *The Journal of Pharmacy and Pharmacology*, *69*(9), 1191–1207. DOI: 10.1111/jphp.12763 PMID: 28631819

Colombo, R., Moretto, G., Pellicorio, V., & Papetti, A. (2024). Globe Artichoke (Cynara scolymus L.) By-Products in Food Applications: Functional and Biological Properties. *Foods*, *13*(10), 1427. Advance online publication. DOI: 10.3390/foods13101427 PMID: 38790727

Dalibalta, S., Majdalawieh, A. F., & Manjikian, H. (2020). Health benefits of sesamin on cardiovascular disease and its associated risk factors. *Saudi Pharmaceutical Journal : SPJ : the Official Publication of the Saudi Pharmaceutical Society*, *28*(10), 1276–1289. DOI: 10.1016/j.jsps.2020.08.018 PMID: 33132721

Dehghani, S., Mehri, S., & Hosseinzadeh, H. (2019). The effects of Crataegus pinnatifida (Chinese hawthorn) on metabolic syndrome: A review. *Iranian Journal of Basic Medical Sciences.*, *22*(5), 460–468. DOI: 10.22038/IJBMS.2019.31964.7678 PMID: 31217924

Dong, X., Zhou, M., Li, Y., Li, Y., Ji, H., & Hu, Q. (2021). Cardiovascular Protective Effects of Plant Polysaccharides: A Review. *Frontiers in Pharmacology*, *12*, 783641. DOI: 10.3389/fphar.2021.783641 PMID: 34867415

Gammone, M. A., Riccioni, G., & D'Orazio, N. (2015). Carotenoids: Potential allies of cardiovascular health? *Food & Nutrition Research*, *59*(1), 26762. DOI: 10.3402/fnr.v59.26762 PMID: 25660385

Ghayur, M. N., & Gilani, A. H. (2005). Ginger lowers blood pressure through blockade of voltage-dependent calcium channels. *Journal of Cardiovascular Pharmacology*, *45*(1), 74–80. DOI: 10.1097/00005344-200501000-00013 PMID: 15613983

Gilani, A. H., Shaheen, E., Saeed, S. A., Bibi, S., Irfanullah, , Sadiq, M., & Faizi, S. (2000). Hypotensive action of coumarin glycosides from Daucus carota. *Phytomedicine*, *7*(5), 423–426. DOI: 10.1016/S0944-7113(00)80064-1 PMID: 11081994

Guo, W., Shao, T., Peng, Y., Wang, H., Chen, Z. S., & Su, H. (2023). Chemical composition, biological activities, and quality standards of hawthorn leaves used in traditional Chinese medicine: A comprehensive review. *Frontiers in Pharmacology*, *14*, 1275244. DOI: 10.3389/fphar.2023.1275244 PMID: 37927599

Huang, Y. L., Cui, S. Y., Cui, X. Y., Cao, Q., Ding, H., Song, J. Z., Hu, X., Ye, H., Yu, B., Sheng, Z.-F., Wang, Z.-J., & Zhang, Y. H. (2016). Tetrandrine, an alkaloid from S. tetrandra exhibits anti-hypertensive and sleep-enhancing effects in SHR via different mechanisms. *Phytomedicine*, *23*(14), 1821–1829. DOI: 10.1016/j.phymed.2016.10.021 PMID: 27912885

Irfan, M., Kwak, Y. S., Han, C. K., Hyun, S. H., & Rhee, M. H. (2020). Adaptogenic effects of Panax ginseng on modulation of cardiovascular functions. *Journal of Ginseng Research*, *44*(4), 538–543. DOI: 10.1016/j.jgr.2020.03.001 PMID: 32617033

Islam, M. R., Dhar, P. S., Akash, S., Syed, S. H., Gupta, J. K., Gandla, K., Akter, M., Rauf, A., Hemeg, H. A., Anwar, Y., Aljohny, B. O., & Wilairatana, P. (2023). Bioactive molecules from terrestrial and seafood resources in hypertension treatment: Focus on molecular mechanisms and targeted therapies. *Natural Products and Bioprospecting*, *13*(1), 45. DOI: 10.1007/s13659-023-00411-1 PMID: 37902881

Kamyab, R., Namdar, H., Torbati, M., Ghojazadeh, M., Araj-Khodaei, M., & Fazljou, S. M. B. (2021). Medicinal Plants in the Treatment of Hypertension: A Review. *Advanced Pharmaceutical Bulletin*, *11*(4), 601–617. DOI: 10.34172/apb.2021.090 PMID: 34888207

Kim, J. H. (2012). Cardiovascular Diseases and Panax ginseng: A Review on Molecular Mechanisms and Medical Applications. *Journal of Ginseng Research*, *36*(1), 16–26. DOI: 10.5142/jgr.2012.36.1.16 PMID: 23717100

Kwak, J. H., Kim, M., Lee, E., Lee, S. H., Ahn, C. W., & Lee, J. H. (2013). Effects of black soy peptide supplementation on blood pressure and oxidative stress: A randomized controlled trial. *Hypertension Research*, *36*(12), 1060–1066. DOI: 10.1038/hr.2013.79 PMID: 23924691

Li, T., Zhang, X., Ren, Y., Zeng, Y., Huang, Q., & Wang, C. (2022). Antihypertensive effect of soybean bioactive peptides: A review. *Current Opinion in Pharmacology*, *62*, 74–81. DOI: 10.1016/j.coph.2021.11.005 PMID: 34929528

Liu, J. C., Hsu, F. L., Tsai, J. C., Chan, P., Liu, J. Y., Thomas, G. N., Tomlinson, B., Lo, M.-Y., & Lin, J. Y. (2003). Antihypertensive effects of tannins isolated from traditional Chinese herbs as non-specific inhibitors of angiontensin converting enzyme. *Life Sciences*, *73*(12), 1543–1555. DOI: 10.1016/S0024-3205(03)00481-8 PMID: 12865094

Liu, Y., Luo, J., Peng, L., Zhang, Q., Rong, X., Luo, Y., & Li, J. (2024). Flavonoids: Potential therapeutic agents for cardiovascular disease. *Heliyon*, *10*(12), e32563. DOI: 10.1016/j.heliyon.2024.e32563 PMID: 38975137

Maaliki, D., Shaito, A. A., Pintus, G., El-Yazbi, A., & Eid, A. H. (2019). Flavonoids in hypertension: A brief review of the underlying mechanisms. *Current Opinion in Pharmacology*, *45*, 57–65. DOI: 10.1016/j.coph.2019.04.014 PMID: 31102958

Marcolongo, P., Gamberucci, A., Tamasi, G., Pardini, A., Bonechi, C., Rossi, C., Giunti, R., Barone, V., Borghini, A., Fiorenzani, P., Frosini, M., Valoti, M., & Pessina, F. (2020). Chemical Characterisation and Antihypertensive Effects of Locular Gel and Serum of Lycopersicum esculentum L. var. "Camone" Tomato in Spontaneously Hypertensive Rats. *Molecules (Basel, Switzerland)*, *25*(16), 3758. Advance online publication. DOI: 10.3390/molecules25163758 PMID: 32824747

Martin, D. S., Breitkopf, N. P., Eyster, K. M., & Williams, J. L. (2001). Dietary soy exerts an antihypertensive effect in spontaneously hypertensive female rats. *American Journal of Physiology. Regulatory, Integrative and Comparative Physiology*, *281*(2), R553–R560. DOI: 10.1152/ajpregu.2001.281.2.R553 PMID: 11448860

Matsutomo, T. (2020). Potential benefits of garlic and other dietary supplements for the management of hypertension. *Experimental and Therapeutic Medicine*, *19*(2), 1479–1484. DOI: 10.3892/etm.2019.8375 PMID: 32010326

Messerli, F. H., Williams, B., & Ritz, E. (2007). Essential hypertension. *Lancet*, *370*(9587), 591–603. DOI: 10.1016/S0140-6736(07)61299-9 PMID: 17707755

Miyawaki, T., Aono, H., Toyoda-Ono, Y., Maeda, H., Kiso, Y., & Moriyama, K. (2009). Antihypertensive effects of sesamin in humans. *Journal of Nutritional Science and Vitaminology*, *55*(1), 87–91. DOI: 10.3177/jnsv.55.87 PMID: 19352068

Moradi, M., Sohrabi, G., Golbidi, M., Yarmohammadi, S., Hemati, N., Campbell, M. S., Moradi, S., Kermani, M. H., & Farzaei, M. H. (2021). Effects of artichoke on blood pressure: A systematic review and meta-analysis. *Complementary Therapies in Medicine*, *57*, 102668. DOI: 10.1016/j.ctim.2021.102668 PMID: 33465383

Nakano, D., Itoh, C., Takaoka, M., Kiso, Y., Tanaka, T., & Matsumura, Y. (2002). Antihypertensive effect of sesamin. IV. Inhibition of vascular superoxide production by sesamin. *Biological & Pharmaceutical Bulletin*, *25*(9), 1247–1249. DOI: 10.1248/bpb.25.1247 PMID: 12230131

Nelson, M. T., & Quayle, J. M. (1995). Physiological roles and properties of potassium channels in arterial smooth muscle. *The American Journal of Physiology*, *268*(4 Pt 1), C799–C822. DOI: 10.1152/ajpcell.1995.268.4.C799 PMID: 7733230

Nomura, S., Monobe, M., Ema, K., Maeda-Yamamoto, M., & Nesumi, A. (2017). Comparison of the Effects of Three Tea Cultivars (Camellia sinensis L.) on Nitric Oxide Production and Aortic Soluble Guanylate Cyclase Expression in High-Salt Diet-Fed Spontaneously Hypertensive Rats. *Journal of Nutritional Science and Vitaminology*, *63*(5), 306–314. DOI: 10.3177/jnsv.63.306 PMID: 29225315

Nugraha, A. S., Agustina, R. P., Mirza, S., Rani, D. M., Winarto, N. B., Triatmoko, B., Pratama, A., Keller, P., & Wangchuk, P. (2022). Phytochemistry and Pharmacology of Medicinal Plants Used by the Tenggerese Society in Java Island of Indonesia. *Molecules (Basel, Switzerland)*, *27*(21), 7532. Advance online publication. DOI: 10.3390/molecules27217532 PMID: 36364351

Nurcahyanti, A. D. R., Cokro, F., Wulanjati, M. P., Mahmoud, M. F., Wink, M., & Sobeh, M. (2022). Curcuminoids for Metabolic Syndrome: Meta-Analysis Evidences Toward Personalized Prevention and Treatment Management. *Frontiers in Nutrition*, *9*, 891339. DOI: 10.3389/fnut.2022.891339 PMID: 35757255

Olas, B. (2024). An Overview of the Versatility of the Parts of the Globe Artichoke (Cynara scolymus L.), Its By-Products and Dietary Supplements. *Nutrients*, *16*(5), 599. Advance online publication. DOI: 10.3390/nu16050599 PMID: 38474726

Oliveira, J. R., Ribeiro, G. H. M., Rezende, L. F., & Fraga-Silva, R. A. (2021). Plant Terpenes on Treating Cardiovascular and Metabolic Disease: A Review. *Protein and Peptide Letters*, *28*(7), 750–760. DOI: 10.2174/0929866528999210128210145 PMID: 33511924

Osinska, A. N., Begier-Krasinska, B., Rzymski, P., Krasinska, A., Tykarski, A., & Krasinski, Z. (2017). The influence of adding tomato extract and acetylsalicylic acid to hypotensive therapy on the daily blood pressure profiles of patients with arterial hypertension and high cardiovascular risk. *Kardiochirurgia i Torakochirurgia Polska = Polish Journal of Cardio-Thoracic Surgery*, *14*(4), 245–252. DOI: 10.5114/kitp.2017.72229 PMID: 29354177

Paran, E., Novack, V., Engelhard, Y. N., & Hazan-Halevy, I. (2009). The effects of natural antioxidants from tomato extract in treated but uncontrolled hypertensive patients. *Cardiovascular Drugs and Therapy*, *23*(2), 145–151. DOI: 10.1007/s10557-008-6155-2 PMID: 19052855

Qiao, Y., Zheng, H., Li, L., Zhang, J., Li, Y., Li, S., Zhu, R., Zhou, J., Zhao, S., Jiang, Y., & Lou, H. (2018). Terpenoids with vasorelaxant effects from the Chinese liverwort Scapania carinthiaca. *Bioorganic & Medicinal Chemistry*, *26*(14), 4320–4328. DOI: 10.1016/j.bmc.2018.07.035 PMID: 30049584

Ramlal, A., Nautiyal, A., Baweja, P., Kumar, V., Mehta, S., Mahto, R. K., Tripathi, S., Shanmugam, A., Pujari Mallikarjuna, B., Raman, P., Lal, S. K., Raju, D., & Rajendran, A. (2022). Angiotensin-converting enzyme inhibitory peptides and isoflavonoids from soybean [Glycine max (L.) Merr.]. *Frontiers in Nutrition*, *9*, 1068388. DOI: 10.3389/fnut.2022.1068388 PMID: 36505231

Romani, A., Ieri, F., Urciuoli, S., Noce, A., Marrone, G., Nediani, C., & Bernini, R. (2019). Health Effects of Phenolic Compounds Found in Extra-Virgin Olive Oil, By-Products, and Leaf of Olea europaea L. *Nutrients*, *11*(8), 1776. Advance online publication. DOI: 10.3390/nu11081776 PMID: 31374907

Romero, M., Toral, M., Gomez-Guzman, M., Jimenez, R., Galindo, P., Sanchez, M., Olivares, M., Gálvez, J., & Duarte, J. (2016). Antihypertensive effects of oleuropein-enriched olive leaf extract in spontaneously hypertensive rats. *Food & Function*, *7*(1), 584–593. DOI: 10.1039/C5FO01101A PMID: 26593388

Rosales-Mendoza, S., & Tello-Olea, M. A. (2015). Carrot cells: A pioneering platform for biopharmaceuticals production. *Molecular Biotechnology*, *57*(3), 219–232. DOI: 10.1007/s12033-014-9837-y PMID: 25572939

Ryu, J. H., & Kang, D. (2017). Physicochemical Properties, Biological Activity, Health Benefits, and General Limitations of Aged Black Garlic: A Review. *Molecules (Basel, Switzerland)*, *22*(6), 919. Advance online publication. DOI: 10.3390/molecules22060919 PMID: 28587168

Saibandith, B., Spencer, J. P. E., Rowland, I. R., & Commane, D. M. (2017). Olive Polyphenols and the Metabolic Syndrome. *Molecules (Basel, Switzerland)*, *22*(7), 1082. Advance online publication. DOI: 10.3390/molecules22071082 PMID: 28661446

Salaramoli, S., Mehri, S., Yarmohammadi, F., Hashemy, S. I., & Hosseinzadeh, H. (2022). The effects of ginger and its constituents in the prevention of metabolic syndrome: A review. *Iranian Journal of Basic Medical Sciences.*, *25*(6), 664–674. DOI: 10.22038/IJBMS.2022.59627.13231 PMID: 35949312

San Cheang, W., Yuen Ngai, C., Yen Tam, Y., Yu Tian, X., Tak Wong, W., Zhang, Y., Wai Lau, C., Chen, Z. Y., Bian, Z.-X., Huang, Y., & Ping Leung, F. (2015). Black tea protects against hypertension-associated endothelial dysfunction through alleviation of endoplasmic reticulum stress. *Scientific Reports*, *5*(1), 10340. DOI: 10.1038/srep10340 PMID: 25976123

Sanchez, M., Gonzalez-Burgos, E., Iglesias, I., Lozano, R., & Gomez-Serranillos, M. P. (2020). The Pharmacological Activity of Camellia sinensis (L.) Kuntze on Metabolic and Endocrine Disorders: A Systematic Review. *Biomolecules*, *10*(4), 603. Advance online publication. DOI: 10.3390/biom10040603 PMID: 32294991

Silva, E. A. P., Carvalho, J. S., Guimaraes, A. G., Barreto, R. S. S., Santos, M. R. V., Barreto, A. S., & Quintans-Junior, L. J. (2019). The use of terpenes and derivatives as a new perspective for cardiovascular disease treatment: A patent review (2008-2018). *Expert Opinion on Therapeutic Patents*, *29*(1), 43–53. DOI: 10.1080/13543776.2019.1558211 PMID: 30583706

Sohrabi, F., Niazmand, S., Mahmoudabady, M., & Niazmand, M. J. (2021). The vasodilatory effect of Apium graveolens L (celery) seed in isolated rat aorta: The roles of endothelium, calcium and potassium channels. *Avicenna Journal of Phytomedicine*, *11*(1), 44–53. https://www.ncbi.nlm.nih.gov/pubmed/33628719 PMID: 33628719

Soleti, R., Coue, M., Trenteseaux, C., Hilairet, G., Fizanne, L., Kasbi-Chadli, F., Mallegol, P., Chaigneau, J., Boursier, J., Krempf, M., Geoffriau, E., Andriantsitohaina, R., & Ouguerram, K. (2021). Carrot Supplementation Improves Blood Pressure and Reduces Aortic Root Lesions in an Atherosclerosis-Prone Genetic Mouse Model. *Nutrients*, *13*(4), 1181. Advance online publication. DOI: 10.3390/nu13041181 PMID: 33918417

Song, X., Kong, J., Song, J., Pan, R., & Wang, L. (2021). Angelica sinensis Polysaccharide Alleviates Myocardial Fibrosis and Oxidative Stress in the Heart of Hypertensive Rats. *Computational and Mathematical Methods in Medicine*, *6710006*, 1–10. Advance online publication. DOI: 10.1155/2021/6710006 PMID: 34527077

Sultana, S., & Asif, H. M. (2017). Review: Medicinal plants combating against hypertension: A green antihypertensive approach. *Pakistan Journal of Pharmaceutical Sciences*, *30*(6), 2311–2319. https://www.ncbi.nlm.nih.gov/pubmed/29175804 PMID: 29175804

Sun, W., Yan, C., Frost, B., Wang, X., Hou, C., Zeng, M., Gao, H., Kang, Y., & Liu, J. (2016). Pomegranate extract decreases oxidative stress and alleviates mitochondrial impairment by activating AMPK-Nrf2 in hypothalamic paraventricular nucleus of spontaneously hypertensive rats. *Scientific Reports*, *6*(1), 34246. DOI: 10.1038/srep34246 PMID: 27713551

Sundar Dhilip Kumar, S., Houreld, N. N., & Abrahamse, H. (2018). Therapeutic Potential and Recent Advances of Curcumin in the Treatment of Aging-Associated Diseases. *Molecules (Basel, Switzerland)*, *23*(4), 835. Advance online publication. DOI: 10.3390/molecules23040835 PMID: 29621160

Tabassum, N., & Ahmad, F. (2011). Role of natural herbs in the treatment of hypertension. *Pharmacognosy Reviews*, *5*(9), 30–40. DOI: 10.4103/0973-7847.79097 PMID: 22096316

Turgut Cosan, D., Saydam, F., Ozbayer, C., Doganer, F., Soyocak, A., Gunes, H. V., Değirmenci, İ., Kurt, H., Üstüner, M. C., & Bal, C. (2015). Impact of tannic acid on blood pressure, oxidative stress and urinary parameters in L-NNA-induced hypertensive rats. *Cytotechnology*, *67*(1), 97–105. DOI: 10.1007/s10616-013-9661-4 PMID: 24306272

Vafaeipour, Z., Razavi, B. M., & Hosseinzadeh, H. (2022). Effects of turmeric (Curcuma longa) and its constituent (curcumin) on the metabolic syndrome: An updated review. *Journal of Integrative Medicine*, *20*(3), 193–203. DOI: 10.1016/j.joim.2022.02.008 PMID: 35292209

Wang, D., Ozen, C., Abu-Reidah, I. M., Chigurupati, S., Patra, J. K., Horbanczuk, J. O., Jóźwik, A., Tzvetkov, N. T., Uhrin, P., & Atanasov, A. G. (2018). Vasculoprotective Effects of Pomegranate (Punica granatum L.). *Frontiers in Pharmacology*, *9*, 544. DOI: 10.3389/fphar.2018.00544 PMID: 29881352

Wang, J., Xiong, X., & Feng, B. (2013). Effect of crataegus usage in cardiovascular disease prevention: An evidence-based approach. *Evidence-Based Complementary and Alternative Medicine : eCAM*, *149363*, 1–16. Advance online publication. DOI: 10.1155/2013/149363 PMID: 24459528

Widmer, R. J., Flammer, A. J., Lerman, L. O., & Lerman, A. (2015). The Mediterranean diet, its components, and cardiovascular disease. *The American Journal of Medicine*, *128*(3), 229–238. DOI: 10.1016/j.amjmed.2014.10.014 PMID: 25447615

Wolak, T., Sharoni, Y., Levy, J., Linnewiel-Hermoni, K., Stepensky, D., & Paran, E. (2019). Effect of Tomato Nutrient Complex on Blood Pressure: A Double Blind, Randomized Dose(-)Response Study. *Nutrients*, *11*(5), 950. Advance online publication. DOI: 10.3390/nu11050950 PMID: 31035474

Xie, M., Tao, W., Wu, F., Wu, K., Huang, X., Ling, G., Zhao, C., Lv, Q., Wang, Q., Zhou, X., Chen, Y., Yuan, Q., & Chen, Y. (2021). Anti-hypertensive and cardioprotective activities of traditional Chinese medicine-derived polysaccharides: A review. *International Journal of Biological Macromolecules*, *185*, 917–934. DOI: 10.1016/j.ijbiomac.2021.07.008 PMID: 34229020

Zhao, T., Li, C., Wang, S., & Song, X. (2022). Green Tea (Camellia sinensis): A Review of Its Phytochemistry, Pharmacology, and Toxicology. *Molecules (Basel, Switzerland)*, *27*(12), 3909. Advance online publication. DOI: 10.3390/molecules27123909 PMID: 35745040

Zheng, W., Huang, T., Tang, Q. Z., Li, S., Qin, J., & Chen, F. (2021). Astragalus Polysaccharide Reduces Blood Pressure, Renal Damage, and Dysfunction Through the TGF-beta1-ILK Pathway. *Frontiers in Pharmacology*, *12*, 706617. DOI: 10.3389/fphar.2021.706617 PMID: 34690754

Zhou, P., Xie, W., He, S., Sun, Y., Meng, X., Sun, G., & Sun, X. (2019). Ginsenoside Rb1 as an Anti-Diabetic Agent and Its Underlying Mechanism Analysis. *Cells*, *8*(3), 204. Advance online publication. DOI: 10.3390/cells8030204 PMID: 30823412

Chapter 8
Millet in Cancer Therapy: An Emerging Wonder Grain in Cancer Therapeutics

Shalini Mani
https://orcid.org/0000-0003-2500-6962
Jaypee Institute of Information Technology, Noida, India

Aanchal Verma
Jaypee Institute of Information Technology, Noida, India

ABSTRACT

Millet, an ancient whole grain, has a variety of health benefits. Its minerals support bone health. Incorporating millet into a healthy diet can improve overall health and provide a flexible and nutritious grain alternative. Despite its role in providing essential nutrients to the body, millet also has anticancer properties which make it an essential grain for the treatment of different types of cancer. Antioxidants of millets such as flavonoids and phenolic compounds, may help prevent oxidative stress and cellular damage, both of which have been associated with cancer formation. Its high fiber content promotes healthy digestion and intestinal regularity, potentially lowering the risk of colorectal cancer. Certain millet varieties also include lignans, which may alter hormone metabolism, potentially lowering the incidence of hormone-related malignancies such as breast cancer. This chapter will explain the role of different natural compounds and phytochemicals from varieties of millet in the treatment of these two main cancers

DOI: 10.4018/979-8-3693-9112-9.ch008

1. INTRODUCTION

Millet belongs to the Poaceae family and encompasses grains from various forage grasses. Due to their grain texture, these grains are categorized as "coarse cereals" similar to sorghum, which makes them less convenient to process and prepare than rice and wheat (Subba Rao et al. 2002; Hassan and Zahra Mohammed 2021). The distinctive qualities of millet make it desirable for both agricultural production and human consumption. In terms of agricultural output, it is ranked as the sixth-largest cereal crop in the world. The crop is more advantageous than most major cereals in several ways, making it especially desirable in regions with difficult agricultural conditions. The resistance of millet to pests and pathogens is one of its important characteristics. Because of this resilience, farmers have a less harmful choice that requires less frequent use of pesticides. Additionally, millet has a shorter growing season than other grains, which enables farmers to cultivate it more effectively and harvest it earlier. Moreover, millet produces well even in dry conditions, which is crucial in areas where a lack of water is a regular problem (Belton et al. 2002; Ajiboye et al. 2017; Devi et al. 2014; Michaelraj et al. 2013). Due to these positive traits, developing nations have expressed a strong interest in using millet as a food source, while some wealthy nations are looking into its potential for the production of bioethanol and biofilms (Li, Jingjun, et al. 2008). Millets can be used as a food source to give human populations nutritional and economic security, particularly in dryland areas of rural India (Pradhan et al. 2010). Millet is a crucial component of the staple diet in many African and Asian nations, especially for the less affluent sections of the population (Chandrasekara et al. 2011). In these regions, millet is frequently used to make traditional dishes and drinks, including bread, porridge, and snack items, whether they are fermented or not (Chandrasekara et al. 2012; Blandino et al. 2003). Millet has different varieties such as proso millet (*Penicum miliaceum*), little millet (*Panicum sumatrense*), kodo millet (*Paspalum setaceum*), pearl millet (*Pennisetum glaucum*), foxtail millet (*Setaria italic*), finger millet (*Eleusine coracana*), sorghum (*Sorghum bicolor*), oats (*Avena sativa*), barnyard millet (*Echinochloa utilis*), proso millet (*Penicum miliaceum*), barley (*Hordeum vulgare*) (Bouis and Howarth E 2000; Kaur et al. 2014). Statistical analysis conducted by the Agricultural and processed food products export development authority (APEDA) found that India is the world's greatest producer of millet with pearl millet being the leading type in India among all the varieties that account for 40.51% of the total production of millet in the whole world in 2020 (https://apeda.gov.in/milletportal/Production.html).

In the coming decades, it is anticipated that climate change will significantly reduce the world's production of wheat, rice, and maize, by anywhere between 13% and 20%, according to a recent study by the Consultative Group for International

Agricultural Research (CGIAR) and the Consortium's Climate Change, Agriculture, and Food Security (CCAFS) (Bossuet J. 2012). It is extremely difficult to meet the estimated food demands of 9 billion people by 2050 with current agricultural output levels, which must be increased by almost 70%. CGIAR experts have suggested that farmers may need to switch their attention to developing crops that demonstrate greater tolerance to drought and heat to overcome this probable loss in agricultural yield. Barley, sorghum, and millet are a few examples of these hardy plants (Bossuet J. 2012). Millets may thus soon overtake other cereal crops as the dominant crop in the fields of national and international agriculture, food and health systems, value chains, and markets.

Apart from serving as an everyday meal, millet is considered to be highly nutritional and found to have the potential to prevent cardiovascular diseases and cancer. Additionally, it has been connected to decreasing cholesterol levels, blood pressure, the risk of heart disease, and the rate of fat absorption (Truswell and A. S 2002; Gupta et al. 2012). Research has revealed that certain whole grain millet types are particularly rich in several healthy substances, which include minerals, protein, unsaturated fatty acids, insoluble dietary fiber, and phenolic acids. Additionally, the majority of millet varieties have low anticipated Glycemic Index (GI) values, indicating that they have hypoglycemic qualities. Because of these properties millet is capable of being utilized as functional food however further in vitro investigations are required in this area (Bora et al. 2019). In this chapter, we have highlighted how millet is a wonderful grain that provides us with different types of nutrients and phytochemicals and the important therapeutic role of millet in the treatment of two different types of cancer that is colorectal cancer and breast cancer.

2. IMPORTANT NUTRIENT AND PHYTOCHEMICAL COMPOSITION OF MILLET

The nutritional value of food is very important for preserving a person's overall physical health. Maximizing human genetic potential, long-term health, and development all depend on good nutrition. Dietary quality must be prioritized to solve the persistent problems of food insecurity and malnutrition (Pragya et al. 2012). India has the highest rates of malnutrition in the world (15.2% of the total population), making it a country that struggles greatly with hunger and malnutrition. Given the severity of the hunger and malnutrition crisis, India was placed 100th out of 119 nations in the Global Hunger Index for 2017 (Von Grebmer K et al. 2017). Along with deficiencies in important micronutrients including iodine, iron, and vitamin A, protein energy malnutrition (PEM) is a major contributor to illness and mortality in

India (Lozano et al. 2012). These dietary deficits cause a variety of health problems and add to the nation's food shortages.

Millets have been discovered to offer excellent nutritional content equivalent to main cereals like wheat and rice, in addition to their agricultural benefits (Parameswaran et al. 1994). Except for lysine and threonine, these grains provide good supplies of vital amino acids in addition to being high in macronutrients like carbs. However, millets have a comparatively high methionine content, a crucial amino acid for several bodily physiological processes (Mal et al. 2010; Pragya et al. 2012). Plants contain bioactive substances called phytochemicals, which are linked to several health advantages and vitamins are also present in millet. They have anti-inflammatory and antioxidant properties and can guard against chronic illnesses. Millets are a potent weapon against nutrient shortages since they are a rich source of phytonutrients, vitamins, and minerals. Millets can be a part of a healthy diet and can be used to combat issues like malnutrition, hunger, and micronutrient deficiencies. This is true, especially in areas where millets are already staple foods (Mal et al. 2010; Pragya et al. 2012; Meena et al. 2021).

2.1 Micronutrients

Minerals are very essential and play a variety of roles in the body's physiological functions, such as bone growth, blood clotting, cell signaling, heart rate regulation, metabolism of cell energy, transport of oxygen, protein, and fat metabolism, and coenzyme function in the nervous system and body immunity (Soetan et al. 2010). Millets provide a substantial benefit in addressing these nutritional needs because they are rich in minerals. Millets have a much higher mineral content per 100g (varying from 1.7% to 4.3%) than other cereals like rice (0.6%) and wheat (1.5%). Osteoporosis is a frequent ailment in India with calcium and iron shortages are widespread in poor nations. Finger millet is a great way to prevent osteoporosis because of its high calcium concentration (340 mg/100 g, roughly) (Puranik et al. 2017; Sharma et al. 2017). Due to their high iron content, pearl millet and barnyard millet are advantageous in preventing anemia. The high zinc concentration of foxtail millet (4.1 mg/100 g) aids in the prevention of disorders linked to low zinc intake and give strength to the immune system (Kulkarni et al. 2018; Kumar et al. 2018; Kumar et al. 2021). Additionally, millets are an excellent provider of water-soluble vitamins including niacin (B3), riboflavin (B2), and folic acid, which must be consumed through diet as they are unable to be stored by the body. Millets are a great approach to improving nutritional security and balance in the diet (Girish et al. 2014).

2.2 Macronutrients

Millets are good for our health since they are rich in fiber, antioxidants, and gluten-free proteins. These grains are loaded with biologically active substances and have a low glycemic index (Kannan et al. 2013). Millets excel way of getting protein, energy, and important minerals like trace elements, according to their nutritional profile. Millets are a great nutritional choice because they are mostly composed of dietary fiber and soluble carbohydrates, making up about 65% of their total carbohydrates. Genotypes of pearl millet include between 62.8% and 70.5% starch, while some studies estimate that the total starch content is between 71.82% and 81.02% (Ouattara-Cheik et al. 2006). According to research, the amount of soluble sugars in pearl millet ranges from 1.2% to 2.6%, and the amount of amylose varies from 21.9% to 28.8%. According to (Bhatt et al.2003), The overall carbohydrate amount in finger millet falls between 72 to 79.5%. Between 59.5% and 61.2% of the samples contained starch, 1.4%–1.8% of cellulose, 6.2%–7.2% of pentosans, and 0.04%–0.6% of lignin (Wankhede et al. 1979).

Millets are an excellent choice for protein, with pearl millet having a protein level that is greater at roughly 11.6% than that of rice (7.2%), barley (11.5%), maize (11.1%), and sorghum (10.4%) (Jha et al. 2013). In contrast, finger millet has a protein content of 5-8% (Adeola et al. 1995). In contrast to wheat, barley, and rice, pearl millet has an amino acid profile that is high in important amino acids including lysine, threonine, methionine, and cysteine (Chethan et al. 2007; Adeola et al. 1995; Rooney et al. 1981). In terms of how proteins are distributed, pearl millet is compared to maize and is an appropriate choice for both protein and energy for people. The necessary amino acids are more easily digested in pearl millet than in maize. In terms of essential amino acid balance, finger millet is superior to other millet varieties because it has higher concentrations of lysine, threonine, and valine (Hoseney and R. C 1994).

Table 1. Comparision of nutritional composition in different varieties of millet

Variety	Carbohydrate (g)	Protein (g)	Fat (g)	Ash (g)	Fibre (g)	Ca (mg)	Fe (mg)	Zn (mg)	Thiamine (mg)	Riboflavin (mg)	Niacin (mg)	Energy (kcal)
Sorghum	71	10.4	3.1	1.8	2.0	25	5.4	3.1	0.38	0.15	4.3	329
Finger Millet	59-75	6.9-10.9	1.5	2.6	15.2	350	3.9	3.13	0.42	0.19	1.1	336
Kodo Millet	72-76	6.2-13.1	3.2-4.9	3.3	5.2	35	1.7	1.9-2.4	0.15	0.09	2.0	353
Foxtail Millet	55-69	11.2	4.0	3.3	9.4	31	2.8	2.92	0.59	0.11	3.2	351

continued on following page

Table 1. Continued

Variety	Carbohydrate (g)	Protein (g)	Fat (g)	Ash (g)	Fibre (g)	Ca (mg)	Fe (mg)	Zn (mg)	Thiamine (mg)	Riboflavin (mg)	Niacin (mg)	Energy (kcal)
Fonio Millet	68-75	8.4	3.3	3.4	18.2	20	2.1	1.5	0.17	0.22	1.15	379
Little Millet	76	15	4.5	3.4	2.5	17	9.3	5.25	0.30	0.09	3.2	329
Barnyard	74	11.0	5.2	4.5	13.6	22	18.6	3	0.33	0.10	4.2	300
Pearl Millet	67-72	11.8	5.1	2.2	13.8	42	11.0	3.29	0.38	0.21	2.8	363
Proso Millet	64-76	12.6	2.9-11.6	2.7	13.1	15	2.2	2.36	0.41	0.28	4.54	316

Adapted from (Kumar, Anil, et al, 2021)

Pearl millet is advantageous for gut health and enhancing bowel motions since it is high in dietary fiber (Hassan et al. 2021). Pearl millet is suitable for non-insulin-dependent diabetic individuals due to the fiber's slow-digesting characteristics that assist control blood glucose levels (McIntosh et al. 2003). Diabetes incidence has been connected to millet consumption (McIntosh et al. 2003). Additionally, The high fiber content of millet may help reduce harmful cholesterol and prevent gall-stone formation. Because millet contains fiber, eating it can help prevent obesity because food moves more slowly through the digestive system. For the farming of livestock, pearl millet is a rich source of both neutral detergent fiber (NDF) and acid detergent fiber (ADF), as chickens have a hard time digesting fibrous diets (Shobana et al. 2009).

Pearl millet has a higher fat content than maize at about 5-7% (Mustafa et al. 2008). It contains a lot of fatty acids including palmitic, stearic, and linoleic acids, but less oleic acid than maize does (Gopalan et al. 1971). The free and bound non-polar lipid components in pearl millet have been characterized as triglycerides, diglycerides, and monoglycerides, which have an overall lipid content that ranges from 1.5 to 6.8%. The primary fatty acids in finger millet, however, are oleic, palmitic, and linoleic acids, with a total lipid content of about 5.2% (Kunyanga et al 2013). The total fatty acid composition of finger millet is composed of 74.4% unsaturated fatty acids and 25.6% saturated fatty acids (Kunyanga et al 2013). Table 1: Nutritional composition of different varieties of millet

2.3 Phytochemicals

A class of naturally occurring secondary metabolites known as polyphenols are distinguished by the presence of numerous phenol rings (Pandey et al. 2009; Manuja et al. 2013). They are categorized based on the number of phenol rings present in them and their binding patterns and are produced from phenylalanine or shikimic acid. The common categories of polyphenols are lignans, stilbenes, flavonoids, and phenolic acids. Millets are full of polyphenols including phenolic acids and tannins, which strengthen the immune system and serve as antioxidants (Chandrasekara et al. 2010). These substances contain antibacterial, antiviral, and anti-inflammatory activities, among other health advantages (Devi et al. 2014). Inhibiting carbohydrate-digesting enzymes is another benefit of millet phenolics, which helps to lower postprandial hyperglycemia (Shobana et al. 2009). Ferulic acid, which has been recognized for having antioxidant qualities, is the most prevalent phenolic acid found in millets. Proanthocyanidins and flavonoids are also present in millets, adding to their antioxidant capacity (Dykes et al. 2006). However, the bioavailability of proteins and minerals may be impacted by the presence of condensed tannins in colored millet cultivars. Overall, millets are beneficial in boosting health and preventing several ailments due to their polyphenol content.

The majority of the tannins in sorghum are phenolic chemicals, which are significant Phytochemicals found in plants (Hahn et al. 1984). These tannins help to safeguard the grain and preserve its quality by acting as a barrier against mold growth and fungal infections (Waniska et al. 1989). The amount of tannins in sorghum can vary greatly depending on how it is processed into food products. For instance, when sorghum was used to make bread and cookies, the tannin concentration was reduced by 72% and 52%, respectively (Awika et al. 2003).

3. HEALTH BENEFITS OF MILLET

Millets' nutraceutical qualities and high nutrient content make them an excellent source of health benefits. In particular, for those with diabetes, their high fiber content and low glycemic index make them a good option for controlling blood sugar levels (Lakshmi Kumari et al. 2002). Furthermore, millet's high magnesium content helps lower the incidence of heart attacks and migraines. Niacin, a nutrient found in millets, helps to lower cholesterol levels, and eating millets may also lower C-reactive protein and harmful lipids, potentially reducing the risk of cardiovascular disease. Phosphorus, which is crucial for determining cell structure and producing ATP, the energy currency of cells, is abundant in millets. Additionally, millets include anti-aging and antioxidant characteristics that can help control oxidative stress and lessen the effects of several health problems, including diabetes, cancer, neurological disorders, cardiovascular troubles, and age-related diseases (Chandrasekara et al. 2010). Whole grains were first believed to have health benefits because of the vitamins, minerals, vital fatty acids, and fiber they contained. However, more recent research has revealed the significance of other bioactive compounds that interact to produce beneficial effects. These molecules include hormone-active elements like lignans and phytosterols, antinutrients like phytic acid and tannins, resistant starch, oligosaccharides, lipids, antioxidants such phenolic acids, avenanthramides, and flavonoids. Therefore this chapter we will particularly discuss the beneficiary effects of millet on colorectal cancer and breast cancer treatment.

3.1 Colorectal Cancer

Colorectal Cancer (CRC) is a common and fatal digestive system cancer that was reported in 2018 approx 9.6 million deaths (Bray et al. 2018). Due to medication resistance, both traditional and cutting-edge therapies, such as the usage of oxaliplatin (OXA), frequently suffer from decreased efficacy (Liu et al. 2014). A breakthrough medication with strong anticancer efficacy and few adverse side effects is urgently needed to address this issue. An important risk factor for CRC development has been identified as inflammatory bowel disease (IBD). IBD patients are more likely to develop CRC, and the severity of IBD is strongly connected with cancer incidence (Zhang et al. 2014; Nadeem et al. 2020). Both spontaneous and colitis-related CRC are significantly influenced by chronic inflammation and modified signaling pathways related to IBD (Liu et al. 2014). Intervention techniques that target intestinal inflammation and early-stage carcinogenesis are vital for lowering CRC morbidity and death, particularly in developing countries where the condition is growing more common. With their wide variety of bioactive components, whole grains have the potential to help prevent and treat CRC. Understanding the mechanisms underlying these effects will allow for the development of novel treatments and medications that effectively harness the potential of whole grains to fight CRC.

3.2 Millet: A New Age Therapeutic of Colorectal Cancer

A wound healing experiment was conducted to determine that FMBP, a novel peroxidase present in foxtail millet, might prevent colon cancer cells (DLD1 cells), from migrating while not affecting healthy colon epithelial cells (FHC cells). In their test, a "wound" was made on a layer of cells, and when the wound heals over time, cell migration was detected. The results showed that FMBP had a considerable dose-dependent inhibitory effect on the migration of colon cancer cells (DLD1 cells) with a negligible effect on normal epithelial cells (FHC cells), indicating that the inhibition of DLD1 cell migration was more pronounced at higher FMBP concentrations (Shan et al. 2014). MTT experiment was also performed to further validate and results showed that FMBP administration had no appreciable impact on the proliferation of both DLD1 and FHC cells at the tested dosages. This is an important piece of proof since it shows that FMBP's inhibition of DLD1 cell migration is not caused by altered cell proliferation. This indicates that rather than having an indirect impact through alterations in the migration process, FMBP's effect on cancer cell migration is probably due to its direct influence on the migration process. Researchers further found that FMBP inhibits epithelial–mesenchymal transition (EMT), which suppresses mesenchymal characteristics by the decrease in N- cadherin and vimentin expression while promoting an epithelial-like state by inducing E- cadherin expression, to cause its anti-migration actions in colon cancer cells. FMBP prevents cancer cells from migrating and invading, which are crucial steps in the metastatic progression of tumors. This is done by preserving an epithelial phenotype and boosting cell-cell adhesion (Shan et al. 2014). In another experiment, findings offer proof that FMBP targets the JAK/STAT3 signaling pathway to exert its anti-EMT actions in colorectal cancer cells. The EMT process is inhibited by FMBP therapy because it lowers the levels of phosphorylated STAT3, which in turn impacts downstream targets like c-Myc and Snail1. An in vivo research was done using xenografted tumor models to ascertain how FMBP interferes with the STAT3 signaling pathway. To do this, the researchers used histology analysis and western blotting to analyze the STAT3 and its downstream proteins expression linked to EMT. The outcomes of the in vivo trial supported the conclusions drawn from the in vitro tests. Particularly, when compared to the control group, STAT3, and phosphorylated STAT3 levels in the cellular matrix and nucleus were considerably lower in mice treated with FMBP. This decrease in STAT3 activity suggests that FMBP effectively prevents the STAT3 signaling pathway from being activated in a tumor context. These results demonstrate the potential of FMBP to be a successful therapeutic drug in the setting of cancer metastasis by inhibiting key signaling pathways related to tumor invasion and EMT (Shan et al. 2014).

Another group of scientists has investigated the potential of foxtail millet's soluble dietary fiber (FMB-SDF). The study used the MTT assay to examine how FMB-SDF affected the activity of colorectal cancer cells (HT-29, and HCT116) and normal human cells (HCT-8, LS-174 T). The rcsults showed that FMB-SDF had no effect on the proliferation of HCT-8 and LS-174 T cells within the examined concentration range of 0-20 mg/mL but had a dose-dependent inhibitory effect on the proliferation of HT-29 and HCT116 cells (Ren et al.2023). This shows that FMB-SDF specifically inhibits HT-29 and HCT116 cell proliferation, two colorectal cancer cell lines. Using HCT116 and HT-29 cells, the researchers carried out cell cloning and development tests to learn more about the anti-colorectal cancer action of FMB-SDF. The outcomes supported the conclusions drawn from the MTT experiment, showing that FMB-SDF significantly inhibited the growth of both HCT116 and HT-29 cells (Ren et al. 2023; Yang et al. 2021). These outcomes bolster FMB-SDF's potential as a powerful drug for the treatment of colorectal cancer. Studies have demonstrated that under normal circumstances, the equilibrium between oxidation and anti-oxidation is maintained (Sun et al. 2013). However, compared to normal cells, tumor cells have a higher baseline level of oxidative stress, which makes them more vulnerable to extra ROS production, which might result in apoptosis (Maillet et al. 2013). The researchers employed a ROS fluorescent probe called dihydroethyl (DHE) to examine how FMB-SDF affected the formation of ROS in colorectal cancer cells. The findings demonstrate that FMB-SDF treatment of HCT116 and HT-29 cells increased the levels of ROS. The data suggest that in comparison to the control group, the increase in ROS levels was very significant in HCT116 cells (with **P 0.01) and substantial in HT-29 cells (with *P 0.05) (Ren et al. 2023). According to these results, FMB-SDF causes excessive ROS generation in both HCT116 and HT-29 cells, which may help explain some of its anti-cancer actions. Tumour cells have a greater baseline level of oxidative stress, which makes them more susceptible to further ROS generation brought on by FMB-SDF. In cancer cells, excessive ROS production can cause oxidative damage and activate apoptotic pathways, thereby inhibiting their ability to proliferate and causing them to die. Mouse model studies have also been done to test the anti-cancer properties of FMB-SDF, the findings imply that the CS7BL/6 mice colon cancer model of FMB-SDF shows strong anti-colon cancer potential. It enhances the mice's general health and body weight and seems to guard against colon tissue damage brought on by the cancer model. These results confirm FMB-SDF's potential as a strong therapeutic agent for the treatment of colon cancer. To completely comprehend its methods of action and its potential efficacy and safety in patients with human colon cancer, however, more investigation and clinical studies are required (Ren et al. 2023).

There are many phytochemicals in millet bran, however, polyphenols stand out for having a wide range of therapeutic and pharmacological effects. In millet bran, polyphenols are present in both free and bound forms which is a very noteworthy quality of millet bran. Free polyphenols are freely soluble in water and quickly absorbed by the body, whereas bound polyphenols are joined to other plant cell wall elements, which reduces their bioavailability during digestion. Research has been done to assess the impact of bound polyphenols in the inner shells (BPIS) on the proliferation of human colon cancer cells (HCT -116) using an MTT assay. The outcomes showed that BPIS suppressed HCT-116 cell proliferation in a way that was both time-dependent as well as dose-dependent. For HCT-116 cells, the BPIS IC50 value was discovered to range between 0.8 and 0.05 mg/ml after treatment for 24 hours with various dosages of BPIS (range from 0 to 1.43 mg/ml) (Shi et al. 2015). This shows that colon adenocarcinoma cells' ability to grow and proliferate is effectively hampered by BPIS. To confirm the antiproliferative effect of BPIS on cancer cells, the scientists further perform the clonogenic assay, which assessed a cell's capacity to form a surviving colony. This assay's outcomes showed that BPIS administration causes HCT-116 cell clonogenic survival to be markedly reduced. The cell clonogenicities were lowered by around 50% at a dosage of 0.30 mg/ml.

This shows that BPIS not only prevents cell proliferation but also affects HCT-116 cells' capacity to form colonies, which is crucial for tumor development and growth (Shi et al. 2015).

It has been already reported that polyphenols cause the generation of ROS and generate fierce oxidative stress which can be the cause of cell death of cancer cells induced by BPIS (Bonilla-Porras et al. 2011). To understand the mechanism or the process behind BPIS-induced cancer cell death they performed an experiment using the DCFH-DA stain via microplate spectrophotometer, the intracellular ROS levels in BPIS-treated and untreated HCT116 cells were examined. The results showed that dose-dependent variations in intracellular ROS levels were caused by BPIS administration at various doses, ranging from 0 to 0.88 mg/ml (Shi et al. 2015). ROS levels significantly increased after 0.71 mg/ml BPIS was applied to HCT-116 cells for 24 hours. The rise in ROS levels was, however, reversed when the culture media is supplemented with ROS scavenger NAC (N-acetyl-cysteine). This shows that the chemical did facilitate the increase in intracellular ROS brought on by BPIS. Apoptosis, a process of programmed cell death, is necessary for maintaining tissue homeostasis. The triggering of apoptosis has been linked to the production of reactive oxygen species (ROS) (Suma et al. 2012). Hoechst 33342 staining was used to look at typical morphological alterations indicative of apoptosis to evaluate the apoptotic effects of BPIS. Following BPIS treatment, the cells exhibited typical apoptotic characteristics with no evident apoptotic characteristics seen when BPIS and NAC (a ROS scavenger) were combined, demonstrating that apoptosis induced by BPIS was facilitated by increased ROS levels (Shi et al. 2015). It was also found the elevated level of ROS reduces mitochondrial membrane potential and results from Western blotting revealed that Bcl-2 protein levels decreased while Bax protein levels rose in BPIS-treated cells, changing the Bcl-2/Bax ratio. The drop in mitochondrial membrane potential brought on by BPIS may be related to these changes in the Bcl-2/Bax ratio (Shi et al. 2015). The altered Bcl-2/Bax ratio and disrupted mitochondrial membrane potential brought on by the higher ROS levels ultimately result in the activation of apoptotic pathways. These results clarify the potential anticancer mechanism of BPIS and support the possibility of using it as an antitumor drug in cancer therapy.

In some studies, it was found that BPIS has remarkable potential in reversing oxaliplatin (OXA) chemo-resistance in colorectal cancer (CRC) both in vitro and in vivo (Zhang et al. 2021). Additionally, scientists have assessed the individual effects of ferulic acid (FA) and p-coumaric acid (p-CA), the effects of the two primary active components of BPIS on OXA chemo-resistance in CRC. The findings showed that, interestingly, FA and p-CA's combined inhibitory effects at their natural proportion as seen in BPIS were less potent than BPIS's at the same dose (Zhang et al. 2021). In colorectal cancer (CRC) patients, the up-regulation of P-gp in cancer tissues is a key cause of chemotherapy failure because it results in higher drug efflux and decreased drug accumulation in cancer cells (Catanzaro et al. 2016). Rho-123, a fluorescent dye frequently used to measure P-gp activity, was utilized to determine the efflux function of P-gp to determine the functional influence of BPIS on P-gp. Results showed that drug-resistant HCT-116/L cells treated with BPIS significantly increased the mean Rho-123 fluorescence intensity. This shows that BPIS improves drug-resistant cells' vulnerability to OXA by decreasing P-gp expression and increasing intracellular accumulation of OXA (Zhang et al. 2021). Drug-resistant HCT-116/L cells have dysregulated levels of the ganglioside GM3 catabolism-related metabolites Cer, GM3, and Gb3 in comparison to HCT-116 cells. The aberrant decrease in Cer and GM3 levels and the increased Gb3 level in drug-resistant HCT-116/L cells were dramatically reversed by BPIS treatment, which is encouraging. Additionally, it was shown that, both in vitro and in vivo, BPIS reduced the expression of NEU3, a crucial enzyme involved in the degradation of ganglioside GM3. These results indicate that BPIS is crucial for the reversal of NEU3-mediated ganglioside GM3 degradation, which helps to reverse chemo-resistance to OXA in CRC (Zhang et al. 2021). The molecular mechanism behind the anti-MDR activity of BPIS in CRC is more understood by the scientists who have found that BPIS, together with its functional components FA and p-CA, epigenetically controls miR-149 production by lowering its methylation. The downregulation of important cell cycle regulators and G2/M phase cell cycle arrest caused by elevated miR-149 expression ultimately boosts the chemosensitivity of CRC cells. These results provide the framework for further BPIS development as a potential anti-MDR agent for the treatment of CRC. BPIS shows promise as a potential therapeutic approach to overcome chemoresistance and enhance the efficacy of chemotherapy in CRC patients by focusing on the epigenetic regulation of miR-149 (Shan et al. 2021).

Researchers have found that foxtail millet consumption had favorable effects in lowering the incidence of colitis-associated CRC and attenuating colonic inflammation in mice produced by a carcinogenic agent (AOM) and inflammatory triggers (DSS) (Zhang et al. 2020). The activation of two important signaling pathways, the Aryl hydrocarbon receptor (AHR) and G-protein-coupled receptors (GPCRs), as well as the reduction of STAT3 phosphorylation, have all been linked to the protective benefits of foxtail millet. These pathways are known to be crucial in controlling inflammation and the growth of tumors. The researchers found that these regulatory effects were mediated by microbial metabolites generated from foxtail millet (Zhang et al. 2020).

Therefore different phytochemicals derived from foxtail millet can be used for the treatment of colorectal cancer (summarised in Table 2). Including foxtail millet in the diet will be beneficial and can be preventive against colorectal cancer.

3.3 Breast Cancer

Breast cancer is a serious global health issue that kills a lot of people every year, mostly women. Approximately 570,000 people died from it worldwide in 2015, and more than 1.5 million women are diagnosed with it each year (Stewart et al. 2003) (https://www.who.int/activities/preventing-cancer). In America, almost 30% of all new instances of cancer among women were breast cancer in 2017 (Siegel et al. 2018). Breast cancer can spread to distant organs, making it difficult to treat at advanced stages, therefore early diagnosis is essential for a better prognosis and greater survival rates. Mammography is a popular screening technique that has significantly decreased mortality. Another screening method is magnetic resonance imaging (MRI), which is renowned for its sensitivity (Drukteinis et al. 2013). Obesity and problems with lipid metabolism, in addition to known risk factors including inheritance, age, menstrual history, marriage, and delivery, also contribute to the development of breast cancer (Shapira and N 2017; Ringel et al. 2020). Lipids are essential to the rapid multiplication of cancer cells, which calls for the synthesis of new cell membranes. Due to their greater fluidity when compared to saturated fatty acids (SFA), monounsaturated fatty acids (MUFA) are frequently used by tumor cells to create cell membranes (Ferreri et al. 2016). There is strong evidence that eating whole grains lowers your chance of developing breast cancer. Whole grains have been noted as potential sources of nutraceutical substances with breast cancer chemopreventive characteristics.

3.4 Millet and Breast Cancer

Multiple experiments have been done to understand the anticancer properties of millet against breast cancer. The triple-negative MDA-MB-231 orthotopic breast cancer model in female BALB/c nude mice was used in the study to examine the anti-tumor effectiveness of BPIS (a compound from the foxtail millet bran). The mice received BPIS (10 mg/kg) over 21 days once the tumors had grown to a size of 80 mm3. According to the findings, BPIS greatly delayed the growth of breast tumors while posing no risk to the heart, liver, spleen, lung, or kidney (Zhang et al. 2021). In vitro tests were also carried out to look into how BPIS affected breast cancer cell lines MDA-MB-231 and MCF-7 as well as healthy mammary gland epithelial cells MCF-10A. In MDA-MB-231 and MCF-7 cells, the administration of BPIS lowered the number of tumor cells and the levels of the cell proliferation indicator ki-67. However, the BPIS therapy did not affect the normal MCF-10A cells (Zhang et al. 2021). Additionally, BPIS reduced the rate of colony development in MDA-MB-231 and MCF-7 cells while having no impact on MCF-10A cell colonies, according to a colony formation experiment (Zhang et al. 2021). In another experiment by the same group of scientists, The outcomes demonstrated that BPIS therapy resulted in G1 phase arrest in breast cancer cells MCF-7 and MDA-MB-231 (Zhang et al. 2021). The production of cell membranes and the growth of new cells both depend heavily on lipids. Surprisingly, BPIS therapy boosted lipid accumulation in both types of breast cancer cells as seen by an increase in lipid droplet size and number. The lipid extraction experiment supported the rise in intracellular lipid accumulation, and this impact was time-dependent (Zhang et al. 2021). In BPIS-treated breast cancer cells, the amount of neutral lipids such as triglycerides (TG) and total cholesterol (TC) also increased dramatically. These results suggest that BPIS may inhibit the production of tumor cells by halting the G1 phase of the cell cycle while concurrently encouraging lipid synthesis in breast cancer cells (Zhang et al. 2021). According to the research, BPIS has the potential to cure breast cancer by focusing on lipid metabolism and the GRP78/SREBP-1 signaling pathway. The discovery of vitexin and syringic acid as the primary active components in charge of the anti-tumor actions of BPIS opened the door for additional investigation and the potential creation of novel breast cancer therapies (Zhang et al. 2021).

In another study, Both FTM-FP (extracting seeds using 70% ethanol) and FTM-BP (extracting seeds using 10% alkali) fractions of foxtail millet have been shown in the study to have antioxidant and antiproliferative properties against breast cancer cells. Their capacity to cause DNA fragmentation and G2/M cell cycle arrest raises the possibility that they play a role in inducing apoptosis, which is a desirable result for prospective cancer therapies (Kuruburu et al. 2022). Red sorghum bran anthocyanins have been found to inhibit the proliferation of breast cancer cells (MCF-7) by inducing apoptosis, or programmed cell death (Devi et al. 2011). A different investigation discovered that a particular 3-deoxyanthocyanin from red sorghum bran reduced the survival of MCF-7 cells by controlling the expression of the proteins p53 and Bcl-2 (Suganyadevi et al. 2013). By causing cell cycle arrest in the G1 phase, sorghum extracts have also been demonstrated to inhibit the proliferation of breast cancer cells (MDA-MB-231 and MCF-7). The extracts accomplished this by downregulating the expression of molecules involved in angiogenesis (VEGF, VEGF-R2) and cell cycle control (cyclin D, cyclin E, p-Rb) as well as influencing particular pathways (JAK/STAT). These extracts greatly outperformed other grains like panicum, millet, and wheat in terms of their anticancer activities (Park et al. 2012). It has been demonstrated that sorghum 3-deoxy anthocyanidins are compared to foods from other diets, more cytotoxic to cancer cells (Shih et al. 2007). Additionally, it has been shown that sorghum tannins, which are contained in the bran, suppress the action of aromatase, an enzyme involved in the manufacture of estrogen and a possible target for the treatment of breast cancer (Hargrove et al. 2011). Recently a new study has been done to find out the anticancer effect of proso millet seeds. The research was carried out meticulously, starting with the extraction of millet seeds in

80% ethanol (EtOH), then sequential fractionation in four different organic solvents (hexane, methylene chloride, ethyl acetate, and butanol). The 80% EtOH extract has a noticeable effect of cytotoxicity on a human breast cancer cell line MDA-MB-231, according to an analysis of its cytotoxicity in comparison to other human cancer cell lines. As a result, the butanol (BuOH) fraction, which was shown to have the highest cytotoxicity among the organic solvent fractions obtained from the EtOH extract, was specifically investigated for its ability to cause apoptotic cell death. Following treatment with the BuOH fraction, the study found several apoptotic events in MDA-MB-231 cells, including the activation of BAK/BAX proteins, disruption of mitochondrial membrane potential (m), mitochondrial cytochrome c release in the cytosol, Caspase-8-9-3 activation, degradation of PARP, and apoptotic DNA fragmentation that was TUNEL-positive (Han et al. 2023). A striking difference in susceptibility between normal human mammary epithelial cells (MCF-10A) and MDA-MB-231 cells revealed that these effects were markedly selective towards the breast cancer cells. Furthermore, the results of the study suggest that the extrinsic apoptotic pathway is not necessary for the apoptotic mechanism induced by the BuOH fraction, as demonstrated by the uniform sensitivity seen in different clones of Jurkat T cells from patients with human acute lymphoblastic leukemia, regardless of Caspase-8 or Fas-associated death domain (FADD) deficiency (Han et al. 2023).

In an experiment, free and bound phenolic compounds were extracted from finger millet seeds via 70% ethanol (FM-FP) and 10% phenol (FM-BP). The research highlighted the antioxidant strength of both fractions, as shown by their robust capacity for DPPH radical scavenging and ferric ion reduction. It's interesting to note that the effect of FM-FP and FM-BP on the proliferation of cells shows significant variation between various cell lines. Particularly, FM-FP outperformed FM-BP in terms of triggering cell death against breast cancer cell lines, exhibiting significant cytotoxic ability (Kuruburu et al. 2022). The insights into cell cycle changes, and additional understandings of the mechanisms behind this cytotoxicity have been gained. Depending on the particular cell line, FM-FP leads to G0/G1 or G2/M phase cell cycle arrest. Additionally, the substantial DNA fragmentation brought on by the cytotoxic FM-FP caused an increase of cells in the Sub-G1 phase, shedding light on the complex mechanisms by which FM phenolic compounds exert their effects (Kuruburu et al. 2022). All the studies showing the effect of millet in the therapy of breast cancer have been summarised in Table 2.

Table 2. Summary of different phytocompounds of millets, used in the treatment of colorectal and breast cancer

S. No	Phytochemical/Natural compound	Type of Millet	Type of Cancer	Effect	Mechanism	Reference
1	Peroxidase	Foxtail Millet	Colorectal cancer	Restrict migration of Colorectal cancer cells	Targets the JAK/ STAT3 signaling pathway to prevent the epithelial-mesenchymal transition.	Shan et al. 2014
2	Soluble Dietary fiber	Foxtail Millet	Colorectal Cancer	Inhibits proliferation of Colorectal cancer cells	It increases the level of ROS in cells which leads to apoptosis.	Ren et al. 2023
3	Polyphenols	Foxtail Millet	Colorectal cancer	Inhibits colorectal cancer cell proliferation	Increases the level of ROS in the cells. Change the Bcl-2/Bax ratio of the cell. It Disrupts mitochondrial membrane potential.	Shi et al. 2015
		Foxtail Millet	Colorectal Cancer	Anti-Multi-drug resistant activity	It regulates the efflux pump of Colorectal cancer cells by decreasing the p-gP expression that leads to reversing the oxaliplatin resistance. It mediates NEU3 mediated gangliosideGM3 degradation. It causes overexpression of miR – 149 leading to an increase in chemosensitivity in colorectal cancer cells.	Zhang et al. 2021

continued on following page

Table 2. Continued

S. No	Phytochemical/Natural compound	Type of Millet	Type of Cancer	Effect	Mechanism	Reference
		Foxtail Millet	Breast Cancer	Inhibits cell proliferation	Reduces the expression of cell proliferation marker Ki-67 Leads to g1 phase cell cycle arrest Lipid accumulation Changes in GRP78/SREBP-1 signalling	Zhang et al. 2021
		Finger Millet	Breast cancer	Cytotoxic Effect	Cell cycle arrest at the G0/G1 or G2/M phase.	Kuruburu et al. 2022
4	Anthocyanin	Red Sorghum	Breast Cancer	Anti proliferative	Causes apoptosis or programmed cell death	Devi et al. 2011

continued on following page

Table 2. Continued

S. No	Phytochemical/Natural compound	Type of Millet	Type of Cancer	Effect	Mechanism	Reference
5	3- deoxyanthocyanin	Red Sorghum	Breast Cancer	Inhibits Cell proliferation	Changing the expression of p53 and Bcl-2 proteins. Causes cell cycle arrest in the G1 phase by downregulation of the expression of VEGF, VEGF-R2 proteins. It causes changes in JALK/STAT signaling	Suganyadevi et al. 2013
6	Seed rich in Phytochemicals	Proso Millet	Breast cancer	Apoptosis and Cytotoxic Effect	Activation of BAK/BAX protein. Disrupts the mitochondrial membrane potential Activation of caspase-8/9/3 PARP degradation	Han et al. 2023

4. CONCLUSION

Cancer is a broad and complex category of illnesses defined by the uncontrollable growth and spread of aberrant cells throughout the body. The prevalence and severity of cancer vary greatly depending on the type of cancer, geographical region, lifestyle factors, genetics, and medical advances. Cancer has become a major global health concern in recent decades, with millions of new cases identified each year. Cancer prevalence has been increasing as a result of causes such as aging populations, carcinogen exposure, bad lifestyles (including tobacco use, poor food, and lack of physical activity), and environmental factors. Cancer treatment with natural products or phytochemicals is a rising field of study that investigates the potential of plant-derived molecules to tackle this complicated disease. According to research, these substances can disrupt important cellular processes involved in cancer development, including angiogenesis (the production of new blood arteries to tumors), apoptosis (programmed cell death), and metastasis. Different varieties of millet are responsible for cancer cell apoptosis and delayed growth. Natural compounds and phytochemicals of foxtail millet such as peroxidases, polyphenols, and dietary fibers can be used as an active compound to develop therapeutics against colorectal cancer. They inhibit the migration of colorectal cancer cells and their proliferation which leads to delayed growth and cell death. Similarly, different varieties of millet such as foxtail millet, proso millet, finger millet, and sorghum millet are has been successful in the treatment of breast cancer. The use of millet in cancer treatment, like any complementary strategy, should be explored with healthcare specialists. Patients must adhere to the traditional therapies prescribed by medical professionals while also evaluating the potential benefits of introducing millet into their diet. More thorough clinical research is required to substantiate millets' unique involvement in cancer therapy and to establish optimal dosage and administration parameters. Millets may offer a fresh pathway for improving general health and potentially promoting the well-being of cancer patients in the context of an integrated and comprehensive treatment plan.

REFERENCES

Adeola, O., & Orban, J. I. (1995). Chemical composition and nutrient digestibility of pearl millet (Pennisetum glaucum) fed to growing pigs. *Journal of Cereal Science*, *22*(2), 177–184. DOI: 10.1016/0733-5210(95)90048-9

Adeola, O., & Orban, J. I. (1995). Chemical composition and nutrient digestibility of pearl millet (Pennisetum glaucum) fed to growing pigs. *Journal of Cereal Science*, *22*(2), 177–184. DOI: 10.1016/0733-5210(95)90048-9

Ajiboye, A. A., Dedeke, O. A., & Adeyemo, F. C. (2017). Investigation on anti-oxidants, free radical scavenger, and lipid peroxidation activities of whole grains finger millet (Eleusine coracana L.). *International Journal of Plant Biology*, *8*(1), 6684. DOI: 10.4081/pb.2017.6684

Awika, J. M., Rooney, L. W., Wu, X., Prior, R. L., & Cisneros-Zevallos, L. (2003). Screening methods to measure antioxidant activity of sorghum (Sorghum bicolor) and sorghum products. *Journal of Agricultural and Food Chemistry*, *51*(23), 6657–6662. DOI: 10.1021/jf034790i PMID: 14582956

Bhatt, A., Singh, V., Shrotria, P. K., & Baskheti, D. C. (2003). Coarse grains of Uttaranchal: ensuring sustainable food and nutritional security. *Indian farmer's digest, 7*(1), 34-38.

Blandino, A. (2003). Al-Aseeri ME Pandiella SS Cantero D. *Webb C. Cereal-Based Fermented Foods and Beverages Food Res.Int*, *36*, 527–543.

Bonilla-Porras, A. R., Jimenez-Del-Rio, M., & Velez-Pardo, C. (2011). Vitamin K3 and vitamin C alone or in combination induced apoptosis in leukemia cells by a similar oxidative stress signalling mechanism. *Cancer Cell International*, *11*(1), 19. DOI: 10.1186/1475-2867-11-19 PMID: 21663679

Bora, P., Ragaee, S., & Marcone, M. (2019). Characterisation of several types of millets as functional food ingredients. *International Journal of Food Sciences and Nutrition*, *70*(6), 714–724. DOI: 10.1080/09637486.2019.1570086 PMID: 30969135

Bossuet, J. 2012. Data from: millet for our bread in 2050? The International Crops Research Institute for the SemiArid Tropics (Library Open Access Repository ICRISAT) [accessed 2018 May 15]. http://www.icrisat.org/ClimateConversations.htm

Bouis, H. E. (2000). Enrichment of food staples through plant breeding: A new strategy for fighting micronutrient malnutrition. *Nutrition (Burbank, Los Angeles County, Calif.)*, *7*(16), 701–704. DOI: 10.1016/S0899-9007(00)00266-5 PMID: 10906604

Bray, F., Ferlay, J., Soerjomataram, I., Siegel, R. L., Torre, L. A., & Jemal, A. (2018). Global cancer statistics 2018: GLOBOCAN estimates of incidence and mortality worldwide for 36 cancers in 185 countries. *CA: a Cancer Journal for Clinicians*, *68*(6), 394–424. DOI: 10.3322/caac.21492 PMID: 30207593

Catanzaro, D., Filippini, R., Vianello, C., Carrara, M., Ragazzi, E., & Montopoli, M. (2016). Chlorogenic Acid Interaction with Cisplatin and Oxaliplatin: Studies in Cervical Carcinoma Cells. *Natural Product Communications*, *11*(4), 499–502. DOI: 10.1177/1934578X1601100421 PMID: 27396204

Chandrasekara, A., & Shahidi, F. (2010). Content of insoluble bound phenolics in millets and their contribution to antioxidant capacity. *Journal of Agricultural and Food Chemistry*, *58*(11), 6706–6714. DOI: 10.1021/jf100868b PMID: 20465288

Chandrasekara, A., & Shahidi, F. (2010). Content of insoluble bound phenolics in millets and their contribution to antioxidant capacity. *Journal of Agricultural and Food Chemistry*, *58*(11), 6706–6714. DOI: 10.1021/jf100868b PMID: 20465288

Chandrasekara, A., & Shahidi, F. (2011). Determination of antioxidant activity in free and hydrolyzed fractions of millet grains and characterization of their phenolic profiles by HPLC-DAD-ESI-MSn. *Journal of Functional Foods*, *3*(3), 144–158. DOI: 10.1016/j.jff.2011.03.007

Chandrasekara, A., & Shahidi, F. (2012). Bioaccessibility and antioxidant potential of millet grain phenolics as affected by simulated in vitro digestion and microbial fermentation. *Journal of Functional Foods*, *4*(1), 226–237. DOI: 10.1016/j.jff.2011.11.001

Chethan, S., & Malleshi, N. G. (2007). Finger millet polyphenols: Optimization of extraction and the effect of pH on their stability. *Food Chemistry*, *105*(2), 862–870. DOI: 10.1016/j.foodchem.2007.02.012

Devi, P. B., Vijayabharathi, R., Sathyabama, S., Malleshi, N. G., & Priyadarisini, V. B. (2014). Health benefits of finger millet (Eleusine coracana L.) polyphenols and dietary fiber: A review. *Journal of Food Science and Technology*, *51*(6), 1021–1040. DOI: 10.1007/s13197-011-0584-9 PMID: 24876635

Devi, P. B., Vijayabharathi, R., Sathyabama, S., Malleshi, N. G., & Priyadarisini, V. B. (2014). Health benefits of finger millet (Eleusine coracana L.) polyphenols and dietary fiber: A review. *Journal of Food Science and Technology*, *51*(6), 1021–1040. DOI: 10.1007/s13197-011-0584-9 PMID: 24876635

Devi, P. S., Kumar, M. S., & Das, S. M. (2011). Evaluation of antiproliferative activity of red sorghum bran anthocyanin on a human breast cancer cell line (mcf-7). *International Journal of Breast Cancer, 2011*, 2011. DOI: 10.4061/2011/891481 PMID: 22312562

Drukteinis, J. S., Mooney, B. P., Flowers, C. I., & Gatenby, R. A. (2013). Beyond mammography: New frontiers in breast cancer screening. *The American Journal of Medicine, 126*(6), 472–479. DOI: 10.1016/j.amjmed.2012.11.025 PMID: 23561631

Dykes, L., & Rooney, L. W. (2006). Sorghum and millet phenols and antioxidants. *Journal of Cereal Science, 44*(3), 236–251. DOI: 10.1016/j.jcs.2006.06.007

Ferreri, C., Masi, A., Sansone, A., Giacometti, G., Larocca, A. V., Menounou, G., Scanferlato, R., Tortorella, S., Rota, D., Conti, M., Deplano, S., Louka, M., Maranini, A., Salati, A., Sunda, V., & Chatgilialoglu, C. (2016). Fatty acids in membranes as homeostatic, metabolic and nutritional biomarkers: Recent advancements in analytics and diagnostics. *Diagnostics (Basel), 7*(1), 1. DOI: 10.3390/diagnostics7010001 PMID: 28025506

Girish, C., Meena, R. K., Mahima, D., & Mamta, K. (2014). Nutritional properties of minor millets: Neglected cereals with potentials to combat malnutrition. *Current Science, 107*(7), 1109–1111.

Gopalan, C., Rama Sastri, B. V., & Balasubramanian, S. C. (1971). *Nutritive value of Indian foods*. No Title.

Gupta, N., Srivastava, A. K., & Pandey, V. N. (2012). Biodiversity and nutraceutical quality of some Indian millets. *Proceedings of the National Academy of Sciences. India. Section B, Biological Sciences, 82*(2), 265–273. DOI: 10.1007/s40011-012-0035-z

Hahn, D. H., Rooney, L. W., & Earp, C. F. (1984). Tannins and phenols of sorghum.

Han, C. R., & Kim, Y. H. (2023). Apoptotic Effect of Proso Millet Grains on Human Breast Cancer MDA-MB-231 Cells Is Exerted by Activation of BAK and BAX, and Mitochondrial Damage-mediated Caspase Cascade Activation. , *33*(1), 15-24.

Hargrove, J. L., Greenspan, P., Hartle, D. K., & Dowd, C. (2011). Inhibition of aromatase and α-amylase by flavonoids and proanthocyanidins from Sorghum bicolor bran extracts. *Journal of Medicinal Food, 14*(7-8), 799–807. DOI: 10.1089/jmf.2010.0143 PMID: 21612457

Hassan, Z. M. (2021). *The nutritional use of millet grain for food and feed* (Doctoral dissertation).

Hassan, Z. M., Sebola, N. A., & Mabelebele, M. (2021). The nutritional use of millet grain for food and feed: A review. *Agriculture & Food Security*, *10*(1), 16. DOI: 10.1186/s40066-020-00282-6 PMID: 33815778

Hoseney, R. C. (1994). *Principles of cereal science and technology* (No. Ed. 2). American Association of Cereal Chemists (AACC).

Jha, A., Tripathi, A. D., Alam, T., & Yadav, R. (2013). Process optimization for manufacture of pearl millet-based dairy dessert by using response surface methodology (RSM). *Journal of Food Science and Technology*, *50*(2), 367–373. DOI: 10.1007/s13197-011-0347-7 PMID: 24425929

Kannan, S. M., Thooyavathy, R. A., Kariyapa, R. T., Subramanian, K., & Vijayalakshmi, K. (2013). Seed production techniques for cereals and millets. *Seed node of the revitalizing rainfed agriculture network Centre for Indian knowledge systems (CIICS)*, 1-39.

Kaur, K. D., Jha, A., Sabikhi, L., & Singh, A. K. (2014). Significance of coarse cereals in health and nutrition: A review. *Journal of Food Science and Technology*, *51*(8), 1429–1441. DOI: 10.1007/s13197-011-0612-9 PMID: 25114333

Kulkarni, D. B., Sakhale, B. K., & Giri, N. A. (2018). A potential review on millet grain processing. *International Journal of Nursing Sciences*, *3*(1), 1018.

Kumar, A., Rani, M., Mani, S., Shah, P., Singh, D. B., Kudapa, H., & Varshney, R. K. (2021). Nutritional significance and antioxidant-mediated antiaging effects of finger millet: Molecular insights and prospects. *Frontiers in Sustainable Food Systems*, *5*, 684318. DOI: 10.3389/fsufs.2021.684318

Kumar, A., Tomer, V., Kaur, A., Kumar, V., & Gupta, K. (2018). Millets: A solution to agrarian and nutritional challenges. *Agriculture & Food Security*, *7*(1), 31. DOI: 10.1186/s40066-018-0183-3

Kunyanga, C. N., Imungi, J. K., & Vellingiri, V. (2013). Nutritional evaluation of indigenous foods with potential food-based solution to alleviate hunger and malnutrition in Kenya. *Journal of Applied Biosciences*, *67*(0), 5277–5288. DOI: 10.4314/jab.v67i0.95049

Kuruburu, M. G., Bovilla, V. R., Leihang, Z., & Madhunapantula, S. V. (2022). Phytochemical-rich Fractions from Foxtail Millet (Setaria italica (L.) P. Beauv) Seeds Exhibited Antioxidant Activity and Reduced the Viability of Breast Cancer Cells In Vitro by Inducing DNA Fragmentation and Promoting Cell Cycle Arrest. *Anti-cancer Agents in Medicinal Chemistry*, *22*(13), 2477–2493. DOI: 10.2174/1871520622666220215122141 PMID: 35168527

Kuruburu, M. G., Bovilla, V. R., Naaz, R., Leihang, Z., & Madhunapantula, S. V. (2022). Variations in the anticancer activity of free and bound phenolics of finger millet (Eleusine coracana (L) Gaertn; variety KMR-301) seeds. *Phytomedicine Plus : International Journal of Phytotherapy and Phytopharmacology*, *2*(2), 100276. DOI: 10.1016/j.phyplu.2022.100276

Lakshmi Kumari, P., & Sumathi, S. (2002). Effect of consumption of finger millet on hyperglycemia in non-insulin-dependent diabetes mellitus (NIDDM) subjects. *Plant Foods for Human Nutrition (Dordrecht, Netherlands)*, *57*(3/4), 205–213. DOI: 10.1023/A:1021805028738 PMID: 12602929

Li, J., Chen, Z., Guan, X., Liu, J., Zhang, M., & Xu, B. (2008). Optimization of germination conditions to enhance hydroxyl radical inhibition by water-soluble protein from stress millet. *Journal of Cereal Science*, *48*(3), 619–624. DOI: 10.1016/j.jcs.2008.01.008

Liu, Y., Wu, W., Hong, W., Sun, X., Wu, J., & Huang, Q. (2014). Raltitrexed-based chemotherapy for advanced colorectal cancer. *Clinics and Research in Hepatology and Gastroenterology*, *38*(2), 219–225. DOI: 10.1016/j.clinre.2013.11.006 PMID: 24388340

Lozano, R., Naghavi, M., Foreman, K., Lim, S., Shibuya, K., Aboyans, V., & Remuzzi, G. (2012). Global and regional mortality from 235 causes of death for 20 age groups in 1990 and 2010: A systematic analysis for the Global Burden of Disease Study 2010. *Lancet*, *380*(9859), 2095–2128. DOI: 10.1016/S0140-6736(12)61728-0 PMID: 23245604

Maillet, A., Yadav, S., Loo, Y. L., Sachaphibulkij, K., & Pervaiz, S. (2013). A novel Osmium-based compound targets the mitochondria and triggers ROS-dependent apoptosis in colon carcinoma. *Cell Death & Disease*, *4*(6), e653–e653. DOI: 10.1038/cddis.2013.185 PMID: 23744353

Mal, B., Padulosi, S., & Bala Ravi, S. (2010). Minor millets in South Asia: learnings from IFAD-NUS Project in India and Nepal.

Manuja, R., Sachdeva, S., Jain, A., & Chaudhary, J. (2013). A comprehensive review on biological activities of p-hydroxy benzoic acid and its derivatives. *International Journal of Pharmaceutical Sciences Review and Research*, *22*(2), 109–115.

McIntosh, G. H., Noakes, M., Royle, P. J., & Foster, P. R. (2003). Whole-grain rye and wheat foods and markers of bowel health in overweight middle-aged men. *The American Journal of Clinical Nutrition*, *77*(4), 967–974. DOI: 10.1093/ajcn/77.4.967 PMID: 12663299

Meena, R. P., Joshi, D., Bisht, J. K., & Kant, L. (2021). Global scenario of millets cultivation. *Millets and millet technology*, 33-50.

Michaelraj, P. S. J., & Shanmugam, A. (2013). A study on millets based cultivation and consumption in India. *International Journal of Marketing. Financial Services & Management Research*, *2*(4), 49–58.

Mustafa, A. F., Seguin, P., Belair, G., & Kumar, A. (2008). Chemical composition and ruminal degradability of grain pearl millet grown in southwestern Quebec. *Canadian Journal of Animal Science*, *88*(1), 71–77. DOI: 10.4141/CJAS07075

Nadeem, M. S., Kumar, V., Al-Abbasi, F. A., Kamal, M. A., & Anwar, F. (2020, August). Risk of colorectal cancer in inflammatory bowel diseases. [). Academic Press.]. *Seminars in Cancer Biology*, *64*, 51–60. DOI: 10.1016/j.semcancer.2019.05.001 PMID: 31112753

Obilana, A. B., & Manyasa, E. (2002). Millets. In Belton, P. S., & Taylor, J. R. N. (Eds.), *Pseudocereals and less common cereals: grain properties and utilization potential* (pp. 177–217). Springerverlag. DOI: 10.1007/978-3-662-09544-7_6

Ouattara-Cheik, A. T., Aly, S., Yaya, B., & Alfred, T. S. (2006). A comparative study on nutritional and technological quality of fourteen cultivars of pearl millets Pennisetum glaucum (L) Leek in Burkina Faso. *Pakistan Journal of Nutrition*, *5*(6), 512–521. DOI: 10.3923/pjn.2006.512.521

Pandey, K. B., & Rizvi, S. I. (2009). Plant polyphenols as dietary antioxidants in human health and disease. *Oxidative Medicine and Cellular Longevity*, *2*(5), 270–278. DOI: 10.4161/oxim.2.5.9498 PMID: 20716914

Parameswaran, K. P., & Sadasivam, S. (1994). Changes in the carbohydrates and nitrogenous components during germination of proso millet, Panicum miliaceum. *Plant Foods for Human Nutrition (Dordrecht, Netherlands)*, *45*(2), 97–102. DOI: 10.1007/BF01088466 PMID: 8153070

Park, J. H., Darvin, P., Lim, E. J., Joung, Y. H., Hong, D. Y., Park, E. U., Park, S. H., Choi, S. K., Moon, E.-S., Cho, B. W., Park, K. D., Lee, H. K., Kim, M.-J., Park, D.-S., Chung, I.-M., & Yang, Y. M. (2012). Hwanggeumchal sorghum induces cell cycle arrest, and suppresses tumor growth and metastasis through Jak2/STAT pathways in breast cancer xenografts. *PLoS One*, *7*(7), e40531. DOI: 10.1371/journal.pone.0040531 PMID: 22792362

Pradhan, A., Nag, S. K., & Patil, S. K. (2010). Dietary management of finger millet (Eleusine coracana L. Gaerth) controls diabetes. *Current Science*, *98*(6), 763–765.

Pragya, S., & Rita, S. R. (2012). Finger millet for food and nutritional security. *African Journal of Food Science*, *6*(4), 77–84. DOI: 10.5897/AJFSX10.010

Puranik, S., Kam, J., Sahu, P. P., Yadav, R., Srivastava, R. K., Ojulong, H., & Yadav, R. (2017). Harnessing finger millet to combat calcium deficiency in humans: Challenges and prospects. *Frontiers in Plant Science*, *8*, 1311. DOI: 10.3389/fpls.2017.01311 PMID: 28798761

Rao, S. (2002). MV; Muralikrishna, G. Evaluation of the antioxidant properties of free and bound phenolic acids from native and malted finger millet (Ragi, Eleusine coracana Indaf-15). *Journal of Agricultural and Food Chemistry*, *50*(4), 889–892. DOI: 10.1021/jf011210d PMID: 11829663

Ren, A., Chen, L., Zhao, W., Shan, S., Li, Z., & Tang, Z. (2023). Extraction optimization and structural characterization of soluble dietary fiber in foxtail millet and its inhibitory activities on colon cancer. *Journal of Functional Foods*, *107*, 105659. DOI: 10.1016/j.jff.2023.105659

Ringel, A. E., Drijvers, J. M., Baker, G. J., Catozzi, A., García-Cañaveras, J. C., Gassaway, B. M., Miller, B. C., Juneja, V. R., Nguyen, T. H., Joshi, S., Yao, C.-H., Yoon, H., Sage, P. T., LaFleur, M. W., Trombley, J. D., Jacobson, C. A., Maliga, Z., Gygi, S. P., Sorger, P. K., & Haigis, M. C. (2020). Obesity shapes metabolism in the tumor microenvironment to suppress anti-tumor immunity. *Cell*, *183*(7), 1848–1866. DOI: 10.1016/j.cell.2020.11.009 PMID: 33301708

Rooney, L. W., Miller, F. R., & Mertin, J. V. (1981, October). Variation in the structure and kernel characteristics of sorghum. In *Proceedings of the international symposium on sorghum grain quality* (Vol. 28, pp. 143-162).

Shan, S., Li, Z., Guo, S., Li, Z., Shi, T., & Shi, J. (2014). A millet bran-derived peroxidase inhibits cell migration by antagonizing STAT3-mediated epithelial-mesenchymal transition in human colon cancer. *Journal of Functional Foods*, *10*, 444–455. DOI: 10.1016/j.jff.2014.07.005

Shan, S., Lu, Y., Zhang, X., Shi, J., Li, H., & Li, Z. (2021). Inhibitory effect of bound polyphenol from foxtail millet bran on miR-149 methylation increases the chemosensitivity of human colorectal cancer HCT-8/Fu cells. *Molecular and Cellular Biochemistry*, *476*(2), 513–523. DOI: 10.1007/s11010-020-03906-4 PMID: 33011952

Shapira, N. (2017). The potential contribution of dietary factors to breast cancer prevention. *European Journal of Cancer Prevention*, *26*(5), 385–395. DOI: 10.1097/CEJ.0000000000000406 PMID: 28746163

Sharma, S., Sharma, N., Handa, S., & Pathania, S. (2017). Evaluation of health potential of nutritionally enriched Kodo millet (Eleusine coracana) grown in Himachal Pradesh, India. *Food Chemistry, 214*, 162–168. DOI: 10.1016/j.foodchem.2016.07.086 PMID: 27507461

Shi, J., Shan, S., Li, Z., Li, H., Li, X., & Li, Z. (2015). Bound polyphenol from foxtail millet bran induces apoptosis in HCT-116 cell through ROS generation. *Journal of Functional Foods, 17*, 958–968. DOI: 10.1016/j.jff.2015.06.049

Shih, C. H., Siu, , Ng, R., Wong, E., Chiu, L. C. M., Chu, I. K., & Lo, C. (2007). Quantitative analysis of anticancer 3-deoxyanthocyanidins in infected sorghum seedlings. *Journal of Agricultural and Food Chemistry, 55*(2), 254–259. DOI: 10.1021/jf062516t PMID: 17227050

Shobana, S., Sreerama, Y. N., & Malleshi, N. G. (2009). Composition and enzyme inhibitory properties of finger millet (Eleusine coracana L.) seed coat phenolics: Mode of inhibition of α-glucosidase and pancreatic amylase. *Food Chemistry, 115*(4), 1268–1273. DOI: 10.1016/j.foodchem.2009.01.042

Siegel, R. L., Miller, K. D., & Jemal, A. (2018). Cancer statistics, 2018. *CA: a Cancer Journal for Clinicians, 68*(1), 7–30. DOI: 10.3322/caac.21442 PMID: 29313949

Soetan, K. O., Olaiya, C. O., & Oyewole, O. E. (2010). The importance of mineral elements for humans, domestic animals and plants: A review. *African Journal of Food Science, 4*(5), 200–222.

Stewart, B. W., & Kleihues, P. (Eds.). (2003). *World cancer report* (Vol. 57). IARC press.

Suganyadevi, P., Saravanakumar, K. M., & Mohandas, S. (2013). The antiproliferative activity of 3-deoxyanthocyanins extracted from red sorghum (Sorghum bicolor) bran through P53-dependent and Bcl-2 gene expression in breast cancer cell line. *Life Sciences, 92*(6-7), 379–382. DOI: 10.1016/j.lfs.2013.01.006 PMID: 23333825

Suma, P. F., & Urooj, A. (2012). Antioxidant activity of extracts from foxtail millet (Setaria italica). *Journal of Food Science and Technology, 49*(4), 500–504. DOI: 10.1007/s13197-011-0300-9 PMID: 23904660

Sun, X., Ai, M., Wang, Y., Shen, S., Gu, Y., Jin, Y., Zhou, Z., Long, Y., & Yu, Q. (2013). Selective induction of tumor cell apoptosis by a novel P450-mediated reactive oxygen species (ROS) inducer methyl 3-(4-nitrophenyl) propiolate. *The Journal of Biological Chemistry, 288*(13), 8826–8837. DOI: 10.1074/jbc.M112.429316 PMID: 23382387

Truswell, A. S. (2002). Cereal grains and coronary heart disease. *European Journal of Clinical Nutrition*, *56*(1), 1–14. DOI: 10.1038/sj.ejcn.1601283 PMID: 11840174

Von Grebmer, K., Bernstein, J., Hossain, N., Brown, T., Prasai, N., & Yohannes, Y. (2017) Global hunger index: the inequalities of hunger. International Food Policy Research Institute. http://www. globalhungerindex.org/pdf/en/2017.pdf. Accessed 21 Jan 2018

Waniska, R. D., Poe, J. H., & Bandyopadhyay, R. (1989). Effects of growth conditions on grain molding and phenols in sorghum caryopsis. *Journal of Cereal Science*, *10*(3), 217–225. DOI: 10.1016/S0733-5210(89)80051-7

Wankhede, D. B., Shehnaj, A., & Raghavendra Rao, M. R. (1979). Carbohydrate composition of finger millet (Eleusine coracana) and foxtail millet (Setaria italica). *Qualitas Plantarum*, *28*(4), 293–303. DOI: 10.1007/BF01095511

Yang, H. L., Feng, P., Xu, Y., Hou, Y. Y., Ojo, O., & Wang, X. H. (2021). The role of dietary fiber supplementation in regulating uremic toxins in patients with chronic kidney disease: A meta-analysis of randomized controlled trials. *Journal of Renal Nutrition*, *31*(5), 438–447. DOI: 10.1053/j.jrn.2020.11.008 PMID: 33741249

Zhang, B., Xu, Y., Liu, S., Lv, H., Hu, Y., Wang, Y., Li, Z., Wang, J., Ji, X., Ma, H., Wang, X., & Wang, S. (2020). Dietary supplementation of foxtail millet ameliorates colitis-associated colorectal cancer in mice via activation of gut receptors and suppression of the STAT3 pathway. *Nutrients*, *12*(8), 2367. DOI: 10.3390/nu12082367 PMID: 32784751

Zhang, L., La, X., Tian, J., Li, H., Li, A., Liu, Y., Wu, C., & Li, Z. (2021). The phytochemical vitexin and syringic acid derived from foxtail fillet bran inhibit breast cancer cells proliferation via GRP78/SREBP-1/SCD1 signaling axis. *Journal of Functional Foods*, *85*, 104620. DOI: 10.1016/j.jff.2021.104620

Zhang, X., Shan, S., Shi, J., Li, H., & Li, Z. (2021). Polyphenol from millet bran increases the sensitivity of colorectal cancer cells to oxaliplatin by blocking the ganglioside GM3 catabolism. *Food & Function*, *12*(1), 291–301. DOI: 10.1039/D0FO02232B PMID: 33300910

Zhang, Y. Z., & Li, Y. Y. (2014). Inflammatory bowel disease: Pathogenesis. *World journal of gastroenterology. World Journal of Gastroenterology*, *20*(1), 91. DOI: 10.3748/wjg.v20.i1.91 PMID: 24415861

Chapter 9
Antimicrobial Properties of Secondary Metabolites

Odangowei Inetiminebi Ogidi
https://orcid.org/0000-0002-9961-893X
Bayelsa Medical University Yenagoa, Nigeria

Happiness Adaekwu Orlu
https://orcid.org/0000-0001-7142-487X
Rivers State University, Port-Harcourt, Nigeria

Imomotimi Timipa Ajoko
https://orcid.org/0000-0002-0486-0644
Niger Delta University, Nigeria

ABSTRACT

Secondary metabolites are highly potent organic compounds that are synthesised by plants, fungi, and bacteria as a defence mechanism against predators. Plants have been employed as traditional remedies for centuries due to their production of a diverse array of secondary metabolites. Many individuals are intrigued by the potential of food and other plant materials to serve as alternative medications due to their bioactive components, which have the ability to suppress microbial proliferation and treat it with minimal adverse effects. The critical function of these components in enhancing the therapeutic efficacy of traditional medications against a diverse array of pathogenic germs was demonstrated by their addition. Additionally, researchers have investigated the use of specific metabolites in conjunction with antimicrobial pharmacological medications to address the issues resulting from drug resistance. Therefore, this chapter examines the antimicrobial properties of secondary metabolites and their role in enhancing drug sensitivity in the presence of pathogenic organisms.

DOI: 10.4018/979-8-3693-9112-9.ch009

INTRODUCTION

Medicinal plants are chiefly regarded for the diverse plant constituents utilised in the treatment of chronic and infectious disorders within the pharmaceutical sector. Prior to humanity's understanding of bacteria, it was already established that such organisms had antibacterial properties that we now recognise. Traditional herbal treatments are rooted in historical and cultural ideas, contributing to their global prevalence (Ogidi & Emaikwu, 2023a, b). In contemporary usage, "herb" denotes both the woody and non-woody components of a plant (Bourinbaiar & Lec-Huang, 1996). The rich origins of antibacterial drugs are derived from medicinal plants. According to the WHO, medicinal plants are the primary source of many pharmacological molecules, with 80 percent of the global population relying on herbal medicine and the use of plant extracts or active ingredients for a significant share of conventional therapies (Ogidi, 2023). Nonetheless, a relatively recent area of study is the research analysis aimed at identifying their antibacterial active components (Anand et al., 2019).

Infectious diseases are common, especially those affecting the skin and mucous membranes. Fungi and bacteria constitute a significant category of skin infections. The most severe inoculation problems encompass dermal irritation, folliculitis, skin degradation, acne, dermatitis, and rosacea, among others. Multi-drug-resistant bacteria have been a major contributor to premium skincare products. A new kind of infectious disease, known as multidrug resistance, has emerged as a result of the widespread and unregulated use of synthetic antimicrobial drugs (Ogidi et al., 2023). It is also known that people with weakened immune systems are more likely to get infections that are difficult to cure. A promising solution to multi-drug resistance bacteria is a new chemical exhibiting diverse mechanisms of antibiotic action against microorganisms. Current medications utilised for the protection of infectious disorders sometimes provoke substantial enquiries concerning their safety. Numerous synthetic pharmaceuticals induce unpleasant responses. Antimicrobial agents derived from potential plants should be investigated to address this issue (Ogidi et al., 2022). These herbal drugs exhibit reduced toxicity; they possess no adverse effects and are cost-effective. They treat infectious illnesses effectively, nearly equivalent to synthetic antimicrobials (Kubo et al., 1994; Ahmed et al., 1993). Plant-dependent antimicrobials provide a significant, underutilised reservoir of pharmaceuticals, necessitating urgent exploration of their potential. Plant-derived antimicrobials possess considerable therapeutic potential. The present study highlights the significant potential of plants as sources of antimicrobial agents (Hunter & Hull, 1993).

The ongoing proliferation of multidrug resistance in various microorganisms has established a formidable obstacle in the fight against infectious diseases (Ferri et al., 2017; Prestinaci et al., 2015). The overuse of antibiotics by humans is one of the reasons that harmful bacteria are developing resistance to them. Nevertheless, it may be crucial to identify new antimicrobial drugs with innovative mechanisms; however, this advancement would be impeded by the ongoing and substantial rise in antimicrobial drug resistance (Amabile-Cuevas, 2003; Rossolini et al., 2014). Numerous reports indicate that this has evolved into a significant threat requiring global attention, necessitating diverse strategies to address this issue. Moreover, due to the harmful consequences of current antibiotics, there has been a surge in interest in investigating the antibacterial capabilities of herbal items that occur naturally (Lee et al., 2013; Michael et al., 2014; Owens, 2008). Drug designers have been offered with several chances by the utilisation of herbal items and the formulation of beneficial combinations (Chandra et al., 2017; Gupta & Birdi, 2017; Mittal et al., 2019; Shin et al., 2018). From ancient times until the turn of the twentieth century, people all over the world have turned to plants and their derivatives to cure a wide range of medical conditions (Greathead, 2003; Patra, 2012; Ramawat et al., 2009).

Nevertheless, the efficacy of allopathic medications garnered significant attention in the 20th century, leading to the replacement of traditional remedies. With the rise in popularity of allopathic antibiotics, fallacies emerged concurrently, portraying them as wonder treatments in many industrialised nations. Nonetheless, the continual exposure to illogical and insufficient dosing regimens of these antimicrobial agents diminished their efficacy. According to findings, one of the most important steps in the development of antibiotic resistance is the spread of drug-resistant genes to different types of microbes (Breithaupt, 1999; Spellberg et al., 2008; Widayati et al., 2012). Mutants that are resistant to more than one antibiotic are known as multi-drug resistant (MDR) or "superbugs" (Bhat et al., 2019). The World Health Organisation (WHO) estimates that more than 80% of the population in developing nations uses naturally occurring herbal treatments since they are inexpensive (Mahady, 2001). Nevertheless, many developing nations continue to use traditional therapeutic approaches (Nair et al., 2005).

Objectives of the Chapter

The aims of this chapter are as follows:

(1) To evaluate the chemistry of secondary metabolites with antibacterial properties.
(2) To discuss the antimicrobial efficacy of phytochemicals.
(3) To discuss the mechanisms of resistance: how bacteria develop resistance to phytochemicals.
(4) To review the synergistic impact of secondary metabolites.
(5) To evaluate biotechnological approaches in antimicrobial drug discovery.

(6) To explore the current status of secondary metabolites in clinical trials and fda-approved usage
(7) To explore the future perspectives of antimicrobial properties of secondary metabolites.

Organization of the Chapter

The rest of this chapter is organized as follows: Section 2 explores the chemistry of secondary metabolites with antibacterial properties. Section 3 discusses discuss the antimicrobial efficacy of phytochemicals. Section 4 discusses the mechanisms of resistance: how bacteria develop resistance to phytochemicals. Section 5 traverse the synergistic impact of secondary metabolites. Section 6 evaluate biotechnological approaches in antimicrobial drug discovery. Section 7 explore the current status of secondary metabolites in clinical trials and fda-approved usage. Section 8 discusses the future perspectives of antimicrobial properties of secondary metabolites. Finally, a concluding section summarizes the antimicrobial properties of secondary metabolites.

THE CHEMISTRY OF SECONDARY METABOLITES WITH ANTIBACTERIAL PROPERTIES

Plants function as innovative chemists (Mann, 2007). They possess a nearly boundless capacity to synthesise chemical compounds. Certain chemical compounds possess nutritional, toxic, hallucinogenic, or medicinal properties. The majority are secondary metabolites that frequently function as defence mechanisms for plants against predation by microbes, insects, and herbivores. Numerous chemicals of this nature contribute to plant taste, such as terpenoids (Cowan, 1999). Although certain chemicals may lack identifiable physiological functions in their respective plants, several ones exert considerable biological impacts on animals. Nonetheless, it is widely acknowledged that they are crucial in plant physiology, encompassing growth, development, reproduction, and the interaction between the plant and its environment (Whiting, 2001). They are, in reality, accountable for the medicinal effects of plants. Certain metabolites have been identified and demonstrated anti-bacterial activity in vitro (Van Etten et al., 1994).

Chemical compounds exhibiting antimicrobial activity are classified as phenols, acids, alkaloids, flavonoids, terpenoids, polyacetylenes, and phenylheptatriyene. The majority of antimicrobial secondary metabolites have a relatively broad spectrum of activity. Numerous antimicrobial investigations have been performed on the extracts of medicinal plants globally, demonstrating herbal medicine as a source of chemotherapeutic drugs with considerable efficacy (Ogidi & Enenebeaku, 2023).

Plant secondary metabolites serve as antimicrobial agents, insecticides, pollinator attractants, growth regulators, feeding deterrents, signalling molecules, and allelopathic agents that affect competition among plant species. The acknowledgement of the biological features and roles of numerous natural products has heightened awareness of metabolites as potential sources for novel pharmaceuticals. In addition to serving as preservatives, flavouring agents, and colours, plant secondary metabolites have been prominently utilised in medicine. A multitude of active principles in folkloric medicine have now been identified. Medicinal plants continue to be an essential component of the daily existence of numerous individuals worldwide due to the numerous benefits they offer (Mann, 2007).

Secondary metabolites are synthesised from primary metabolites. A modest quantity of building blocks can provide a diverse range of secondary metabolites. Primary building blocks for secondary metabolite synthesis come from the intermediates 1-deoxyxylulose-5-phosphate, shikimic acid, mevalonic acid, and acetyl coenzyme A. The mevalonate, acetate, shikimate, and deoxyxylulose phosphate pathways all make use of them in that order. Synthesis of secondary metabolites can involve a combination of many types of elements or a large number of identical ones. Numerous secondary metabolites may incorporate one or more sugar molecules, which can be either basic primary metabolites (such as glucose) or significantly altered and atypical sugars (Ogidi & Ajoko, 2024). Some secondary metabolites with antibacterial properties are shown in Table 1.

Table 1. Chemistry of secondary metabolites with antibacterial properties

Secondary Metabolite	Class	Structure	Antibacterial Activity	Mechanism of Action	Examples of Producing Organisms	Minimum Inhibitory Concentration (MIC)
1. Tetracycline	Polyketide	Multicyclic	Broad-spectrum	Inhibits protein synthesis	*Streptomyces aureofaciens*	0.1-10 µg/mL
2. Penicillin	β-Lactam	β-Lactam ring	Gram-positive	Interferes with cell wall synthesis	*Penicillium chrysogenum*	0.01-1 µg/mL
3. Cephalosporin	β-Lactam	β-Lactam ring	Broad-spectrum	Interferes with cell wall synthesis	*Cephalosporium acremonium*	0.1-10 µg/mL
4. Erythromycin	Macrolide	Macrocyclic lactone	Gram-positive	Inhibits protein synthesis	*Saccharopolyspora erythraea*	0.1-10 µg/mL

continued on following page

Table 1. Continued

Secondary Metabolite	Class	Structure	Antibacterial Activity	Mechanism of Action	Examples of Producing Organisms	Minimum Inhibitory Concentration (MIC)
5. Allicin	Thiosulfinate	Sulfur-containing	Gram-positive, Gram-negative	Disrupts cell membranes	*Allium sativum (Garlic)*	1-10 µg/mL
6. Catechin	Flavonoid	Phenolic	Gram-positive	Inhibits cell division	*Camellia sinensis (Tea)*	10-100 µg/mL
7. Quercetin	Flavonoid	Phenolic	Broad-spectrum	Inhibits DNA gyrase	*Various plant species*	10-100 µg/mL
8. Berberine	Alkaloid	Isoquinoline	Gram-positive, Gram-negative	Inhibits DNA replication	*Berberis vulgaris (Barberry)*	5-50 µg/mL
9. Capsaicin	Alkaloid	Vanilloid	Gram-positive	Disrupts cell membranes	*Capsicum annuum (Chili Pepper)*	10-100 µg/mL
10. Usnic Acid	Lichen acid	Dibenzofuran	Broad-spectrum	Inhibits cell division	*Lichens (e.g., Usnea barbata)*	1-10 µg/mL
11. Chloramphenicol	Amphenicol	Nitrobenzene	Broad-spectrum	Inhibits protein synthesis	*Streptomyces venezuelae*	0.1-10 µg/mL
12. Lincomycin	Lincosamide	Octose sugar	Gram-positive	Inhibits protein synthesis	*Streptomyces lincolnensis*	0.1-10 µg/mL
13. Polymyxin B	Lipopeptide	Cyclic peptide	Gram-negative	Disrupts cell membranes	*Paenibacillus polymyxa*	0.1-10 µg/mL
14. Bacitracin	Lipopeptide	Cyclic peptide	Gram-positive	Interferes with cell wall synthesis	*Bacillus subtilis*	0.1-10 µg/mL
15. Nisin	Lantibiotic	Cyclic peptide	Gram-positive	Disrupts cell membranes	*Lactococcus lactis*	0.1-10 µg/mL

ANTIMICROBIAL EFFICACY OF PHYTOCHEMICALS

Numerous antibiotics have their origins in nature. Tetracycline, penicillin, cephalosporins, and vancomycin comprise this group (Calixto, 2019; Monciardini et al., 2014). The discovery of compounds that can combat antibiotic resistance has been simplified for scientists by the introduction of new instruments for molecular docking and high-throughput screening (Demain, 2014). The therapeutic utility of these compounds is restricted by their inability to access cell membranes, block efflux pumps, or bypass mutational resistance. Researchers are particularly enthusiastic about identifying the most effective plant-based products in terms of their antibacterial properties (Fischbach & Walsh, 2009; Livermore, 2011). Recent developments in synthetic biology, bioinformatics, and genomics have enabled high-throughput screening of botanical products to surpass outdated methodologies (Paytubi et al., 2017; Ogwu et al., 2025). With the current drug discovery techniques, drug designers have the ability to chemically modify the structures of specific bioactive secondary metabolites in order to enhance their efficacy (Amirkia & Heinrich, 2015). Many secondary metabolites, including phenolics, alkaloids, saponins, terpenoids, limonoids, polyacetylenes, and secoiridoids, are responsible for the many biological effects of herbal remedies (Jujjavarapu & Dhaga, 2018). Being byproducts of primary metabolism, these secondary metabolites play a crucial role in plants' inherent defensive mechanisms (Davis et al., 2020; Hatcher et al., 2020). The drugs made from these physiologically active byproducts are considered natural antibiotics because of their link to the breakdown of microbial cell walls and membranes (Kliebenstain & Osbourn, 2012). Cell death is the result of the activation of enzymes, the degradation of the protein binding domain, and the consequent loss of cellular contents (Kroymann, 2011; Pichersky & Gang, 2000). Antimicrobial efficacy of some phytochemicals are shown in Table 2.

Table 2. Antimicrobial efficacy of phytochemicals

Phytochemical	Class	Plant Source	Antimicrobial Activity	MIC (μg/mL)	Target Microorganisms	Mechanism of Action
1. Quercetin	Flavonoid	Apple, Onion	Bacteria, Fungi	10-100	*E. coli, S. aureus, C. albicans*	Inhibits DNA gyrase
2. Catechin	Flavonoid	Green Tea	Bacteria, Viruses	5-50	*E. coli, H. influenzae, HIV*	Interferes with viral replication
3. Allicin	Thiosulfinate	Garlic	Bacteria, Fungi	1-10	*E. coli, S. aureus, C. albicans*	Disrupts cell membranes
4. Berberine	Alkaloid	Barberry	Bacteria, Fungi	5-50	*E. coli, S. aureus, C. albicans*	Inhibits DNA replication
5. Capsaicin	Alkaloid	Chili Pepper	Bacteria	10-100	*E. coli, S. aureus*	Disrupts cell membranes
6. Tannin	Polyphenol	Tea, Grape	Bacteria, Fungi	10-100	*E. coli, S. aureus, C. albicans*	Interferes with enzyme activity
7. Eugenol	Phenol	Clove	Bacteria, Fungi	1-10	*E. coli, S. aureus, C. albicans*	Disrupts cell membranes
8. Thymol	Phenol	Thyme	Bacteria, Fungi	1-10	*E. coli, S. aureus, C. albicans*	Disrupts cell membranes

continued on following page

Table 2. Continued

Phytochemical	Class	Plant Source	Antimicrobial Activity	MIC (µg/mL)	Target Microorganisms	Mechanism of Action
9. Gallic Acid	Phenol	Grape	Bacteria, Fungi	10-100	*E. coli, S. aureus, C. albicans*	Interferes with enzyme activity
10. Curcumin	Polyphenol	Turmeric	Bacteria, Viruses	5-50	*E. coli, H. influenzae, HIV*	Inhibits inflammatory responses
11. Saponin	Glycoside	Ginseng	Bacteria, Fungi	10-100	*E. coli, S. aureus, C. albicans*	Interferes with cell membrane integrity
12. Anthocyanin	Flavonoid	Berries	Bacteria, Fungi	10-100	*E. coli, S. aureus, C. albicans*	Antioxidant and radical scavenging
13. Luteolin	Flavonoid	Spinach	Bacteria, Viruses	5-50	*E. coli, H. influenzae, HIV*	Inhibits DNA gyrase
14. Apigenin	Flavonoid	Parsley	Bacteria, Fungi	10-100	*E. coli, S. aureus, C. albicans*	Interferes with cell cycle regulation
15. Resveratrol	Polyphenol	Grape	Bacteria, Viruses	5-50	*E. coli, H. influenzae, HIV*	Activates cellular defense mechanisms
16. Ellagic Acid	Phenol	Pomegranate	Bacteria, Fungi	10-100	*E. coli, S. aureus, C. albicans*	Interferes with enzyme activity
17. Gingerol	Phenol	Ginger	Bacteria, Fungi	10-100	*E. coli, S. aureus, C. albicans*	Anti-inflammatory and antioxidant
18. Cinnamaldehyde	Aldehyde	Cinnamon	Bacteria, Fungi	1-10	*E. coli, S. aureus, C. albicans*	Disrupts cell membranes
19. Limonene	Terpene	Lemon	Bacteria, Fungi	10-100	*E. coli, S. aureus, C. albicans*	Interferes with cell membrane integrity
20. Ursolic Acid	Triterpenoid	Rosemary	Bacteria, Fungi	10-100	*E. coli, S. aureus, C. albicans*	Anti-inflammatory and antioxidant

Polyphenols

The phenolic compounds found in plants serve as defence mechanisms against microbial infections, ultraviolet radiation, and chemical stressors (Ogidi & Emaikwu, 2024). A large number of polyphenols found in various fruits and vegetables have been studied by the experts for their potential anti-disease properties (Manach et al., 2004; Quideau et al., 2011). Flavonoids and nonflavonoids (phenolic acids) are the usual ways to classify polyphenols. The large amounts of flavonoids and phenolic acids in Salvia officinalis extract provide it antibacterial and bacteriostatic characteristics (Ghorbani & Esmaeilizadeh, 2017). Evidence from phytochemical analyses of four plant extracts—Rosmarinus officinalis, Prunus avium, Mentha piperita, and Eugenia caryophyllata—points to the presence of phenolic acids, flavonoids, and terpenoids with antibacterial effects (Alamri & Moustafa, 2012). The ethanolic extract of A. contains five distinct phenolic components. The antibacterial properties of Ampeloprasum are particularly noteworthy against Prunus aeruginosa and Micrococcus spp., thanks to the presence of phenolic acids such as cinnamic acid, p-coumaric acid, catechin, and sinapic acid. Pomegranate juice contains polyphenols such gallic acid, caffeic acid, and epigalocatechin 3-gallate (EGCG), which have been demonstrated to inhibit the action of several microbes that may be found in dental plaque (Singh et al., 2018; Thangavelu et al., 2017). Several phenolic compounds found in clove oil have shown promising antifungal activity against opportunistic fungal infections, including Aspergillus fumigatus, Candida albicans, and Cryptococcus neoformans (Ahmad et al., 2006). The chemical structure of Polyphenols is shown in Figure 1.

Figure 1. Chemical structure of polyphenols

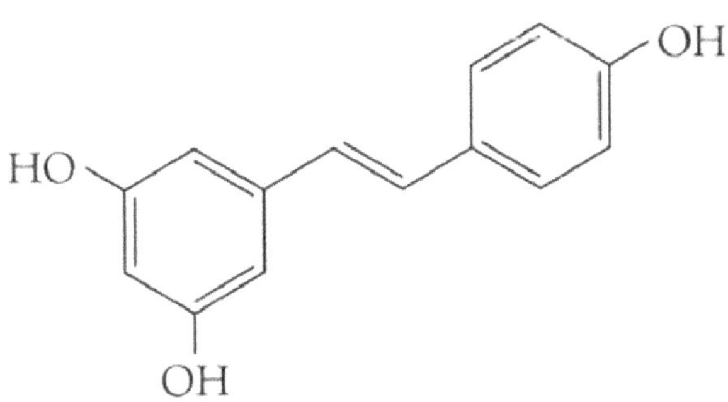

Phenolic Acids

When it comes to phenolic acids, the bacteria that have demonstrated the highest level of antibacterial activity are Gram-positive bacteria, not Gram-negative bacteria. Gram-negative bacteria have a topology that is hydrophobic, which inhibits many hydrophilic antibiotics, such as phenolic acids, from penetrating their outer membrane (Alakomi et al., 2007). To a certain extent, phenolic acids have the ability to inhibit the growth rates of certain Gram-negative bacteria. There are methanolic extracts from the leaves of Matricaria aureus, which are also known as golden chamomile (Cueva et al., 2010). These extracts have the ability to inhibit the growth of a number of bacteria, including Bacillus subtilis, Streptococcus pyogenes, Staphylococcus aureus, and Klebsiella pneumonia (Merkl et al., 2018). Golden chamomile extracts have been proven to be effective against a variety of strains of Aspergillus flavus, Colletotrichum gleosporoides, and Aspergillus niger, according to the results of experiments conducted on their respective strains (Rizwana, 2016). The chemical structure of phenolic acid is shown in Figure 2.

Figure 2. Chemical structure of phenolic acid

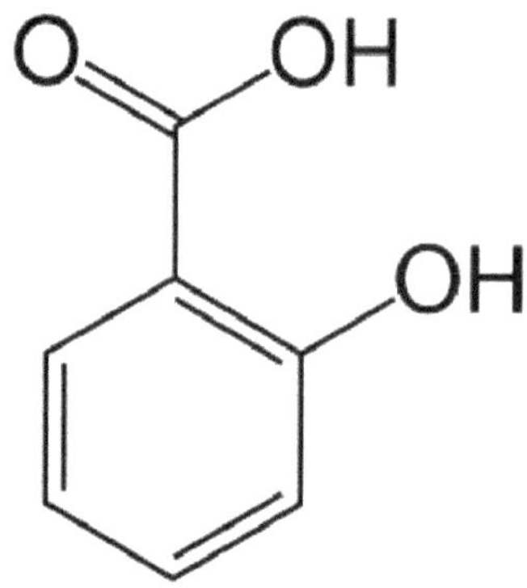

Flavonoids

Vegetables, fruits, nuts, and seeds are the most common plant foods that contain flavonoids. Their main classifications include isoflavones, anthocyanidins, flavonols, flavanones, flavan-3-ols, and flavones. This collection of flavonoids encompasses a diverse array of secondary metabolites, including luteolin, apigenin, diosmetin, chrysoeriol, tangeretin, sinensetin, gardenin, vitexin, baicalein, kaempferol, quercetin, galangin, datiscetin, morin, robinetin, isorhamnetin, tamarixetin, isoctytososide, quercetagetin, myricetin, hesperetin, taxifolin, eriodictyol, naringenin, catechin, epicatechin, genistein, daidzein, coumestrol, cyanidin, delphinidin, pelargonidin, peonidin, among others (Kumar & Pandey, 2013; Sarbu et al., 2019). The antibacterial activities of several flavonoids were tested against Salmonella, Gram-negative Escherichia coli CM 871, and intestinal Gram-positive lactic acid bacteria. While cyanidin-3-glucoside, luteolin, pelargonidin, and delphinidin were efficient against E. coli, myricetin had a strong inhibitory effect on Lactobacillus growth (Puupponen-Pimia et al., 2001). The bioactive compound isocytisoside, derived from the leaves of Aquilegia vulgaris, has demonstrated efficacy against fungi as well as Gram-positive and Gram-negative bacteria (Bylka et al., 2004; Ogidi, 2022). Many components of the Combretum erythrophyllum leaf extract were evaluated for their ability to inhibit the growth of Vibrio cholerae, Enterococcus faecalis, Micrococcus luteus, and Shigella sonnei. Among these ingredients are genkwanin, apigenin, kaempferol, quercetin, and rhamnazin. All of the medications significantly reduced the growth of Vibrio cholerae and Escherichia coli when tested (Martini et al., 2004).

The cases of S. sonei and M. luteus were successfully treated with quercetin and rhamocitrin, though. Marrubium globosum has a long history of usage as a remedy for skin ailments and urinary tract infections (UTIs). Rutin and naringenin, two flavonoids included in the methanolic extract of M. Globosum, were determined to possess an 8 mg/ml MIC against S. Epidermidis and E. Faecalis (Rigano et al., 2007). The increased concentrations of quercetin and kaempferol in the ethylene acetate extract of Argyreia speciosa led to a significant efficacy against Mycobacterium TB and Klebsiella pneumonia (Habbu et al., 2009). Many different types of infections have been shown to be susceptible to kaempferol, including Pseudomonas aeruginosa, Bacillus cereus, and Listeria monocytogenes (Fierascu et al., 2018; Kloucek et al., 2005). Flavone, an extract from Feijoa sellowiana fruits, has been shown to be effective against several bacteria, including Helicobacter pylori, Proteus vulgaris, Pseudomonas aeruginosa, and Pseudomonas mirabilis (Basile et al., 2010). Morin and quercetin, two compounds found in guava (Psidium guajava) fruit, were found to have antibacterial effects against Salmonella enteritidis, Bacillus cereus, and other bacteria that might cause food poisoning, according to the study (Arima & Danno, 2002; Rattanachaikunsopon & Phumkhachorn, 2010). Black cumin, or Nigella sativa, has the antibacterial thymoquinone in its seeds, which is effective against many different types of bacteria (Goyal et al., 2017; Khan, 2018). Figure 3 shows the chemical structure of flavonoids.

Figure 3. Chemical structure of flavonoids

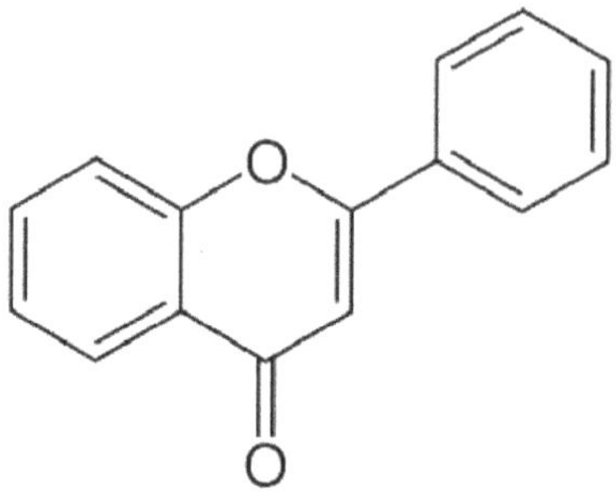

Quinones

A defining feature of quinones is the presence of two ketone replacements in their aromatic rings. In recent years, researchers have identified a minimum of 400 naturally occurring quinones present in all plant organs. With their wide range of biological activities, naphthoquinones are among the most extensive classes of secondary metabolites found in plants. Among the more than twenty plant families that include natural naphthoquinones are the Plumbaginaceae, Ebanaceae, and Boraginaceae. Some of these families' more well-known members include plumbagin, shikonin, alkannin, and derivatives of these (Carson and Hammer, 2010; Savoia, 2012; Ramawat, 2007). Plubagin can be found as an active component of naphthoquinones, in plants belonging to the Plumbaginaceae, Droseraceae, and Ebenaceae families. Plants produce these compounds through a number of different pathways, each tailored to a different quinone. For lawsone and juglone, these pathways include the ortho-succinyl benzoic acid pathway; for shikonin, they include the para-hydroxybenzoic acid-mevalonic acid system; and for plumbagin, they include the acetic acid-mevalonic acid mechanism (Ramawat, 2007). In their study on naphthoquinones as an antibacterial agent, Papageorgious et al. (2008) focused on each enantiomer has two names: alkannin and shikonin. Lithospermum is one of about 150 species that contain alkannins or shikonins; these species are mostly from the Boraginaceae family. Scientific studies on animals and humans have confirmed that histoplastin red, a medical ointment containing alkannins and shikonin esters, is effective. The esters included in 1-Listoplastin Red have anti-inflammatory and antibacterial properties that can help heal wounds and prevent ulcers from forming, according to clinical trials (Papageorgiou et al., 2008).

Furthermore, the effectiveness of Histoplastin Red against Staphylococcus aureus and Staphylococcus epidermidis was assessed. Researchers found that the enantiomer alkannin inhibited the development of both strains of Staphylococcus. In addition, the alkannin ester P-dimethylacryl significantly inhibited the growth of every Staphylococcus (Papageorgiou et al., 2008). According to Papageorgiou et al. (2008), there is clinical evidence that shikonin enantiomers, alkannins, and naphthoquinone derivatives have a wide variety of antibacterial effects. The chemical structure of quinones is shown in Figure 4.

Figure 4. Chemical structure of quinones

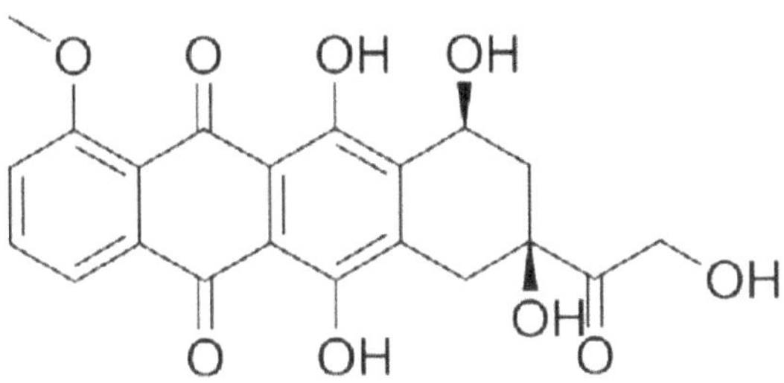

Naphtoquinones

Plants contain naphthoquinones, whereas fungi are known for one of the most extensively researched groups of secondary metabolites regarding their biological functions. The activity of Candida albicans, Candida tropicalis, and Cryptococcus neoformans is inhibited by the naphthoquinones lapachol and β-lapachone (Guiraud et al., 1994). Chemicals were retrieved from species of Tabebuia. The research found that diospyrin and isodiospyrin, two naphthoquinones found in Diospyros picatoria root, were highly effective against a range of harmful bacteria (Adeniye et al., 2000). In addition, anthraquinone-containing extracts from T. impetiginosa bark and lapachol have shown promising results in combating Helicobacter pylori (Park et al., 2006). The minimum inhibitory concentrations (MICs) for Gram-positive Staphylococcus aureus and Gram-negative Escherichia coli were found to be 7.6 and 31.3 mg/ml, respectively, according to the research on 1,4-naphthoquinone sulphides. The antifungal efficacy of 1,4-naphthoquinone sulphides was lower (23.4 mg/ml) than that of Amphotericin B (31.3 mg/ml) in tests conducted against Candida albicans (Wellington et al., 2019). Researchers found that lawsone (2-hydroxy-1,4-naphthoquinone) was more effective than traditional antibiotics at killing methicillin-resistant Staphylococcus aureus (MRSA) in both laboratory and animal trials (Song et al., 2020; Wellington et al., 2019). The chemical structure of naphtoquinones is shown in Figure 5.

Figure 5. Chemical structure of naphtoquinones

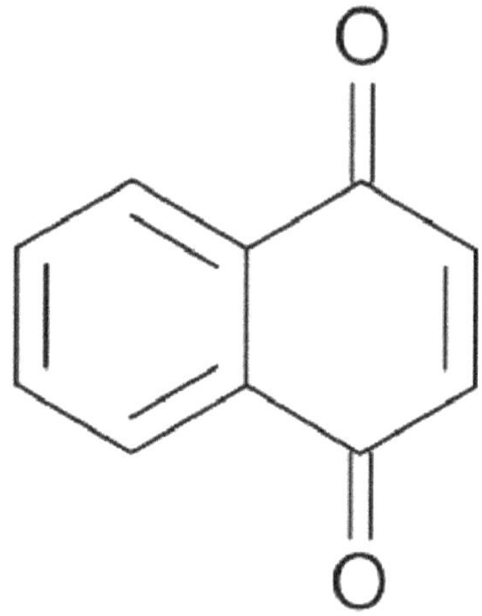

Terpenes

Terpenes are the most extensive class of naturally occurring compounds, with over 30,000 identified structures. A hemiterpene is a compound that contains one isoprene unit, a monoterpene is a complex that contains two isoprene units, and so forth, in accordance with the number of isoprene units present. According to Carson & Hammer (2010), Savoia (2012), and Ramawat (2007), the main components of essential oils are sesquiterpenes and monoterpenes, which are made up of three isoprene units. Two five-carbon isoprene units are combined to make monoterpenes, which have the chemical formula C10H16. Cyclic, linear, regular, and irregular are the four primary varieties of monoterpene structures. Monoterpenes are also present as derivatives in Savoia (2012), Ramawat (2007), and Carson & Hammer (2010), in addition to alcohols, esters, phenols, ketones, and aldehydes. The synthesis of terpenes is influenced by two distinct biological mechanisms. The primary products of the mevalonic acid pathway are sesquiterpenes, sterols, and ubiquinones. Hemiterpenes, monoterpenes, and diterpenes are the most prevalent metabolites of the methyl-erythritol phosphate pathway, as per Carson & Hammer (2010), Savoia (2012), and Ramawat (2007).

Terpenoids are an illustration of a terpene compound. Terpenoids were detected in greater quantities in the ethanol extract than in the water-based extract of Psidium guajava's bark. According to Abdulhamid et al. (2014), this set of compounds showed anti-Streptococcus faecalis activity when mixed with other phytochemicals found in bark. According to the phytochemical examination of Marinda citifolia (Rubiaceae) plant components, the ethanol extract of the leaves also showed a significant content of terpenoids. According to Sibi et al. (2012), this extract showed efficacy against P. aeruginosa and S. epidermidis. Researchers looked explored the antimicrobial properties of three different plant families—Rutaceae, A. mossambicensis (Compositae), and O. gratissimum (Labiatae)—against Pseudomonas aeruginosa and methicillin-resistant Staphylococcus aureus (MRSA). Results showed that the ethanol extract was the most effective antibacterial agent against MRSA. The only plant parts that showed terpenoids in quantifiable amounts were the roots, stem bark, and leaves. In every study, the O. gratissimum extracts had trace amounts of terpenoids. Anthemis mossambicensis and Terminalia asiatica plants were isolated (Enenebeaku et al., 2022b).

According to Munyendo et al. (2011), it may have antibacterial characteristics due to phytochemicals and secondary metabolites. Korir et al. (2012) investigated the antibacterial characteristics of Cyanthula polycephala (Amaranthaceae) and Senna didymobotrya (Caesalpinaceae). The different plant species were extracted using hexane, dichloromethane, and methanol as solvents. Five different bacteria—Staphylococcus aureus, Methicillin-resistant Staphylococcus aureus, Escherichia coli, Pseudomonas aeruginosa, Klebsiella pneumoniae, and Staphylococcus aureus—were used to test the antibacterial capabilities of the plant components. Koorir et al. (2012) conducted an experiment to measure the antibacterial activity by measuring the lengths of inhibitory zones. Compared to water and hexane, dichloromethane and methanol extracts performed better. Korir et al. (2012) used thin layer chromatography to perform phytochemical analysis, and the results showed that both plant extracts contained phenolic chemicals. Researchers found that C. polycephala's methanol extract effectively killed the antibiotic-resistant bacterium methicillin-resistant Staphylococcus aureus. The extract showed an inhibition zone of 16.0 mm, however the positive control medication Gentamicin had an inhibition zone of 9.0 mm. According to Korir et al. (2012), the methanol extract caused a 14 mm inhibitory zone for Staphylococcus aureus and a 10 mm inhibitory zone for Pseudomonas aeruginosa. Figure 6 shows the chemical structure of terpenes.

Figure 6. Chemical structure of terpenes

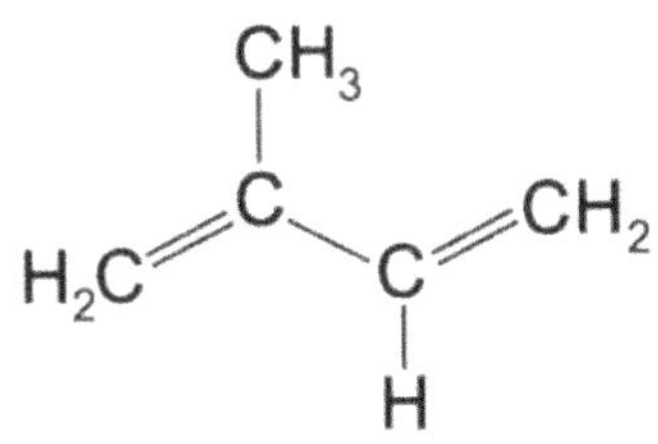

Tannins

Almost every part of a plant contains tannins, which are polymeric phenolic chemicals. Many studies have shown that tannins contain many biological activities, including antibacterial and antifungal effects (Carson & Hammer, 2010; Savoia, 2012; Ramawat, 2007). According to Abdulhamid et al. (2014), a variety of bacteria were tested for their antibacterial properties using ethanol and water-based stem-bark preparations from Psidium guajava (Myrtaceae). The bacteria included Staphylococcus aureus, Streptococcus faecalis, Bacillus subtilis, Escherichia coli, and Salmonella sp. Extracts made with water and those made with ethanol both contained high amounts of tannin. Results showed that ethanol and water-based Psidium guajava bark extracts were effective against all tested microorganisms. When tested against Salmonella species, the ethanol extract showed greater zones of inhibition compared to the water-based extract. This was especially true when testing against S. Faecalis, the kind of Salmonella that was least susceptible (Abdulhamid et al., 2014).

In a distinct experiment, the methanol extract of S. Multiflorus was discovered to possess anti-Mycobacterium fortuitum activity. Actions of Salmonella typhimurium and Staphylococcus aureus. This methanol extract contained substantial concentrations of tannins, as indicated by phytochemical analysis. The A. Nilotica methanol extract was efficacious against Staphylococcus aureus, as indicated by the results. The activities of Pseudomonas aeruginosa were found to contain a significant concentration of tannins. When combined with other phytochemicals, these tannins may exhibit antibacterial properties, as per Mariita et al. (2011). The antimicrobial efficacy of plant components, such as the intact leaves, roots, and stems of Morinda citrifolia (Rubiaceae), was assessed. The antibacterial effects of the ethanol leaf extract were observed to be effective against both Pseudomonas aeruginosa and Staphylococcus epidermidis (Ogidi et al., 2021a,b,c,d). The root and leaf ethanol extracts contained high levels of tannins, which exhibited antibacterial effects, as indicated by phytochemical investigations (Sibi et al., 2012). In a related study, Oboh (2010) collected Ocimum gratissimum L. In Nigeria, herbalists frequently employ leaves from the Labiatae family to address a diverse array of skin conditions, respiratory infections, and migraines. The susceptibility of a variety of microorganisms to an ethanol extract was assessed, including Pseudomonas aeruginosa, Shigella dysenteriae, Escherichia coli, Klebsiella species, Staphylococcus aureus, and Proteus species. The zero. Gratissimum extract exhibited antibacterial activity against S. aureus, Proteus species, S. dysenteriae, and P. aeruginosa. Phytochemical research indicates that the leaves contain a variety of secondary metabolites, including tannins, which may enhance their antibacterial properties (Oboh, 2010). Figure 7 shows the chemical structure of tannins.

Figure 7. Chemical structure of tannins

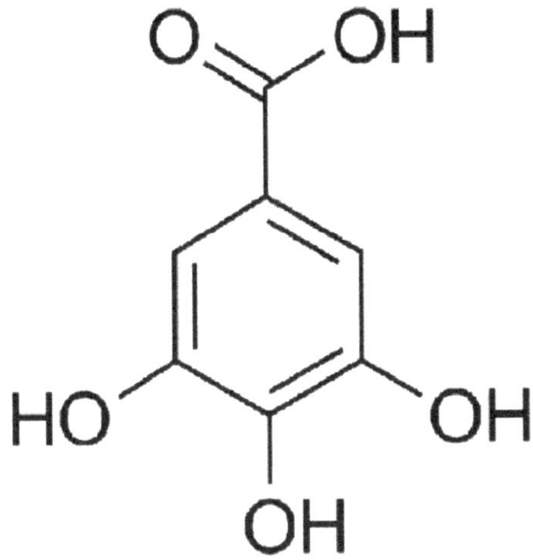

Alkaloids

The plant kingdom is home to a wide variety of alkaloids, according to the research. Terpenoids, quinazoline, indole, pyrrolidine, glyoxaline, lupinane, tropan, phenanthridine, imidazoline, alkaloidal amines, and piperine are only a few examples (among many). Strychnos ptatorum extracts containing indole-type alkaloids inhibited P. vulgaris growth (Othman et al., 2019; Shen et al., 2019). Numerous microorganisms, such as Mycobacterium, Staphylococcus aureus, Salmonella typhimurium, and Vibrio cholerae. C. albicans and Acinetobacter niger tuberculosis at the same time (Yu et al., 2018). The antimicrobial effects of the various alkaloid families are different (Li et al., 2013; Mittal & Jaitak, 2019). Pergularinine and tylophorinidine are alkaloids belonging to the indolizine class that inhibit dihydrofolate reductase, an enzyme involved in the production of nucleic acids (Rao & Venkatachalam, 2000).

Evidence suggests that bisindole alkaloids, including deoxytopsentin and dibromodeoxytopsentin, can block pyruvate kinase, making them effective against methicillin-resistant Staphylococcus aureus (Veale et al., 2015). The Hydrastis candensis is a natural source of alkaloids such candine, berberine, and hydrastine, which were found to suppress bacterial growth via the QQE, according to the study. By inhibiting the production of detrimental genes, QQE regulates the disease rather than killing germs directly (Mohtar et al., 2009). Animal studies showed that a water-based Tinospora cordifoila extract—which contains numerous secondary metabolites, including alkaloids—could cure systemic candidiasis and restore impaired immune systems (Alrumaihi et al., 2019). The Infected mice with Salmonella typhimurium had a lower bacterial load and a higher survival rate after receiving AETC (Alsuhaibani & Khan, 2017). The chemical structure of alkaloids is shown in Figure 8.

Figure 8. Chemical structure of alkaloids

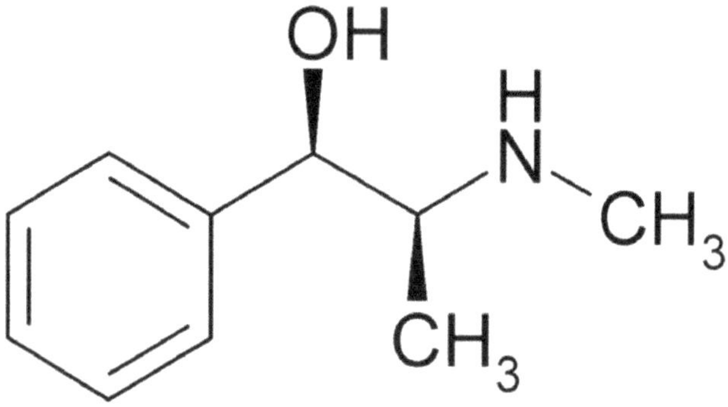

Resins

There are two main types of plant compounds called resins: surface resins and interior resins. Resins are non-volatile. Although some substances do not dissolve in water, they do in organic solvents. Resins are complex plant chemicals that often include lipids, flavonoids, and terpenoids. Plant oil glands are the source of essential oils, which are a type of resin (Carson & Hammer, 2010; Savoia, 2012; Ramawat, 2007). These oils are volatile and dissolve in organic solvents. Diterpenes are a class of phytochemicals that include the anticancer drug taxol (Ogidi, 2024). The initial source of this chemical was found in the bark of the Taxus brevifolia tree. A 30-carbon triterpene is produced by combining two sesquiterpene precursors. Many of these compounds, known as glycosides or saponins, are found in plants. Carron & Hammer (2010), Savoia (2012), and Ramawat (2007) all agree that saponins are carbohydrate-linked steroids or triterpene molecules. The antibacterial activity of an ethanol extract from the leaves of Ocimum gratissimum (Labiatae) was investigated by Oboh (2010).

Staphylococcus aureus, Shigella dysenteriae, Proteus species, and *Pseudomonas aeruginosa* were all effectively inhibited by the ethanol extract's antibacterial properties. Cardiovascular glycosides are among the several chemicals found in O. Gratissimum leaves, according to phytochemical studies (Oboh, 2010). Phytochemical examination of Tamarindus indica's aqueous pulp extract revealed the presence of several phytochemicals, including resins, particularly saponins (2.2%) and glycosides (1.59%). Although it showed minimal sensitivity to S. typhi, the pulp extract was very sensitive to S. aureus (Abukakar et al., 2008). The phytochemical analysis of S. Multiflorus's methanol extract confirmed the presence of abundant saponins. Microorganisms such as M. Fortuitum, S. Aureus, and S. Typhi were successfully combated by the methanol extract. As a result, these secondary metabolites might display these biological activities when combined with other phytochemicals (Mariita et al., 2011). Ocimum gratissimum (Labiatae) leaf ethanol extract was the subject of an experimental study by Oboh (2010) that sought to determine the plant's antibacterial capabilities. Several bacteria, including *P. aeruginosa, S. dysenteriae, Proteus species,* and *S. aureus,* were found to be susceptible to the antibacterial effects of the ethanol extract. According to phytochemical studies, O. Gratissimum leaves contain a number of phytoconstituents, one of which is saponin (Oboh, 2010; Ogidi & Julius, 2021). Figure 9 shows the chemical structure of epoxy resins.

Figure 9. Chemical structure of epoxy resins

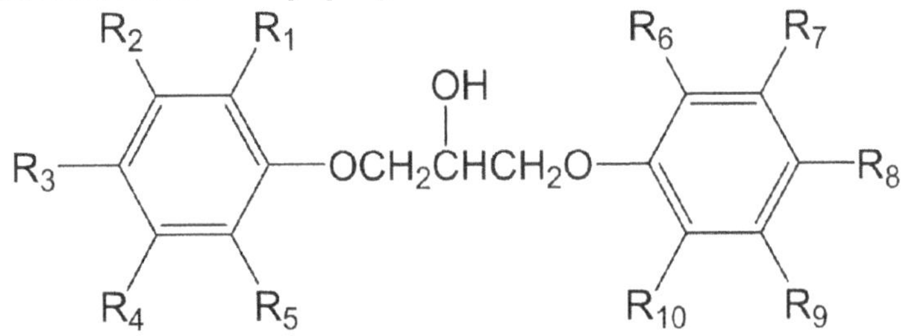

Organosulfur Compounds

Garlic contains organosulfur thiosulfinates, which are its main secondary metabolites. These compounds have shown to be very suppressive against a variety of harmful bacteria and yeast (Rouf et al., 2020; Yamaguchi & Kumagai, 2020). The active ingredient derived from garlic that inhibits microbial development is DADS (Kyung & Lee, 2001). Dimethyl trisulfide, methyl methanethiosulfinate, and methyl methanethiosulfonate are some of the organosulfur compounds found in cabbage that have demonstrated potent anti-growth properties against several bacterial and fungal species (Avato et al., 2000; Kyung & Fleming, 1997). Many plants that can be eaten contain sulfur-containing compounds called glucosinolates (Fahey et al., 2001). White mustard includes p-hydroxybenzyl glucosinolate, while brown mustard contains gluconapin. Horseradish, cabbage, and rapeseed all had high concentrations of allyl, methylthiopropyl, and 2-hydroxy 3-butenyl, respectively (Melrose, 2019; Paul et al., 2019). Hydrolytic derivatives of glucosinolates were the only ones shown to have antibacterial activities. Sulforaphane and benzyl isothiocyanate, in particular, were shown to be potent inhibitors of human pathogenic microbes in a number of investigations. A wide range of microorganisms were effectively inhibited by 4-methyl sulfinyl butylisothiocyanate (Kou et al., 2018; Romeo et al., 2018). Figure 10 shows the chemical structure of garlic organosulfur thiosulfinate.

Figure 10. Chemical structure of garlic organosulfur thiosulfinate

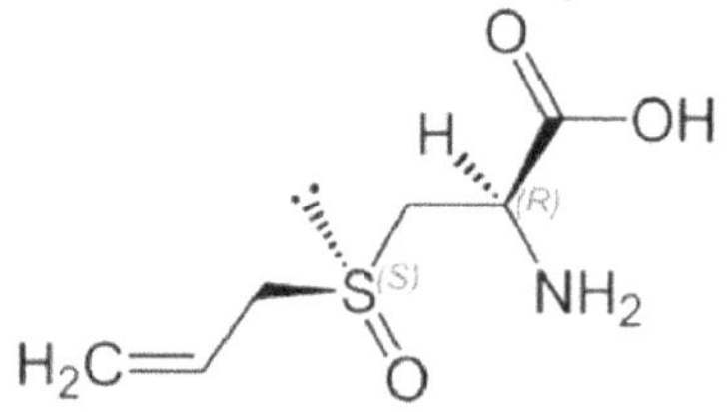

MECHANISMS OF RESISTANCE: HOW BACTERIA DEVELOP RESISTANCE TO PHYTOCHEMICALS

Bacteria can develop resistance to phytochemicals—the bioactive compounds derived from plants—through various adaptive and evolutionary strategies, similar to their resistance mechanisms against synthetic antibiotics. One primary mechanism involves efflux pumps, which are transmembrane proteins that actively expel toxic substances, including phytochemicals, out of bacterial cells. Efflux systems like the AcrAB-TolC in *Escherichia coli* and MexAB-OprM in *Pseudomonas aeruginosa* have been shown to reduce intracellular accumulation of plant-derived antimicrobials such as flavonoids and alkaloids, thus lowering their efficacy (Tegos et al., 2002). These efflux pumps can be either specific to certain phytochemicals or exhibit broad substrate specificity, contributing to multidrug resistance.

Another common mechanism is modification of target sites within bacterial cells. Many phytochemicals exert their antimicrobial action by interfering with bacterial enzymes, ribosomes, or DNA replication machinery. Bacteria can acquire mutations in these target sites, rendering the phytochemical ineffective. For instance, berberine targets DNA and RNA polymerases, but resistant bacteria may develop mutations that alter the binding affinity of these enzymes, reducing berberine's activity (Stermitz et al., 2000). Similarly, bacteria can produce enzymes that degrade or chemically modify phytochemicals before they reach their targets. For example, some bacteria express oxidoreductases that inactivate phenolic compounds, or esterases that hydrolyze antimicrobial terpenes and alkaloids (Cowan, 1999).

Bacteria may also develop resistance by forming biofilms, which are structured communities of bacteria embedded in a protective extracellular matrix. Biofilms significantly increase bacterial tolerance to phytochemicals by limiting their penetration and creating microenvironments that reduce metabolic activity, making bacteria less susceptible to antimicrobial agents. Biofilm-associated resistance is particularly relevant in chronic infections, where plant-based antimicrobials may show diminished efficacy unless used in combination with biofilm-disrupting agents (Khameneh et al., 2019). Moreover, the extracellular matrix can adsorb phytochemicals, reducing their availability to target cells and facilitating the survival of persister cells within the biofilm.

Lastly, bacteria may engage in horizontal gene transfer (HGT) to acquire resistance genes from other microbial species. Plasmids and transposons may carry genes that encode for resistance to specific plant-derived antimicrobials, particularly in environments where phytochemicals are used extensively, such as in herbal treatments or agriculture. Over time, selective pressure from constant phytochemical exposure can lead to the proliferation of resistant strains. This highlights the importance of rational use of phytochemicals and the need for combination therapies that reduce the risk of resistance development (Mandal et al., 2017). A deeper understanding of these resistance mechanisms is essential to enhance the design of more effective phytochemical-based antimicrobial strategies.

SYNERGISTIC IMPACT OF SECONDARY METABOLITES

One successful approach to controlling multidrug resistance (MDR) is the synergistic combination of present antibiotics with plant extracts or secondary metabolites. Multiple studies have shown that traditional antibiotics are more effective when taken with plant-based extracts or bioactive secondary metabolites (Ayaz et al., 2019). A number of studies have put up different theories as to how phytochemicals and antibiotics work together to combat various pathogenic bacteria, including those that are resistant to several drugs (Abreu et al., 2012; Anand et al., 2020).

Synergistic Effects Against Pathogenic Bacteria

Many bacterial species have developed resistance to antibiotics, which they combat by creating new molecules that target them instead. These molecules may function as receptors or enzymes. The binding affinity for β-lactam antibiotics, like penicillin and cephalosporin, was decreased in MRSA due to the synthesis of PB2a and other penicillin-binding proteins (PBPs). So, the cells keep living and keep synthesising peptidoglycan, which could be an alternative way to inhibit additional resistance active sites. When provided concurrently, crude uva-ursi extract decreased the MIC of oxacillin and cefmitazole against MRCA. In a study including multiple b-lactams plus corilagin, the main bioactive secondary metabolite in uva-ursi, the researchers found MIC values for MRSA that were thousands of times higher than those for the b-lactams alone. However, it failed to show a decrease in MIC against Staphylococcus aureus strains that are susceptible to Methicillin. Unlike PBPs, PBP2a was the intended target of uva-ursi or corilagin extracts (Algammal et al., 2020; Leonard & Markey, 2008). Additionally, a number of phenolic compounds, including tiliroside, pinoresinol, magnatriol B, and momorcharaside B, have shown that they work along with β-lactams to combat MRSA by directing their action towards alternate sites, such as PBP2a or PBP4 (Shimizu et al., 2001; Kuok et al., 2017; Li et al., 2018).

Bacterial resistance is greatly exacerbated by b-lactamases, which break down b-lactam antibiotics. To battle drug resistance in Gram-positive and Gram-negative bacterial species, it is crucial to identify secondary metabolites that block drug-metabolizing enzymes. This knowledge can greatly impact the development of successful combinations of phytochemicals and antibiotics. The therapeutic efficiency of certain β-lactam antibiotics can be improved by using clavulanic acid, a possible β-lactamase inhibitor, in combination with them (Yam et al., 1998). Research has shown that bioactive substances derived from green tea can restore antibiotic sensitivity by inhibiting β-lactamase (Livermore, 1995; Susic, 2004). Furthermore, baicalin and silibinin are just two of several flavonoids that have shown synergistic benefits against antibiotic-resistant bacteria, leading to a lower MIC (Kang et al., 2011; Liu et al., 2000). Because certain bacterial strains lack certain D2 porins or include efflux pumps like MexAB-OprM and MexCD-OprJ, the development of multidrug resistance (MDR) makes it more difficult for antibiotics to enter cells (Chopra, 1992; Poole, 2001, 2011).

There have been a lot of studies that point to specific secondary metabolites serving as EPIs. Apocynaceae plant species include the steroidal alkaloid conessine, which has shown efficacy in restoring P. aeruginosa susceptibility to the respective medications by blocking MexAB-OprM expression (Siriyong et al., 2017). Secondary metabolites are known to block efflux pumps, however this effect is antibiotic-dependent and cannot be achieved on their own. It has been demonstrated that the usage of monoterpenes, particularly pinene, significantly enhances the efficacy of various treatments against various strains of Campylobacter jejuni; however, when examined separately, no benefit was noted (Stermitz et al., 2000). Berberine and 5'-methoxyhydnocarpin, two active chemicals found in the barberry plant, worked together to inhibit the efflux pump mechanism, making the bacteria more sensitive to the antibiotic (Kovac et al., 2015). Additional phytochemicals that can block the efflux transporter NorA of Staphylococcus aureus include kaempferol 3 O α L (2,4 bis E p coumaroyl) rhamnoside, capsaicin, reserpine, carnosol, and carnosic acid (Holler et al., 2012). Several studies have shown that caffeic acid can penetrate the Gram-negative bacteria's oily outer membrane, increasing permeability and allowing the drug to enter the cells at higher concentrations (Kalia et al., 2012; Oluwatuyi et al., 2004; Ponnusamy et al., 2010; Schmitz et al., 1998).

Synergistic Effects Against Fungal Infections

Biofilm formation and overexpression of efflux pump proteins are two major causes of resistance, both of which phytochemicals have shown to effectively combat. Because antifungal medications are in short supply, scientists have been looking into several bioactive substances found in nature as potential solutions to the problem of fungus resistance. It has been found that garlic extracts have a synergistic effect that increases the effectiveness of treatments against Candida albicans (Movahed et al., 2016; Ngo et al., 2016). When the phenolic compound punicalagin was added to fluconazole, the minimum inhibitory concentration (MIC) against Candida albicans was cut in half. Essential oil from Pelargonium graveolens has shown promise in boosting etoconazole's effectiveness against a variety of trematodes (Salih, 2016; Zainal et al., 2020). Also, studies have looked at how different combinations of fluconazole and nystatin can work synergistically with caffeic acid and its derivatives to make them more effective against Candida albicans (Shin & Lim, 2004; Sardi et al., 2016; Khan et al., 2018). It was observed that fluconazole had an increased sensitivity to C. When administered to diabetic mice, thymoquinone and antifungal medications had an effect on Candida albicans. Multiple studies have shown that the active ingredient in Berberis vulgaris, berberine, increases the effectiveness of fluconazole in killing drug-resistant Candida albicans. The CDR1 gene, which is involved in fluphenazine-activated drug resistance, has its expression downregulated (Dhamgaye et al., 2014; Li et al., 2013; Xu et al., 2009). The antifungal characteristics and synergistic impact with azoles have been demonstrated by nyasol, a main component of the Chinese herb Anemarrhena asphodeloides (Iida et al., 2000; Park et al., 2003). The anti-disease effects of curcumin, a component of turmeric, have been the subject of substantial scientific investigation. When a combination of azoles and polyenes is applied to Candida albicans, it has been found to increase the generation of ROS and induce cell death (Sharma et al., 2010). Lots of research have shown that eugenol, the main ingredient in clove essential oils, can make fluconazole work better against fungal infections that are resistant to other drugs (Ahmad et al., 2010).

BIOTECHNOLOGICAL APPROACHES IN ANTIMICROBIAL DRUG DISCOVERY

Biotechnological advancements have significantly transformed the landscape of antimicrobial drug discovery, offering innovative strategies to identify novel compounds and overcome antibiotic resistance. Genome mining is one such approach that involves exploring the genetic material of microorganisms to uncover biosynthetic gene clusters (BGCs) responsible for producing secondary metabolites, many of which have antimicrobial properties. Advances in sequencing technologies have made it possible to analyze microbial genomes for "silent" or "cryptic" BGCs that are not expressed under standard laboratory conditions. These clusters often encode novel antibiotics that have yet to be discovered through traditional culturing methods (Ziemert et al., 2016). Tools like antiSMASH and PRISM facilitate the annotation and prediction of these gene clusters, accelerating the discovery pipeline.

Metabolomics, another powerful biotechnological tool, involves the comprehensive analysis of small-molecule metabolites in biological samples. In the context of antimicrobial research, metabolomics helps in identifying and characterizing bioactive compounds produced by microorganisms and understanding their mechanisms of action. By profiling metabolite changes in response to pathogen exposure or genetic manipulation, researchers can pinpoint potential antimicrobial agents and assess their biosynthetic pathways (Pang et al., 2021). Coupled with mass spectrometry and nuclear magnetic resonance (NMR) techniques, metabolomics enables high-throughput screening of microbial libraries and natural product extracts for novel antibiotic candidates.

Synthetic biology plays a crucial role by enabling the design and engineering of microorganisms to produce desired antimicrobial compounds or enhance the yield of existing ones. Through genetic circuit engineering, researchers can activate silent biosynthetic pathways or reprogram metabolic networks to generate new-to-nature molecules with improved efficacy and reduced toxicity (Smanski et al., 2016). Additionally, synthetic biology allows the heterologous expression of BGCs from uncultivable or slow-growing microbes in well-characterized host organisms like *Escherichia coli* or *Streptomyces*, facilitating the production and optimization of antimicrobial agents under controlled conditions. The integration of genome mining, metabolomics, and synthetic biology represents a synergistic platform for modern antimicrobial drug discovery. These approaches not only expand the chemical space for antibiotic development but also provide tools for understanding resistance mechanisms and developing next-generation therapeutics. As microbial resistance continues to threaten global health, the use of these biotechnological tools offers a promising pathway for sustainable and efficient discovery of novel antimicrobials.

CURRENT STATUS OF SECONDARY METABOLITES IN CLINICAL TRIALS AND FDA-APPROVED USAGE

Secondary metabolites—natural compounds not directly involved in the normal growth, development, or reproduction of organisms—have long served as rich sources for drug discovery. Many clinically used antibiotics, anticancer agents, immunosuppressants, and antiparasitic drugs originate from microbial and plant secondary metabolites. For example, penicillin, erythromycin, and tacrolimus were all derived from microbial sources. Recent advancements in biotechnology have rejuvenated interest in these compounds, with several secondary metabolites either progressing through clinical trials or already approved for therapeutic use (Newman & Cragg, 2020). These metabolites continue to be vital in addressing complex diseases and emerging drug resistance.

Several secondary metabolites are currently in clinical trials for a wide range of indications, including cancer, bacterial infections, and neurodegenerative diseases. For instance, Plitidepsin, a marine-derived cyclic depsipeptide, has shown promise in clinical trials for multiple myeloma and viral infections like COVID-19 (Varona et al., 2021). Similarly, Bryostatin-1, derived from marine bryozoans, is under investigation for treating Alzheimer's disease and HIV latency reversal. The rich chemical diversity and unique mechanisms of action of these metabolites often give them an advantage in targeting previously undruggable sites, making them valuable candidates in modern therapeutic development pipelines (Atanasov et al., 2021). In terms of FDA-approved drugs, several secondary metabolites have seen clinical success. Paclitaxel (Taxol®), derived from the Pacific yew tree, remains a cornerstone in chemotherapy for breast, lung, and ovarian cancers. Artemisinin, a sesquiterpene lactone from *Artemisia annua*, is the backbone of artemisinin-based combination therapies (ACTs) for malaria. These examples highlight the continued clinical relevance and potential of secondary metabolites, especially when supported by advances in synthetic biology, fermentation technology, and combinatorial biosynthesis, which enhance their production and structural optimization (Newman & Cragg, 2020).

FUTURE PERSPECTIVES

The future of secondary metabolites as antimicrobial agents is both promising and strategically vital, especially in light of rising antimicrobial resistance (AMR). With advancements in genome mining and metagenomics, scientists can now explore unculturable or rare microorganisms for novel bioactive compounds that were previously inaccessible (Yasmeen et al., 2025). These technologies will likely lead to the discovery of new classes of secondary metabolites with unique modes of action that can bypass existing resistance mechanisms. Moreover, synthetic biology and metabolic engineering offer powerful tools to optimize the production and modification of antimicrobial secondary metabolites. By reconstructing or enhancing biosynthetic pathways in heterologous hosts, researchers can improve yield, stability, and specificity, making these compounds more suitable for pharmaceutical development. This opens the door for the custom design of next-generation antibiotics, tailored to target multidrug-resistant pathogens (Barwant et al., 2025a, b).

In order to determine the antibacterial capabilities and secondary metabolites of various plant families, a large number of scientists have conducted research on these groupings. In subsequent study, experimental investigations should be conducted in order to evaluate the biological characteristics of a variety of plant groups (Enenebeaku et al., 2022a). A substantial number of potential medical applications of the antibacterial characteristics have been identified. To proceed with the process of gaining a grasp of how these secondary metabolites are processed, the next step is to be aware of the processes themselves. Furthermore, later researchers ought to isolate all compounds from plants in order to exactly establish the individual component that is responsible for the antibacterial activity. Researchers have been prompted to explore a wide variety of secondary metabolites as a result of the numerous studies that have been published demonstrating that plant extracts possess antibacterial capabilities (Ogidi et al., 2019a,b; Akpan et al., 2020). As a consequence of this, there is a possibility that a number of secondary metabolites are present, which results in a lack of clarity regarding the determination of whether specific components are responsible for the observed activity or whether a synergistic impact among different molecules is involved. In a nutshell, the future of ethnopharmacology appears to be bright, with potential strategies proposed to combat germs that are resistant to antibiotics through the utilisation of phytochemicals (Enenebeaku et al., 2022a).

The integration of nanotechnology and advanced drug delivery systems may further enhance the efficacy and bioavailability of secondary metabolites, enabling targeted therapy and reducing toxicity. Additionally, the development of synergistic formulations, combining secondary metabolites with conventional antibiotics or adjuvants, holds promise for reviving the efficacy of existing drugs and mitigating resistance. Finally, global collaboration in open-access compound libraries, bioinformatics databases, and artificial intelligence (AI)-driven screening tools will accelerate the identification and optimization of promising antimicrobial metabolites (Ogidi et al., 2025). The future lies in a multidisciplinary approach that leverages chemistry, microbiology, data science, and clinical medicine to fully realize the antimicrobial potential of secondary metabolites.

CONCLUSION

In the course of various investigations into possible remedies for a wide variety of diseases, researchers have discovered a large number of secondary metabolites. It has also been established that a number of phytochemicals have the potential to either inhibit the growth of bacteria or destroy them. Secondary metabolites have been shown to be effective against microbial infections in vivo, and several studies have proven that they do so while also maintaining the beneficial bacteria that are found in the gut. The phytochemicals, when combined with standard antibiotics, proved to be effective against a wide variety of bacterial strains. In addition, secondary metabolites have the capacity to collaborate with less potent antibiotics in order to enhance the efficacy of the latter against a wide variety of diseases, including those that are brought on by bacteria that are resistant to several drugs. Due to the fact that the potential implications of pharmaceutical interactions with secondary metabolites have not been thoroughly proved, there has been a lack of focus on this subject. When taken as a whole, the findings indicate that secondary metabolites have the potential to play a significant part in the creation of drugs in the 21st century, either as an alternative or in conjunction with the antimicrobial therapies that are already in use.

Abbreviations

WHO: World Health Organization
MDR: Multi-Drug Resistant
EGCG: Epigalocatechin-3-Gallate
UTIs: Urinary Tract Infections
TB: Tuberculosis
MICs: Minimum Inhibitory Concentrations
MRSA: Methicillin-Resistant Staphylococcus Aureus
QQE: Quorum Quenching Enzyme
AETE: Aqueous Extract of Tagetes Erecta
DADS: Diallyl Disulfide
PBPs: Penicillin-Binding Proteins
ROS: Reactive Oxygen Species
B: Beta
A: Alpha

REFERENCES

Abdulhamid, A., Fakai, J. M., Sani, I., Argungu, A. U., & Bello, F. (2014). Preliminary phytochemical and antibacterial activity of ethanolic and aqueous stem bark extracts of *Psidium guajava.Am. J. Drug Discovery Dev*, *4*(1), 85–89. DOI: 10.3923/ajdd.2014.85.89

Abreu, A. C., McBain, A. J., & Simões, M. (2012). Plants as sources of new antimicrobials and resistance-modifying agents. *Natural Product Reports*, *29*(9), 1007–1021. DOI: 10.1039/c2np20035j PMID: 22786554

Abukakar, M. G., Ukwuani, A. N., & Shehu, R. A. (2008). Phytochemical screening and antibacterial activity of *Tamarindus indica* pulp extract. *Asian J. Biochem.*, *3*(2), 134–138. DOI: 10.3923/ajb.2008.134.138

Adeniyi, B. A., Fong, H. H., Pezzuto, J. M., Luyengi, L., & Odelola, H. A. (2000). Antibacterial activity of diospyrin, isodiospyrin and bisisodiospyrin from the root of Diospyros piscatoria (Gurke) (Ebenaceae). *Phytotherapy Research*, *14*(2), 112–117. DOI: 10.1002/(SICI)1099-1573(200003)14:2<112::AID-PTR488>3.0.CO;2-T PMID: 10685108

Ahmad, A., Khan, A., Khan, L. A., & Manzoor, N. (2010). In vitro synergy of eugenol and methyleugenol with fluconazole against clinical Candida isolates. *Journal of Medical Microbiology*, *59*(Pt 10), 1178–1184. DOI: 10.1099/jmm.0.020693-0 PMID: 20634332

Ahmad, N., Alam, M. K., Shehbaz, A., Khan, A., Mannan, A., Hakim, S. R., Bisht, D., & Owais, M. (2005). Antimicrobial activity of clove oil and its potential in the treatment of vaginal candidiasis. *Journal of Drug Targeting*, *13*(10), 555–561. DOI: 10.1080/10611860500422958 PMID: 16390816

Ahmed, A. A., Mahmoud, A. A., Williams, H. J., Scott, A. I., Reibenspies, J. H., & Mabry, T. J. (1993). New sesquiterpene alpha-methylene lactones from the Egyptian plant Jasonia candicans. *Journal of Natural Products*, *56*(8), 1276–1280. DOI: 10.1021/np50098a011 PMID: 8229012

Akpan, U. M., Ogidi, O. I., Wodu, P. D., & Kanu, J. S. (2020). Antimicrobial Potency of Palm Kernel oil against selected clinical isolates in Abak Local Government Area of Akwa Ibom State, Nigeria. [APJOCASR]. *Akwapoly Journal of Communication and Scientific Research*, *5*(1), 65–72.

Alakomi, H. L., Puupponen-Pimiä, R., Aura, A. M., Helander, I. M., Nohynek, L., Oksman-Caldentey, K. M., & Saarela, M. (2007). Weakening of salmonella with selected microbial metabolites of berry-derived phenolic compounds and organic acids. *Journal of Agricultural and Food Chemistry*, *55*(10), 3905–3912. DOI: 10.1021/jf070190y PMID: 17439151

Alamri, S. A., & Moustafa, M. F. (2012). Antimicrobial properties of 3 medicinal plants from Saudi Arabia against some clinical isolates of bacteria. *Saudi Medical Journal*, *33*(3), 272–277. PMID: 22426907

Algammal, A. M., Hetta, H. F., Elkelish, A., Alkhalifah, D. H. H., Hozzein, W. N., Batiha, G. E., El Nahhas, N., & Mabrok, M. A. (2020). Methicillin-Resistant *Staphylococcus aureus* (MRSA): One Health Perspective Approach to the Bacterium Epidemiology, Virulence Factors, Antibiotic-Resistance, and Zoonotic Impact. *Infection and Drug Resistance*, *13*, 3255–3265. DOI: 10.2147/IDR.S272733 PMID: 33061472

Alrumaihi, F., Allemailem, K. S., Almatroudi, A., Alsahli, M. A., Khan, A., & Khan, M. A. (2019). Tinospora cordifolia Aqueous Extract Alleviates Cyclophosphamide-Induced Immune Suppression, Toxicity and Systemic Candidiasis in Immunosuppressed Mice: In vivo Study in Comparison to Antifungal Drug Fluconazole. *Current Pharmaceutical Biotechnology*, *20*(12), 1055–1063. DOI: 10.2174/1389201019666190722151126 PMID: 31333126

Alsuhaibani, S., & Khan, M. A. (2017). Immune-Stimulatory and Therapeutic Activity of *Tinospora cordifolia*: Double-Edged Sword against Salmonellosis. *Journal of Immunology Research*, *1787803*, 1–9. Advance online publication. DOI: 10.1155/2017/1787803 PMID: 29318160

Amábile-Cuevas, C. F. (2003). New antibiotics and new resistance: In many ways, the fight against antibiotic resistance is already lost; Preventing bacterial disease requires thoughtful new approaches. *American Scientist*, *91*(2), 138–149. DOI: 10.1511/2003.12.138

Amirkia, V., & Heinrich, M. (2015). Natural products and drug discovery: A survey of stakeholders in industry and academia. *Frontiers in Pharmacology*, *6*, 237. DOI: 10.3389/fphar.2015.00237 PMID: 26578954

Anand, U., Jacobo-Herrera, N., Altemimi, A., & Lakhssassi, N. (2019). A Comprehensive Review on Medicinal Plants as Antimicrobial Therapeutics: Potential Avenues of Biocompatible Drug Discovery. *Metabolites*, *9*(11), 258. DOI: 10.3390/metabo9110258 PMID: 31683833

Anand, U., Nandy, S., Mundhra, A., Das, N., Pandey, D. K., & Dey, A. (2020). A review on antimicrobial botanicals, phytochemicals and natural resistance modifying agents from Apocynaceae family: Possible therapeutic approaches against multidrug resistance in pathogenic microorganisms. *Drug resistance updates: reviews and commentaries in antimicrobial and anticancer chemotherapy, 51*, 100695. https://doi.org/DOI: 10.1016/j.drup.2020.100695

Arima, H., & Danno, G. (2002). Isolation of antimicrobial compounds from guava (Psidium guajava L.) and their structural elucidation. *Bioscience, Biotechnology, and Biochemistry*, *66*(8), 1727–1730. DOI: 10.1271/bbb.66.1727 PMID: 12353635

Atanasov, A. G., Zotchev, S. B., Dirsch, V. M., & Supuran, C. T. (2021). Natural products in drug discovery: Advances and opportunities. *Nature Reviews. Drug Discovery*, *20*(3), 200–216. DOI: 10.1038/s41573-020-00114-z PMID: 33510482

Avato, P., Tursil, E., Vitali, C., Miccolis, V., & Candido, V. (2000). Allylsulfide constituents of garlic volatile oil as antimicrobial agents. *Phytomedicine*, *7*(3), 239–243. DOI: 10.1016/S0944-7113(00)80010-0 PMID: 11185736

Ayaz, M., Ullah, F., Sadiq, A., Ullah, F., Ovais, M., Ahmed, J., & Devkota, H. P. (2019). Synergistic interactions of phytochemicals with antimicrobial agents: Potential strategy to counteract drug resistance. *Chemico-Biological Interactions*, *308*, 294–303. DOI: 10.1016/j.cbi.2019.05.050 PMID: 31158333

Barwant, M. M., Ogidi, O. I., Singh, S., & Singh, B. (2025a). Novel Drug Delivery Methods for Herbal Medicine. In: Farid, A. (Ed.). (2025). Herbal Pharmacopeia: Nanotechnology and Advancing Drug Discovery (1st ed.). CRC Press. https://doi.org/DOI: 10.1201/9781003544418-15

Barwant, M. M., Singh, S., Singh, B., Sharma, A., & Ogidi, O. I. (2025b). Nanotechnology-Enhanced Delivery of Herbal Extract: Formulation, Preclinical and Clinical Efficiency. In: Farid, A. (Ed.). (2025). Herbal Pharmacopeia: Nanotechnology and Advancing Drug Discovery (1st ed.). CRC Press. https://doi.org/DOI: 10.1201/9781003544418

Basile, A., Conte, B., Rigano, D., Senatore, F., & Sorbo, S. (2010). Antibacterial and antifungal properties of acetonic extract of Feijoa sellowiana fruits and its effect on Helicobacter pylori growth. *Journal of Medicinal Food*, *13*(1), 189–195. DOI: 10.1089/jmf.2008.0301 PMID: 20136454

Bhat, B. B., Udupa, N., & Sreedhar, D. (2019). Herbal Products Regulations in a Few Countries-A Brief Overview. *Current Drug Discovery Technologies*, *16*(4), 368–371. DOI: 10.2174/1570163815666181105091254 PMID: 30394210

Bourinbaiar, A. S., & Lee-Huang, S. (1996). The activity of plant-derived antiretroviral proteins MAP30 and GAP31 against herpes simplex virus in vitro. *Biochemical and Biophysical Research Communications*, *219*(3), 923–929. DOI: 10.1006/bbrc.1996.0334 PMID: 8645280

Breithaupt, H. (1999). The new antibiotics. *Nature Biotechnology*, *17*(12), 1165–1169. DOI: 10.1038/70705 PMID: 10585711

Bylka, W., Szaufer-Hajdrych, M., Matławska, I., & Goślińska, O. (2004). Antimicrobial activity of isocytisoside and extracts of Aquilegia vulgaris L. *Letters in Applied Microbiology*, *39*(1), 93–97. DOI: 10.1111/j.1472-765X.2004.01553.x PMID: 15189294

Calixto, J. B. (2019). The role of natural products in modern drug discovery. *Anais da Academia Brasileira de Ciências*, *91*(Suppl 3), e20190105. DOI: 10.1590/0001-3765201920190105 PMID: 31166478

Carson, C. F., & Hammer, K. A. (2010). Chemistry and Bioactivity of Essential Oils. In Thormar, H. (Ed.), *Lipids and Essential Oils as Antimicrobial Agents* (pp. 203–238). John Wiley & Sons.

Chandra, H., Bishnoi, P., Yadav, A., Patni, B., Mishra, A. P., & Nautiyal, A. R. (2017). Antimicrobial Resistance and the Alternative Resources with Special Emphasis on Plant-Based Antimicrobials-A Review. *Plants*, *6*(2), 16. DOI: 10.3390/plants6020016 PMID: 28394295

Chopra, I. (1992). Efflux-based antibiotic resistance mechanisms: The evidence for increasing prevalence. *The Journal of Antimicrobial Chemotherapy*, *30*(6), 737–739. DOI: 10.1093/jac/30.6.737 PMID: 1289349

Cowan, M. M. (1999). Plant products as antimicrobial agents. *Clinical Microbiology Reviews*, *12*(4), 564–582. DOI: 10.1128/CMR.12.4.564 PMID: 10515903

Cowan, M. M. (1999). Plant products as antimicrobial agents. *Clinical Microbiology Reviews*, *12*(4), 564–582. DOI: 10.1128/CMR.12.4.564 PMID: 10515903

Cueva, C., Moreno-Arribas, M. V., Martín-Alvarez, P. J., Bills, G., Vicente, M. F., Basilio, A., Rivas, C. L., Requena, T., Rodríguez, J. M., & Bartolomé, B. (2010). Antimicrobial activity of phenolic acids against commensal, probiotic and pathogenic bacteria. *Research in Microbiology*, *161*(5), 372–382. DOI: 10.1016/j.resmic.2010.04.006 PMID: 20451604

Davies, K. M., Jibran, R., Zhou, Y., Albert, N. W., Brummell, D. A., Jordan, B. R., Bowman, J. L., & Schwinn, K. E. (2020). The Evolution of Flavonoid Biosynthesis: A Bryophyte Perspective. *Frontiers in Plant Science*, *11*, 7. DOI: 10.3389/fpls.2020.00007 PMID: 32117358

Demain, A. L. (2014). Importance of microbial natural products and the need to revitalize their discovery. *Journal of Industrial Microbiology & Biotechnology*, *41*(2), 185–201. DOI: 10.1007/s10295-013-1325-z PMID: 23990168

Dhamgaye, S., Devaux, F., Vandeputte, P., Khandelwal, N. K., Sanglard, D., Mukhopadhyay, G., & Prasad, R. (2014). Molecular mechanisms of action of herbal antifungal alkaloid berberine, in Candida albicans. *PLoS One*, *9*(8), e104554. DOI: 10.1371/journal.pone.0104554 PMID: 25105295

Endo, E. H., Cortez, D. A., Ueda-Nakamura, T., Nakamura, C. V., & Dias Filho, B. P. (2010). Potent antifungal activity of extracts and pure compound isolated from pomegranate peels and synergism with fluconazole against Candida albicans. *Research in Microbiology*, *161*(7), 534–540. DOI: 10.1016/j.resmic.2010.05.002 PMID: 20541606

Enenebeaku, C.K., Ogukwe, C.E., Nweke, C.O., Anyado-Nwadike, S.O., Obi, M. Duru, I.K., Enenebeaku, U.E., & Ogidi, O.I. (2022a). Antiplasmodial and in vitro antioxidant potentials of crude aqueous and methanol extracts of *Chasmanthera dependens* (Hochst). *Bulletin of the National Research Centre, (Springer Open)* 46(33), 1-12. https://doi.org/DOI: 10.1186/s42269-022-00721-3

Enenebeaku, U. E., Duru, C. E., Okotcha, E. N., Ogidi, O. I., Mgbemena, I. C., Nwigwe, H. C., & Enenebeaku, C. K. (2022b). Phytochemical analysis and Antioxidant Evaluation of Crude Extracts from the Roots, Stem and Leaves of Dictyandraarborescens (Welw.). *Tropical Journal of Natural Product Research*, *6*(1), 62–70. DOI: 10.26538/tjnpr/v6i1.12

Fahey, J. W., Zalcmann, A. T., & Talalay, P. (2001). The chemical diversity and distribution of glucosinolates and isothiocyanates among plants. *Phytochemistry*, *56*(1), 5–51. DOI: 10.1016/S0031-9422(00)00316-2 PMID: 11198818

Ferri, M., Ranucci, E., Romagnoli, P., & Giaccone, V. (2017). Antimicrobial resistance: A global emerging threat to public health systems. *Critical Reviews in Food Science and Nutrition*, *57*(13), 2857–2876. DOI: 10.1080/10408398.2015.1077192 PMID: 26464037

Fierascu, R. C., Georgiev, M. I., Fierascu, I., Ungureanu, C., Avramescu, S. M., Ortan, A., Georgescu, M. I., Sutan, A. N., Zanfirescu, A., Dinu-Pirvu, C. E., Velescu, B. S., & Anuta, V. (2018). Mitodepressive, antioxidant, antifungal and anti-inflammatory effects of wild-growing Romanian native Arctium lappa L. (Asteraceae) and Veronica persica Poiret (Plantaginaceae). *Food and chemical toxicology: an international journal published for the British Industrial Biological Research Association, 111*, 44–52. https://doi.org/DOI: 10.1016/j.fct.2017.11.008

Fischbach, M. A., & Walsh, C. T. (2009). Antibiotics for emerging pathogens. *Science, 325*(5944), 1089–1093. DOI: 10.1126/science.1176667 PMID: 19713519

Ghorbani, A., & Esmaeilizadeh, M. (2017). Pharmacological properties of *Salvia officinalis* and its components. *Journal of Traditional and Complementary Medicine, 7*(4), 433–440. DOI: 10.1016/j.jtcme.2016.12.014 PMID: 29034191

Goyal, S. N., Prajapati, C. P., Gore, P. R., Patil, C. R., Mahajan, U. B., Sharma, C., Talla, S. P., & Ojha, S. K. (2017). Therapeutic Potential and Pharmaceutical Development of Thymoquinone: A Multitargeted Molecule of Natural Origin. *Frontiers in Pharmacology, 8*, 656. DOI: 10.3389/fphar.2017.00656 PMID: 28983249

Greathead, H. (2003). Plants and plant extracts for improving animal productivity. *The Proceedings of the Nutrition Society, 62*(2), 279–290. DOI: 10.1079/PNS2002197 PMID: 14506875

Guiraud, P., Steiman, R., Campos-Takaki, G. M., Seigle-Murandi, F., & Simeon de Buochberg, M. (1994). Comparison of antibacterial and antifungal activities of lapachol and beta-lapachone. *Planta Medica, 60*(4), 373–374. DOI: 10.1055/s-2006-959504 PMID: 7938274

Gupta, P. D., & Birdi, T. J. (2017). Development of botanicals to combat antibiotic resistance. *Journal of Ayurveda and Integrative Medicine, 8*(4), 266–275. DOI: 10.1016/j.jaim.2017.05.004 PMID: 28869082

Habbu, P. V., Mahadevan, K. M., Shastry, R. A., & Manjunatha, H. (2009). Antimicrobial activity of flavanoid sulphates and other fractions of Argyreia speciosa (Burm.f) Boj. *Indian Journal of Experimental Biology, 47*(2), 121–128. PMID: 19374167

Hatcher, C. R., Ryves, D. B., & Millett, J. (2020). The function of secondary metabolites in plant carnivory. *Annals of Botany, 125*(3), 399–411. DOI: 10.1093/aob/mcz191 PMID: 31760424

Holler, J. G., Christensen, S. B., Slotved, H. C., Rasmussen, H. B., Gúzman, A., Olsen, C. E., Petersen, B., & Mølgaard, P. (2012). Novel inhibitory activity of the Staphylococcus aureus NorA efflux pump by a kaempferol rhamnoside isolated from Persea lingue Nees. *The Journal of Antimicrobial Chemotherapy*, *67*(5), 1138–1144. DOI: 10.1093/jac/dks005 PMID: 22311936

Hunter, M. D., & Hull, L. A. (1993). Variation in concentrations of phloridzin and phloretin in apple foliage. *Phytochemistry*, *34*(5), 1251–1254. DOI: 10.1016/0031-9422(91)80010-X

Iida, Y., Oh, K. B., Saito, M., Matsuoka, H., & Kurata, H. (2000). In vitro synergism between nyasol, an active compound isolated from Anemarrhena asphodeloides, and azole agents against Candida albicans. *Planta Medica*, *66*(5), 435–438. DOI: 10.1055/s-2000-8589 PMID: 10909263

Jujjavarapu, S. E., & Dhagat, S. (2018). In Silico Discovery of Novel Ligands for Antimicrobial Lipopeptides for Computer-Aided Drug Design. *Probiotics and Antimicrobial Proteins*, *10*(2), 129–141. DOI: 10.1007/s12602-017-9356-9 PMID: 29218506

Kalia, N. P., Mahajan, P., Mehra, R., Nargotra, A., Sharma, J. P., Koul, S., & Khan, I. A. (2012). Capsaicin, a novel inhibitor of the NorA efflux pump, reduces the intracellular invasion of Staphylococcus aureus. *The Journal of Antimicrobial Chemotherapy*, *67*(10), 2401–2408. DOI: 10.1093/jac/dks232 PMID: 22807321

Kang, H. K., Kim, H. Y., & Cha, J. D. (2011). Synergistic effects between silibinin and antibiotics on methicillin-resistant Staphylococcus aureus isolated from clinical specimens. *Biotechnology Journal*, *6*(11), 1397–1408. DOI: 10.1002/biot.201000422 PMID: 21491604

Khameneh, B., Iranshahy, M., Soheili, V., & Bazzaz, B. S. F. (2019). Review on plant antimicrobials: A mechanistic viewpoint. *Antimicrobial Resistance and Infection Control*, *8*(1), 118. DOI: 10.1186/s13756-019-0559-6 PMID: 31346459

Khan, M. A. (2018). Antimicrobial action of thymoquinone. In Younus, H. (Ed.), *Molecular and Therapeutic actions of Thymoquinone: Actions of Thymoquinone* (pp. 57–64). Springer. DOI: 10.1007/978-981-10-8800-1_5

Khan, M. A., Aldebasi, Y. H., Alsuhaibani, S. A., AlSahli, M. A., Alzohairy, M. A., Khan, A., & Younus, H. (2018). Therapeutic potential of thymoquinone liposomes against the systemic infection of Candida albicans in diabetic mice. *PLoS One*, *13*(12), e0208951. DOI: 10.1371/journal.pone.0208951 PMID: 30589842

Kliebenstein, D. J., & Osbourn, A. (2012). Making new molecules - evolution of pathways for novel metabolites in plants. *Current Opinion in Plant Biology*, *15*(4), 415–423. DOI: 10.1016/j.pbi.2012.05.005 PMID: 22683039

Kloucek, P., Polesny, Z., Svobodova, B., Vlkova, E., & Kokoska, L. (2005). Antibacterial screening of some Peruvian medicinal plants used in Callería District. *Journal of Ethnopharmacology*, *99*(2), 309–312. DOI: 10.1016/j.jep.2005.01.062 PMID: 15894143

Korir, R. K., Mutai, C., Kiiyukia, C., & Bii, C. (2012). Antimicrobial activity and safety of two medicinal plants traditionally used in bomet district of Kenya. *Research Journal of Medicinal Plant*, *6*(5), 370–382. DOI: 10.3923/rjmp.2012.370.382

Kou, X., Li, B., Olayanju, J. B., Drake, J. M., & Chen, N. (2018). Nutraceutical or Pharmacological Potential of Moringa oleifera Lam. *Nutrients*, *10*(3), 343. DOI: 10.3390/nu10030343 PMID: 29534518

Kovač, J., Šimunović, K., Wu, Z., Klančnik, A., Bucar, F., Zhang, Q., & Možina, S. S. (2015). Antibiotic resistance modulation and modes of action of (-)-α-pinene in Campylobacter jejuni. *PLoS One*, *10*(4), e0122871. DOI: 10.1371/journal.pone.0122871 PMID: 25830640

Kroymann, J. (2011). Natural diversity and adaptation in plant secondary metabolism. *Current Opinion in Plant Biology*, *14*(3), 246–251. DOI: 10.1016/j.pbi.2011.03.021 PMID: 21514879

Kubo, I., Muroi, H., & Kubo, A. (1994). Naturally occurring antiacne agents. *Journal of Natural Products*, *57*(1), 9–17. DOI: 10.1021/np50103a002 PMID: 8158169

Kumar, S., & Pandey, A. K. (2013). Chemistry and biological activities of flavonoids: An overview. *TheScientificWorldJournal*, *162750*(1), 162750. Advance online publication. DOI: 10.1155/2013/162750 PMID: 24470791

Kuok, C. F., Hoi, S. O., Hoi, C. F., Chan, C. H., Fong, I. H., Ngok, C. K., Meng, L. R., & Fong, P. (2017). Synergistic antibacterial effects of herbal extracts and antibiotics on methicillin-resistant Staphylococcus aureus: A computational and experimental study. *Experimental Biology and Medicine (Maywood, N.J.)*, *242*(7), 731–743. DOI: 10.1177/1535370216689828 PMID: 28118725

Kyung, K. H., & Fleming, H. P. (1997). Antimicrobial activity of sulfur compounds derived from cabbage. *Journal of Food Protection*, *60*(1), 67–71. DOI: 10.4315/0362-028X-60.1.67 PMID: 10465044

Kyung, K. H., & Lee, Y. C. (2001). Antimicrobial activities of sulfur compounds derived from s-alk (en)yl-l-cysteine sulfoxides in allium and brassica. *Food Reviews International, 17*(2), 183–198. DOI: 10.1081/FRI-100000268

Lee, C. R., Cho, I. H., Jeong, B. C., & Lee, S. H. (2013). Strategies to minimize antibiotic resistance. *International Journal of Environmental Research and Public Health, 10*(9), 4274–4305. DOI: 10.3390/ijerph10094274 PMID: 24036486

Leonard, F. C., & Markey, B. K. (2008). Meticillin-resistant Staphylococcus aureus in animals: a review. *Veterinary journal (London, England: 1997), 175*(1), 27–36. https://doi.org/DOI: 10.1016/j.tvjl.2006.11.008

Li, D. D., Xu, Y., Zhang, D. Z., Quan, H., Mylonakis, E., Hu, D. D., Li, M. B., Zhao, L. X., Zhu, L. H., Wang, Y., & Jiang, Y. Y. (2013). Fluconazole assists berberine to kill fluconazole-resistant Candida albicans. *Antimicrobial Agents and Chemotherapy, 57*(12), 6016–6027. DOI: 10.1128/AAC.00499-13 PMID: 24060867

Li, D. D., Xu, Y., Zhang, D. Z., Quan, H., Mylonakis, E., Hu, D. D., Li, M. B., Zhao, L. X., Zhu, L. H., Wang, Y., & Jiang, Y. Y. (2013). Fluconazole assists berberine to kill fluconazole-resistant Candida albicans. *Antimicrobial Agents and Chemotherapy, 57*(12), 6016–6027. DOI: 10.1128/AAC.00499-13 PMID: 24060867

Li, X., Deng, Y., Zheng, Z., Huang, W., Chen, L., Tong, Q., & Ming, Y. (2018). Corilagin, a promising medicinal herbal agent. *Biomedicine & pharmacotherapy = Biomedecine & pharmacotherapie, 99*, 43–50. https://doi.org/DOI: 10.1016/j.biopha.2018.01.030

Liu, I. X., Durham, D. G., & Richards, R. M. (2000). Baicalin synergy with beta-lactam antibiotics against methicillin-resistant Staphylococcus aureus and other beta-lactam-resistant strains of S. aureus. *The Journal of Pharmacy and Pharmacology, 52*(3), 361–366. DOI: 10.1211/0022357001773922 PMID: 10757427

Livermore, D. M. (1995). beta-Lactamases in laboratory and clinical resistance. *Clinical Microbiology Reviews, 8*(4), 557–584. DOI: 10.1128/CMR.8.4.557 PMID: 8665470

Livermore, D. M., Blaser, M., Carrs, O., Cassell, G., Fishman, N., Guidos, R., Levy, S., Powers, J., Norrby, R., Tillotson, G., Davies, R., Projan, S., Dawson, M., Monnet, D., Keogh-Brown, M., Hand, K., Garner, S., Findlay, D., Morel, C., & White, T. (2011). Discovery research: The scientific challenge of finding new antibiotics. *The Journal of Antimicrobial Chemotherapy, 66*(9), 1941–1944. DOI: 10.1093/jac/dkr262 PMID: 21700626

Mahady, G. B. (2001). Global harmonization of herbal health claims. *The Journal of Nutrition, 131*(3, 3s), 1120S–1123S. DOI: 10.1093/jn/131.3.1120S PMID: 11238830

Manach, C., Scalbert, A., Morand, C., Rémésy, C., & Jiménez, L. (2004). Polyphenols: Food sources and bioavailability. *The American Journal of Clinical Nutrition, 79*(5), 727–747. DOI: 10.1093/ajcn/79.5.727 PMID: 15113710

Mandal, S. M., Chakraborty, D., & Dey, S. (2017). Phenolic acids act as signaling molecules in plant-microbe symbioses. *Plant Signaling & Behavior, 5*(4), 359–368. DOI: 10.4161/psb.5.4.10871 PMID: 20400851

Mann, A. (2007). *Survey of Ethnomedicine for the treatment of Tuberculosis: Chemistry Perspective. Ayanwola Printing Works*. Minna.

Mariita, R. M., Ogol, C. K. P. O., Oguge, N. O., & Okemo, P. O. (2011). Methanol extract of three medicinal plants from samburu in northern kenya show significant antimycobacterial, antibacterial and antifungal properties. *Research Journal of Medicinal Plant, 5*(1), 54–64. DOI: 10.3923/rjmp.2011.54.64

Martini, N. D., Katerere, D. R., & Eloff, J. N. (2004). Biological activity of five antibacterial flavonoids from Combretum erythrophyllum (Combretaceae). *Journal of Ethnopharmacology, 93*(2-3), 207–212. DOI: 10.1016/j.jep.2004.02.030 PMID: 15234754

Melrose, J. (2019). The Glucosinolates: A Sulphur Glucoside Family of Mustard Anti-Tumour and Antimicrobial Phytochemicals of Potential Therapeutic Application. *Biomedicines, 7*(3), 62. DOI: 10.3390/biomedicines7030062 PMID: 31430999

Merkl, R., Hradkova, I., Filip, V., & Smidrkal, J. (2018). Antimicrobial and antioxidant properties of phenolic acids alkyl esters. *Czech Journal of Food Sciences, 28*(4), 275–279. DOI: 10.17221/132/2010-CJFS

Michael, C. A., Dominey-Howes, D., & Labbate, M. (2014). The antimicrobial resistance crisis: Causes, consequences, and management. *Frontiers in Public Health, 2*, 145. DOI: 10.3389/fpubh.2014.00145 PMID: 25279369

Mittal, R. P., & Jaitak, V. (2019). Plant-Derived Natural Alkaloids as New Antimicrobial and Adjuvant Agents in Existing Antimicrobial Therapy. *Current Drug Targets, 20*(14), 1409–1433. DOI: 10.2174/1389450120666190618124224 PMID: 31215387

Mittal, R. P., Rana, A., & Jaitak, V. (2019). Essential Oils: An Impending Substitute of Synthetic Antimicrobial Agents to Overcome Antimicrobial Resistance. *Current Drug Targets, 20*(6), 605–624. DOI: 10.2174/13894501196661810311 22917 PMID: 30378496

Mohtar, M., Johari, S. A., Li, A. R., Isa, M. M., Mustafa, S., Ali, A. M., & Basri, D. F. (2009). Inhibitory and resistance-modifying potential of plant-based alkaloids against methicillin-resistant Staphylococcus aureus (MRSA). *Current Microbiology, 59*(2), 181–186. DOI: 10.1007/s00284-009-9416-9 PMID: 19475447

Monciardini, P., Iorio, M., Maffioli, S., Sosio, M., & Donadio, S. (2014). Discovering new bioactive molecules from microbial sources. *Microbial Biotechnology, 7*(3), 209–220. DOI: 10.1111/1751-7915.12123 PMID: 24661414

Movahed, E., Tan, G. M., Munusamy, K., Yeow, T. C., Tay, S. T., Wong, W. F., & Looi, C. Y. (2016). Triclosan Demonstrates Synergic Effect with Amphotericin B and Fluconazole and Induces Apoptosis-Like Cell Death in Cryptococcus neoformans. *Frontiers in Microbiology, 7*, 360. DOI: 10.3389/fmicb.2016.00360 PMID: 27047474

Munyendo, W. L. L., Orwa, J. A., Rukunga, G. M., & Bii, C. C. (2011). Bacteriostatic and bactericidal activities of *Aspilia mossambicensis, Ocimum gratissimum* and *Toddalia asiatica* extracts on selected pathogenic bacteria. *Research Journal of Medicinal Plant, 5*(6), 717–727. DOI: 10.3923/rjmp.2011.717.727

Nair, R., Kalariya, T., & Chanda, S. (2005). Antibacterial activity of some selected Indian medicinal flora. *Turkish Journal of Biology = Türk Biyoloji Dergisi, 29*, 41–47.

Newman, D. J., & Cragg, G. M. (2020). Natural products as sources of new drugs over the nearly four decades from 01/1981 to 09/2019. *Journal of Natural Products, 83*(3), 770–803. DOI: 10.1021/acs.jnatprod.9b01285 PMID: 32162523

Ngo, H. X., Garneau-Tsodikova, S., & Green, K. D. (2016). A complex game of hide and seek: The search for new antifungals. *MedChemComm, 7*(7), 1285–1306. DOI: 10.1039/C6MD00222F PMID: 27766140

Oboh, G. (2010). Antioxidant and antimicrobial properties of ethanolic extract of *Ocimum gratissimum* leaves. *J. Pharmacol. Toxicol., 5*(7), 396–402. DOI: 10.3923/jpt.2010.396.402

Ogidi, O. I. (2022). Phytochemicals of Bioactive compounds of Brassica Juncea (Brown Mustard) Seeds. In: Medicinal and Aromatic Plants of the World. Published by *Encylopedia of Life Support Systems (EOLSS).* http://www.eolss.net/Eloss-sampleAllChapter.aspx

Ogidi, O. I. (2023). Chapter 12: Sustainable Utilization of Important Medicinal Plants in Africa. In: Sustainable Utilization and Conservation of Africa's Biological Resources and Environment, Sustainable Development and Biodiversity. *Springer Nature Singapore Pte Ltd.* https://doi.org/DOI: 10.1007/978-981-19-6974-4_12

Ogidi, O. I. (2024). Recent advances in anticancer activity and Bioinformatics Approach from Potential Plants. In: Computational Approaches in Biomaterials, Bioinformatics and Biomedical Engineering Applications. *CRC Press, Taylor and Francis Group, Florida, USA*. DOI: 10.1201/9781003354437-3

Ogidi, O. I., & Ajoko, I. (2024). Neuroprotective Potentials of Phytochemicals. In: M.S. Rajput, T. Sarachana, P.D. Sarkar, M. Raval (eds) NeuroPhytomedicine. *CRC Press, Routledge Taylor and Francis Group.*

Ogidi, O. I., Alfred-Ugbenbo, D., & Ebitimitula, O. (2025). Drug Discovery and Development with Generative Artificial Intelligence. In Gupta, S., Gupta, U., Sharma, M., & Malik, K. (Eds.), *Generative Intelligence in Healthcare: Transforming Patient Care with AI Creativity* (1st ed.). CRC Press., DOI: 10.1201/9781003539483-1

Ogidi, O. I., Ayebabogha, M. N., Eze, P. U., Omu, O., & Okafor, C. E. (2021d). Determination of Phytoconstituents and Antimicrobial activities of aqueous and methanol extracts of neem (*Azadirachtaindica*) leaves. *International Journal of Pharmacy and Chemistry*, *2*(2), 60–67. DOI: 10.46796/ijpc.vi.155

Ogidi, O. I., Carbom, H. E., & Tawariowei, A. M. (2023). Effects of Methanol and N-hexane Extracts of *Raphia vinifera* Fruit and *Elaeis guineensis* Seeds against *Staphylococcus aureus* and *Escherichia coli.International Journal of Applied Sciences & Development*, *2*, 177–187. DOI: 10.37394/232029.2023.2.19

Ogidi, O. I., Chukwudi, P., Ibe, A. I., Eze, P. U., & Canus, T. N. (2021a). Preliminary phytochemical profile and antimicrobial potentials of white-green African garden egg (*solanum macrocarpon*) fruits obtained from Yenagoa. *ASIO Journal of Pharmaceutical & Herbal Medicines Research (ASIO-JPHMR),* 7(2), 01-05. https://doi-ds.org/doilink/06.2021-76274373/10.2016-19146535/ASIO-JPHMR/2021/457

Ogidi, O. I., & Emaikwu, N. G. (2023). Chapter 1: Adoption and Application of Biotechnology in Herbal Medicine Practices. In: Reference Series in Phytochemistry. Herbal Medicine Phytochemistry. *Springer Nature Singapore Pte Ltd.*

Ogidi, O. I., & Emaikwu, N. G. (2023a). Utilization methods and Practices of herbal Medicine in Africa. In: Reference Series in Phytochemistry. Herbal Medicine Phytochemistry. *Springer Nature Singapore Pte Ltd.* DOI: 10.1007/978-3-031-21973-3_7-1

Ogidi, O. I., & Emaikwu, N. G. (2024). Plant Phenolic compound isolation and its Bioinformatics Approaches of Molecular Mechanisms in Antimicrobial activities and Resistance. In: Computational Approaches in Biomaterials, Bioinformatics and Biomedical Engineering Applications. *CRC Press, Taylor and Francis Group, Florida, USA*. DOI: 10.1201/9781003354437-8

Ogidi, O. I., & Enenebeaku, U. E. (2023b). Chapter 11: Medicinal Potentials of Aloe Vera (*Aloe barbadensis* Miller): Technologies for the Production of Therapeutics. In: Sustainable Utilization and Conservation of Africa's Biological Resources and Environment, Sustainable Development and Biodiversity. *Springer Nature Singapore Pte Ltd.* https://doi.org/DOI: 10.1007/978-981-19-6974-4_11

Ogidi, O. I., Esie, N. G., & Dike, O. G. (2019b). Phytochemical, Proximate and Mineral compositions of *Bryophyllum Pinnatum* (Never die) medicinal plant. *Journal of Pharmacognosy and Phytochemistry*, *8*(1), 629–635.

Ogidi, O. I., George, D. G., & Esie, N. G. (2019a). Ethnopharmacological properties of *Vernonia amygdalina* (Bitter Leave) Medicinal plant. *Journal of Medicinal Plants Studies.*, *7*(2), 175–181.

Ogidi, O. I., & Julius, J. C. (2021). Assessment of Ethno-pharmacological Compounds and Antimicrobial efficacy of white Onion (*Allium cepa*) Bulb Extracts against Pathogenic microbial isolates. *PhytoChem & BioSub Journal.*, *15*(2), 167–174. DOI: 10.163.pcbsj/2021.15.-2-167

Ogidi, O. I., Oguoma, L. M. O., Adigwe, P. C., & Anthony, B. B. (2021c). Phytochemical properties and in-vitro antimicrobial Potency of Wild Edible Mushrooms (*Pleurotusostreatus*) obtained from Yenagoa, Nigeria. *The Journal of Phytopharmacology*, *10*(3), 180–184. DOI: 10.31254/phyto.2021.10306

Ogidi, O. I., Okore, C. C., Akpan, U. M., Ayebabogha, M. N., & Onukwufo, C. J. (2021b). Evaluation of Antimicrobial Activity and Bioactive Phytochemical Properties of Mango (*Mangifera Indica*) Stem-Bark Extracts. *International Journal of Pharmacognosy : a Journal of Crude Drug Research*, *8*(5), 189–195. http://dx.org/10.13040/IJPSR.0975-8232.IJP.8(5).189-95

Ogidi, O. I., Tobia, P. S., Ijere, D. N., Akpan, U. M., Omu, O., Carbom, H. E., & Iyosayi, A. R. (2022). Investigation of Bioactive compounds and antimicrobial sensitivity of pawpaw (*caricapapaya*) leave extracts against morbific microorganisms. *Journal of Applied Pharmaceutical Research*, *10*(1), 21–28. DOI: 10.18231/J.JOAPR.2020.21.28

Ogwu, M. C., Ogidi, O. I., Izah, S. C., & Odubo, T. C. (2025). Therapeutic and Preventive Effects of Natural Compounds Derived from Microbes. In Ramawat, K. G., & Mérillon, J. M. (Eds.), *Natural Products*. Springer., DOI: 10.1007/978-3-642-36202-6_287-1

Oluwatuyi, M., Kaatz, G. W., & Gibbons, S. (2004). Antibacterial and resistance modifying activity of Rosmarinus officinalis. *Phytochemistry*, *65*(24), 3249–3254. DOI: 10.1016/j.phytochem.2004.10.009 PMID: 15561190

Othman, L., Sleiman, A., & Abdel-Massih, R. M. (2019). Antimicrobial Activity of Polyphenols and Alkaloids in Middle Eastern Plants. *Frontiers in Microbiology*, *10*, 911. DOI: 10.3389/fmicb.2019.00911 PMID: 31156565

Owens, R. C.Jr. (2008). Antimicrobial stewardship: Concepts and strategies in the 21st century. *Diagnostic Microbiology and Infectious Disease*, *61*(1), 110–128. DOI: 10.1016/j.diagmicrobio.2008.02.012 PMID: 18384997

Pang, Z., Chong, J., Zhou, G., de Lima Morais, D. A., Chang, L., Barrette, M., Gauthier, C., Jacques, P.-É., Li, S., & Xia, J. (2021). MetaboAnalyst 5.0: Narrowing the gap between raw spectra and functional insights. *Nucleic Acids Research*, *49*(W1), W388–W396. DOI: 10.1093/nar/gkab382 PMID: 34019663

Papageorgiou, V. P., Assimopoulou, A. N., & Ballis, A. C. (2008). Alkannins and shikonins: A new class of wound healing agents. *Current Medicinal Chemistry*, *15*(30), 3248–3267. DOI: 10.2174/092986708786848532 PMID: 19075667

Park, B. S., Lee, H. K., Lee, S. E., Piao, X. L., Takeoka, G. R., Wong, R. Y., Ahn, Y. J., & Kim, J. H. (2006). Antibacterial activity of Tabebuia impetiginosa Martius ex DC (Taheebo) against Helicobacter pylori. *Journal of Ethnopharmacology*, *105*(1-2), 255–262. DOI: 10.1016/j.jep.2005.11.005 PMID: 16359837

Park, H. J., Lee, J. Y., Moon, S. S., & Hwang, B. K. (2003). Isolation and anti-oomycete activity of nyasol from Anemarrhena asphodeloides rhizomes. *Phytochemistry*, *64*(5), 997–1001. DOI: 10.1016/S0031-9422(03)00462-X PMID: 14561517

Patra, A. K. (2012). An Overview of Antimicrobial Properties of Different Classes of Phytochemicals. *Dietary Phytochemicals and Microbes*, 1–32. https://doi.org/ DOI: 10.1007/978-94-007-3926-0_1

Paul, S., Geng, C. A., Yang, T. H., Yang, Y. P., & Chen, J. J. (2019). Phytochemical and Health-Beneficial Progress of Turnip (Brassica rapa). *Journal of Food Science*, *84*(1), 19–30. DOI: 10.1111/1750-3841.14417 PMID: 30561035

Paytubi, S., de La Cruz, M., Tormo, J. R., Martín, J., González, I., González-Menendez, V., Genilloud, O., Reyes, F., Vicente, F., Madrid, C., & Balsalobre, C. (2017). A High-Throughput Screening Platform of Microbial Natural Products for the Discovery of Molecules with Antibiofilm Properties against *Salmonella.Frontiers in Microbiology*, *8*, 326. DOI: 10.3389/fmicb.2017.00326 PMID: 28303128

Pichersky, E., & Gang, D. R. (2000). Genetics and biochemistry of secondary metabolites in plants: An evolutionary perspective. *Trends in Plant Science*, *5*(10), 439–445. DOI: 10.1016/S1360-1385(00)01741-6 PMID: 11044721

Ponnusamy, K., Ramasamy, M., Savarimuthu, I., & Paulraj, M. G. (2010). Indirubin potentiates ciprofloxacin activity in the NorA efflux pump of Staphylococcus aureus. *Scandinavian Journal of Infectious Diseases, 42*(6-7), 500–505. DOI: 10.3109/00365541003713630 PMID: 20380543

Poole, K. (2001). Multidrug efflux pumps and antimicrobial resistance in Pseudomonas aeruginosa and related organisms. *Journal of Molecular Microbiology and Biotechnology, 3*(2), 255–264. PMID: 11321581

Poole, K. (2011). Pseudomonas aeruginosa: Resistance to the max. *Frontiers in Microbiology, 2*, 65. DOI: 10.3389/fmicb.2011.00065 PMID: 21747788

Prestinaci, F., Pezzotti, P., & Pantosti, A. (2015). Antimicrobial resistance: A global multifaceted phenomenon. *Pathogens and Global Health, 109*(7), 309–318. DOI: 10.1179/2047773215Y.0000000030 PMID: 26343252

Puupponen-Pimiä, R., Nohynek, L., Meier, C., Kähkönen, M., Heinonen, M., Hopia, A., & Oksman-Caldentey, K. M. (2001). Antimicrobial properties of phenolic compounds from berries. *Journal of Applied Microbiology, 90*(4), 494–507. DOI: 10.1046/j.1365-2672.2001.01271.x PMID: 11309059

Quideau, S., Deffieux, D., Douat-Casassus, C., & Pouységu, L. (2011). Plant polyphenols: Chemical properties, biological activities, and synthesis. *Angewandte Chemie International Edition, 50*(3), 586–621. DOI: 10.1002/anie.201000044 PMID: 21226137

Ramawat, K. G. (2007). Secondary Plant Products in Nature. In Ramawat, K. G., & Merillon, J. M. (Eds.), *Biotechnology: Secondary Metabolites; Plants and Microbes* (pp. 21–57). Science Publishers.

Ramawat, K. G., Dass, S., & Mathur, M. (2009). The chemical diversity of bioactive molecules and therapeutic potential of medicinal plants. In Ramawat, K. G. (Ed.), *Herbal Drugs: Ethnomedicine to Modern Medicine* (pp. 7–32). Springer. DOI: 10.1007/978-3-540-79116-4_2

Rao, K. N., & Venkatachalam, S. R. (2000). Inhibition of dihydrofolate reductase and cell growth activity by the phenanthroindolizidine alkaloids pergularinine and tylophorinidine: the in vitro cytotoxicity of these plant alkaloids and their potential as antimicrobial and anticancer agents. *Toxicology in vitro: an international journal published in association with BIBRA, 14*(1), 53–59. https://doi.org/DOI: 10.1016/S0887-2333(99)00092-2

Rattanachaikunsopon, P., & Phumkhachorn, P. (2010). Contents and antibacterial activity of flavonoids extracted from leaves of Psidium guajava. *Journal of Medicinal Plants Research*, *4*, 393–396.

Rigano, D., Formisano, C., Basile, A., Lavitola, A., Senatore, F., Rosselli, S., & Bruno, M. (2007). Antibacterial activity of flavonoids and phenylpropanoids from Marrubium globosum ssp. libanoticum. *Phytotherapy Research*, *21*(4), 395–397. DOI: 10.1002/ptr.2061 PMID: 17186490

Rizwana, H., Alwhibi, M. S., & Soliman, D. A. (2016). Antimicrobial activity and chemical composition of flowers of matricaria aurea a native herb of Saudi Arabia. *International Journal of Pharmacology*, *12*(6), 576–586. DOI: 10.3923/ijp.2016.576.586

Romeo, L., Iori, R., Rollin, P., Bramanti, P., & Mazzon, E. (2018). Isothiocyanates: An Overview of Their Antimicrobial Activity against Human Infections. *Molecules (Basel, Switzerland)*, *23*(3), 624. DOI: 10.3390/molecules23030624 PMID: 29522501

Rossolini, G. M., Arena, F., Pecile, P., & Pollini, S. (2014). Update on the antibiotic resistance crisis. *Current Opinion in Pharmacology*, *18*, 56–60. DOI: 10.1016/j.coph.2014.09.006 PMID: 25254623

Rouf, R., Uddin, S. J., Sarker, D. K., Islam, M. T., Ali, E. S., Shilpi, J. A., Nahar, L., Tiralongo, E., & Sarker, S. D. (2020). Antiviral potential of garlic (*Allium sativum*) and its organosulfur compounds: A systematic update of pre-clinical and clinical data. *Trends in Food Science & Technology*, *104*, 219–234. DOI: 10.1016/j.tifs.2020.08.006 PMID: 32836826

Salih, K. (2016). Synergistic effects of plant extracts and antifungal drugs on C. albicans. *Journal of Developing Drugs*, *5*(3), 1–15. DOI: 10.4172/2329-6631.1000165

Sarbu, L. G., Bahrin, L. G., Babii, C., Stefan, M., & Birsa, M. L. (2019). Synthetic flavonoids with antimicrobial activity: A review. *Journal of Applied Microbiology*, *127*(5), 1282–1290. DOI: 10.1111/jam.14271 PMID: 30934143

Sardi, J. C., Gullo, F. P., Freires, I. A., Pitangui, N. S., Segalla, M. P., Fusco-Almeida, A. M., Rosalen, P. L., Regasini, L. O., & Mendes-Giannini, M. J. (2016). Synthesis, antifungal activity of caffeic acid derivative esters, and their synergism with fluconazole and nystatin against Candida spp. *Diagnostic Microbiology and Infectious Disease*, *86*(4), 387–391. DOI: 10.1016/j.diagmicrobio.2016.08.002 PMID: 27638348

Savoia, D. (2012). Plant-derived antimicrobial compounds: Alternatives to antibiotics. *Future Microbiology*, *7*(8), 979–990. DOI: 10.2217/fmb.12.68 PMID: 22913356

Schmitz, F. J., Fluit, A. C., Lückefahr, M., Engler, B., Hofmann, B., Verhoef, J., Heinz, H. P., Hadding, U., & Jones, M. E. (1998). The effect of reserpine, an inhibitor of multidrug efflux pumps, on the in-vitro activities of ciprofloxacin, sparfloxacin and moxifloxacin against clinical isolates of Staphylococcus aureus. *The Journal of Antimicrobial Chemotherapy*, *42*(6), 807–810. DOI: 10.1093/jac/42.6.807 PMID: 10052906

Sharma, M., Manoharlal, R., Negi, A. S., & Prasad, R. (2010). Synergistic anticandidal activity of pure polyphenol curcumin I in combination with azoles and polyenes generates reactive oxygen species leading to apoptosis. *FEMS Yeast Research*, *10*(5), 570–578. DOI: 10.1111/j.1567-1364.2010.00637.x PMID: 20528949

Shen, Y., Chen, B. L., Zhang, Q. X., Zheng, Y. Z., & Fu, Q. (2019). Traditional uses, secondary metabolites, and pharmacology of Celastrus species - a review. *Journal of Ethnopharmacology*, *241*, 111934. DOI: 10.1016/j.jep.2019.111934 PMID: 31129308

Shimizu, M., Shiota, S., Mizushima, T., Ito, H., Hatano, T., Yoshida, T., & Tsuchiya, T. (2001). Marked potentiation of activity of beta-lactams against methicillin-resistant Staphylococcus aureus by corilagin. *Antimicrobial Agents and Chemotherapy*, *45*(11), 3198–3201. DOI: 10.1128/AAC.45.11.3198-3201.2001 PMID: 11600378

Shin, J., Prabhakaran, V. S., & Kim, K. S. (2018). The multi-faceted potential of plant-derived metabolites as antimicrobial agents against multidrug-resistant pathogens. *Microbial Pathogenesis*, *116*, 209–214. DOI: 10.1016/j.micpath.2018.01.043 PMID: 29407230

Shin, S., & Lim, S. (2004). Antifungal effects of herbal essential oils alone and in combination with ketoconazole against Trichophyton spp. *Journal of Applied Microbiology*, *97*(6), 1289–1296. DOI: 10.1111/j.1365-2672.2004.02417.x PMID: 15546420

Sibi, G., Chatly, P., Adhikari, S., & Ravikumar, K. R. (2012). Phytoconstituents and their influence on antimicrobial properties of *Marinda citrifolia* L. *Research Journal of Medicinal Plant*, *6*(6), 441–448. DOI: 10.3923/rjmp.2012.441.448

Singh, B., Singh, J. P., Kaur, A., & Singh, N. (2018). Phenolic compounds as beneficial phytochemicals in pomegranate (Punica granatum L.) peel: A review. *Food Chemistry*, *261*, 75–86. DOI: 10.1016/j.foodchem.2018.04.039 PMID: 29739608

Siriyong, T., Srimanote, P., Chusri, S., Yingyongnarongkul, B. E., Suaisom, C., Tipmanee, V., & Voravuthikunchai, S. P. (2017). Conessine as a novel inhibitor of multidrug efflux pump systems in Pseudomonas aeruginosa. *BMC Complementary and Alternative Medicine, 17*(1), 405. DOI: 10.1186/s12906-017-1913-y PMID: 28806947

Smanski, M. J., Zhou, H., Claesen, J., Shen, B., Fischbach, M. A., & Voigt, C. A. (2016). Synthetic biology to access and expand nature's chemical diversity. *Nature Reviews. Microbiology, 14*(3), 135–149. DOI: 10.1038/nrmicro.2015.24 PMID: 26876034

Song, R., Yu, B., Friedrich, D., Li, J., Shen, H., Krautscheid, H., Huang, S. D., & Kim, M. H. (2020). Naphthoquinone-derivative as a synthetic compound to overcome the antibiotic resistance of methicillin-resistant S. aureus. *Communications Biology, 3*(1), 529. DOI: 10.1038/s42003-020-01261-0 PMID: 32973345

Spellberg, B., Guidos, R., Gilbert, D., Bradley, J., Boucher, H. W., Scheld, W. M., Bartlett, J. G., & Edwards, J.Jr. (2008). The epidemic of antibiotic-resistant infections: A call to action for the medical community from the Infectious Diseases Society of America. *Clinical Infectious Diseases, 46*(2), 155–164. DOI: 10.1086/524891 PMID: 18171244

Stermitz, F. R., Lorenz, P., Tawara, J. N., Zenewicz, L. A., & Lewis, K. (2000). Synergy in a medicinal plant: Antimicrobial action of berberine potentiated by 5′-methoxyhydnocarpin, a multidrug pump inhibitor. *Proceedings of the National Academy of Sciences of the United States of America, 97*(4), 1433–1437. DOI: 10.1073/pnas.030540597 PMID: 10677479

Stermitz, F. R., Lorenz, P., Tawara, J. N., Zenewicz, L. A., & Lewis, K. (2000). Synergy in a medicinal plant: Antimicrobial action of berberine potentiated by 5′-methoxyhydnocarpin, a multidrug pump inhibitor. *Proceedings of the National Academy of Sciences of the United States of America, 97*(4), 1433–1437. DOI: 10.1073/pnas.030540597 PMID: 10677479

Susić E. (2004). Mehanizmi rezistencije enterobakterija prema beta-laktamskim antibioticima [Mechanisms of resistance in Enterobacteriaceae towards beta-lactamase antibiotics]. *Acta medica Croatica: casopis Hravatske akademije medicinskih znanosti, 58*(4), 307–312.

Tegos, G., Stermitz, F. R., Lomovskaya, O., & Lewis, K. (2002). Multidrug pump inhibitors uncover remarkable activity of plant antimicrobials. *Antimicrobial Agents and Chemotherapy, 46*(10), 3133–3141. DOI: 10.1128/AAC.46.10.3133-3141.2002 PMID: 12234835

Thangavelu, A., Elavarasu, S., Sundaram, R., Kumar, T., Rajendran, D., & Prem, F. (2017). Ancient Seed for Modern Cure - Pomegranate Review of Therapeutic Applications in Periodontics. *Journal of Pharmacy & Bioallied Sciences*, *9*(5, Suppl 1), S11–S14. DOI: 10.4103/jpbs.JPBS_101_17 PMID: 29284927

VanEtten, H. D., Mansfield, J. W., Bailey, J. A., & Farmer, E. E. (1994). Two Classes of Plant Antibiotics: Phytoalexins versus "Phytoanticipins". *The Plant Cell*, *6*(9), 1191–1192. DOI: 10.2307/3869817 PMID: 12244269

Varona, J. F., Landete, P., López-Martínez, A., Álvarez-Sala, R., Lora-Tamayo, J., & Arenas-Jiménez, J.Plitidepsin Clinical Study Group. (2021). Plitidepsin has potent preclinical efficacy against SARS-CoV-2 through inhibition of the host protein eEF1A. *Science*, *372*(6549), 89–93. DOI: 10.1126/science.abf4058

Veale, C. G., Zoraghi, R., Young, R. M., Morrison, J. P., Pretheeban, M., Lobb, K. A., Reiner, N. E., Andersen, R. J., & Davies-Coleman, M. T. (2015). Synthetic analogues of the marine bisindole deoxytopsentin: Potent selective inhibitors of MRSA pyruvate kinase. *Journal of Natural Products*, *78*(3), 355–362. DOI: 10.1021/np500755v PMID: 25372480

Wellington, K. W., Nyoka, N. B. P., & McGaw, L. J. (2019). Investigation of the antibacterial and antifungal activity of thiolated naphthoquinones. *Drug Development Research*, *80*(3), 386–394. DOI: 10.1002/ddr.21512 PMID: 30609114

Whiting, D. A. (2001). Natural phenolic compounds 1900-2000: A bird's eye view of a century's chemistry. *Natural Product Reports*, *18*(6), 583–606. DOI: 10.1039/b003686m PMID: 11820759

Widayati, A., Suryawati, S., de Crespigny, C., & Hiller, J. E. (2012). Knowledge and beliefs about antibiotics among people in Yogyakarta City Indonesia: A cross sectional population-based survey. *Antimicrobial Resistance and Infection Control*, *1*(1), 38. DOI: 10.1186/2047-2994-1-38 PMID: 23176763

Xu, Y., Wang, Y., Yan, L., Liang, R. M., Dai, B. D., Tang, R. J., Gao, P. H., & Jiang, Y. Y. (2009). Proteomic analysis reveals a synergistic mechanism of fluconazole and berberine against fluconazole-resistant Candida albicans: Endogenous ROS augmentation. *Journal of Proteome Research*, *8*(11), 5296–5304. DOI: 10.1021/pr9005074 PMID: 19754040

Yam, T. S., Hamilton-Miller, J. M., & Shah, S. (1998). The effect of a component of tea (Camellia sinensis) on methicillin resistance, PBP2′ synthesis, and beta-lactamase production in Staphylococcus aureus. *The Journal of Antimicrobial Chemotherapy*, *42*(2), 211–216. DOI: 10.1093/jac/42.2.211 PMID: 9738838

Yamaguchi, Y., & Kumagai, H. (2020). Characteristics, biosynthesis, decomposition, metabolism and functions of the garlic odour precursor, *S*-allyl-L-cysteine sulfoxide. *Experimental and Therapeutic Medicine, 19*(2), 1528–1535. DOI: 10.3892/etm.2019.8385 PMID: 32010334

Yasmeen, M., Barwant, M. M., Balwant Singh, B., & Ogidi, O. I. (2025). Present Challenges and Future Perspective of the Herbal Drug Industry. In: Farid, A. (Ed.). (2025). Herbal Pharmacopeia: Nanotechnology and Advancing Drug Discovery (1st ed.). CRC Press. https://doi.org/DOI: 10.1201/9781003544418-22

Yu, H. F., Qin, X. J., Ding, C. F., Wei, X., Yang, J., Luo, J. R., Liu, L., Khan, A., Zhang, L. C., Xia, C. F., & Luo, X. D. (2018). Nepenthe-Like Indole Alkaloids with Antimicrobial Activity from Ervatamia chinensis. *Organic Letters, 20*(13), 4116–4120. DOI: 10.1021/acs.orglett.8b01675 PMID: 29927253

Zainal, M., Mohamad Zain, N., Mohd Amin, I., & Ahmad, V. N. (2021). The antimicrobial and antibiofilm properties of allicin against *Candida albicans* and *Staphylococcus aureus* - A therapeutic potential for denture stomatitis. *The Saudi Dental Journal, 33*(2), 105–111. DOI: 10.1016/j.sdentj.2020.01.008 PMID: 33551624

Ziemert, N., Alanjary, M., & Weber, T. (2016). The evolution of genome mining in microbes – a review. *Natural Product Reports, 33*(8), 988–1005. DOI: 10.1039/C6NP00025H PMID: 27272205

Chapter 10
Nature's Cure: Harnessing the Therapeutic Power of Secondary Metabolites in Medicine

Simran Jatwani
Department of Biotechnology, Bennett University, India

Deepa Khare
https://orcid.org/0000-0002-6931-7183
Department of Biotechnology, Bennett University, India

ABSTRACT

Secondary metabolites are organic compounds produced by microorganisms, higher plants, and fungi, with significant ecological and human health relevance. This chapter explores their biological activities, types, and biosynthesis, emphasizing their applications in disease prevention and control. It highlights the pharmacological properties of key compounds, including phenolics, alkaloids, flavonoids, terpenoids, glycosides, and polyketides, in treating and preventing cancer, diabetes, heart diseases, infections, mental disorders, and immune system dysfunctions. Their roles in combating aging, inflammation, oxidative stress, neurodegeneration, malaria, and modulating immunity are also discussed.

DOI: 10.4018/979-8-3693-9112-9.ch010

1. INTRODUCTION: THE HIDDEN POWER OF SECONDARY METABOLITES

The story of secondary metabolites began in 1891 when A. Kossel introduced the term, recognizing their significance beyond the primary processes of life. Nearly two decades later, in 1910, his groundbreaking work earned him the Nobel Prize in Medicine or Physiology. Secondary metabolites, though not essential for the immediate survival of an organism, are indispensable for long-term success. Their absence may not curtail life but can severely impair an organism's ability to thrive, (Thirumurugan *et al.,* 2018a).

Derived from primary metabolic pathways, secondary metabolites are found across diverse life forms—plants, bacteria, fungi, and marine organisms like sponges, tunicates, and corals. Unlike primary metabolites, which are fundamental to cellular functions and energy production, secondary metabolites excel in specialized roles. They bolster defense against biotic and abiotic stresses, paint the vibrant hues of fruits and flowers, and aid in pollination, (Andryukov, Mikhailov, & Besednova, 2019).

Scientists have cataloged approximately 2.14 million secondary metabolites, classified based on their structure, function, and synthesis. Intriguingly, about 80% of these compounds are derived from plants, with the rest originating from microbes and marine life. Secondary metabolites in plants and microorganisms are classified into six major groups, showcasing their diversity and complexity. These include alkaloids (e.g., morphine and nicotine), terpenoids (e.g., menthol and carotenoids), phenolics (e.g., flavonoids and lignin), polyketides (e.g., erythromycin), glycosides (e.g., digitoxin), and non-protein amino acids (e.g., canavanine). Each class plays unique roles in ecological interactions, defense mechanisms, and has significant applications in medicine and industry **(Figure 1)**. This remarkable diversity has allowed secondary metabolites to find extensive use in pharmaceuticals, agriculture, and beyond, (Demain, 1999).

The versatility of secondary metabolites makes them invaluable to humankind. In medicine, they serve as antimicrobial agents, enzyme inhibitors, immunomodulators, and anti-tumor compounds. In agriculture, their properties such as insecticides, pesticides, and pheromones enhance crop productivity while maintaining ecological balance, (Microbial Secondary Metabolites, 2021). These compounds also play vital ecological roles, fostering symbiotic relationships between plants and other organisms and aiding in sporulation and germination, (Griesbach, 2010).

Plants dominate the production of secondary metabolites, contributing approximately 80% of the known compounds. This dominance stems from their evolutionary need to interact dynamically with their environment. The remaining metabolites come from other natural sources such as bacteria, fungi, and marine organisms, underscoring the collaborative ingenuity of nature, (Thirumurugan *et al.,* 2018a).

Secondary metabolites represent a fascinating intersection of biology and chemistry, with their applications ranging from healing humans to protecting crops. As we continue to uncover their secrets, these compounds remind us of nature's ingenuity and its enduring capacity to inspire innovation (**Table 1**).

Table 1. Diverse sources of secondary metabolites, bioactive compounds and antibiotics

Sources	**All known compounds**	**Bio actives**	**Antibiotics**
Natural Products	over one million	200000 to 250000	30000
Plant Kingdom	600000 to 700000	150000 to 200000	~25000
Microbes	Over 50000	22000 to 23000	~17000
Algae, Lichens	3000 to 5000	1500 to 2000	~1000
Higher Plants	500000 to 600000	~100000	10000 to 12000
Animal Kingdom	300000 to 400000	50000 to 100000	~5000
Protozoa	several hundreds	100 to 200	~50
Invertebrates:	~100000	NA	~500
Marine animals	20000 to 25000	7000 to 8000	3000 to 4000
Insects/worms/etc.	8000 to 10000	800 to 1000	150 to 200
Vertebrates (mammals, fishes, amphibians, etc.)	200000 to 250000	50000 to 70000	~1000

Figure 1. Classification of plant secondary metabolites. Plant secondary metabolites are categorized into six major classes: Alkaloids (e.g., morphine, nicotine), Terpenoids (e.g., menthol, carotenoids), Phenolics (e.g., flavonoids, lignin), Polyketides (e.g., resveratrol, curcumin), Glycosides (e.g., digitoxin, saponins), and Non-protein Amino Acids (e.g., canavanine).

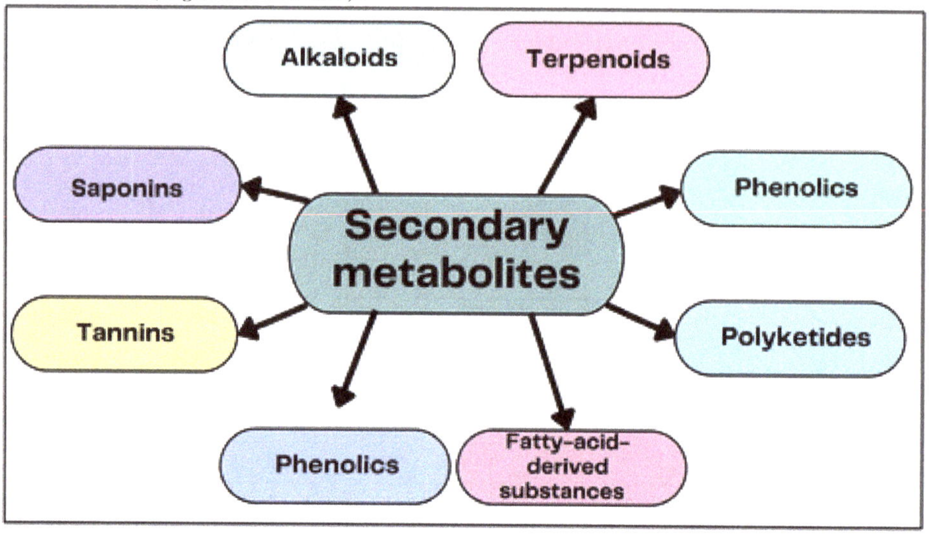

These compounds contribute to plant defense, pigmentation, and ecological interactions, as well as serving as therapeutic agents for various diseases

The Fascinating World of Plant Secondary Metabolites

Secondary metabolites, unique to the plant kingdom, are nature's hidden arsenal, designed not only for survival but also to enrich our lives. These specialized compounds play pivotal roles in plant development, structure, and environmental interactions. From defending against pests to adding vibrant colors to fruits and vegetables, secondary metabolites are integral to a plant's success in adapting to its surroundings, (Erb & Kliebenstein, 2020).

For centuries, humans have tapped into the power of these compounds, weaving them into traditional medicine systems like Ayurveda in India, Traditional Chinese Medicine (TCM), and the ancient practices of Egypt and Greece. Remarkable herbs such as garlic (*Allium sativum*), ginseng (*Panax ginseng*), and turmeric (*Curcuma longa*) have been used to treat ailments ranging from digestive issues to immune deficiencies. These remedies often worked without the knowledge of their intricate chemical compositions, relying instead on observations passed down through generations, (Crozier, Clifford, & Ashihara, 2007).

The mid-20th century marked a dramatic shift in medical practice with the advent of synthetic drugs. After World War II, the pharmaceutical industry embraced synthetic medications for their consistency, mass production capabilities, and standardization. Beyond efficacy, economics played a critical role—synthetic compounds could be patented, granting manufacturers exclusive rights to their sale. In contrast, herbal medicines, with their natural origins and historical usage, lacked such patentability, making attractive, (Twaji & Hasan, 2022).

This shift marginalized the use of plant-based remedies, despite their rich therapeutic properties. Traditional herbal medicines, often complex mixtures of secondary metabolites, offer a broader spectrum of effects, such as anti-inflammatory, analgesic, and anti-tumor benefits. In contrast, synthetic drugs, typically based on single active ingredients, dominate due to their easier regulation and profitability, (Twaji & Hasan, 2022) (Hussein *et al.,* 2018).

Despite their historical sidelining, the intricate molecular interactions of herbal medicines with biological targets, such as enzymes and receptors, hint at untapped potential. Modern healthcare is beginning to re-evaluate the role of these natural compounds, recognizing the need for a more integrative approach that blends the strengths of both synthetic and herbal paradigms. This renewed interest could lead to better patient outcomes and a richer understanding of holistic health, (Crozier, Clifford, & Ashihara, 2007).

Plants are master chemists, producing an astonishing variety of secondary metabolites. These include alkaloids, steroids, tannins, glycosides, terpenoids, phenolics, and essential oils. Unlike primary metabolites, which support basic growth and nutrition, secondary metabolites serve as guardians and communicators, aiding in defense, pollination, and even seed germination. Phenolic compounds, for instance, are known for their aromatic properties and potential health benefits, ranging from antioxidant effects to cardiovascular protection, (Thirumurugan *et al.,* 2018b).

The diversity of secondary metabolites is a testament to plants' evolutionary ingenuity. By deriving these compounds from primary metabolites, plants enhance their resilience and adaptability, offering not only survival advantages but also therapeutic benefits for humans, (Erb & Kliebenstein, 2020).

As we continue to explore these natural compounds, the potential for new discoveries grows. With greater scientific understanding and a shift towards integrative healthcare, the forgotten treasures of herbal medicine may once again take their rightful place alongside modern synthetic innovations.

2. SECONDARY METABOLITES AND THEIR THERAPEUTIC APPLICATIONS

2.1. Phenolic Compounds: Guardians of Human Health and Plant Defense

Phenolic compounds form one of the largest and most significant groups of secondary metabolites, distinguished by their hydroxyl (-OH) groups attached to aromatic rings. These versatile compounds are biosynthesized mainly through the shikimate pathway in plants, playing crucial roles in their physiology and defense mechanisms. Structurally, phenolic compounds range from simple molecules like phenol to complex polymers such as lignin, (Mamari, 2021).

In plants, phenolics are integral to the formation of structural components like lignin, suberin, and cutin, which strengthen cell walls and provide resilience. Additionally, these compounds serve as biochemical shields, protecting plants against microbial attacks and environmental stressors. Beyond their importance in plant health, phenolics are renowned for their therapeutic potential, particularly in human health, (Lin *et al.,* 2016).

Phenolic compounds are broadly classified into three major categories: flavonoids, polyphenols, and simple phenolics, each contributing distinctively to their bioactivity. Among these, flavonoids have emerged as the most extensively studied group, owing to their structural diversity and wide-ranging pharmacological properties.

Flavonoids: The Therapeutic Powerhouses

Flavonoids, with their polyphenolic structure, are abundant in fruits, vegetables, herbs, nuts, and seeds, contributing to their vibrant colors and health benefits. Chemically, flavonoids consist of a benzopyrone backbone with phenolic and non-phenolic substitutions that influence their biological activity.

Biological and Pharmacological Activities

Flavonoids have garnered significant attention for their diverse therapeutic properties, which include:

1. **Antioxidant Potential:** Flavonoids such as quercetin and catechins combat oxidative stress by scavenging reactive oxygen species (ROS) and stabilizing free radicals. This antioxidant activity underlies their protective role in conditions like cardiovascular diseases and neurodegeneration, (Takahashi & Ohnishi, 2004).

2. **Anti-inflammatory Effects:** These compounds inhibit key inflammatory mediators, reducing risks associated with chronic conditions such as arthritis and inflammatory bowel disease, (Tungmunnithum *et al.*, 2018) (Berk *et al.*, 2022).
3. **Anticancer Activity:** Flavonoids like apigenin and kaempferol demonstrate anticancer properties by modulating cell signaling pathways, inducing apoptosis, and inhibiting tumor angiogenesis, (Kopustinskiene *et al.*, 2020).
4. **Cardioprotective Effects:** Flavonoids contribute to vascular health by improving endothelial function, reducing oxidative stress, and modulating lipid metabolism. Compounds like anthocyanins and flavanols have shown promise in preventing atherosclerosis and hypertension, (Kris-Etherton *et al.*, 2002).

FDA-Approved Applications and Beyond

Several flavonoid-based compounds have transitioned from research to practical applications. Notable examples include:

a. **Silymarin:** A flavonolignan derived from milk thistle, approved for managing liver disorders.
b. **Rutin:** A flavonoid is used in treatments for chronic venous insufficiency and capillary fragility.
c. **Hesperidin:** Found in citrus fruits, this flavonoid is used in dietary supplements for improving vascular health.

Diverse Subcategories of Flavonoids

They are classified into various subcategories:

1. **Flavonols:** Commonly found in onions, kale, and tomatoes, flavonols like quercetin and kaempferol offer antioxidant and anti-inflammatory benefits, (Hernaez, Xu, & Dashwood, 1998) (Kager *et al.*, 2010) (Forester & Lambert, 2011) (Choudhary *et al.*, 2012).
2. **Flavanones:** Predominantly present in citrus fruits, flavanones such as naringenin and hesperetin exhibit radical-scavenging properties and contribute to metabolic health. E.g. (Balakrishnan & Menon, 2007) (Ahmadi *et al.*, 2008) (Ganapathy *et al.*, 2008) (Kamaraj *et al.*, 2009) (Yeh *et al.*, 2009) (Bodduluru *et al.*, 2016).
3. **Anthocyanins:** Responsible for the vivid colors of berries and red grapes, these compounds act as potent antioxidants and anti-inflammatory agents. E.g. Delphinidin, (Kang *et al.*, 2020) (Iqbal *et al.*, 2024).

4. **Isoflavonoids:** Found in soy products, isoflavonoids like genistein and diadzens exhibit phytoestrogenic properties and play a role in hormone-dependent conditions, (Khan *et al.,* 2009) (Coward *et al.*, 2009) (Stagos *et al.,* 2012) (Spagnuolo *et al.*, 2015) (Tuli *et al.,* 2019) **(Figure 2).**
5. **Chalcones:** Open-chain flavonoids like phloridzin and chalconaringenin are known for their anti-inflammatory and antimicrobial effects.

Figure 2. Flavonoids are subclassified into flavones, flavonols, flavanones, isoflavonoids, anthocyanins, and chalcones.

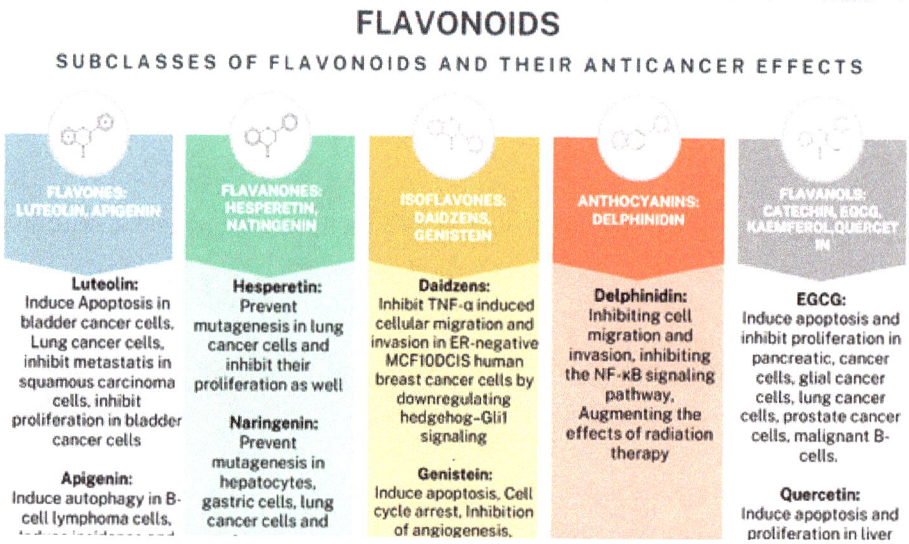

Each subclass encompasses distinct compounds with diverse biological activities, particularly in anticancer therapy. These compounds exert therapeutic effects through mechanisms such as antioxidant activity, inhibition of tumor growth, modulation of cell signaling pathways, induction of apoptosis, and reduction of oxidative stress. The classification highlights their significant role in cancer prevention and treatment, showcasing their potential as natural agents in therapeutic applications

Polyphenols: The Versatile Protectors

Polyphenols are a diverse group of compounds characterized by multiple hydroxyl groups on aromatic rings. Resveratrol, a well-known polyphenol found in red wine, exemplifies their therapeutic potential, showing benefits in cardiovascular health, aging, and cancer prevention.

Phenolic compounds, especially flavonoids, represent a cornerstone of plant-based bioactivity with significant implications for human health. Their diverse pharmacological properties and widespread occurrence in nature make them a vital focus of therapeutic research and application.

Among various polyphenol-rich sources, mulberries, especially the wild varieties found in India, stand out due to their high anthocyanin content and potent antioxidant properties. Research has shown that mulberries exhibit anticancer effects by inhibiting tumor growth and metastasis, with promising potential in fighting lung and breast cancers, (Ahmed *et al.,* 2022).

Phenolic Acids: A Multifaceted Group with Therapeutic Potential

Phenolic acids are a remarkable and diverse group of plant-based compounds, primarily categorized into two major groups: hydroxycinnamic acids and hydroxybenzoic acids. These natural compounds are found in a wide array of fruits, vegetables, grains, and herbs, offering more than just flavor and color. They are packed with health benefits, making them an exciting area of research in both nutrition and medicine. Known for their antimicrobial, antioxidant, and anti-inflammatory properties, phenolic acids also show great promise in the treatment and prevention of a variety of chronic conditions, including cancer, cardiovascular diseases, and type 2 diabetes, (Okunade *et al.,* 1997) (Nichenametla *et al.,* 2006) (Prats *et al.,* 2007) (Kumar *et al.,* 2021).

Among the most studied phenolic acids are caffeic acid, ferulic acid, and cinnamic acid, each of which plays a significant role in both plant biology and human health. These compounds are potent bioactive molecules with the ability to act as fungicides, bactericides, and neuroprotectants, and they hold substantial potential in the prevention and treatment of a range of diseases

Caffeic Acid: A Cancer Fighter

Caffeic acid, a polyphenolic compound widely present in foods like coffee, apples, pears, and herbs such as basil and thyme, is emerging as a potent natural agent in cancer prevention and therapy. With its robust antioxidant properties, caffeic acid combats the damaging effects of reactive oxygen species (ROS) in cancer cells, reducing oxidative stress and mitigating DNA damage that contributes to tumor progression, (Oršolić *et al.,* 2016) (Jin *et al.*, 2021).

One of its remarkable anticancer mechanisms is its ability to reduce angiogenesis, the process by which tumors develop their blood supply to sustain growth. In hepatocellular carcinoma (HCC) cells, caffeic acid inhibits the phosphorylation of JNK-1, suppressing the activity of hypoxia-inducible factor 1-alpha (HIF-1α) (**Figure 3**). This inhibition leads to a reduction in vascular endothelial growth factor (VEGF) expression, effectively cutting off the nutrient and oxygen supply tumors needed for survival and metastasis, (Monteiro *et al.,* 2019) (Okla *et al.,* 2021).

Additionally, caffeic acid promotes apoptosis, or programmed cell death, in cancer cells. It activates pro-apoptotic pathways while suppressing anti-apoptotic factors, ensuring the selective elimination of malignant cells, (Jawhari *et al.,* 2021) (Didehdar *et al.,* 2022). This mechanism disrupts tumor growth and offers a natural approach to targeted cancer therapy.

Another critical role of caffeic acid lies in its ability to regulate the glycolytic phenotype of tumor cells. Cancer cells typically shift to aerobic glycolysis (Warburg effect) to support their high metabolic demands. Caffeic acid interferes with this metabolic adaptation, thereby starving tumor cells of the energy required for proliferation, (El-Seedi *et al.,* 2017) (Mingoia *et al.,* 2022).

Caffeic acid also acts as a protector against carcinogenic nitrogen compounds by neutralizing nitrosamines, which are known to induce DNA mutations leading to cancer. This chemopreventive property makes caffeic acid a valuable agent for reducing cancer risk at the dietary level, (Jawhari *et al.*, 2021).

With its multifaceted mechanisms, including reducing angiogenesis, inducing apoptosis, regulating tumor metabolism, and preventing carcinogen formation, caffeic acid represents a promising natural compound in the fight against cancer. Its inclusion in the diet or therapeutic interventions may pave the way for safer and more effective strategies to combat malignancies, (Oršolić *et al.,* 2016) (Didehdar *et al.,* 2022) (Mingoia *et al.,* 2022).

Figure 3. The role of caffeic acid in modulating angiogenesis in hepatocellular carcinoma (HCC) cells.

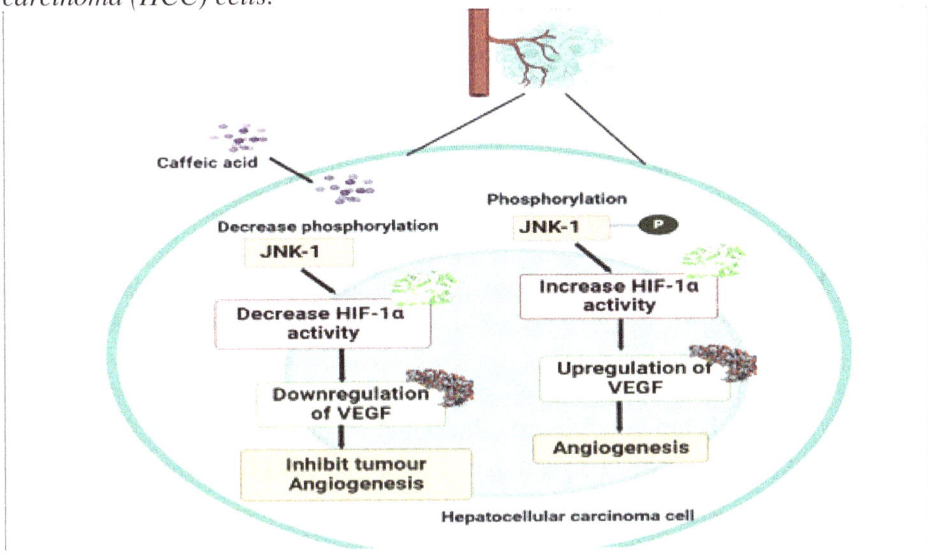

In the absence of caffeic acid, tumor cells stimulate angiogenesis through the phosphorylation of JNK-1, which activates hypoxia-inducible factor 1-alpha (HIF-1α). This, in turn, leads to the upregulation of vascular endothelial growth factor (VEGF), a key mediator in the formation of new blood vessels to support tumor growth. In the presence of caffeic acid, the phosphorylation of JNK-1 is reduced, leading to decreased activation of HIF-1α and subsequent downregulation of VEGF. As a result, angiogenesis is inhibited, limiting the tumor's blood supply and potentially slowing its growth

Ferulic Acid: A Multitasking Natural Protector

Ferulic acid, a potent phenolic compound found in whole grains, fruits, and vegetables, offers a spectrum of health benefits thanks to its remarkable antioxidant, anti-inflammatory, and protective properties. By neutralizing free radicals, it shields cells from oxidative damage, which is a significant driver of aging and chronic diseases, including cardiovascular and neurodegenerative disorders. Its cardioprotective effects further solidify its role as a key component of a heart-healthy diet.

One of ferulic acid's standout therapeutic roles lies in glucose metabolism. In individuals with type 2 diabetes, ferulic acid enhances insulin sensitivity by promoting GLUT4 translocation to the cell membrane via a PI3K-dependent pathway, boosting glucose uptake in muscle and fat cells, (Prabhakar & Doble, 2011). Additionally, it helps manage postprandial hyperglycemia by inhibiting GLUT2, a key intestinal glucose transporter. By limiting glucose absorption in the gut, ferulic acid prevents sudden blood sugar spikes after meals, (Malunga, Eck, & Beta, 2016). This dual regulatory action on glucose makes ferulic acid a promising candidate for both acute and long-term blood sugar control.

The benefits of ferulic acid extend beyond glucose management. Its anti-inflammatory effects make it valuable in reducing the risk of chronic diseases, including diabetes, cancer, and cardiovascular disorders. Ferulic acid's ability to modulate inflammation complements its antioxidant capacity in protecting against cellular and organ damage. Furthermore, its neuroprotective and hepatoprotective properties highlight their potential in preventing neurological decline and supporting liver health.

From managing blood sugar to reducing oxidative stress and supporting heart, brain, and liver health, ferulic acid is a multitasking natural compound with promising therapeutic applications. Its diverse range of benefits makes it an essential focus of ongoing research into natural remedies for chronic diseases.

Cinnamic Acid: A Versatile Therapeutic Agent

Cinnamic acid, a phenolic compound naturally found in various plants, exhibits a wide range of therapeutic properties, including antimicrobial, antifungal, antioxidant, and anti-inflammatory effects. These characteristics make cinnamic acid a valuable compound for combating oxidative stress, preventing infections, and managing chronic diseases. Its antioxidant capacity plays a crucial role in reducing oxidative damage, which is implicated in aging and numerous health conditions, including cardiovascular diseases and renal dysfunction, (Jawhari *et al.,* 2021) (Didehdar *et al.,* 2022) (El-Seedi *et al.*, 2017).

One of cinnamic acid's most notable benefits lies in its potential for managing type 2 diabetes. It enhances glucose uptake in muscle and fat cells by promoting GLUT4 translocation via the PPARγ pathway, thereby improving blood sugar regulation and insulin sensitivity, (Prabhakar & Doble, 2011). This mechanism is particularly beneficial in addressing insulin resistance, a key factor in type 2 diabetes.

Beyond its effects on glucose metabolism, cinnamic acid demonstrates protective actions against renal and cardiovascular dysfunction, owing to its potent antioxidant and anti-inflammatory properties. Its hepatoprotective benefits also suggest a role in supporting liver health, while its neuroprotective effects make it a candidate for managing conditions like Alzheimer's disease, (Okla *et al.,* 2021) (Jawhari *et al.,* 2021) (Didehdar *et al.,* 2022) (El-Seedi *et al.*, 2017) (Mingoia *et al.,* 2022) (Li *et al.,* 2021).

Cinnamic acid's versatility extends to its anticancer potential, with studies suggesting its ability to inhibit tumor growth and combat oxidative stress associated with cancer progression. Its antimicrobial and antifungal properties further enhance its therapeutic profile, making it a promising natural compound for both preventive and therapeutic applications.

From improving glucose metabolism to preventing oxidative stress and chronic inflammation, cinnamic acid is a multifunctional agent with significant potential for treating and managing various diseases. Its diverse range of benefits highlights its importance in ongoing medical research.

Mechanisms in Diabetes Management

Ferulic acid can help manage postprandial hyperglycemia (high blood sugar after meals) by reducing the absorption of glucose from the intestine. Normally, glucose from food is absorbed through the small intestine by two key transporters: the sodium-dependent glucose co-transporter-1 (SGLT1), which brings glucose into the enterocyte cells, and the glucose transporter 2 (GLUT2), which moves glucose from the enterocyte into the bloodstream. Ferulic acid interferes with GLUT2, reducing glucose absorption and lowering blood sugar levels after meals. It also inhibits other transporters that help glucose and monosaccharides enter the bloodstream, making it beneficial for controlling blood sugar, especially in individuals with type 2 diabetes.

In addition to its effect on glucose absorption in the intestine, phenolic acids like caffeic acid, cinnamic acid, and isoferulic acid have shown potential in improving the management of Type 2 diabetes by enhancing the action of key glucose transporters, GLUT4 and GLUT2. GLUT4 plays a crucial role in the uptake of glucose into muscle and fat cells. These compounds help increase GLUT4 translocation to the cell membrane, improving glucose absorption from the blood. By improving GLUT4 function, these acids enhance the body's ability to take up glucose, further contributing to lower blood glucose levels.

Thus, by improving the function of both GLUT4 and GLUT2, these phenolic acids help lower blood glucose levels, support better insulin sensitivity (which is often impaired in Type 2 diabetes), and improve overall glucose homeostasis (**Figure 4**). This dual action makes ferulic acid, cinnamic acid, and isoferulic acid particularly valuable for managing blood sugar levels and improving insulin sensitivity in diabetic patients, (Prabhakar & Doble, 2011) (Liu *et al.*, 2001).

Figure 4. The management of Type 2 diabetes through ferulic acid, cinnamic acid, and isoferulic acid.

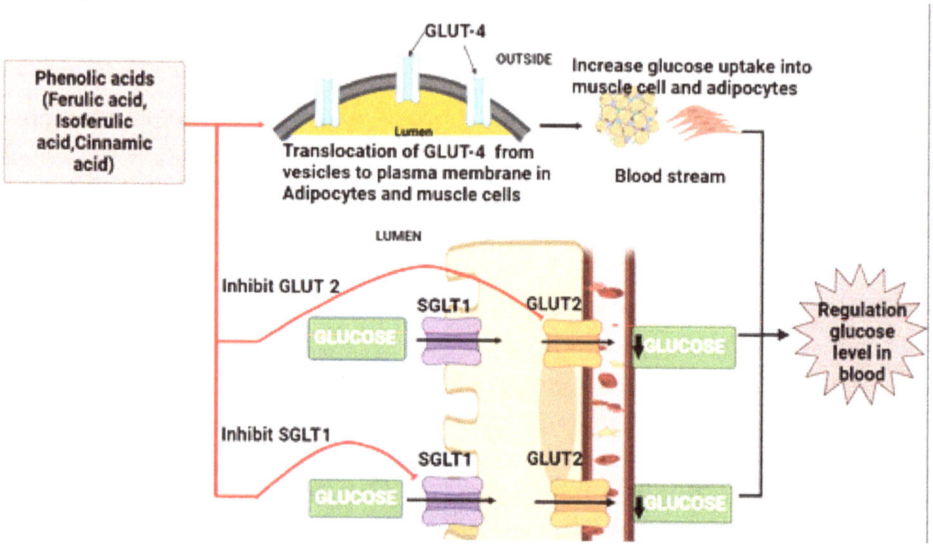

These compounds enhance glucose uptake by promoting GLUT4 translocation to the cell membrane, improving insulin sensitivity. Additionally, ferulic acid and cinnamic acid reduce postprandial hyperglycemia by inhibiting GLUT2-mediated glucose absorption in the intestines. Together, these mechanisms contribute to better glucose regulation and improved control of blood sugar levels in Type 2 diabetes. Phenolic acids exert dual action by reducing glucose absorption in the intestine (through GLUT2 and SGLT1 inhibition) and enhancing glucose uptake into peripheral tissues (via GLUT4 translocation), making them valuable in the management of Type 2 diabetes and blood glucose homeostasis

A Promising Future for Phenolic Acids

The potential of phenolic acids like caffeic, ferulic, and cinnamic acids in both preventing and treating chronic diseases is vast. Their antioxidants, anti-inflammatory, and glucose-regulating properties make them prime candidates for inclusion in therapeutic strategies aimed at managing cancer, diabetes, cardiovascular diseases, and other health conditions. Ongoing research is uncovering more about how these compounds work at the molecular level, providing deeper insights into their therapeutic mechanisms and potential for clinical application.

Incorporating phenolic acids into our diets, whether through food sources or supplements, may help improve overall health and prevent the onset of many chronic diseases. As the scientific community continues to explore the many ways these compounds interact with our bodies, it is likely that phenolic acids will play an increasingly prominent role in modern medicine and wellness.

2.2. Tannins: Unlocking Nature's Therapeutic Potential

Tannins, a diverse group of polyphenolic compounds, are found in many plant-based foods and beverages, including grapes, persimmons, blueberries, tea, chocolate, and legume forages, (Serrano *et al.*, 2009). Known for their astringent taste, tannins have long been recognized for their ability to bind and precipitate proteins, which not only affects the flavor and texture of foods but also grants them significant therapeutic properties (**Figure 5).** While tannins are widely consumed in everyday items such as wine, tea, and chocolate, recent research has shifted focus to their medicinal uses, highlighting their potential in the treatment and prevention of various diseases, including cancer and viral infections like HIV.

Tannins are primarily classified into two types: hydrolysable tannins and non-hydrolysable (condensed) tannins. Hydrolysable tannins are predominantly found in plant families like Leguminosae, Fabaceae, Combretaceae, and Anacardiaceae, often in the seeds, bark, and wood of plants. Meanwhile, condensed tannins are abundant in foods such as fruits, vegetables, cocoa, red wine, and even some grains like sorghum and millet. These tannins are not only valued for their role in flavor enhancement but also for their potent health-promoting properties.

Therapeutic Uses of Tannins

Antiviral Properties

Tannins, plant-derived polyphenols, show promise as natural anti-HIV agents due to their ability to disrupt key steps in the viral life cycle. They bind to viral glycoproteins, such as gp120, preventing HIV from attaching to CD4 receptors on host cells and inhibiting viral entry. Additionally, certain tannins, like punicalagin from pomegranate, inhibit HIV reverse transcriptase, blocking the synthesis of viral DNA. Tannins may also destabilize the viral envelope and enhance antiviral immune responses. Despite challenges like poor bioavailability, their multi-target mechanism and low cytotoxicity make them a potential adjunct in HIV therapy, (Sanna *et al.*, 2021).

Antimicrobial Properties

Tannins exhibit significant antimicrobial activity against bacteria and fungi. Their action involves binding microbial cell walls and membranes, disrupting their integrity and inhibiting microbial growth. Tannins can destabilize bacterial cell walls, interfering with nutrient uptake and metabolic processes, as seen in their effectiveness against *Staphylococcus aureus* and *Escherichia coli*. They also inhibit fungal growth by disrupting cell membrane integrity and preventing spore germination, showing strong activity against *Candida albicans* and other pathogenic fungi.

Anticancer Effects

The anticancer potential of tannins is one of the most exciting areas of research. These compounds work through several mechanisms to target cancer cells and inhibit tumor growth:

a. **Antioxidant Activity**: Tannins neutralize free radicals, reducing oxidative stress, which is a precursor to DNA damage and cancer progression. For example, ellagic acid, a tannin derivative, has shown potent antioxidant properties that protect cells from carcinogenic mutations, (Chen *et al.,* 2007). The use of Indian gooseberry, also known as amla, rich source of vitamin C and polyphenols, making it a powerful antioxidant. Studies suggest that amla helps reduce oxidative stress, a key contributor to cancer development. Amla's ellagic acid content has shown promise in inducing apoptosis (programmed cell death) in various cancer cells, particularly breast and colorectal cancers. It also enhances the activity of detoxifying enzymes and acts as an immune booster, supporting overall health and well-being in cancer patients, (Poltanov *et al.,* 2009) (Mohamed *et al.,* 2016). Indian black raspberries, known for their high content of ellagic acid and anthocyanins, have been linked to anticancer effects, particularly in colon cancer. These bioactive compounds help inhibit cancer cell migration and invasion. Research has shown that black raspberries can reduce the size of tumors by interfering with various molecular pathways associated with cancer cell proliferation and spread, (Kresty, Mallery, & Stoner, 2016). The use of Indian berries in cancer treatment presents a promising avenue for natural and complementary therapeutic options. From Indian gooseberry to wild mulberries, these fruits offer a variety of bioactive compounds that work through multiple mechanisms to combat cancer. While the current evidence is promising, further clinical research is needed to confirm the effectiveness of these berries as part of cancer treatment protocols. Integrating these berries into conventional therapies could provide a natural, adjunctive approach to managing cancer and improving patient outcomes.

b. **Induction of Apoptosis:** Tannins like tannic acid can trigger programmed cell death in cancer cells by modulating apoptotic pathways. They increase pro-apoptotic factors (e.g., Bax) and suppress anti-apoptotic proteins (e.g., Bcl-2), effectively halting tumor growth. Studies have demonstrated that tannic acid induces apoptosis in leukemia cells and other cancer types, (Youness *et al.*, 2021).
c. **Cell Cycle Arrest:** Certain tannins, such as gallotannins, interrupt the cell cycle, especially in the G2/M phase, thereby inhibiting cancer cell proliferation. For instance, corilagin, found in *Phyllanthus niruri*, arrests the cell cycle and promotes apoptosis in ovarian cancer cells via modulation of signaling pathways like TGF-β and AKT/ERK, (Gupta *et al.*, 2019).
d. **Anti-inflammatory Effects:** By suppressing inflammatory pathways, tannins reduce chronic inflammation, a key factor in cancer development. Corilagin, a hydrolysable tannin from *Phyllanthus species*, exerts anti-inflammatory effects by modulating TGF-β and NF-κB signaling pathways, thereby reducing the secretion of pro-inflammatory cytokines like TNF-α, (Zhao *et al.*, 2021).
e. **Specific Examples:** Tannins from sources like pomegranate (*Punica granatum*) inhibit proliferation in colon, prostate, and oral cancer cells, while ellagitannins from *Geranium wilfordii* show cytotoxicity against various cancer lines, including lung and ovarian cancers. Additionally, tannic acid has been found to synergize with chemotherapy agents like cisplatin, enhancing their anticancer effects, (Syed *et al.*, 2013).

The therapeutic potential of tannins extends beyond their ability to enhance flavor in foods and beverages. These natural compounds emerge as key players in the fight against viral infections and cancer. Their ability to combat oxidative stress, induce cell death in cancer cells, and regulate immune responses opens exciting possibilities for their use in medicinal treatments. As research continues to explore their benefits, tannins could play a pivotal role in developing new therapies for conditions like HIV, cancer, and even chronic inflammation-related diseases.

By tapping into the therapeutic power of tannins, we may unlock a natural and accessible avenue for managing complex diseases, all while making use of the compounds naturally found in our diets. With ongoing research, tannins could soon become a cornerstone in both preventative health and clinical therapies, offering a safer and more holistic approach to disease management.

Figure 5. Therapeutic uses of tannins showcasing their diverse medicinal applications including antioxidant, anti-inflammatory, anticancer, antiviral, and antimicrobial properties.

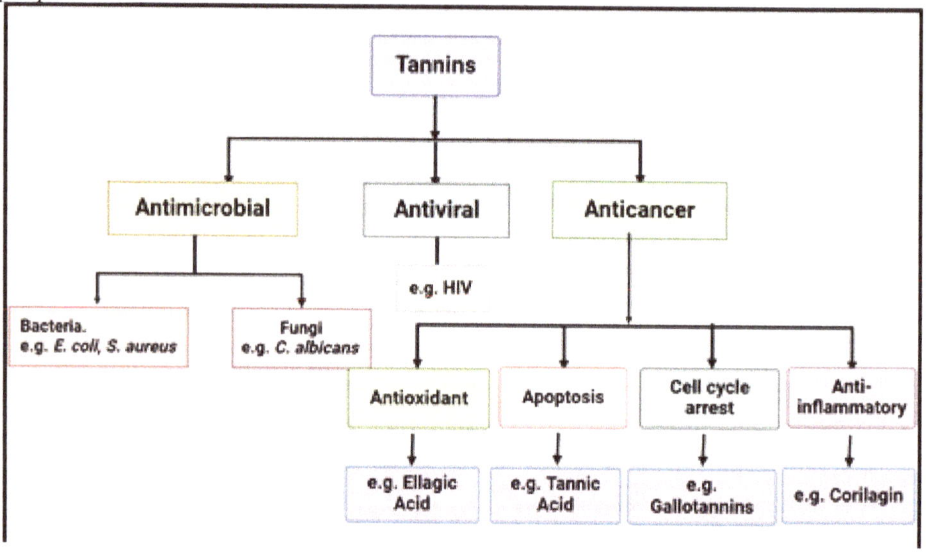

Tannins are effective in reducing oxidative stress, modulating inflammatory cytokines, inducing apoptosis in cancer cells, inhibiting HIV replication, and preventing microbial growth. These therapeutic effects make tannins valuable in treating diseases like cancer, HIV, inflammation-related conditions, and infections

2.3. Alkaloids

Alkaloids are a diverse group of naturally occurring compounds that contain nitrogen and exhibit alkaline properties. Produced primarily as secondary metabolites in plants, mammals, fungi and bacteria, they play significant roles in various physiological processes and have gained prominence for their therapeutic applications in human medicine.

Classification of Alkaloids

Alkaloids can be categorized based on their biogenesis into three main classes:

1. **True Alkaloids**: Containing a heterocyclic ring, these compounds are primarily derived from amino acids and are known for their strong biological activity. Common examples include morphine, cocaine, and quinine.

2. **Protoalkaloids**: These lack a heterocyclic ring but contain nitrogen sourced from amino acids. Examples include hordenine and mescaline, which are used to treat various ailments.
3. **Pseudoalkaloids**: Not directly derived from amino acids, these compounds have different carbon skeletons and include substances like caffeine and capsaicin (Hotti & Rischer, 2017) **(Figure 6).**

Alkaloids as Biopesticides

The growing interest in alkaloids such as botanical pesticides is due to their effectiveness and environmental safety. With the Food and Agriculture Organization (FAO) reporting that pests account for approximately 20-40% of global crop yield loss each year, the need for organic pest management solutions is critical. Alkaloids, being naturally occurring compounds, offer a promising alternative to synthetic pesticides, (Lengai, Muthomi, & Mbega, 2020).

Advantages of Alkaloids

a. Low Toxicity and Degradability: Alkaloids typically have low toxicity to non-target organisms and break down easily in the environment, making them more sustainable compared to chemical pesticides, (Wu *et al.*, 2021).
b. Modification Potential: Alkaloids can be chemically modified to enhance their effectiveness, leading to the development of more potent pest control agents.
c. Diverse Applications: They can function as insecticides, acaricides, fungicides, virucides, and herbicides, broadening their utility in agricultural practices.

Alkaloids are versatile compounds with significant ecological roles and potential applications in agriculture and medicine. Their ability to protect plants, deter pests, and serve as bioactive agents makes them valuable resources in the quest for sustainable pest management and effective treatments for human diseases. As research continues to explore their complexities, alkaloids may play an increasingly important role in both ecological balance and agricultural productivity, reinforcing their significance in modern science.

Figure 6. Alkaloids are classified biogenetically based on their biosynthetic origins and structural features.

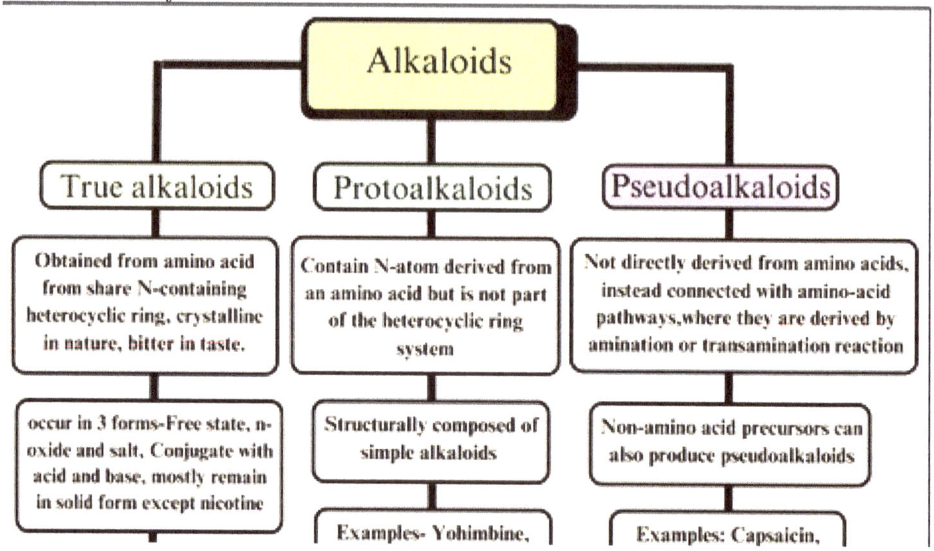

True alkaloids are synthesized from amino acids and have nitrogen within a heterocyclic ring, like morphine. Protoalkaloids also derive from amino acids but lack nitrogen in the ring, such as mescaline. Pseudoalkaloids originate from non-amino acid precursors, such as steroids or terpenoids, exemplified by caffeine. Lastly, non-heterocyclic alkaloids like colchicine lack cyclic nitrogen structures, showcasing the diversity of this natural product group

Therapeutic Uses in Human Medicine

a. **Pain Management**: One of the most famous alkaloids, morphine, derived from the opium poppy, is a powerful analgesic used to manage severe pain, particularly in cancer patients and during postoperative recovery. It works by binding to opioid receptors in the brain, altering the perception of pain, (Dewey, 2007).
b. **Malaria Treatment**: Quinine, another well-known alkaloid, has been used for centuries to treat malaria by interfering with the growth of the malaria parasite in red blood cells. Although newer medications have emerged, quinine remains an important treatment option, (Achan *et al.*, 2011).

c. **Cardiovascular Health**: Alkaloids like caffeine, found in coffee and tea, improve alertness and cognitive function. In moderate amounts, caffeine may also have protective effects against certain cardiovascular diseases, (Turnbull *et al.*, 2017).

d. **Mental Health Disorders**: Yohimbine, derived from the Yohimbe tree, is used to treat erectile dysfunction and may also aid in managing depression and anxiety by stimulating the nervous system, (Jabir *et al.*, 2022).

e. **Anticancer Properties**: Alkaloids such as vincristine and vinblastine, derived from the Madagascar periwinkle, are used in chemotherapy to treat various cancers. They inhibit cell division, preventing cell proliferation. Additionally, colchicine, an alkaloid derived from the *autumn crocus*, has shown potential as an anticancer agent. It inhibits cell division by disrupting microtubule dynamics, particularly targeting cancer cells with rapid division, and is researched for its role in managing solid tumors and hematological malignancies, (Alam *et al.*, 2017). Ber, or jujube, is an important berry native to India, rich in flavonoids, alkaloids, and saponins. Ber has shown potential for anticancer, especially in lung and liver cancers. Alkaloids in berberries have been observed to inhibit the proliferation of cancer cells. Additionally, ber's high vitamin C content contributes to its antioxidant and anti-inflammatory actions, which help reduce oxidative stress and prevent cancer initiation, (Hussain *et al.*, 2021).

f. **Antibiotic, Antimicrobial, and Antiviral Activity**: Berberine, found in goldenseal, exhibits antibacterial, antifungal, and antiviral properties. It is effective against infections caused by bacteria like *Staphylococcus aureus* and viruses such as hepatitis B and herpes simplex virus (HSV). Colchicine, while mainly used for treating gout and inflammation, also shows antiviral effects, particularly against viruses like COVID-19, by interfering with viral replication and disrupting the microtubules that assist in viral transport within host cells, (Wojtyczka *et al.*, 2014).

g. **Neurological Benefits**: Alkaloids like scopolamine and hyoscyamine are used to treat motion sickness and as sedatives, working by blocking certain neurotransmitters in the brain, (Spinks & Wasiak, 2011) (Hwang *et al.*, 2011) **(Figure 7)**.

Figure 7. Alkaloids offer diverse therapeutic actions in human medicine.

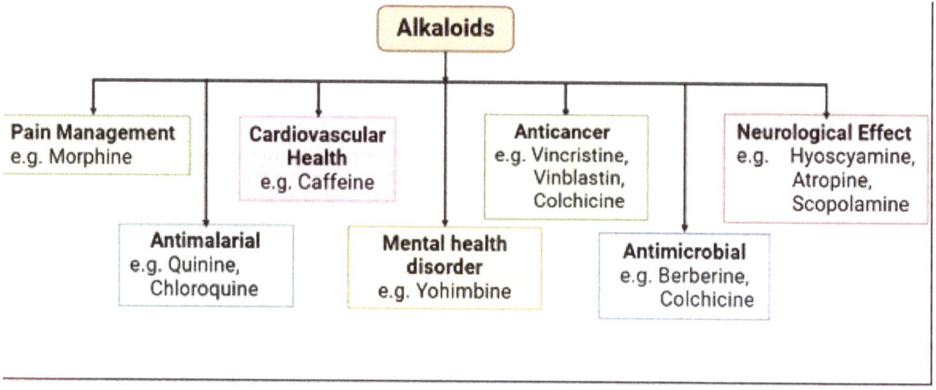

Morphine is used for pain management by binding to opioid receptors. Quinine treats malaria by inhibiting parasite growth in red blood cells. Caffeine improves cognitive function and may protect against cardiovascular diseases. Yohimbine helps treat erectile dysfunction and mental health issues like depression and anxiety. Vincristine and vinblastine are chemotherapy agents that inhibit cancer cell division. Berberine has antibiotic and antifungal properties, while scopolamine and hyoscyamine treat motion sickness and act as sedatives by blocking neurotransmitters

Mechanism of Action of Important Alkaloids

1. **Alkaloids as Antimalarial agents: Quinine, chloroquine**

Chloroquine and quinine are both alkaloids used in the treatment of malaria, though they have slightly different mechanisms of action. Both drugs work by interfering with the *Plasmodium* parasite's ability to metabolize hemoglobin in red blood cells. Quinine, derived from the cinchona tree, interferes with the *Plasmodium* parasite's ability to digest hemoglobin into heme and globin. Globin is utilized by parasites as a source of essential amino acids and heme get polymerized to hemozoin that is non-toxic to parasites, (Achan *et al.*, 2011) (Foley & Tilley, 1997). Quinine inhibits heme polymerization by inhibiting enzyme heme polymerase, leading to the buildup of toxic free heme and eventually killing the parasite. Chloroquine also interferes with the parasite's ability to detoxify the free heme, disrupting its metabolic processes and leading to parasite death. Additionally, chloroquine can increase the pH within the acidic food vacuole, impairing the parasite's ability to process hemoglobin properly, (Jha, Trivedi, & Deshmukh, 2022) **(Figure 8).**

Figure 8. Mechanism of action of Quinine and chloroquine in malaria parasite: Both antimalarial drugs, disrupt the malaria parasite's ability to digest hemoglobin within red blood cells.

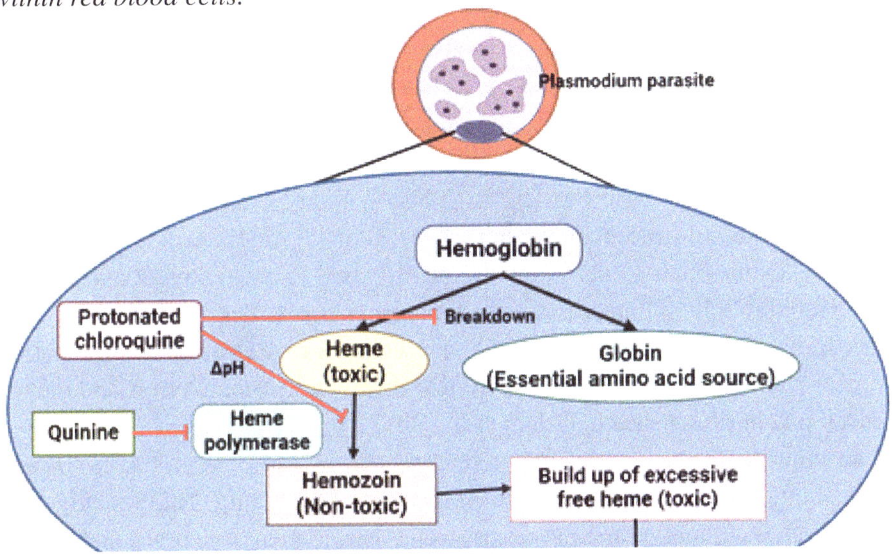

They accumulate in the parasite's food vacuole, inhibiting the polymerization of toxic heme into hemozoin. This results in the buildup of free heme, which is toxic to the parasite, leading to its death. Both drugs also increase the pH of the vacuole, further hindering the parasite's digestive function. Their combined actions prevent the parasite from effectively processing hemoglobin, thus inhibiting its growth and replication

2. Alkaloids with anticancer activity: Vincristine and vinblastine

Vincristine and vinblastine are both FDA-approved chemotherapy drugs derived from the *Catharanthus roseus* plant (Madagascar periwinkle). These drugs belong to the class of vinca alkaloids and are widely used in the treatment of various cancers, including leukemia, lymphoma, breast cancer, and testicular cancer. They have become essential components of combination chemotherapy regimens due to their ability to target rapidly dividing cancer cells, (Alam *et al.,* 2017) (Puri *et al.,* 2023).

Both vincristine and vinblastine exert their antitumor effects by disrupting the mitotic spindle during cell division. They bind to tubulin, a protein that forms microtubules, which are vital for chromosome separation during mitosis. By binding to tubulin, these drugs prevent the polymerization of microtubules, thus inhibiting the formation of the mitotic spindle (**Figure 9**). Without proper spindle formation, cells cannot complete mitosis, leading to cell cycle arrest in the M phase and eventually causing cell death. This mechanism is particularly effective for treating cancers with rapid cell division, such as leukemia and lymphoma. While both drugs share a similar mechanism of action, they have distinct clinical uses based on their unique pharmacological profiles, (Jha, Trivedi, & Deshmukh, 2022) (Puri *et al.,* 2023).

Vincristine is commonly used in combination chemotherapy regimens for cancers such as Hodgkin's lymphoma, non-Hodgkin's lymphoma, and childhood cancers like acute lymphoblastic leukemia (ALL), (Arrillaga-Romany, Monje, & Wen, 2016). Its effectiveness in treating these cancers has made it a cornerstone of pediatric oncology. Vinblastine, on the other hand, is more frequently used in the treatment of testicular cancer, Hodgkin's lymphoma, and breast cancer. Despite the differences in their specific indications, both vincristine and vinblastine are often used in combination with other chemotherapy agents to maximize therapeutic effectiveness and reduce the development of resistance, (Alam *et al.,* 2017).

Both vincristine and vinblastine were approved by the FDA in the 1960s and have been integral to cancer treatment for decades. These drugs are typically used alongside other chemotherapeutic agents to improve patient outcomes and reduce the risk of drug resistance. However, they do come with side effects, including neurotoxicity (especially with vincristine), myelosuppression (a reduction in bone marrow activity), and nausea. Neurotoxicity with vincristine can lead to peripheral neuropathy, which limits its use in higher doses. Managing these side effects is crucial to maintaining the drugs' effectiveness in cancer therapy. Ongoing research aims to enhance the efficacy of vincristine and vinblastine, especially in the face of emerging resistance, particularly in solid tumors, (Alam *et al.,* 2017) (Puri *et al.,* 2023).

Figure 9. Mechanism of action of Vinca alkaloids in cancer cell: Vinblastine and vincristine, both vinca alkaloids, exert their antitumor effects by binding to tubulin, a protein essential for microtubule formation.

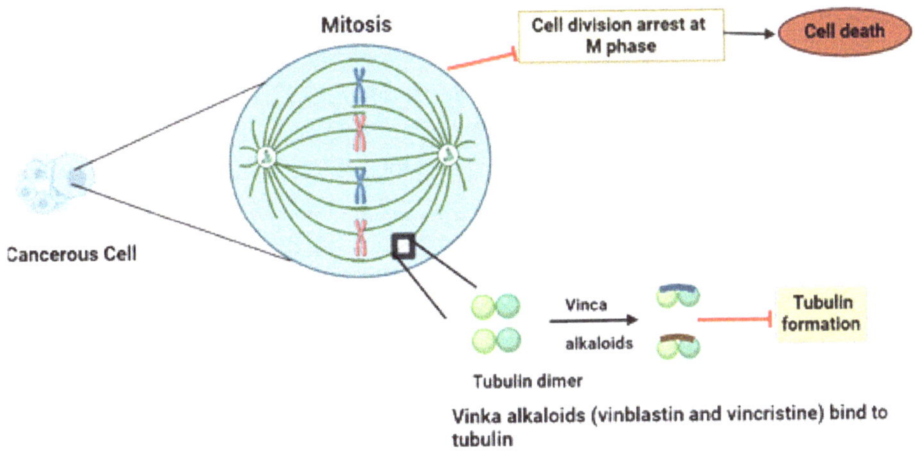

This binding inhibits the polymerization of tubulin into microtubules, disrupting the formation of the mitotic spindle during cell division. As a result, mitosis is arrested in the M phase, leading to cell cycle blockade and eventual cell death. These drugs are particularly effective against rapidly dividing cancer cells, and they are used in the treatment of cancers such as lymphoma, leukemia, and testicular cancer

3. Alkaloid with anti-inflammatory and antiviral properties: Colchicine

Colchicine is an alkaloid derived from the *Autumn crocus* plant, widely known for its use in treating gout and inflammation and is also being explored for its potential effects in managing COVID-19, (Schlesinger, Firestein, & Brunetti, 2020) (Kamel *et al.*, 2022).

In the context of gout, colchicine works by inhibiting the formation of microtubules and disrupting cellular processes in the inflammatory response. Specifically, colchicine prevents the assembly of tubulin into microtubules, which are essential for cell movement and function. In gout, this action reduces the migration of inflammatory cells (neutrophils) to the affected area (usually joints), which in turn reduces the inflammatory response caused by the buildup of uric acid crystals. This results in less pain, swelling, and tissue damage associated with gout attacks. Colchicine also inhibits the release of pro-inflammatory cytokines such as interleukin-1

(IL-1), contributing to a reduction in overall inflammation and easing symptoms, (Schlesinger, Firestein, & Brunetti, 2020) (Leung, Yao Hui, & Kraus, 2015).

In the case of COVID-19, colchicine's potential benefits have been studied due to its anti-inflammatory properties. Researchers have suggested that colchicine might help reduce the cytokine storm, a hyper-inflammatory response seen in severe COVID-19 cases. By inhibiting microtubule formation, colchicine may prevent the activation of inflammasomes and reduce the production of excessive inflammatory cytokines such as IL-1 and TNF-α. This can potentially lessen lung damage and other complications related to severe viral infections. Colchicine is thought to reduce vascular inflammation and prevent excessive clot formation, which is a key complication in COVID-19. However, clinical evidence for its efficacy in COVID-19 is still under investigation, and its use remains under scrutiny in large-scale trials, (Schlesinger, Firestein, & Brunetti, 2020) (Kamel *et al.,* 2022) (**Figure 10**).

Figure 10. Mechanism of dual action of colchicine in gout and COVID-19. In gout, colchicine inhibits microtubule formation by binding to tubulin, which prevents neutrophil migration and activation at inflammation sites, reducing pain and swelling.

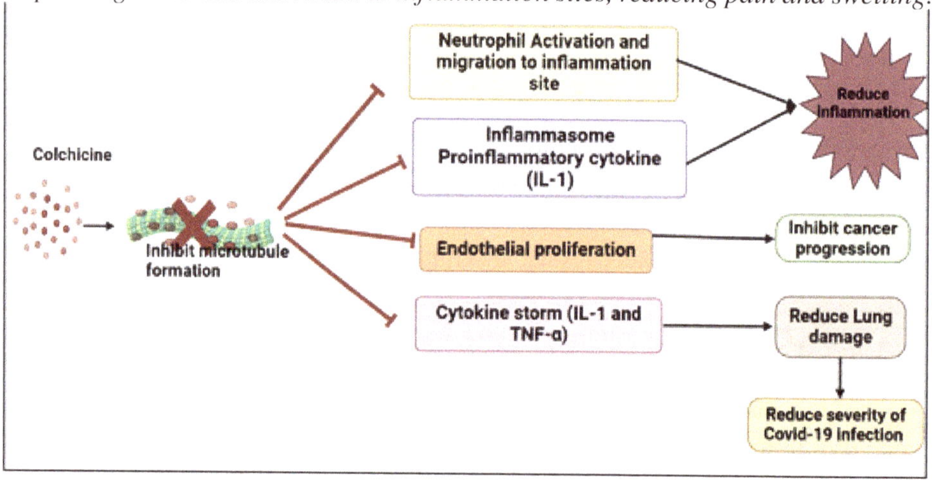

It also blocks the release of interleukin-1 (IL-1), mitigating inflammatory cytokine production. In COVID-19, colchicine disrupts microtubule-dependent inflammasome activation, decreasing cytokines like IL-1 and TNF-α, which can help manage the hyper-inflammatory "cytokine storm." Additionally, colchicine reduces vascular inflammation and minimizes thrombotic complications in severe cases

4. Tropane Alkaloids in Neurology, Gastroenterology, and Cardiology

Scopolamine, hyoscyamine, and atropine are tropane alkaloids derived from plants of the Solanaceae family, including *Atropa belladonna*, *Datura stramonium*, and *Hyoscyamus niger*. These compounds are renowned for their pharmacological effects mediated through their role as competitive antagonists of muscarinic acetylcholine receptors (mAChRs). By inhibiting acetylcholine binding, they suppress parasympathetic nervous system activity, leading to diverse therapeutic effects, (Kohnen-Johannsen & Kayser, 2019).

Scopolamine works primarily by inhibiting the binding of acetylcholine to muscarinic receptors in the vestibular system, a part of the inner ear involved in balance and spatial orientation. The vestibular system sends signals to the brain that can cause nausea when there is a mismatch between visual input and motion perception, such as during travel (motion sickness). By blocking acetylcholine's action on the muscarinic receptors, scopolamine reduces the overstimulation of the vestibular system, and the nausea associated with it. This mechanism makes scopolamine an effective treatment for motion sickness and post-operative nausea. It is often administered as a transdermal patch, which allows for controlled release of the drug over several hours. Scopolamine's ability to modify cholinergic transmission in the brain's nausea pathways is also what makes it useful in treating other conditions involving excessive acetylcholine activity, such as some types of vertigo or certain post-surgical complications, (Kohnen-Johannsen & Kayser, 2019) (Christen, 2000).

Hyoscyamine acts on smooth muscles of the gastrointestinal tract, reducing spasm and offering relief in conditions like irritable bowel syndrome (IBS). In addition to its use in gastrointestinal conditions, hyoscyamine has also been explored for its potential benefits in Parkinson's disease, particularly for managing the motor symptoms of the disease, such as tremors and rigidity. In Parkinson's, there is an imbalance between acetylcholine and dopamine due to dopamine depletion. By inhibiting acetylcholine's action, hyoscyamine can help restore this balance and improve symptoms, particularly tremors. However, its use in Parkinson's is less common today due to the availability of other treatments such as dopamine replacement therapy (e.g., levodopa). Nonetheless, anticholinergics like hyoscyamine may still play a role in combination therapies for some patients with Parkinson's, especially for those who experience tremors as a dominant symptom. While hyoscyamine provides therapeutic benefits in both gastrointestinal and neurological contexts, it should be used cautiously due to potential side effects like dry mouth, blurred vision, and confusion, particularly in older adults with Parkinson's, (Christen, 2000) (Lazaraki, Chatzimavroudis, & Katsinelos, 2014).

Atropine is also a critical antidote for poisoning by acetylcholinesterase inhibitors, such as organophosphates or certain nerve agents, by reversing the excessive accumulation of acetylcholine at receptor sites. This helps alleviate symptoms like muscle weakness, respiratory distress, and convulsions caused by the toxicity of these substances. Additionally, atropine causes pupil dilation (mydriasis) by blocking the action of acetylcholine on the iris sphincter muscle, leading to muscle relaxation and opening of the pupil. This effect is useful in ophthalmology for diagnostic procedures and for treating certain eye conditions, such as uveitis, where reducing the muscle spasm of the iris is necessary. These diverse actions make atropine a versatile drug in both emergencies and clinical settings, (Eddleston *et al.*, 2008) (Robb, Regina, & Baker, 2023) **(Figure 11)**.

FDA-Approved and Applications:

Scopolamine: Approved as a **transdermal patch** for **motion sickness** and post-operative nausea management.

Hyoscyamine: Utilized for gastrointestinal conditions such as **IBS** and as an antispasmodic agent.

Atropine: Used in **emergency treatment of bradycardia**, as an antidote for **organophosphate poisoning**, and in ophthalmology for diagnostic pupil dilation.

These alkaloids play crucial roles in managing neurological, gastrointestinal, and cardiovascular conditions. However, due to side effects like dry mouth, blurred vision, tachycardia, and central nervous system disturbances, careful dosing and monitoring are essential to maximize their benefits while minimizing risks.

Figure 11. Mechanism and FDA-approved applications of tropane alkaloids. Scopolamine, hyoscyamine, and atropine, derived from the Solanaceae family, act as muscarinic acetylcholine receptor antagonists, suppressing parasympathetic activity.

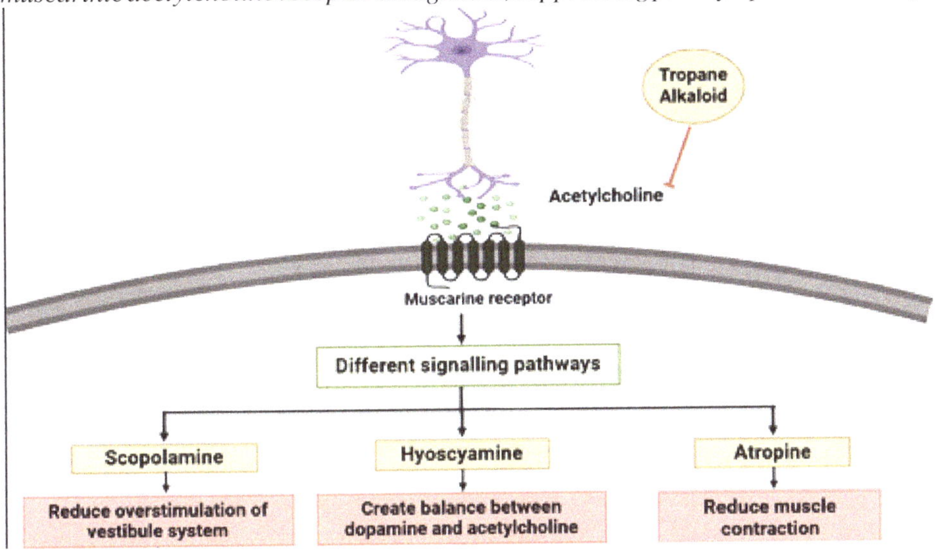

Scopolamine prevents nausea by modulating cholinergic transmission in the vestibular system. Hyoscyamine relaxes gastrointestinal muscles, aiding in IBS management. Atropine increases heart rate, treats organophosphate poisoning, and induces pupil dilation. These alkaloids are FDA-approved for neurological, gastrointestinal, and cardiovascular conditions, demonstrating diverse therapeutic applications

2.4. Terpenoids: Diversity, Classification, and Therapeutic Potential

Terpenoids, a vast group of natural compounds, are biosynthesized by plants and microbes, with over 80,000 distinct types identified to date, (Christianson, 2017) (Cseke, 2006). These secondary metabolites are crucial for ecological interactions, functioning as herbivore repellents, pollinator attractants, and mediators of stress responses, (Gershenzon & Dudareva, 2007) (Bohlmann & keeling, 2008). Structurally, terpenoids are composed of isoprene (C5) units, which categorize them based on the number of carbon atoms: monoterpenes (C10), sesquiterpenes (C15), diterpenes (C20), triterpenes (C30), tetraterpenes (C40) and polyterpenoids (>C40) (90–93) **Table 2.**

Their biosynthesis occurs through the mevalonate (MVA) or 1-deoxy-D-xylulose-5-phosphate (DXP) pathways, (Moses *et al.,* 2013). This structural diversity translates into a wide range of biological activities, making terpenoids indispensable for therapeutic applications, such as anti-inflammatory, antimicrobial, and anticancer properties. For example, monoterpenes like menthol serve as analgesics, while sesquiterpenes like artemisinin are antimalarial agents.

Table 2. Types of terpenoids and their medicinal property

S. No.	Terpenes	Plant Sources	Effects
1	**Monoterpenes**		
	Limonene	Bitter orange (*Citrus aurantium*), lemon (*Citrus limon*), Orange Maltaise (*Citrus sinensis*), and Mandarin (*Citrus reticulate*) (Bourgou *et al.*, 2012)	Antifungal, anti-inflammatory (chronic inflammation), antimicrobial, antispasmodic, Carminative, spasmolytic, choleretic, Sedative, analgetic, Diuretic, Antiseptic, Expectorant.
	Myrcene	Hops, Cannabis, Lemongrass, Verbena and Bay (The Terpenes, n.d.) (Guenther, n.d.)	Antifungal, antibacterial properties, Cytotoxic effects on cancer cell lines, Reduced DNA damage, Diuretic, Antiseptic, anti-inflammatory, Expectorant, secretomotoric, spasmolytic, anti-inflammatory, Diuretic, anti-inflammatory
	Sabinene	Juniper (*Juniperus Sabina*), marjoram (*Origanum majorana)*, Holm oak (*Quercus ilex*), Norway spruce (*Picea abies*), Douglas fir (*Pseudotsuga menziesii*), Spearmint (*Mentha spicata*), Angelica (*Angelica archangelica, Apiaceae*), Carrots (*Daucus Carota*), Black pepper (*Piperaceae*) (Jirovetz *et al.*, 2000) (Verma *et al.*, 2016) (Abdel-Kader *et al.*, 2019) (Dallali *et al.*, 2021)	Digestive, carminative
	Menthol	Cornmint (*Mentha canadensis* L.) and Peppermint (*M. x piperita L.*) (Kamatou *et al.*, 2013)	Digestive, carminative, anti-spasmolytic, choleretic, antimicrobial
	Sabinol	Savin Juniper (*Juniperus sabina*), American Beautyberry (*Callicarpa americana*), Common Sage (*Salvia officinalis*), Chinese weeping cypress (*Cupressus mollissima*) (Craig *et al.*, 2004) (Jantan & Goh, n.d.) (Roe, 1964)	Anti-oral bacterial.

continued on following page

Table 2. Continued

S. No.	Terpenes	Plant Sources	Effects
1	**Monoterpenes**		
	Carvone	Caraway (*Carum carvi* L.), Dill (*Anethum graveolens L.*), Cumin (*Cuminum cyminum L.*), Fennel (*Foeniculum vulgare Mill*) (Bhatia *et al.*, 2008) (Bouyahya *et al.*, 2021)	Carminative, antispasmodic, antimicrobial, virucidal, anticancer
	Pinene	Frankincense *(Boswellia frereana)*, Mastic tree *(Pistacia lentiscus)*, Myrtle *(Myrtus communis* and *Leptospermum ericoides*), Rock rose *(Cistus reticus* and *salviifolius)*, Juniper *(Juniperus communis)*, Camphor *(Cinnamomum camphora)*, and Conifers *(Pinaceae* family) (Silva *et al.*, 2012) (Tisserand & Young, 2014)	Anti-inflammatory, Antioxidant, and Neuroprotective Properties, Reduced cell viability, induced apoptosis, reduce ROS production, and cell cycle arrest, Antiseptic, carminative, expectorant, Diuretic, Digestive, Carminative, spasmolytic, antiviral, Analgesic, antiseptic, expectorant, antioxidant, anticancer, Anti-inflammatory, estrogenic, antiChE, crminative, antimicrobial, antihidrotic
2	**Sesquiterpene**		
	Elemenes	Turmeric *(Curcumae Rhizoma, Curcuma longa)*(Chen *et al.*, 2021) (Chen, Feng, & Liu, 2022)	Restores functions of nervous system Increases fertiltity Used to treat asthma and cold
	Valencene	Grapefruit, Tangerine (*Citrus tangerine*), Orange (Citrus sinensis), Nectarines *(Prunus persica)*, and Mangoes (*Mangifera indica*) (Song *et al.*, 2024)	Reduced cellular proliferation and acted efficiently synergistically with doxorubicin
	β-sesquiphellandrene	Flossflower (*Ageratum houstonianum),* Wild pepper *(Piper mullesua*), Ginger *(Zingiber officinale),* Turmeric *(Curcuma longa),* and Wild pepper *(Alpinia conchigera)*(Onyenekwe & Hashimoto, 1999) (Ibrahim *et al.*, 2009) (Tyagi *et al.*, 2015)	Digestive, carminative, anti-inflammatory, antiemetic
	Nerolidol	Lemongrass *(Cymbopogon citratus),* Palmarosa *(Cymbopogon martini),* Jasmine *(Jasminum grandiflorum)* (Terpenes and Testing Magazine, n.d.)	Strong antiseptic, Exhibited cytotoxic effects and induced apoptosis and cell cycle arrest. Acted synergistically with doxorubicin
	Zingiberene	Ginger *(Zingiber officinale)* (Ivanović, Makoter, & Razboršek, 2021)	Digestive, carminative, anti-inflammatory, antiemetic
3	**Diterpene**		
	Artemisinin (earlier-Qinghaosu)	Sweet wormwood *(Artemisia annua* L.) (Liao, 2009)	Antimalarial, treatment of bacterial infections, migraines, and to improve skin
	Triptolide	Thunder God Vine (*Tripterygium wilfordii, Tripterygium hypoglaucum*), yellow vine *(Tripterygium regelii)* (Tong *et al.*, 2021) (Gao *et al.*, 2021)	Anticancer, anti-inflammatory, immune modulation, antiproliferative, and proapoptotic activity

continued on following page

Table 2. Continued

S. No.	Terpenes	Plant Sources	Effects
1	**Monoterpenes**		
	Andrographolide	Kalmegh/ King of Bitters, (*Andrographis paniculata), False* waterwillow (*Andrographis echioides, Andrographis alata)* (Li *et al.*, 2022) (Yadav & Karuppusamy, 2024)	Anti-diabetic, ayurvedic (digestive problems, Joint pain and air sickness)
4	**Triterpene**		
	Oleanolic acid	Lantana *(Lantana camara),* Glossy privet *(Lisgustrum lucidum),* Garden thyme (*Thymus vulgaris)* and Clove plants *(Syzygium aromaticum),* Apple *(Malus),* Loquat (*Eriobotrya japonica*), Grape *(Vitis),* Elderberry *(Sambucus)* and Sage *(Salvia officinalis)* (Jäger *et al.*, 2009) (*Xia et al.*, 2011)	Anti-inflammatory, estrogenic, antiChE, crminative, antimicrobial, antihidrotic, Expectorant, secretomotoric, spasmolytic.

Therapeutic Uses and Mechanisms of Terpenoids

1. **Anti-inflammatory Agents:** Terpenoids such as oleanolic acid (triterpene) and boswellic acids (pentacyclic triterpenes) exhibit potent anti-inflammatory activities. Their mechanisms include the inhibition of pro-inflammatory mediators like cyclooxygenase (COX) enzymes and lipoxygenases (LOX). Oleanolic acid suppresses the nuclear factor kappa B (NF-κB) signaling pathway, reducing cytokine production and oxidative stress. Boswellic acids block leukotriene synthesis, mitigating inflammation associated with arthritis and chronic inflammatory conditions, (Dewick, 2002) (Siddiqui & Serrata, 2011).
2. **Antimicrobial Properties:** Farnesol (sesquiterpenoid) disrupts biofilm formation in Candida albicans, thereby reducing its virulence. Farnesol also interferes with quorum sensing, a bacterial communication mechanism, enhancing the efficacy of antifungal treatments, (Ramage *et al.,* 2002). Whereas Tea Tree Oil contains monoterpenes like terpinen-4-ol, which *combat Staphylococcus aureus* and methicillin-resistant *S. aureus* (MRSA). These compounds disrupt bacterial cell membranes and inhibit biofilm formation, making them effective in treating skin infections, (Kairey *et al.*, 2023).
3. **Anticancer Applications:** Artemisinin (sesquiterpene lactone) from Artemisia annua generates reactive oxygen species (ROS) by reacting with iron in tumor cells. This oxidative stress leads to cell membrane damage and apoptosis in cancerous cells, (Pacios-Michelena *et al.,* 2021). Triptolide (diterpene) suppresses tumor growth by inducing apoptosis and inhibiting angiogenesis. It

targets molecular pathways like NF-κB and PI3K/Akt, disrupting cancer cell proliferation, (Zhang *et al.*, 2012).

4. **Analgesic and Sedative Effects:** Menthol (monoterpene) derived from peppermint, provides analgesic and antispasmodic effects through its multifaceted mechanisms. It activates TRPM8 cold-sensing ion channels, inducing a cooling sensation and reducing pain perception by limiting excitatory neurotransmitter release. Its antispasmodic effects are mediated by the inhibition of voltage-dependent L-type calcium channels, which decreases intracellular calcium levels, preventing the activation of myosin light-chain kinase (MLCK) necessary for muscle contraction. Simultaneously, menthol activates potassium channels, such as BK channels, leading to hyperpolarization of the cell membrane, reducing muscle excitability. Additionally, menthol enhances intracellular cyclic adenosine monophosphate (cAMP) levels, activating protein kinase A (PKA). PKA inactivates MLCK through phosphorylation and activates protein phosphatases that dephosphorylate myosin light chains, promoting muscle relaxation, (Liu *et al.*, 2013). These actions collectively make menthol effective in topical formulations for pain relief and as an antispasmodic agent for conditions like irritable bowel syndrome (IBS), respiratory spasms, and uterine cramps **(Figure 12).** Eugenol (phenylpropene, related to terpenoids) from clove oil inhibits pain signals by acting on vanilloid receptors and is highly effective for dental pain relief.
5. **Respiratory Relief:** Eucalyptus oil (monoterpenes like eucalyptol) acts as an antispasmodic and mucolytic agent. It relaxes airway smooth muscles by modulating calcium ion channels, making it beneficial for conditions like bronchitis and asthma, (Salvatori *et al.*, 2023).
6. **Cardiovascular and Antidiabetic Benefits:** Tanshinones (diterpenes) from *Salvia miltiorrhiza* improve cardiac function by reducing oxidative stress and neuroinflammation. They also inhibit platelet aggregation, protecting against cardiovascular diseases, (Zhang *et al.*, 2012). Andrographolide (diterpene lactone) from Andrographis paniculata enhances glucose uptake in cells and protects pancreatic β-cells, aiding in glycemic control, (Cho *et al.*, 2017).
7. **Neuroprotective Roles:** Linalool (monoterpenol) exhibits anxiolytic and antidepressive effects by modulating the GABAergic system. It also reduces oxidative stress and inflammation, showing potential for treating neurodegenerative diseases like Alzheimer's and Parkinson's, (Pereira *et al.*, 2018).
8. **Antioxidant and Photoprotective Effects (Tetraterpenes):** β-Carotene: Functions as an antioxidant and vitamin A precursor, enhancing vision and immunity. Lycopene: Reduces oxidative stress, supporting cardiovascular health and cancer prevention. Astaxanthin: Protects against UV damage, reduces inflammation, and benefits skin and eye health, (Grune *et al.*, 2010). Building on the antioxidant and immune-boosting properties of carotenoids,

Goji berries are particularly rich in β-carotene, vitamin C, and polysaccharides, all of which contribute to their potent anticancer effects. Studies suggest that goji berries can help prevent the spread of cancer cells, particularly in liver and lung cancers. The unique combination of bioactive compounds in goji berries strengthens the immune system, enhancing the body's natural defenses against cancer progression. Furthermore, the high levels of vitamin C in these berries support antioxidant activities, reducing oxidative stress that is often associated with cancer development, (Vidović *et al.,* 2022). This makes goji berries not only beneficial for boosting immunity but also for improving overall health and potentially preventing cancer.

9. **Biomedical and Functional Applications (Polyterpenes):** Rubber (Polyisoprene): Used in medical-grade latex products for flexibility and durability. Gutta-percha is utilized in dentistry for root canal procedures as biocompatible material. Polyprenols exhibit antiviral and immunomodulatory effects, with potential roles in liver and metabolic health, (Combe, Cohen, & Cummings, 2001) (Vishwanath & Rao, 2019). These diverse terpenoid classes demonstrate their wide-ranging therapeutic potential, driven by their complex chemical structures and precise modes of action.

Figure 12. Mechanisms underlying the antispasmodic effects of Menthol (essential oil), particularly focusing on three major pathways. (a) inhibition of voltage-dependent calcium channels, leading to a reduction in intracellular calcium levels; (b) modulation of potassium channels resulting in membrane hyperpolarization and decreased muscle excitability; and (c) modulation of intracellular cyclic adenosine monophosphate (cAMP) levels.

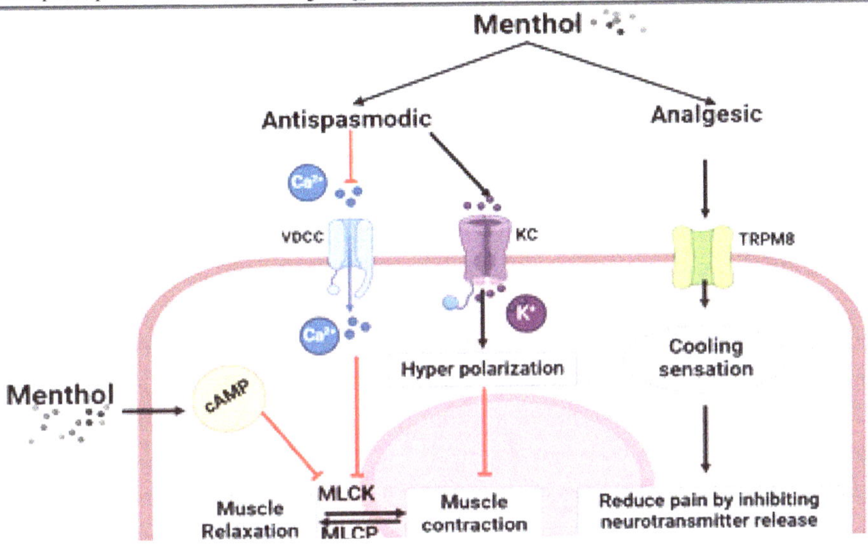

These mechanisms collectively reduce muscle contractions and promote relaxation. Key components involved include voltage-dependent calcium channels (VDCC), potassium channels (KC), Transient Receptor Potential Melastatin 8 cold-sensing ion channels (TRPM8), myosin light-chain kinase (MLCK), myosin light-chain phosphatase (MLCP), and cAMP demonstrating the integrated signaling pathways that contribute to the antispasmodic effects

2.5. Fatty-Acid-Derived Substances and Polyketides: Natural Powerhouses with Diverse Therapeutic Effects

Fatty-acid-derived substances and polyketides from plants exhibit diverse biological and therapeutic properties. Jasmonic acid and methyl jasmonate, derived from plant fatty acids, play crucial roles in plant defense and stress responses and have been explored for their potential in cancer therapy due to their ability to induce apoptosis in tumor cells, (Jarocka-Karpowicz & Markoswka, 2021). Cutin and suberin, protective biopolymers in plant cell walls, contribute to wound healing and antimicrobial resistance in plants, with emerging applications in biomaterials, (Grabarczyk *et al.,* 2024a). Green leaf volatiles (GLVs), such as hexenal and hexenol, act as insect repellents and have potential in agriculture as natural pest control agents, (Wei *et al.,* 2007). Additionally, prostaglandin-like compounds found in certain algae and higher plants exhibit anti-inflammatory properties, like their animal counterparts, (Groenewald & Van Der Westhuizen, 1997).

Among polyketides, resveratrol, a polyphenol found in grapes, peanuts, and berries, is well known for its antioxidant, anti-inflammatory, and cardioprotective effects, making it a potential therapeutic agent for cardiovascular diseases and neurodegenerative disorders. Curcumin, the active component of turmeric, has demonstrated powerful anti-inflammatory, anticancer, and neuroprotective effects, with applications in managing conditions like arthritis, Alzheimer's disease, and various cancers, (Grabarczyk *et al.,* 2024a). Additionally, flavonoids, such as quercetin and genistein, are synthesized via polyketide pathways and offer antioxidant, anti-inflammatory, and immune-boosting benefits, contributing to their role in preventing chronic diseases, including diabetes and cardiovascular conditions These plant-derived fatty-acid-related substances and polyketides highlight nature's potential in drug discovery and therapeutic applications (**Figure 13).**

Plant-derived fatty-acid-related substances and polyketides exhibit a range of therapeutic properties:

Jasmonic Acid and Methyl Jasmonate: These compounds, derived from plant fatty acids, are recognized for their anti-inflammatory and anticancer activities. Their structural similarity to prostaglandins allows them to modulate inflammatory responses and induce apoptosis in cancer cells, (Jarocka-Karpowicz & Markoswka, 2021).

Resveratrol: A polyphenol found in grapes, peanuts, and berries, resveratrol is noted for its antioxidant and anti-inflammatory effects. It has been studied for potential benefits in cardiovascular health and neuroprotection, (Grabarczyk *et al.*, 2024b).

Curcumin: The active component of turmeric, curcumin exhibits anti-inflammatory and anticancer properties. It has been explored for its role in managing conditions like arthritis and various cancers, (Grabarczyk *et al.*, 2024b).

Flavonoids: Compounds such as quercetin and genistein, synthesized via polyketide pathways, offer antioxidant and anti-inflammatory benefits. They contribute to the prevention of chronic diseases, including diabetes and cardiovascular conditions, (Mutha, Tatiya, & Surana, 2021).

These examples highlight the therapeutic potential of plant-derived fatty-acid-related substances and polyketides.

Figure 13. Therapeutic uses of fatty acid derived substances and polyketides from plants

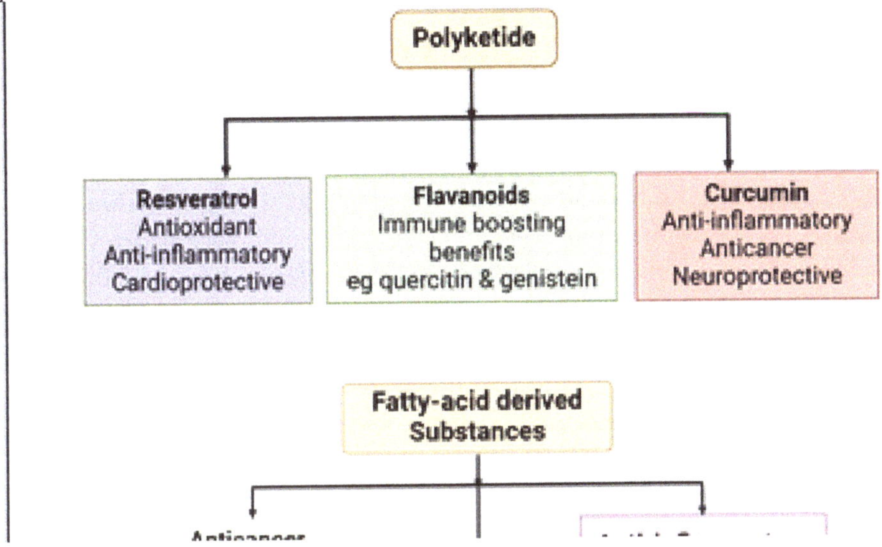

3. CONCLUDING REMARKS

Secondary metabolites, such as alkaloids, terpenoids, polyketides, and non-ribosomal peptides, have long been recognized for their profound therapeutic potential. These naturally occurring compounds, produced by plants, fungi, and microorganisms, have shown remarkable efficacy in the treatment of various diseases, including cancer, infectious diseases, autoimmune disorders, and cardio-vascular conditions. They provide unique modes of action that are often not found in conventional synthetic drugs, making them indispensable in the pharmaceutical industry. Furthermore, their bioactive properties, such as anti-inflammatory, anti-microbial, and anticancer effects, continue to drive research into their applications as effective treatment options.

The discovery of novel secondary metabolites and the advancement of bio-technology techniques, such as genetic manipulation and biosynthetic pathway engineering, hold promise for overcoming current limitations in drug development. By harnessing the natural diversity of these compounds, we can potentially address drug resistance, reduce side effects, and create more targeted therapies.

4. FUTURE PERSPECTIVES

Looking ahead, the future of secondary metabolites in disease treatment is incredibly promising. Advances in synthetic biology and metabolic engineering will allow for the more efficient production of these compounds, increasing yield and lowering costs. Furthermore, the application of computational tools to predict and design novel secondary metabolites could greatly expand the scope of natural product-based drugs. Additionally, there is growing interest in personalized medicine, where secondary metabolites could be tailored to individual patients' needs, enhancing therapeutic efficacy and reducing adverse effects, (Su *et al.*, 2024).

Research into drug resistance, particularly in the context of antimicrobial and anticancer agents, will be a major focus. As resistance continues to rise, secondary metabolites could play a crucial role in developing new drugs capable of overcoming resistant strains. Moreover, the synergistic effects of combining secondary metabolites with conventional therapies are expected to gain more attention, providing more potent and holistic treatment regimens for complex diseases, (Muteeb *et al.*, 2023).

In summary, while secondary metabolites have already demonstrated vast therapeutic applications, their full potential remains largely untapped. As our understanding of their mechanisms and biosynthesis deepens, the development of novel, effective, and sustainable therapies will be increasingly within reach. Their future as a cornerstone of medical treatment looks brighter than ever.

ACKNOWLEDGEMENT

We sincerely thank Bennett University for the continuous support during the preparation of this chapter.

REFERENCES

Abad Martínez, M. J., Del Olmo, L. M. B., Ticona, L. A., & Benito, P. B. (2012). The *Artemisia* L. genus: A review of bioactive sesquiterpene lactones. In Atta-ur-Rahman (Ed.), *Studies in Natural Products Chemistry* (Vol. 37, pp. 43–65). Elsevier.

Abdel-Kader, M. S., Soliman, G. A., Alqarni, M. H., Hamad, A. M., Foudah, A. I., & Alqasoumi, S. I. (2019). Chemical composition and protective effect of *Juniperus sabina* L. essential oil against CCl4 induced hepatotoxicity. *Saudi Pharmaceutical Journal : SPJ : the Official Publication of the Saudi Pharmaceutical Society*, *27*(7), 945–951. DOI: 10.1016/j.jsps.2019.07.003 PMID: 31997901

Achan, J., Talisuna, A. O., Erhart, A., Yeka, A., Tibenderana, J. K., Baliraine, F. N., Rosenthal, P. J., & D'Alessandro, U. (2011). Quinine, an old anti-malarial drug in a modern world: Role in the treatment of malaria. *Malaria Journal*, *10*(1), 144. https://pmc.ncbi.nlm.nih.gov/articles/PMC3121651/. DOI: 10.1186/1475-2875-10-144 PMID: 21609473

Ahmadi, A., Hosseinimehr, S. J., Naghshvar, F., Hajir, E., & Ghahremani, M. (2008). Chemoprotective effects of hesperidin against genotoxicity induced by cyclophosphamide in mice bone marrow cells. *Archives of Pharmacal Research*, *31*(6), 794–797. https://link.springer.com/article/10.1007/s12272-001-1228-z. DOI: 10.1007/s12272-001-1228-z PMID: 18563363

Ahmed, S. A., Mendonca, P., Elhag, R., & Soliman, K. F. A. (2022). Anticancer effects of fucoxanthin through cell cycle arrest, apoptosis induction, angiogenesis inhibition, and autophagy modulation. *International Journal of Molecular Sciences*, *23*(24), 16091. DOI: 10.3390/ijms232416091 PMID: 36555740

Al Mamari, H. H. (2021, July 19). Phenolic compounds: Classification, chemistry, and updated techniques of analysis and synthesis. https://www.intechopen.com/chapters/77604

Alam, M. M., Naeem, M., Masroor, M. A. K., & Uddin, M. (2017). Vincristine and vinblastine anticancer *Catharanthus* alkaloids: Pharmacological applications and strategies for yield improvement. In *Catharanthus roseus: Current research and future prospects* (pp. 277–307).

Andryukov, B., Mikhailov, V., & Besednova, N. (2019, June 3). The biotechnological potential of secondary metabolites from marine bacteria. *Journal of Marine Science and Engineering*, *7*(6), 176. https://www.mdpi.com/2077-1312/7/6/176/htm. DOI: 10.3390/jmse7060176

Arrillaga-Romany, I., Monje, M., & Wen, P. Y. (2016). Neurologic complications of oncologic therapy. In *Handbook of neuro-oncology neuroimaging* (2nd ed., pp. 125–142). DOI: 10.1016/B978-0-12-800945-1.00015-X

Balakrishnan, A., & Menon, V. P. (2007). Effect of hesperidin on matrix metalloproteinases and antioxidant status during nicotine-induced toxicity. *Toxicology*, *238*(2–3), 90–98. DOI: 10.1016/j.tox.2007.04.022 PMID: 17643689

Berk, Ş., Kaya, S., Akkol, E. K., & Bardakçı, H. (2022). A comprehensive and current review on the role of flavonoids in lung cancer–Experimental and theoretical approaches. *Phytomedicine*, *98*, 153938. DOI: 10.1016/j.phymed.2022.153938 PMID: 35123170

Bhatia, S. P., McGinty, D., Letizia, C. S., & Api, A. M. (2008). Fragrance material review on carveol. *Food and Chemical Toxicology, 46*(Suppl. 11). https://pubmed.ncbi.nlm.nih.gov/18640224/

Bodduluru, L. N., Kasala, E. R., Madhana, R. M., Barua, C. C., Hussain, M. I., Haloi, P., & Borah, P. (2016). Naringenin ameliorates inflammation and cell proliferation in benzo(a)pyrene induced pulmonary carcinogenesis by modulating CYP1A1, NFκB and PCNA expression. *International Immunopharmacology*, *30*, 102–110. DOI: 10.1016/j.intimp.2015.11.036 PMID: 26655880

Bohlmann, J., & Keeling, C. I. (2008). Terpenoid biomaterials. *The Plant Journal*, *54*(4), 656–669. https://onlinelibrary.wiley.com/doi/full/10.1111/j.1365-313X.2008.03449.x. DOI: 10.1111/j.1365-313X.2008.03449.x PMID: 18476870

Bourgou, S., Rahali, F. Z., Ourghemmi, I., & Tounsi, M. S. (2012). Changes of peel essential oil composition of four Tunisian citrus during fruit maturation. *TheScientificWorldJournal*, *2012*, 528593. Advance online publication. DOI: 10.1100/2012/528593 PMID: 22645427

Bouyahya, A., Mechchate, H., Benali, T., Ghchime, R., Charfi, S., Balahbib, A., Burkov, P., Shariati, M. A., Lorenzo, J. M., & Omari, N. E. (2021). Health benefits and pharmacological properties of carvone. *Biomolecules*, *11*(12), 1872. https://pubmed.ncbi.nlm.nih.gov/34944447/. DOI: 10.3390/biom11121803 PMID: 34944447

Chen, C. H., Liu, T. Z., Chen, C. H., Wong, C. H., Chen, C. H., Lu, F. J., & Chen, S. C. (2007). The efficacy of protective effects of tannic acid, gallic acid, ellagic acid, and propyl gallate against hydrogen peroxide-induced oxidative stress and DNA damages in IMR-90 cells. *Molecular Nutrition & Food Research, 51*(8), 962–968. https://pubmed.ncbi.nlm.nih.gov/17628875/. DOI: 10.1002/mnfr.200600230 PMID: 17628875

Chen, W., Feng, Z., & Liu, Q. (2022). Asymmetric total synthesis of (1S,2S,4S)-β-elemene. *RSC Advances, 12*(13), 8249–8255. https://www.ncbi.nlm.nih.gov/pmc/articles/PMC8982354/. DOI: 10.1039/D2RA01408D PMID: 35424753

Chen, X., Chen, X., Chen, X., Zou, N., Liang, L., & Liang, L.. (2021). Submarine cable monitoring system based on enhanced COTDR with simultaneous loss measurement and vibration monitoring ability. *Optics Express, 29*(9), 13115–13128. https://opg.optica.org/viewmedia.cfm?uri=oe-29-9-13115&seq=0&html=true. DOI: 10.1364/OE.418920 PMID: 33985053

Cho, K. S., Lim, Y. R., Lee, K., Lee, J., Lee, J. H., & Lee, I. S. (2017). Terpenes from forests and human health. *Toxicological Research, 33*(2), 97–106. DOI: 10.5487/TR.2017.33.2.097 PMID: 28443180

Choudhary, S., Sood, S., Donnell, R. L., & Wang, H. C. R. (2012). Intervention of human breast cell carcinogenesis chronically induced by 2-amino-1-methyl-6-phenylimidazo[4,5-b]pyridine. *Carcinogenesis, 33*(4), 876–885. DOI: 10.1093/carcin/bgs097 PMID: 22307971

Christen, P. (2000). Tropane alkaloids: Old drugs used in modern medicine. In Atta-ur-Rahman (Ed.), *Studies in Natural Products Chemistry* (Vol. 22, Part C, pp. 717–749). Elsevier.

Christianson, D. W. (2017). Structural and chemical biology of terpenoid cyclases. *Chemical Reviews, 117*(17), 11570–11648. https://pubmed.ncbi.nlm.nih.gov/28841019/. DOI: 10.1021/acs.chemrev.7b00287 PMID: 28841019

Combe, E. C., Cohen, B. D., & Cummings, K. (2001). Alpha- and beta-forms of gutta-percha in products for root canal filling. *International Endodontic Journal, 34*(6), 447–451. DOI: 10.1046/j.1365-2591.2001.00415.x PMID: 11556511

Coward, L., Barnes, N. C., Setchell, K. D. R., & Barnes, S. (2009). Genistein, daidzein, and their beta-glycoside conjugates—Antitumor isoflavones in soybean foods from American and Asian diets. *Journal of Agricultural and Food Chemistry, 41*(11), 1961–1967. DOI: 10.1021/jf00035a027

Cox-Georgian, D., Ramadoss, N., Dona, C., & Basu, C. (2019). Therapeutic and medicinal uses of terpenes. In *Medicinal Plants* (p. 333). https://www.ncbi.nlm.nih.gov/pmc/articles/PMC7120914/

Craig, A. M., Karchesy, J. J., Blythe, L. L., González-Hernández, M. D. P., & Swan, L. R. (2004). Toxicity studies on western juniper oil (*Juniperus occidentalis*) and Port-Orford-cedar oil (*Chamaecyparis lawsoniana*) extracts utilizing local lymph node and acute dermal irritation assays. *Toxicology Letters*, *154*(3), 217–224. DOI: 10.1016/j.toxlet.2004.08.004 PMID: 15501613

Crozier, A., Clifford, M. N., & Ashihara, H. (2007, November 12). *Plant secondary metabolites: Occurrence, structure and role in the human diet.* Wiley. https://onlinelibrary.wiley.com/doi/book/10.1002/9780470988558

Cseke, L. J., & Kirakosyan, A. (2006). How and why these compounds are synthesized by plants. In *Natural products from plants* (pp. 51–100). https://scholar.google.com/scholar_lookup?title=How%20and%20why%20these%20compounds%20are%20synthesized%20by%20plants&author=L.J.%20Cseke&publication_year=2006&pages=51-100

da Silva, A. C. R., Lopes, P. M., de Azevedo, M. M. B., Costa, D. C. M., Alviano, C. S., & Alviano, D. S. (2012). Biological activities of α-pinene and β-pinene enantiomers. *Molecules (Basel, Switzerland)*, *17*(6), 6305–6316. https://www.mdpi.com/1420-3049/17/6/6305. DOI: 10.3390/molecules17066305 PMID: 22634841

Dallali, S., Zouaoui, R., Dallali, D., Jdidi, S., & Toumi, L. (2021). Determination of some biochemical parameters from leaves of *Quercus ilex* L. (Fagaceae), collected in Djabel Zagouan (Tunisia). *Arabian Journal of Medicinal and Aromatic Plants,* *7*(1), 1–28. https://revues.imist.ma/index.php/AJMAP/article/view/24994

Demain, A. L. (1999). Pharmaceutically active secondary metabolites of microorganisms. *Applied Microbiology and Biotechnology*, *52*(4), 455–463. https://pubmed.ncbi.nlm.nih.gov/10570792/. DOI: 10.1007/s002530051546 PMID: 10570792

Dewey, W. (2007). Morphine. In *xPharm: The Comprehensive Pharmacology Reference* (pp. 1–6). Elsevier.

Dewick, P. (2002). *Medicinal natural products: A biosynthetic approach.* Retrieved October 20, 2024, from https://www.just.edu.jo/FacultiesandDepartments/FacultyofPharmacy/Documents/Syllabus_PharD332_Spring_2019.pdf

Didehdar, M., Chegini, Z., Tabaeian, S. P., Razavi, S., & Shariati, A. (2022). *Cinnamomum*: The new therapeutic agents for inhibition of bacterial and fungal biofilm-associated infection. *Frontiers in Cellular and Infection Microbiology*, *12*, 9309250. DOI: 10.3389/fcimb.2022.930624 PMID: 35899044

Eddleston, M., Buckley, N. A., Eyer, P., & Dawson, A. H. (2008). Management of acute organophosphorus pesticide poisoning. *Lancet*, *371*(9612), 597–607. https://pmc.ncbi.nlm.nih.gov/articles/PMC2493390/. DOI: 10.1016/S0140-6736(07)61202-1 PMID: 17706760

El-Seedi, H. R., Taher, E. A., Sheikh, B. Y., Anjum, S., Saeed, A., & AlAjmi, M. F.. (2017). Hydroxycinnamic acids: Natural sources, biosynthesis, possible biological activities, and roles in Islamic medicine. In Rahman, A. (Ed.), *Studies in Natural Products Chemistry* (Vol. 55, pp. 269–292). Elsevier., DOI: 10.1016/B978-0-444-63933-8.00009-6

Erb, M., & Kliebenstein, D. J. (2020). Plant secondary metabolites as defenses, regulators, and primary metabolites: The blurred functional trichotomy. *Plant Physiology*, *184*(1), 39–52. DOI: 10.1104/pp.20.00433 PMID: 32636341

Foley, M., & Tilley, L. (1997). Quinoline antimalarials: Mechanisms of action and resistance. *International Journal for Parasitology*, *27*(2), 231–240. https://pubmed.ncbi.nlm.nih.gov/9088993/. DOI: 10.1016/S0020-7519(96)00152-X PMID: 9088993

Forester, S. C., & Lambert, J. D. (2011). The role of antioxidant versus pro-oxidant effects of green tea polyphenols in cancer prevention. *Molecular Nutrition & Food Research*, *55*(6), 844–854. https://onlinelibrary.wiley.com/doi/full/10.1002/mnfr.201000641. DOI: 10.1002/mnfr.201000641 PMID: 21538850

Ganapathy, E., Peramaiyan, R., Rajasekaran, D., Venkataraman, M., & Dhanapal, S. (2008). Modulatory effect of naringenin on N-methyl-N′-nitro-N-nitrosoguanidine- and saturated sodium chloride-induced gastric carcinogenesis in male Wistar rats. *Clinical and Experimental Pharmacology & Physiology*, *35*(10), 1190–1196. https://onlinelibrary.wiley.com/doi/full/10.1111/j.1440-1681.2008.04987.x. DOI: 10.1111/j.1440-1681.2008.04987.x PMID: 18565195

Gao, J., Zhang, Y., Liu, X., Wu, X., Huang, L., & Gao, W. (2021). Triptolide: Pharmacological spectrum, biosynthesis, chemical synthesis and derivatives. *Theranostics*, *11*(15), 7199–7221. http://www.thno.org. DOI: 10.7150/thno.57745 PMID: 34158845

Gershenzon, J., & Dudareva, N. (2007). The function of terpene natural products in the natural world. *Nature Chemical Biology*, *3*(7), 408–414. https://pubmed.ncbi.nlm.nih.gov/17576428/. DOI: 10.1038/nchembio.2007.5 PMID: 17576428

Grabarczyk, M., Justyńska, W., Czpakowska, J., Smolińska, E., Bielenin, A., Glabinski, A., & Szpakowski, P. (2024). Role of plant phytochemicals: Resveratrol, curcumin, luteolin and quercetin in demyelination, neurodegeneration, and epilepsy. *Antioxidants*, *13*(11), 1364. https://www.mdpi.com/2076-3921/13/11/1364/htm. DOI: 10.3390/antiox13111364 PMID: 39594506
Grabarczyk, M., Justyńska, W., Czpakowska, J., Smolińska, E., Bielenin, A., Glabinski, A., & Szpakowski, P. (2024). Role of plant phytochemicals: Resveratrol, curcumin, luteolin and quercetin in demyelination, neurodegeneration, and epilepsy. *Antioxidants*, *13*(11), 1364. https://www.mdpi.com/2076-3921/13/11/1364/htm. DOI: 10.3390/antiox13111364 PMID: 39594506
Griesbach, R. J. (2010, June 23). Biochemistry and genetics of flower color. In *Plant Breeding Reviews* (Vol. 25, pp. 89–114). https://onlinelibrary.wiley.com/doi/full/10.1002/9780470650301.ch4

Groenewald, E. G., & Van Der Westhuizen, A. J. (1997). Prostaglandins and related substances in plants. *Botanical Review*, *63*(3), 199–220. DOI: 10.1007/BF02857948

Grune, T., Lietz, G., Palou, A., Ross, A. C., Stahl, W., Tang, G., Thurnham, D., Yin, S., & Biesalski, H. K. (2010). β-Carotene is an important vitamin A source for humans. *The Journal of Nutrition*, *140*(12), 2268S–2285S. https://pmc.ncbi.nlm.nih.gov/articles/PMC3139236/. DOI: 10.3945/jn.109.119024 PMID: 20980645

Guenther, E. (n.d.). *Essential oils (Vol. II)*. [Scribd]. Retrieved February 3, 2025, from https://www.scribd.com/document/477436004/ernest-guenther-Essential-oils-vol-II-pdf

Gupta, A., Singh, A. K., Kumar, R., Ganguly, R., Rana, H. K., Pandey, P. K., Sethi, G., Bishayee, A., & Pandey, A. K. (2019). Corilagin in cancer: A critical evaluation of anticancer activities and molecular mechanisms. *Molecules (Basel, Switzerland)*, *24*(18), 3399. https://pubmed.ncbi.nlm.nih.gov/31546767/. DOI: 10.3390/molecules24183399 PMID: 31546767

Hernaez, J. F., Xu, M., & Dashwood, R. H. (1998). Antimutagenic activity of tea towards 2-hydroxyamino-3-methylimidazo[4,5-f]quinoline: Effect of tea concentration and brew time on electrophile scavenging. *Mutation Research. Fundamental and Molecular Mechanisms of Mutagenesis*, *402*(1–2), 299–306. DOI: 10.1016/S0027-5107(97)00309-6 PMID: 9675318

Hotti, H., & Rischer, H. (2017). The killer of Socrates: Coniine and related alkaloids in the plant kingdom. *Molecules (Basel, Switzerland)*, *22*(11), 1962. https://pmc.ncbi.nlm.nih.gov/articles/PMC6150177/. DOI: 10.3390/molecules22111962 PMID: 29135964

Hussain, S. Z., Naseer, B., Qadri, T., Fatima, T., & Bhat, T. A. (2021). Ber/jujube (*Ziziphus mauritiana*): Morphology, taxonomy, composition and health benefits. In *Fruits grown in highland regions of the Himalayas* (pp. 157–168).

Hussein, R. A., & El-Anssary, A. A. (2018, November 5). Plants secondary metabolites: The key drivers of the pharmacological actions of medicinal plants. In *Herbal Medicine*. IntechOpen. https://www.intechopen.com/chapters/61866

Hwang, Y. P., Oh, K. N., Yun, H. J., & Jeong, H. G. (2011). The flavonoids apigenin and luteolin suppress ultraviolet A-induced matrix metalloproteinase-1 expression via MAPKs and AP-1-dependent signaling in HaCaT cells. *Journal of Dermatological Science*, *61*(1), 23–31. DOI: 10.1016/j.jdermsci.2010.10.016 PMID: 21112745

Ibrahim, H., Aziz, A. N., Syamsir, D. R., Ali, N. A. M., Mohtar, M., Ali, R. M., & Awang, K. (2009). Essential oils of *Alpinia conchigera* Griff. and their antimicrobial activities. *Food Chemistry*, *113*(2), 575–577. DOI: 10.1016/j.foodchem.2008.08.033

Iqbal, S., Omara, T., Kahwa, I., & Khan, U. M. (2024). Anticancer potential of delphinidin and its derivatives: Therapeutic and mechanistic insights. *Medicinal Chemistry Research*, *33*(10), 1769–1786. DOI: 10.1007/s00044-024-03296-y

Ivanović, M., Makoter, K., & Razboršek, M. I. (2021). Comparative study of chemical composition and antioxidant activity of essential oils and crude extracts of four characteristic Zingiberaceae herbs. *Plants*, *10*(3), 501. https://www.mdpi.com/2223-7747/10/3/501/htm. DOI: 10.3390/plants10030501 PMID: 33800364

Jabir, N. R., Firoz, C. K., Zughaibi, T. A., Alsaadi, M. A., Abuzenadah, A. M., Al-Asmari, A. I., Alsaieedi, A., Ahmed, B. A., Ramu, A. K., & Tabrez, S. (2022). A literature perspective on the pharmacological applications of yohimbine. *Annals of Medicine*, *54*(1), 2861. https://pmc.ncbi.nlm.nih.gov/articles/PMC9590431/. DOI: 10.1080/07853890.2022.2131330 PMID: 36263866

Jäger, S., Trojan, H., Kopp, T., Laszczyk, M. N., & Scheffler, A. (2009). Pentacyclic triterpene distribution in various plants – Rich sources for a new group of multi-potent plant extracts. *Molecules (Basel, Switzerland)*, *14*(6), 2016–2031. https://www.mdpi.com/1420-3049/14/6/2016/htm. DOI: 10.3390/molecules14062016 PMID: 19513002

Jantan, I., & Goh, S. H. (n.d.). The essential oils of *Cinnamomum mollissimum* as natural sources of safrole and benzyl benzoate. *Journal information not available*.

Jarocka-Karpowicz, I., & Markowska, A. (2021). Therapeutic potential of jasmonic acid and its derivatives. *International Journal of Molecular Sciences*, *22*(16), 8437. https://www.mdpi.com/1422-0067/22/16/8437/htm. DOI: 10.3390/ijms22168437 PMID: 34445138

Jawhari, F. Z., Moussaoui, A. E. L., Bourhia, M., Imtara, H., Saghrouchni, H., Ammor, K., Ouassou, H., Elamine, Y., Ullah, R., Ezzeldin, E., Mostafa, G. A. E., & Bari, A. (2021). *Anacyclus pyrethrum* var. *pyrethrum* (L.) and *Anacyclus pyrethrum* var. *depressus* (Ball) Maire: Correlation between total phenolic and flavonoid contents with antioxidant and antimicrobial activities of chemically characterized extracts. *Plants*, *10*(1), 19. DOI: 10.3390/plants10010149 PMID: 33451098

Jha, S., Trivedi, V., & Deshmukh, R. (2022). Approaches and molecular tools for targeted drug delivery in malaria infected red blood cells. In *Combination drug delivery approach as an effective therapy for various diseases* (pp. 149–172). DOI: 10.1016/B978-0-323-85873-1.00014-9

Jin, X., Guo, J. L., Wang, L., Zhong, X., Yao, W. F., Gao, H., & Liu, M.-Y. (2021). Natural products as pharmacological modulators of mitochondrial dysfunctions for the treatments of Alzheimer's disease: A comprehensive review. *European Journal of Medicinal Chemistry*, *218*, 113351. DOI: 10.1016/j.ejmech.2021.113401 PMID: 33831779

Jirovetz, L., Buchbauer, G., Stoyanova, A., & Metodiev, S. (2000). Seasonal depending variations of the composition and biological activities of Douglas Fir (Pseudotsuga menziesii) essential oils from Bulgaria. *Scientia Pharmaceutica*, *68*(3), 323–328. DOI: 10.3797/scipharm.aut-00-30

Kager, N., Ferk, F., Kundi, M., Wagner, K. H., Mišík, M., & Knasmüller, S. (2010). Prevention of oxidative DNA damage in inner organs and lymphocytes of rats by green tea extract. *European Journal of Nutrition*, *49*(4), 227–234. https://link.springer.com/article/10.1007/s00394-009-0068-0. DOI: 10.1007/s00394-009-0068-0 PMID: 19851801

Kairey, L., Agnew, T., Bowles, E. J., Barkla, B. J., Wardle, J., & Lauche, R. (2023). Efficacy and safety of *Melaleuca alternifolia* (tea tree) oil for human health—A systematic review of randomized controlled trials. *Frontiers in Pharmacology*, *14*, 1116077. DOI: 10.3389/fphar.2023.1116077 PMID: 37033604

Kamaraj, S., Ramakrishnan, G., Anandakumar, P., Jagan, S., & Devaki, T. (2009). Antioxidant and anticancer efficacy of hesperidin in benzo(a)pyrene induced lung carcinogenesis in mice. *Investigational New Drugs*, *27*(3), 214–222. https://link.springer.com/article/10.1007/s10637-008-9159-7. DOI: 10.1007/s10637-008-9159-7 PMID: 18704264

Kamatou, G. P. P., Vermaak, I., Viljoen, A. M., & Lawrence, B. M. (2013). Menthol: A simple monoterpene with remarkable biological properties. *Phytochemistry*, *96*, 15–25. DOI: 10.1016/j.phytochem.2013.08.005 PMID: 24054028

Kamel, N. A., Ismail, N. S. M., Yahia, I. S., & Aboshanab, K. M. (2022). Potential role of colchicine in combating COVID-19 cytokine storm and its ability to inhibit protease enzyme of SARS-CoV-2 as conferred by molecular docking analysis. *Medicina*, *58*(1), 1–16. PMID: 35056328

Kang, S. H., Bak, D. H., Chung, B. Y., Bai, H. W., & Kang, B. S. (2020). Delphinidin enhances radio-therapeutic effects via autophagy induction and JNK/MAPK pathway activation in non-small cell lung cancer. *The Korean Journal of Physiology & Pharmacology; Official Journal of the Korean Physiological Society and the Korean Society of Pharmacology*, *24*(5), 413–422. DOI: 10.4196/kjpp.2020.24.5.413 PMID: 32830148

Khan, M. T. H., Orhan, I., Şenol, F. S., Kartal, M., Şener, B., Dvorská, M., Šmejkal, K., & Šlapetová, T. (2009). Cholinesterase inhibitory activities of some flavonoid derivatives and chosen xanthone and their molecular docking studies. *Chemico-Biological Interactions*, *181*(3), 383–389. DOI: 10.1016/j.cbi.2009.06.024 PMID: 19596285

Kohnen-Johannsen, K. L., & Kayser, O. (2019). Tropane alkaloids: Chemistry, pharmacology, biosynthesis and production. *Molecules (Basel, Switzerland)*, *24*(4), 796. https://pmc.ncbi.nlm.nih.gov/articles/PMC6412926/. DOI: 10.3390/molecules24040796 PMID: 30813289

Kopustinskiene, D. M., Jakstas, V., Savickas, A., & Bernatoniene, J. (2020). Flavonoids as anticancer agents. *Nutrients*, *12*(2), 457. https://pubmed.ncbi.nlm.nih.gov/32059369/. DOI: 10.3390/nu12020457 PMID: 32059369

Kresty, L. A., Mallery, S. R., & Stoner, G. D. (2016). Black raspberries in cancer clinical trials: Past, present and future. *Journal of Berry Research*, *6*(2), 251–261. https://pmc.ncbi.nlm.nih.gov/articles/PMC5008867/. DOI: 10.3233/JBR-160125 PMID: 27594930

Kris-Etherton, P. M., Hecker, K. D., Bonanome, A., Coval, S. M., Binkoski, A. E., Hilpert, K. F., Griel, A. E., & Etherton, T. D. (2002). Bioactive compounds in foods: Their role in the prevention of cardiovascular disease and cancer. *The American Journal of Medicine*, *113*(9, Suppl 2), 71–88. DOI: 10.1016/S0002-9343(01)00995-0 PMID: 12566142

Kumar, M., Singh, S. K., Singh, P. P., Singh, V. K., Rai, A. C., Srivastava, A. K., Shukla, L., Kesawat, M. S., Kumar Jaiswal, A., Chung, S.-M., & Kumar, A. (2021). Potential anti-mycobacterium tuberculosis activity of plant secondary metabolites: Insight with molecular docking interactions. *Antioxidants*, *10*(12), 1911. DOI: 10.3390/antiox10121990 PMID: 34943093

Lazaraki, G., Chatzimavroudis, G., & Katsinelos, P. (2014). Recent advances in pharmacological treatment of irritable bowel syndrome. *World Journal of Gastroenterology*, *20*(27), 8867–8885. https://pmc.ncbi.nlm.nih.gov/articles/PMC4112893/ PMID: 25083060

Lengai, G. M. W., Muthomi, J. W., & Mbega, E. R. (2020). Phytochemical activity and role of botanical pesticides in pest management for sustainable agricultural crop production. *Scientific African*, *7*, e00239. DOI: 10.1016/j.sciaf.2019.e00239

Leung, Y. Y., & Hui, Y. L. L., & Kraus, V. B. (2015). Colchicine — Update on mechanisms of action and therapeutic uses. *Seminars in Arthritis and Rheumatism*, *45*(3), 341–350. https://pmc.ncbi.nlm.nih.gov/articles/PMC4656054/

Li, X., Yuan, W., Wu, J., Zhen, J., Sun, Q., & Yu, M. (2022). Andrographolide, a natural anti-inflammatory agent: An update. [http://www.symmap]. *Frontiers in Pharmacology*, *13*, 920435. DOI: 10.3389/fphar.2022.920435 PMID: 36238575

Li, Y., Zhou, Y., Wu, J., Li, J., & Yao, H. (2021). Phelligridin D from *Inonotus obliquus* attenuates oxidative stress and accumulation of ECM in mesangial cells under high glucose via activating Nrf2. *Journal of Natural Medicines*, *75*(4), 1021–1029. DOI: 10.1007/s11418-021-01534-w PMID: 34052991

Liao, F. (2009). Discovery of artemisinin (Qinghaosu). *Molecules (Basel, Switzerland)*, *14*(12), 5362–5366. https://www.mdpi.com/1420-3049/14/12/5362/htm. DOI: 10.3390/molecules14125362

Lin, D., Xiao, M., Zhao, J., Li, Z., Xing, B., Li, X., Kong, M., Li, L., Zhang, Q., Liu, Y., Chen, H., Qin, W., Wu, H., & Chen, S. (2016). An overview of plant phenolic compounds and their importance in human nutrition and management of type 2 diabetes. *Molecules (Basel, Switzerland)*, *21*(10), 1374. https://pmc.ncbi.nlm.nih.gov/articles/PMC6274266/. DOI: 10.3390/molecules21101374 PMID: 27754463

Liu, B., Fan, L., Balakrishna, S., Sui, A., Morris, J. B., & Jordt, S. E. (2013). TRPM8 is the principal mediator of menthol-induced analgesia of acute and inflammatory pain. *Pain, 154*(10), 2169–2177. https://pmc.ncbi.nlm.nih.gov/articles/PMC3778045/ . DOI: 10.1016/j.pain.2013.06.043 PMID: 23820004

Liu, I. M., Tsai, C. C., Lai, T. Y., & Cheng, J. T. (2001). Stimulatory effect of isoferulic acid on α1A-adrenoceptor to increase glucose uptake into cultured myoblast C2C12 cell of mice. *Autonomic Neuroscience, 88*(3), 175–180. DOI: 10.1016/S1566-0702(01)00241-7 PMID: 11474559

Malunga, L. N., Eck, P., & Beta, T. (2016). Inhibition of intestinal α-glucosidase and glucose absorption by feruloylated arabinoxylan mono- and oligosaccharides from corn bran and wheat aleurone. *Journal of Nutrition and Metabolism, 2016*, 1932532. Advance online publication. DOI: 10.1155/2016/1932532 PMID: 27073693

Mingoia, M., Conte, C., Di Rienzo, A., Dimmito, M. P., Marinucci, L., Magi, G., Turkez, H., Cufaro, M. C., Del Boccio, P., Di Stefano, A., & Cacciatore, I. (2022). Synthesis and biological evaluation of novel cinnamic acid-based antimicrobials. *Pharmaceuticals (Basel, Switzerland), 15*(2), 219. DOI: 10.3390/ph15020228 PMID: 35215340

Mohamed, M. A., Mahdy, E. S. M. E., Ghazy, A. E. H. M., Ibrahim, N. M., El-Mezayen, H. A., & Ghanem, M. M. E. (2016). The activity of detoxifying enzymes in the infective juveniles of *Heterorhabditis bacteriophora* strains: Purification and characterization of two acetylcholinesterases. *Comparative Biochemistry and Physiology. Toxicology & Pharmacology : CBP, 180*, 11–22. https://pubmed.ncbi.nlm.nih.gov/26545490/. DOI: 10.1016/j.cbpc.2015.10.014 PMID: 26545490

Monteiro Espíndola, K. M., Ferreira, R. G., Mosquera Narvaez, L. E., Rocha Silva Rosario, A. C., Machado Da Silva, A. H., & Bispo Silva, A. G.. (2019). Chemical and pharmacological aspects of caffeic acid and its activity in hepatocarcinoma. *Frontiers in Oncology, 9*, 467241. DOI: 10.3389/fonc.2019.00541 PMID: 31293975

Moses, T., Pollier, J., Thevelein, J. M., & Goossens, A. (2013). Bioengineering of plant (tri)terpenoids: From metabolic engineering of plants to synthetic biology in vivo and in vitro. *The New Phytologist, 200*(1), 27–43. DOI: 10.1111/nph.12325 PMID: 23668256

Muteeb, G., Rehman, M. T., Shahwan, M., & Aatif, M. (2023). Origin of antibiotics and antibiotic resistance, and their impacts on drug development: A narrative review. *Pharmaceuticals (Basel, Switzerland), 16*(11), 1615. DOI: 10.3390/ph16111615 PMID: 38004480

Mutha, R. E., Tatiya, A. U., & Surana, S. J. (2021). Flavonoids as natural phenolic compounds and their role in therapeutics: An overview. *Future Journal of Pharmaceutical Sciences*, *7*(1), 1–13. DOI: 10.1186/s43094-020-00161-8 PMID: 33495733

Nichenametla, S. N., Taruscio, T. G., Barney, D. L., & Exon, J. H. (2006). A review of the effects and mechanisms of polyphenolics in cancer. *Critical Reviews in Food Science and Nutrition*, *46*(2), 161–183. DOI: 10.1080/10408390591000541 PMID: 16431408

Okla, M. K., Alatar, A. A., Al-Amri, S. S., Soufan, W. H., Ahmad, A., & Abdel-Maksoud, M. A. (2021). Antibacterial and antifungal activity of the extracts of different parts of *Avicennia marina* (Forssk.) Vierh. *Plants*, *10*(2), 380. DOI: 10.3390/plants10020252 PMID: 33525519

Okunade, A. L., Hufford, C. D., Clark, A. M., & Lentz, D. (1997). Antimicrobial properties of the constituents of *Piper aduncum.Phytotherapy Research*, *11*(2), 142–144. DOI: 10.1002/(SICI)1099-1573(199703)11:2<142::AID-PTR61>3.0.CO;2-Y

Onyenekwe, P. C., & Hashimoto, S. (1999). The composition of the essential oil of dried Nigerian ginger (*Zingiber officinale* Roscoe). *European Food Research and Technology*, *209*(6), 407–410. DOI: 10.1007/s002170050517

Oršolić, N., Kunštić, M., Kukolj, M., Gračan, R., & Nemrava, J. (2016). Oxidative stress, polarization of macrophages and tumour angiogenesis: Efficacy of caffeic acid. *Chemico-Biological Interactions*, *256*, 111–124. DOI: 10.1016/j.cbi.2016.06.027 PMID: 27378625

Owen, L. N. (1947). *The Terpenes.: The Simpler Acyclic and Monocyclic Terpenes & Their Derivatives*. University Press.

Pacios-Michelena, A., Kasaragod, V. B., & Schindelin, H. (2021). Artemisinins and their impact on inhibitory neurotransmission. *Current Opinion in Pharmacology*, *59*, 19–25. DOI: 10.1016/j.coph.2021.04.008 PMID: 34051675

Pereira, I., Severino, P., Santos, A. C., Silva, A. M., & Souto, E. B. (2018). Linalool bioactive properties and potential applicability in drug delivery systems. *Colloids and Surfaces. B, Biointerfaces*, *171*, 566–578. DOI: 10.1016/j.colsurfb.2018.08.001 PMID: 30098535

Poltanov, E. A., Shikov, A. N., Dorman, H. J. D., Pozharitskaya, O. N., Makarov, V. G., Tikhonov, V. P., & Hiltunen, R. (2009). Chemical and antioxidant evaluation of Indian gooseberry (*Emblica officinalis* Gaertn., syn. *Phyllanthus emblica* L.) supplements. *Phytotherapy Research, 23*(9), 1309–1315. DOI: 10.1002/ptr.2775 PMID: 19172666

Prabhakar, P. K., & Doble, M. (2011). Interaction of cinnamic acid derivatives with commercial hypoglycemic drugs on 2-deoxyglucose uptake in 3T3-L1 adipocytes. *Journal of Agricultural and Food Chemistry*, *59*(18), 9835–9844. DOI: 10.1021/jf2015717 PMID: 21870829

Prats, E., Galindo, J. C., Bazzalo, M. E., León, A., Macías, F. A., Rubiales, D., & Jorrín, J. V. (2007). Antifungal activity of a new phenolic compound from capitulum of a head rot-resistant sunflower genotype. *Journal of Chemical Ecology*, *33*(12), 2245–2253. DOI: 10.1007/s10886-007-9388-9 PMID: 18034282

Puri, S., Hegde, N., Sawant, S., Latambale, G., & Juvale, K. (2023). Applications of phytochemicals in cancer therapy and anticancer drug development. In *Recent frontiers of phytochemicals: Applications in food, pharmacy, cosmetics, and biotechnology* (pp. 335–351). DOI: 10.1016/B978-0-443-19143-5.00026-8

Ramage, G., Saville, S. P., Wickes, B. L., & López-Ribot, J. L. (2002). Inhibition of *Candida albicans* biofilm formation by farnesol, a quorum-sensing molecule. *Applied and Environmental Microbiology*, *68*(11), 5459–5463. https://pmc.ncbi.nlm.nih.gov/articles/PMC129887/. DOI: 10.1128/AEM.68.11.5459-5463.2002 PMID: 12406738

Robb, E. L., Regina, A. C., & Baker, M. B. (2023). Organophosphate toxicity. In *StatPearls*. https://www.ncbi.nlm.nih.gov/books/NBK470430/

Roe, F. J. (1964). The chronic toxicity of naturally-occurring substances. Essential oils. *Food and Cosmetics Toxicology*, *2*, 681–682. DOI: 10.1016/S0015-6264(64)80059-0 PMID: 14282280

Salvatori, E. S., Morgan, L. V., Ferrarini, S., Zilli, G. A. L., Rosina, A., Almeida, M. O. P., Hackbart, H. C. S., Rezende, R. S., Albeny-Simões, D., Oliveira, J. V., Gasparetto, A., Müller, L. G., & Dal Magro, J. (2023). Anti-inflammatory and antimicrobial effects of *Eucalyptus* spp. essential oils: A potential valuable use for an industry byproduct. *Evidence-Based Complementary and Alternative Medicine : eCAM*, *2023*(1), 2582698. https://pmc.ncbi.nlm.nih.gov/articles/PMC10322318/. DOI: 10.1155/2023/2582698 PMID: 37416804

Sanna, C., Marengo, A., Acquadro, S., Caredda, A., Lai, R., Corona, A., Tramontano, E., Rubiolo, P., & Esposito, F. (2021). In vitro, anti-HIV-1 reverse transcriptase and integrase properties of *Punica granatum* L. leaves, bark, and peel extracts and their main compounds. *Plants*, *10*(10), 2124. https://pubmed.ncbi.nlm.nih.gov/34685933/ . DOI: 10.3390/plants10102124 PMID: 34685933

Schlesinger, N., Firestein, B. L., & Brunetti, L. (2020). Colchicine in COVID-19: An old drug, new use. *Current Pharmacology Reports*, *6*(4), 137–145. https://link.springer.com/article/10.1007/s40495-020-00225-6. DOI: 10.1007/s40495-020-00225-6 PMID: 32837853

Serrano, J., Puupponen-Pimiä, R., Dauer, A., Aura, A. M., & Saura-Calixto, F. (2009). Tannins: Current knowledge of food sources, intake, bioavailability and biological effects. *Molecular Nutrition & Food Research*, *53*(S2, Suppl. 2), S310–S329. DOI: 10.1002/mnfr.200900039 PMID: 19437486

Siddiqui, M. Z. (2011). *Boswellia serrata*, a potential anti-inflammatory agent: An overview. *Indian Journal of Pharmaceutical Sciences*, *73*(3), 255. https://pmc.ncbi.nlm.nih.gov/articles/PMC3309643/ PMID: 22457547

Song, Y., Liu, H., Quax, W. J., Zhang, Z., Chen, Y., Yang, P., Cui, Y., Shi, Q., & Xie, X. (2024). Application of valencene and prospects for its production in engineered microorganisms. *Frontiers in Microbiology*, *15*, 1444099. https://www.basf.com/jp/en/media/news-releases/. DOI: 10.3389/fmicb.2024.1444099 PMID: 39171255

Spagnuolo, C., Russo, G. L., Orhan, I. E., Habtemariam, S., Daglia, M., Sureda, A., Nabavi, S. F., Devi, K. P., Loizzo, M. R., Tundis, R., & Nabavi, S. M. (2015). Genistein and cancer: Current status, challenges, and future directions. *Advances in Nutrition*, *6*(4), 408–419. DOI: 10.3945/an.114.008052 PMID: 26178025

Spinks, A., & Wasiak, J. (2011). Scopolamine (hyoscine) for preventing and treating motion sickness. *Cochrane Database of Systematic Reviews*, *2011*(6), CD002851. https://pmc.ncbi.nlm.nih.gov/articles/PMC7138049/. DOI: 10.1002/14651858.CD002851.pub4 PMID: 21678338

Stagos, D., Amoutzias, G. D., Matakos, A., Spyrou, A., Tsatsakis, A. M., & Kouretas, D. (2012). Chemoprevention of liver cancer by plant polyphenols. *Food and Chemical Toxicology*, *50*(6), 2155–2170. DOI: 10.1016/j.fct.2012.04.002 PMID: 22521445

Su, J., Yang, L., Sun, Z., & Zhan, X. (2024). Personalized drug therapy: Innovative concept guided with proteoformics. *Molecular & Cellular Proteomics*, *23*(3), 100737. DOI: 10.1016/j.mcpro.2024.100737 PMID: 38354979

Syed, D., Chamcheu, J. C., Adhami, V., & Mukhtar, H. (2013). Pomegranate extracts and cancer prevention: Molecular and cellular activities. *Anti-cancer Agents in Medicinal Chemistry, 13*(8), 1149–1161. https://pubmed.ncbi.nlm.nih.gov/23094914/ . DOI: 10.2174/1871520611313080003 PMID: 23094914

Takahashi, A., & Ohnishi, T. (2004). The significance of the study about the biological effects of solar ultraviolet radiation using the exposed facility on the International Space Station. *Uchu Seibutsu Kagaku, 18*(4), 255–260. DOI: 10.2187/bss.18.255 PMID: 15858393

Thirumurugan, D., Cholarajan, A., Raja, S. S., & Vijayakumar, R. (2018). An introductory chapter: secondary metabolites. Secondary metabolites-sources and applications, 1, 13.

Thirumurugan, D., Cholarajan, A., Raja, S. S. S., & Vijayakumar, R. (2018, September 5). An introductory chapter: Secondary metabolites. In *Secondary metabolites - Sources and applications*. IntechOpen. DOI: 10.5772/intechopen.79766

Tisserand, R., & Young, R. (2014). *Essential oil safety: A guide for health care professionals* (2nd ed.). Elsevier.

Tong, L., Zhao, Q., Datan, E., Lin, G. Q., Minn, I., Pomper, M. G., Yu, B., Romo, D., He, Q.-L., & Liu, J. O. (2021). Triptolide: Reflections on two decades of research and prospects for the future. *Natural Product Reports, 38*(4), 843–860. https://pubs.rsc.org/en/content/articlehtml/2021/np/d0np00054j. DOI: 10.1039/D0NP00054J PMID: 33146205

Tuli, H. S., Tuorkey, M. J., Thakral, F., Sak, K., Kumar, M., Sharma, A. K., Sharma, U., Jain, A., Aggarwal, V., & Bishayee, A. (2019). Molecular mechanisms of action of genistein in cancer: Recent advances. *Frontiers in Pharmacology, 10*, 489844. DOI: 10.3389/fphar.2019.01336 PMID: 31866857

Tungmunnithum, D., Thongboonyou, A., Pholboon, A., & Yangsabai, A. (2018). Flavonoids and other phenolic compounds from medicinal plants for pharmaceutical and medical aspects: An overview. *Medicines (Basel, Switzerland), 5*(3), 93. https://pmc.ncbi.nlm.nih.gov/articles/PMC6165118/. DOI: 10.3390/medicines5030093 PMID: 30149600

Turnbull, D., Rodricks, J. V., Mariano, G. F., & Chowdhury, F. (2017). Caffeine and cardiovascular health. *Regulatory Toxicology and Pharmacology, 89*, 165–185. DOI: 10.1016/j.yrtph.2017.07.025 PMID: 28756014

Twaij, B. M., & Hasan, M. N. (2022). Bioactive secondary metabolites from plant sources: Types, synthesis, and their therapeutic uses. *International Journal of Plant Biology, 13*(1), 4–14. https://www.mdpi.com/2037-0164/13/1/3/htm. DOI: 10.3390/ijpb13010003

Tyagi, A. K., Prasad, S., Yuan, W., Li, S., & Aggarwal, B. B. (2015). Identification of a novel compound (β-sesquiphellandrene) from turmeric (*Curcuma longa*) with anticancer potential: Comparison with curcumin. *Investigational New Drugs, 33*(6), 1175–1186. DOI: 10.1007/s10637-015-0296-5 PMID: 26521943

Verma, R. S., Padalia, R. C., Chauhan, A., Verma, R. K., ur Rahman, L., & Singh, A. (2016). Changes in the essential oil composition of *Origanum majorana* L. during post-harvest drying. *Journal of Essential Oil-Bearing Plants, 19*(6), 1547–1552. DOI: 10.1080/0972060X.2014.935039

Vidović, B. B., Milinčić, D. D., Marčetić, M. D., Djuriš, J. D., Ilić, T. D., Kostić, A., & Pešić, M. B. (2022). Health benefits and applications of goji berries in functional food products development: A review. *Antioxidants, 11*(2), 248. https://pmc.ncbi.nlm.nih.gov/articles/PMC8868247/. DOI: 10.3390/antiox11020248 PMID: 35204130

Vishwanath, V., & Rao, H. M. (2019). Gutta-percha in endodontics - A comprehensive review of material science. *Journal of Conservative Dentistry : JCD, 22*(3), 216. https://pmc.ncbi.nlm.nih.gov/articles/PMC6632621/. DOI: 10.4103/JCD.JCD_420_18 PMID: 31367101

Wei, J., Wang, L., Zhu, J., Zhang, S., Nandi, O. I., & Kang, L. (2007). Plants attract parasitic wasps to defend themselves against insect pests by releasing hexenol. *PLoS One, 2*(9), e852. https://journals.plos.org/plosone/article?id=10.1371/journal.pone.0000852. DOI: 10.1371/journal.pone.0000852 PMID: 17786223

Wojtyczka, R. D., Dziedzic, A., K pa, M., Kubina, R., Kabała-Dzik, A., Mularz, T., & Idzik, D. (2014). Berberine enhances the antibacterial activity of selected antibiotics against coagulase-negative *Staphylococcus* strains *in vitro.Molecules (Basel, Switzerland), 19*(5), 6583–6596. https://pmc.ncbi.nlm.nih.gov/articles/PMC6272005/. DOI: 10.3390/molecules19056583 PMID: 24858093

Wu, Y., Ren, D., Gao, C., Li, J., Du, B., Wang, Z., & Qian, S. (2021). Recent advances for alkaloids as botanical pesticides for use in organic agriculture. *International Journal of Pest Management, 69*(3), 288–298. https://www.tandfonline.com/doi/abs/10.1080/09670874.2021.1917723. DOI: 10.1080/09670874.2021.1917723

Xia, E., Wang, B., Xu, X., Zhu, L., Song, Y., & Li, H. B. (2011). Microwave-assisted extraction of oleanolic acid and ursolic acid from *Ligustrum lucidum* Ait. *International Journal of Molecular Sciences*, *12*(8), 5319–5329. https://www.mdpi.com/1422-0067/12/8/5319. DOI: 10.3390/ijms12085319 PMID: 21954361

Yadav, P. B. S., & Karuppusamy, S. (2024). Botany of *Andrographis wall. ex Nees* (Andrographinae: Acanthaceae). In *Andrographolide and its analogs: Botanical sources, phytochemistry, pharmacology, and biotechnology* (pp. 10–29). Bentham Science Publishers.

Yang, W., Chen, X., Li, Y., Guo, S., Wang, Z., & Yu, X. (2020). Advances in pharmacological activities of terpenoids. *Natural Product Communications*, *15*(3), 1934578X20903555. Advance online publication. DOI: 10.1177/1934578X20903555

Yeh, M. H., Kao, S. T., Hung, C. M., Liu, C. J., Lee, K. H., & Yeh, C. C. (2009). Hesperidin inhibited acetaldehyde-induced matrix metalloproteinase-9 gene expression in human hepatocellular carcinoma cells. *Toxicology Letters*, *184*(3), 204–210. DOI: 10.1016/j.toxlet.2008.11.018 PMID: 19110045

Youness, R. A., Kamel, R., Elkasabgy, N. A., Shao, P., & Farag, M. A. (2021). Recent advances in tannic acid (gallotannin) anticancer activities and drug delivery systems for efficacy improvement: A comprehensive review. *Molecules (Basel, Switzerland)*, *26*(5). Advance online publication. https://pubmed.ncbi.nlm.nih.gov/33803294/. DOI: 10.3390/molecules26051486 PMID: 33803294

Zhang, Y., Jiang, P., Ye, M., Kim, S. H., Jiang, C., & Lü, J. (2012). Tanshinones: Sources, pharmacokinetics and anti-cancer activities. *International Journal of Molecular Sciences*, *13*(10), 13621–13666. https://pmc.ncbi.nlm.nih.gov/articles/PMC3497345/. DOI: 10.3390/ijms131013621 PMID: 23202971

Zhao, H., Wu, L., Yan, G., Chen, Y., Zhou, M., Wu, Y., & Li, Y. (2021). Inflammation and tumor progression: Signaling pathways and targeted intervention. *Signal Transduction and Targeted Therapy*, *6*(1), 1–46. https://www.nature.com/articles/s41392-021-00658-5. DOI: 10.1038/s41392-021-00658-5 PMID: 34248142

Chapter 11
Secondary Metabolites of Carob Tree (Ceratonia siliqua L.): Potential Applications

Yassine Mouniane
https://orcid.org/0000-0002-6037-5301
Laboratory of Natural Resources and Sustainable Development, Faculty of Sciences, Ibn Tofaïl University, Morocco

Yassine Kadmi
LASIRE, Equipe Physico-Chimie de l'Environnement, CNRS UMR 8516, Université Lille, France

Meryem Doubi
https://orcid.org/0009-0000-3812-316X
Faculty of Sciences, Ibn Tofail University, Kenitra, Morocco

Salma Tabi
Department of Life Sciences, Faculty of Science and Technology, Sultan Moulay Slimane University, Morocco

Issam El-Khadir
https://orcid.org/0000-0002-3970-2865
Faculty of Sciences, Ibn Tofail University, Kenitra, Morocco

Ahmed Chriqui
Faculty of Sciences, Ibn Tofail University, Kenitra, Morocco

Abdelaati Soufiani
https://orcid.org/0000-0002-5164-7707
Faculty of Sciences, Ibn Tofail University, Kenitra, Morocco

Brahim El Ouardi
https://orcid.org/0009-0000-4559-6141
Faculty of Sciences, Ibn Tofail University, Kenitra, Morocco

Khawla Rachmoune
https://orcid.org/0009-0001-6483-1060
Interdisciplinary Laboratory of Research in Bio-Resources, Environment and Materials, Higher Normal School, Cadi Ayyad University, 40000 Marrakech, Morocco

DOI: 10.4018/979-8-3693-9112-9.ch011

Amir Souissi
https://orcid.org/0000-0002-4418-5807
Swift Current Research and Development Centre, Agriculture and Agrifood Canada, Canada

Arpit Sharma
CHEORS, RWE, India

Shelika Joshi
Walden University, Canada

Mohammed Choukri Belkadi
https://orcid.org/0009-0009-7628-8358
Faculty of Medicine and Pharmacy, University Mohammed the First, Oujda, Morocco

Driss Hmouni
https://orcid.org/0000-0001-7598-6204
Faculty of Sciences, Ibn Tofail University, Kenitra, Morocco

ABSTRACT

Research into these bioactive compounds will allow us to better understand their contribution to health benefits. Carob (Ceratonia siliqua L.) is a Mediterranean species rich in secondary metabolites such as polyphenols, flavonoids, and other bioactive compounds. These secondary metabolites confer important antioxidants, anti-inflammatory, and antimicrobial properties to carob, offering multiple applications in the food and pharmaceutical industries. This chapter reviews the main secondary metabolites present in carob fruits and leaves and their potential applications.

1. INTRODUCTION

Secondary metabolites are a class of organic compounds that are not essentially involved in or necessary for survival, growth or reproduction, although often crucial to the plants' own metabolism and thereby a key element in ecological systems. The familiar adage that 'Plants produce primary metabolites to grow and reproduce but synthesize secondary metabolites to survive and adapt' is a useful simplification but an overstatement of the issue, given that many secondary metabolites contribute to the health of an organism and its offspring (Lv et al., 2024) .Bioactive compounds of different classes, such as polyphenols, flavonoids, tannins, alkaloids and terpenes, play specific roles in the protection mechanisms of plants like defense against herbivores and pests, tolerance of environmental stresses, and adaptation to environmental change (Lv et al., 24). Plants often create secondary metabolites because of their defensive function or other interaction with other organisms in their environment, including pathogens, herbivorous animals, or competing plants. However, in recent years, increasing attention is being paid to these phytochemicals for their important pharmacological food and cosmetic properties (Zhu et al. 2019; Ahanger et al. 2020).

The bioactive compounds present in plants offer a wide array of properties, including antioxidant, anti-inflammatory, antimicrobial and anticancer among many others, become very important, as they form the basis of many new medicines introduced to the market (Fogarasi et al., 2024). Carob tree, *Ceratonia siliqua* L. an evergreen tree is famous not only for its numerous traditional uses but is also recognized for its health and nutritional benefits, as it is rich in phenolic compounds and especially witnessed in antioxidant properties, which has supported and increased its reputation worldwide. This nutrient-dense superfood is from the pea family and originates from the Mediterranean area where its pods have been harvested for thousands of years as medicine and food. Botanically, carob is in the subfamily Caesalpinioideae and is part of the legume family, Fabaceae. This plant thrives in extremely dry areas with low quality soils (Mouniane et al., 2024). The carob tree is a native to the Mediterranean countries where it is used for centuries for its fruits that are edible directly from the trees, are used to prepare lots of dishes or are used to prepare a flour substitute which is becoming very popular in bakery goods. This valuable and drought-tolerant plant is also widely used in land rehabilitation and afforestation programs (Batlle & Tous, 1997). The carob tree is grown commercially in several Mediterranean countries, the major supply of bioactive compounds of the plant are in good quantities in its pods, seeds, and leaves. These bioactive compounds are what give carob powder a high antioxidant capacity and its ability to confer anti-inflammatory and antioxidant activity on both humans and animals.

Thus, carob powder may have numerous cardiac health advantages along with other national disease risk factors and added value to longevity. Multiple research publications validate this. (Ben Ayache et al., 2020; Brassesco et al., 2021). In this chapter, I will discuss the secondary metabolites of carob and their bioactive properties and provide a slight overview on their major application constituents.

2. SECONDARY METABOLITES OF CAROB

Active components like polyphenols, flavonoids, and tannins with positive impacts on our bodies are present in carob leaves. These leaves have been known for their medicinal qualities (Ghanemi et al., 2017; Ghanemi & Belarbi, 2021). Flavonols are, however, the most abundant in carob including carob's richest flavonoids – quercetin, myricetin, camphirose and their glycosidic derivatives such as rhamnoside quercetin and rhamnoside myricetin. Quercetin, myricetin and kaempferol are flavonols, apigenin, chrysoeriol and luteolin are flavones, naringenin and havanensin are from flavanones, and genistein is an isoflavone. Usually, these components have a negligible presence. (Owen et al., 2003; Papagiannopoulos et al., 2004; Ortega et al., 2009) which suggests that – Leaves. Perhaps a valuable and natural supplier of biologically beneficial constituents. However, for the *C. siliqua* sample assessed, no aglycones were found (Abidar et el., 2020). Indeed, very few studies connected with possible carob is have been assumed that the leaves of carob are treated as an industrial waste in the processing of carob fruit (Elbouzidi et al., 2023).

Figure 1. Chemical structures of major phenolic compounds from carob pods and leaves (Rtibi et al., 2017)

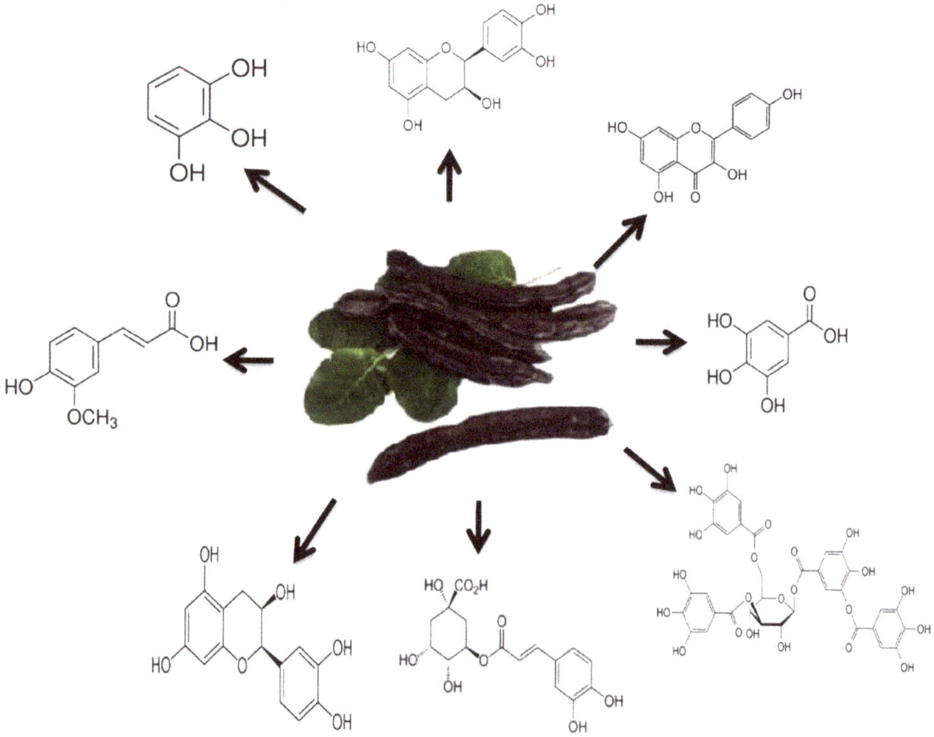

2.1. Polyphenols

The study conducted by Dallali et al. (2018) has highlighted the potential presence of total phenolic content in carob tree leaves ranging from a low of 2.50 and a variable high of 6.45 mg EGA/g DW, this indicates a high concentration of bioactive compounds which emphasizes the antioxidant potential of the leaves and therefore, their potential in health-promoting applications owing to their role in the scavenging of free radicals. The leaves of the carob tree are high in polyphenols, essentially there is found an average of total polyphenols (GAE) per 100 g of dry material in male carob trees at 28.8 g, for the female trees at 30.7 g, and the hermaphrodite tree averaged 12.3 g (Custódio et al., 2007). Elbouzidi et al. (2023) concluded that the phenolic content in carob leaves is high, especially total phenolics, as it was found to contain an average of about 96.98 mg GAE (gallic acid equivalents) per 100 g of dry weight. The total polyphenolic content regarding the leaves of *Ceratonia siliqua* was markedly greater in ethanolic extracts with total polyphenolic content of 60.09 ± 0.23 grams gallic acid equivalent per 100 g of dry weight (g GAE/100 g DW) than in the aqueous extract of carob leaves, which contained only 28.67 ± 0.09 g GAE/100 g DW of total polyphenolic content. This clearly illustrates how much more efficient ethanol is at extracting phenolic substances from carob leaves (Othmen et al., 2020).

2.2. Flavonoids

Dallali et al. (2018) studied the leaves of carob (*Ceratonia siliqua* L.) and its extracts for antioxidant activity via methanolic extraction and its chemical constituents. It was reported that the total flavonoid content in the leaves of the carob tree *C. siliqua* ranged from 1.75 to 4.20 mg QE/g DW which further corroborates the significant contribution of flavonoids as an antioxidant to withstand environmental stress and stressors and underlines its possible role in efficacious health impacts. The concentration of the carob leaves flavonoids as well as their possible biological importance as an antioxidant, antimicrobial, and anticancer agent activity was reported in a study by Elbouzidi et al. 2023 which also set out to describe the profile of flavonoids from carob leaves. Metabolites showed a range of 5.92 ± 0.06 mg RE/100 g DW as total flavonoids in the leaves, thus indicating the moderate amount of flavonoids identified in the methanolic extracts. In his 2007 work, Custódio et al. (2007) concluded that the leaf extract of *C. siliqua* yielded considerable amounts of flavonoids, with the predominant sex determined to be the male at 7.0 ± 1.0 g of rutin equivalents (RE)/100 g of dry weight. The female leaves displayed the next highest RS at 5.8 ± 0.6 g RE/100 g dry weight, whilst the hermaphrodite leaves possessed the least amount with 1.6 ± 0.1 RE per 100 grams (Elbouzidi et al., 2023). As noted, the tree's sex did indeed have a noted impact on the relative concentration of its flavonoids. The value of leaf flavonoid content for the ethanolic extract was significantly higher (4.00 ± 0.02 g RE/100 g DW) compared to the aqueous extract (1.43 ± 0.00 g RE/100 g DW) which demonstrates the increased extraction capability of ethanol. Ethanol can extract and solubilizing much higher quantities of flavonoids such as apigenin, chrysoeriol, and/or quercetin unlike water (Othmen et al., 2020).

2.3. Condensed Tannis

The study conducted by Elbouzidi et al. (2023) revealed that the condensed tannins in the carob leaves extracted 29.61 mg catechin equivalents (CE) per 100 g dry weight; among the extracts in the study. Another effort also revealed that there are differences in the condensed tannins based on sex. In their study they used both the vanillin method and DMACA method to analyze the material. In accordance to the vanillin method, male trees yielded 4.4 grams of CE per 100 grams of dry material and hermaphrodite trees produced 9.7 grams of CE per 100 grams (Custódio et al., 2007). Female trees yielded 2.1 grams of CE per 100 grams. The leaves, (*Ceratonia siliqua*), contained condensed tannins, which varied in relation to the collection location. Dallali et al. (2018) reported the values of tannin as EAG per dry weight in the range of 2.50 ± 0.14 mg EAG/g and 6.45 ± 0.22 mg EAG/g, which indicates lower and upper limits. This disparity in concentration suggests an environmental cause, perhaps starker environmental conditions at certain sites which resulted in higher concentrations of tannins. The results of the study (Othmen et al., 2020) showed that condensed tannins were 18.52 ± 0.03 grams catechin equivalent of condensed tannins per 100 grams of dry weight (g CE/100 g of DW) just in the ethanolic extract, while the aqueous extract only had 2.42 ± 0.10 g CE/100 g of DW a 7.66 increase in the ethanolic extract.

3. BIOLOGICAL ACTIVITY AND THERAPEUTIC POTENTIAL OF CAROB

Phytotherapy products typically include carob for many reasons, such as its benefits for lungs and respiratory issues, including asthma and bronchitis, as it works by inducing relaxation in the upper respiratory tract, and so forth. Notably, carob can help with the risk of lung cancer promotion as OGG1 (the DNA repair protein) is improved with the use of dietary carob, also considered an antioxidant and anti-allergic because it inhibits inflammatory mediators such as histamine and cytokines. Carob is also recognized for having many vitamins and minerals, in addition, carob improves many systems in the body, including the immune system and the digestive system. The phytochemical of concern is not present in carob, which would include the toxins (such as caffeine) that could cause asthma. Thus, it is a safer ingredient to consume for treatment of asthma and cold allergies. A thickener made from locust bean gum which is carob seeds will also help provide thickeners for food products as well as added nutritional value. (Aboura et al., 2017; Azab, 2022; Dahmani et al., 2023).

Table 1. Carob parts and extraction methods for treating conditions like diabetes, cough, and cancer

Health Conditions and Therapeutic Activities	Part used	Extraction method
Diarrhea	Fruit	barks
Diabetes	Seeds or leaves	Infusion, powder
Cough	Leaves	Decoction cold or hot beverage of the pods
Antibacterial	The table details plant parts and extraction methods for treating conditions like diabetes, cough, and cancer.seeds	Alcohol or aqueous solvent
Anti-oxidant activity	Pulp	Water extraction
Anticancer, antiproliferative and related activities	Pods	Ethanolic and ethyl acetate extracts
Anxiolytic-sedative and antiproliferative	leaves and pods	Methanolic extract

Carob is a significant source of phenolic compounds that encompass phenolic acids, flavonoids, condensed tannins, and hydrolysable tannins. When absorbed in the gastrointestinal tract, carob phenolic extract will combine/disassociate with the gut microbiota and digestive enzymes that may also convert some phenolics to smaller metabolites impacting the bioactivities and subsequent health-related properties (Ydjedd et al., 2017). In addition, the monofloral carob samples from Morocco analysis mentioned potassium (K) as the major mineral element found, followed by sodium (Na); calcium (Ca) and magnesium (Mg). The concentration of these mineral elements was higher in carob honey and adds to its unique nutritional profile and its potential to offer a health benefit to humans, especially in terms of electrolytes and essential nutrients serving functions in human physiology (Boublenza et al., 2017; Ben Tahar et al., 2024).

3.1. Antioxidant Properties

3.1.1 Carob Polyphenols and Flavonoids

Polyphenols and flavonoids extracted from carob (*Ceratonia siliqua L.*) include compounds such as tannins, flavanols and anthocyanins (Brassesco et al., 2021). A new study has found that carob pod extracts contain up to 19.2% polyphenols, with high amounts of gallic acid and ellagic acid. Antioxidant activity tests, using DPPH (2,2-diphenyl-1-picrylhydrazyl) and the β-carotene-linoleic acid system, found that carob extracts are excellent at neutralizing free radicals and preventing lipid oxidation. For example, extracts with 25ug/mL concentration exhibited greater free radical scavenging capacity than some of the individual polyphenols like (+)-catechin and (-)-epicatechin (Stavrou et al., 2018). And that pods which are not frequently studied can also qualify as a functional food due to their antioxidant activity (Rico et al., 2019). Free radical scavenging activities (DPPH, hydroxyl, and nitric oxide) of CPAE were evaluated and it was found that the extract greatly suppressed the free radicals and possessed remarkable antioxidant activity (Darwish et al., 2021). Carob's methanolic extract is highly rich in polyphenolic compounds, gallic acid and catechin might be some of them which possibly averts oxidative damage by free radical neutralization and thus mitigates resulting oxidative damage. These results suggest that CPAE might be useful for future strategies aimed at combating oxidative stress. The antioxidant potential of methanolic extract of carob maybe is be by neutralizing reactive oxygen molecules and myeloperoxidase (Rtibi et al., 2017; Ioannou et al., 2023). However, the *in vitro/in vivo* antioxidant activity of most plants had not been fully aligned. As a result, the effect of methanolic extract of carob on in vivo antioxidant enzyme systems using pancreatic homogenate should be investigated dimensionality. Many useful parts of the carob tree were used in extensive testing with antioxidants and great antioxidant results were seen (Table 2). Overall, these results indicate that the carob tree has great potential for viably using it as a natural antioxidant source with exciting possibilities for in the health, food and cosmetics applications.

Table 2. Antioxidant effect of different parts of the carob tree

Part of plant used	**Results**	**Reference**
Carob pods	Roasting carob powder under specific conditions markedly increases its antiradical activity and reducing power. FRAP values rise from 20.87 mg TE/g and 0.966 mmol $FeSO_4$/g, respectively, in ABTS native carob to 36.46 mg TE/g and 2.265 mmol $FeSO_4$/g after roasting at 130°C for 30 minutes.	**Čepo et al. (2014)**
Carob pods and seeds	Roasting reduces the moisture content of carob powder from 7.90% to 1.25%, with this decrease varying according to the roasting temperature. Total phenolic content (TPC) also increases with roasting, rising from 0.570 to 1.131 g/100 g dry matter, peaking at 75 minutes before decreasing slightly. Antioxidant activity increases in parallel with phenol concentration up to the optimum temperature. Furthermore, the increase in browning index reflects the chemical changes occurring during roasting, while the slight decrease in pH suggests a change in the powder's chemical composition.	**Şahin et al. (2009)**
Carob pods	Values ranged from 1.57 to 23.48 mmol AAE/L, indicating a wide range of antioxidant capacity among the samples. Values range from 210.83 to 2277.19 µmol TE/L, also showing significant variation in antioxidant capacity.	**Rodríguez-Solana et al. (2019a)**

continued on following page

Table 2. Continued

Part of plant used	Results	Reference
Carob pods	The results indicate that the DPPH radical-scavenging capacity of CF extracts ranges from 49.68 to 155.19 μM TE/g, while for ABTS radicals it ranges from 56.24 to 200.26 μM TE/g. The reducing power, assessed by FRAP assay, ranges from 22.85 to 57.68 μM Fe^{2+}/g.	**Rašković et al. (2023)**
carob pulp	The study revealed that the antioxidant activity of carob extracts, measured by the DPPH method, improved with roasting. IC50 values decreased from 0.06 for the unroasted sample to 0.01 for the sample roasted at 150°C. In addition, total polyphenol content (TPC) increased from 0.51%, indicating that roasting improves both TPC and antioxidant activity of carob extracts.	**Boublenza et al. (2017)**
Carob pulp	Significant increase: 31x (DPPH), 1.7x (FRAP), 2.3x (ABTS) compared with control sample.	**Zahorec et al. (2024)**

3.1.2 Mechanisms of Antioxidant Properties

Free radicals, specifically reactive oxygen species, can create cellular damage through oxidative stress, which can cause cellular dysfunctions and be responsible for chronic diseases such as cardiovascular disease, type 2 diabetes, and various cancers (Reuter et al., 2010). The antioxidant actions of flavonoids can be as effective as synthetic antioxidants, promoting their inclusion into health and disease prevention formulations, assuming the flavonoids could be extracted from inexpensive sources using effective methods. The polyphenols and flavonoids in carob play a critical role in combating the free radicals. They perform their antioxidant actions by donating electrons to free radicals, forming stable complexes and diminishing harmful effects. Additionally, the antioxidants may regulate endogenous antioxidant enzymes, which enhance cellular defense against cellular oxidative stress (Sęczyk et al., 2016; Ben Ayache et al., 2020).

3.1.3 Therapeutic Applications

Carob is known to have health benefits from its high content in polyphenols and flavonoids that may play a relevant role in preventing many chronic diseases. In fact, recent research suggests that polyphenols and flavonoids present in carob be potent agents with health benefits against a range of ailments as atherosclerosis and cardiovascular diseases by inhibiting low-density lipoprotein oxidation and reducing the oxidative damage which is responsible for the onset of heart disease. For this reason, foods or plants, as carob, which are rich in polyphenols may have an important role in diseases prevention as well. As cardiovascular diseases are an important cause of death, the use of food polyphenols could be an effective dietary modification for the treatment and prevention of cardiovascular diseases, thus reducing deaths from coronary artery heart disease, particularly in developing countries (Rico et al., 2019). One other recent study has shown that carob-polyphenols can be used in functional foods and nutraceuticals to reduce oxidative stress and inflammation and lipid profile without causing overall weight gain, and hence they can be very favorable and part of a cost-effective measure of the public health policies aimed to the reduction of chronic diseases and their complications

3.2. Antimicrobial Effect

Carob is said to have antimicrobial activity, based largely on the presence of bioactive compounds that contain antimicrobial properties. In particular, these bioactive compounds include tannins, flavonoids, polyphenols and saponins, and this means carob is efficacious against a diverse array of bacterial and fungal strains (Dahmani al., 2023). Tannins, especially hydrolyzable tannins and gallotannins are phenolic compounds present in all plants. Carob contains essential phytocompounds, mainly polyphenols, including condensed and hydrolyzable tannins, phenolic acids, flavonoids and flavonoid glycosides, with potential antibacterial and cytotoxic activities (Dahmani et al., 2023). A study utilizing an aqueous extract of carob pods and the disk diffusion assay, determined that the aqueous extract had maximum antibacterial activity, with an inhibition rate of up to 100% against *Escherichia coli* and an inhibition zone diameter greater than 25 mm, emphasizing the potential of synergistic properties of *Ceratonia siliqua* L. extracts with antibiotics. Additionally, a study was conducted on the antimicrobial activity of various types of carob extracts (pulp, seeds and Rob) against different pathogenic strains such as *E. coli*, *Staphylococcus aureus*, and *Pseudomonas aeruginosa*, and certain fungal strains in terms of pathogenicity. The extracts have varied efficiency and potential against the microorganism tested with more efficacy against gram-positive bacteria, likely due to higher penetration of bioactive compounds across the cell walls of gram-positive bacteria in comparison to gram-negative bacteria. Rob, which is abundant in phenolic compounds and other antimicrobial metabolites was the most efficacious, indicating carob products could be a possible alternative natural antimicrobial product to current antimicrobial therapies for treating and preventing bacterial and fungal infections.

Some flavonoids found in carob, including rutin, naringin and apigenin, have shown antimicrobial activity (Ullah et al., 2020). This variety of antimicrobial activities produced by the tannins and flavonoids in carob supports the fact that these compounds may contribute meaningfully to food safety and extended shelf life of products in light of the increased demand for natural alternatives.

The antimicrobial activity of tannins and flavonoids include, but are not limited to, inhibition of pathogen growth, they also include antioxidant and anti-inflammatory activity which could offer different advantages towards human health. In analyzing these compounds for formulations regarding food, we can think of methods to better the safety and quality of food products. This study demonstrated that the ethanolic extract of carob pulp has a moderate antimicrobial activity with inhibition zones from 6-25 mm against five microorganisms it highlighted its potential as a natural antimicrobial agent (Khelouf et al., 2023). Other studies show that carob phenolics could inhibit growth of relatively pathogenic bacteria, such as L. monocytogenes and S. aureus mainly maintaining probiotic bacteria. This selective inhibition is enhanced post-digestion providing greater inhibition towards pathogens (Chaalal et al., 2023). CPAE has also been evaluated for its antimicrobial activities against several pathogens including *Staphylococcus aureus*, *Escherichia coli*, *Candida albicans*, and herpes simplex virus type I (HSV-I). The study found significant inhibition against each pathogen with differing zones of inhibition for the different microorganisms confirming the potential for CPAE to act as an antimicrobial agent (Darwish et al., 2021). This could be attributed to polyphenols and flavonoids reported in the extract that have recognized antimicrobial activities; that evidence supports the potential of CPAE as a natural preservative in pharmaceutical and food products. Comprehensive research has been undertaken on several useful components of the carob tree, reporting a fifty strong potentially powerful high-quality antimicrobial effect against several types of bacteria studied (Table 3). This study also examined the carob tree's ability as a potent food source and a natural source for addressing bacterial infection and promote engagement with the commercialization of new solutions in the health and pharmaceutical arena.

Table 3. Antibacterial activity of carob parts against various bacterial strains

Part of plant used	**Results**	**Reference**
carob leaves and carob pods	The Gram (-) bacteria *P.atrosepticum* (Pca, CFBP-3584) was determined in this study. The leaf extracts showed strong inhibitory activity against Pca with MIC50 values between 1.5 and 2.4 mg/ml	**Meziani et al. (2015)**
Carob pulp	Phenolic extracts from carob inhibit pathogenic bacteria while preserving probiotics, promoting balanced intestinal health.	**Chaalal et al. (2023)**
Carob pulp	Carob flour extracts, rich in gallic acid, are effective against Gram-positive bacteria but show limited activity on Gram-negative strains and fungi, warranting further research.	**Rašković et al. (2023)**

continued on following page

Table 3. Continued

Part of plant used	Results	Reference
Carob leaves	The ethanolic extract of *C. siliqua* shows broad antimicrobial activity, highlighting its potential for developing natural treatments amid rising antibiotic resistance.	**Elbouzidi et al. (2023)**
carob leaves	The methanolic extract of locust bean leaves shows strong activity against *Listeria monocytogenes*, but no effect on other strains, indicating specific antimicrobial potential. Further studies are needed to assess its broader effectiveness for food safety applications.	**Nadhem et al. (2012)**
Carob pods	Zinc oxide nanoparticles exhibit selective antimicrobial activity, effectively inhibiting certain bacterial, yeast, and fungal strains. Their strain-specific action suggests potential as antimicrobial agents, requiring further investigation for optimized application.	**Karmous et al. (2022)**

3.3. Anti-Diabetic Effect

Carob, rich in D-Pinitol, has well-documented anti-diabetic effects. This compound acts as a natural insulin regulator, improving insulin sensitivity and reducing blood glucose levels. Studies have shown that D-Pinitol activates metabolic pathways essential for glucose absorption, making carob a potential adjunct to diabetes treatments, particularly beneficial for Mediterranean populations. Compared with other insulin-regulating plant products, D-Pinitol and carob-derived products offer several advantages, as presented in Table 4 to the right.

Table 4. Advantages of D-Pinitol and carob-derived products

Advantage	Description	Reference
High concentration	Carob pods contain the highest concentration of D-Pinitol of all the plants studied.	**Kim et al. (2005)**
Bienfaits des produits dérivés	Carob products rich in D-Pinitol, such as carob molasses, provide important health benefits.	**Papaefstathiou et al. (2018)**
Active transformation	D-Pinitol, in the case of methoxy group hydrolysis, transforms into chiro-inositol, another active insulin regulator.	**Kim et al. (2021)**
Synergistic effect	D-Pinitol's activity is significantly enhanced when it acts synergistically with other natural products, although few studies have explored this.	**Tewari et al. (2017)**
Therapeutic versatility	D-Pinitol is a multifunctional natural product, enhancing its potential as a drug for a variety of medical uses.	**Azab. (2022)**

The essential idea of these studies is that carob pods, rich in D-pinitol, can improve insulin sensitivity thanks to the insulin-like effects of D-pinitol (Tetik et al., 2011). However, studies show that an insulin-deficient model (streptozotocin- and nicotinamide-induced diabetes) was used, not an insulin-resistant model (Furman, 2015). Furthermore, the slight increase in insulin observed in the glibenclamide (GD)-treated group is expected, as glibenclamide is known to stimulate insulin secretion (Chan and Colagiuri, 2015). Interestingly, the slight increase in insulin in the high-dose carob (CS1000)-treated group could occur via an insulin-independent mechanism (Papakonstantinou et al., 2017). The anti-diabetic effect of CPAE was tested via its inhibitory action on several key digestive enzymes, including amylase, maltase, sucrase and lactase, which are involved in the breakdown of carbohydrates into simple sugars (Darwish et al., 2021). Those enzymes that may increase post-meal glucose level surges and worsen glycemic control were significantly inhibited by CPAE. The range of effects observed with CPAE would make it suitable for developing products that aid in diabetes management or for inclusion in products designed to lower glycemic response. The studies on carob pulp also attempt to investigate its anti-obesity and anti-dyslipidemic effects. The studies also suggested that the carob pulp synergistically with simvastatin aids in the cessation of weight gain while improving lipid profile through increased HDL cholesterol and decrease in leptin levels.

Furthermore, considering the potential use of carob pulp for natural obesity treatments helps in understanding how effective these treatments might be for lipid adoption (Rašković et al., 2023). The studies referenced in Table 4 outline the findings on the anti-diabetic properties of the various parts of the carob tree. Extracts from the carob has shown high potential for lowering blood sugar levels and improving the functionality of the pancreas. These studies suggest the potential for treatment options available from the carob tree as a source of natural agents to assist with and prevent diabetes. The studies that were performed open up new avenues for the use of carob extracts for the development of -anti diabetic treatments to use as adjuncts to conventional therapy. Rtibi et al. (2017) found evidence for the anti-diabetic effects of aqueous extracts of immature locust bean pods (*Ceratonia siliqua* L.) in an isolated mouse jejunum model when using a Ussing chamber method; they found a dose-dependent inhibition of intestinal glucose absorption by sodium-glucose cotransporter SGLT1. The research established that immature pods exhibit more effective inhibition of glucose transport - immature pods have more polyphenols and flavonoids than mature pods which are primarily composed of fiber (~30% depending on some definitions) and total sugars (~60%), and while some of the specific qualities of the immature pod including chlorogenic acid and epicatechin (which also were present at greater amounts in immature pods) could be responsible for these effects. The antihyperglycemic activity of carob (*Ceratonia siliqua*) will be explored in an *in vitro* experiment analyzing the inhibitory effect of a methanolic extract of carob pods on α-amylase and α-glucosidase enzymes, and the in vivo glycemic effects of the extract on streptozotocin and nicotineamide-induced diabetic rats. The researchers also hope to explore the antioxidant effects of this extract and assess the acute oral toxicity to rats to determine if it is safe to use (Qasem et al., 2018).

Table 5. Antidiabetic effect of the different parts of the carob

Part of the plant	Results	Reference
Carob pods	D-Pinitol enhances insulin sensitivity, lowers blood glucose, and protects tissues from oxidative damage, showing strong potential for diabetes management.	**Azab. (2022)**
Carob fruits	CSAT+® carob extract has shown promising effects in the treatment of diabetes-related conditions, improving insulin sensitivity and reducing inflammation, which could make it a useful adjunct in the management of type 2 diabetes.	**De La Fuente-Fernández et al. (2022)**
Carob pods	Extract has shown promising effects in the treatment of glycemia, insulinemia and HOMA-β	**Macho-González et al. (2020b)**
Carob pods	A high dose of carob exhibits an in vivo antihyperglycemic activity and warrants further in-depth study to identify the potential carob extract composition.	**Qasem et al. (2018)**
Carob fruit	Carob powder has great potential as a food or feed due to their high content of fiber which reduced the levels of blood gloucose in diabetic rats and useful for human nutrition	**Hussein et al. (2022)**

3.3. Anti-Inflammatory Effect

Carob extract Shows promise as an anti-inflammatory remedy because it markedly reduced the production of inflammatory mediators such as nitric oxide (NO) and prostaglandin D2 (PGD2). Carob pod, seed skin, and germ extracts were also reported to reduce NO production in LPS-treated Raw 264.7 macrophages, which raises the potential of these carob by-products as bioactive ingredients to help mitigate metabolic syndrome (MetS) (Rico et al., 2019). Strikingly, these findings suggest that carob extract may serve as a promising complementary treatment to counterbalance the metabolic consequences of obesity and metabolic syndrome. A preclinical study investigated the impact of CSAT+® carob extract supplementation on mice with metabolic syndrome. Findings showed that CSAT+® supplementation, regardless of combined aerobic training, alleviated some of the insulin resistance and inflammation-related metabolic complications. Moreover, CSAT+® supplementation significantly reduced blood pressure even without exercise (De La Fuente-Fernández et al., 2022). The research conducted on carob extracts as seen in Table 6 proves that unique sections of the carob tree possess advanced anti-inflammatory abilities and serve to suppress inflammatory markers, symptoms, and signs associated with the varying stages of inflammation. In general, the above statements suggest that the carob tree- in all its parts, has great prowess as a natural remedy for chronic and acute inflammatory diseases. The present findings open new avenues to further investigate carob's possible uses in anti-inflammatory medicines. Recent work has started to focus on studying the mechanism that mediates the anti-inflammatory effect of carob and has shed more light on bioactive compounds. It is almost predictable that investigators are focusing on the effects of carob polyphenols on various key pro-inflammatory enzymes such as cyclooxygenase-2 and lipoxygenase because carobcontains a significant number of polyphenols, flavonoids, and tannins and exerts an inhibitory effect on the various pathways of pro-inflammatory mediators throughout the inflammation cascade.

Table 6. Anti-inflammatory effect of the different parts of the carob tree

Part of the plant used	Results	Reference
Carob leaves	Carob leaf extract reduce inflammation by inhibiting pro-inflammatory markers, showing promise for managing inflammatory conditions through natural therapies.	**Aboura et al. (2017)**
Carob pods	carob extract has a strong capacity to inhibit hyaluronidase activity, suggesting significant anti-inflammatory potential.	**Elaoufi et al. (2022)**
Carob seed peel, germ and pod	Carob extracts, particularly those from the pod and germ, have notable anti-inflammatory properties, attributed to their phenolic compound content.	**Rico et al. (2019)**
Carob pods and seeds	A blend of cocoa and carob flavonoids reduces diabetes-related cardiac inflammation, suggesting a promising dietary approach for improving heart health and managing complications.	**García-Díez et al. (2022)**

4. CLINICAL APPLICATIONS OF CAROB EXTRACTS

Carob is a source of carbohydrates, fats, and minerals, including potassium, calcium, and phosphorus. Carob leaves and pods are rich in polyphenols and antioxidants, so it's considered healthy. Carob gum is used in pharmaceuticals for formulations, including pomade, anti-celiac agent, pills, and dental paste. From a clinical perspective, carob has demonstrated anti-cancer, anti-reflux, anti-diabetic, anti-diarrheal, anti-hyperlipidemia, antibacterial, antimicrobial, and anti-fungal qualities. Dallali et al. (2018) found that methanolic carob leaves DPPH radical scavenging activity of the average ranged from 40.32% to 75.89%. The results indicate the high antioxidant capacity of carob leaves and the ability to counter stress by the scavenging of free radical. The antioxidant activity of (*Ceratonia siliqua*) leaf extracts by DPPH radical scavenging method were of more value when using the ethanolic extract at 178.33 ± 2.12 g Trolox equivalent: 100 g dry weight (g TE/100 g DW), however, when using the aqueous extract compared to the ethanolic extract, was lower. The outcome suggests the more efficient extraction of antioxidant compounds using ethanol instead of water from carob leaves (Othmen et al., 2020). The ethanolic extract showed good antioxidant activity. DPPH radical scavenging of the ethanolic extract produced an IC50 of 302.78 ± 7.55 μg/mL, exposing a good radical scavenging ability but slightly reduced ascorbic acid IC50 of 260.24 ± 6.45 μg/mL. β-carotene bleaching assay indicated the ethanolic extract was 352.06 ± 12.16 μg/mL (Elbouzidi et al., 2023). Cegledi et al. (2024) reported that carob leaf extracts had high antioxidant activity for all extraction methods. In the DPPH assay, the antioxidant activities were between 0.50 and 0.58 mmol Trolox Equivalents (TE) per gram of dry leaf. The FRAP assay values for carob leaf extracts ranged from 0.46 to 1.02 mmol TE/g. This study emphasizes the potential that carob leaf has as a natural antioxidant source.

Table 7. Therapeutic potential of carob in the management of pathological conditions

Pathological	Role	Chemotherapeutic agent	References
Infections (bacteria, virus, fungi)	Antibacterial	Polyphenols	**Roseiro et al. (2013)**
	Antiviral	Gallic acid	**Meziani et al. (2015)**
	Antifungal	Epigallocatechin	**Abulyazid et al. (2017)**
Inflammation	Anti-inflammatory	Catechin	**Rico et al. (2019)**
Oxidative stress	Antioxidant	Quercetin	**Rodríguez-Solana et al. (2019b)**
		Myricetin	**Atta et al. (2023)**
		Kaempferol	**Ikram et al. (2023)**
		Rutin	**Elbouzidi et al. (2023)**
		Cinnamic acid	
		Polyphenols	**Ben Tahar et al. (2024)**
Cancer	Anticancer	Gallic acid	**Christou et al. (2019)**
	Antiproliferative	Phenolic compounds	**Gregoriou et al. (2021)**
		D-pinitol	**Khazaei et al. (2023)**

continued on following page

Table 7. Continued

Pathological	Role	Chemotherapeutic agent	References
Diabetes	Antidiabetic	D-pinitol	**Abu Hafsa et al. (2017)**
		Chlorogenic acid	**Qasem et al. (2018)**
		Epicatechin	**Macho-González et al. (2020a)**
Digestive system problems	Antidiarrheal	Tannins	**Gruendel et al. (2007)**
		Galactomannan	**Sigge et al. (2011)**
		Flavonol glycosides	**Xie et al. (2020)**

4.1. Treatment of Gastrointestinal Disorders

Carob offers a range of health benefits, including anti-diarrheal, anti-bacterial, anti-inflammatory, anti-ulcer, and anti-diabetic properties. Extracts from carob leaves have been shown to inhibit the growth of harmful bacteria such as *Escherichia coli* and *Staphylococcus*, which can help manage bacterial infections and diarrhea. Carob also demonstrates significant anti-inflammatory effects, reducing inflammation markers in the colon and aiding in the prevention of conditions like inflammatory bowel disease. In studies involving rats, carob extracts have been found to reverse gastric damage caused by ethanol, promoting ulcer healing and protecting against Helicobacter pylori infections. Additionally, carob helps manage diabetes by inhibiting enzymes like alpha-amylase and alpha-glucosidase, reducing postprandial hyperglycemia and lowering glucose absorption, making it a natural option for diabetes management. Carob has shown benefits in managing hypercholesterolemia and diarrhea. Studies found that carob fiber reduced total cholesterol, LDL, and triglycerides in people with hypercholesterolemia, with more significant effects in women. For diarrhea, carob bean juice (CBJ) combined with oral rehydration solution (ORS) reduced the duration of diarrhea by 45% in children compared to ORS alone. Carob fractions also improved symptoms in infants with diarrhea, though its effectiveness in treating traveler's diarrhea was limited. Overall, carob helps improve lipid profiles and treat diarrhea, particularly in children. A study on *Ceratonia siliqua* (carob) showed that carob extract (CE) protects the liver in a paracetamol-induced toxicity model in mice. CE reduced liver damage, restored antioxidant enzyme activities, and minimized histopathological changes. Carob bean gum is a polysaccharide used for drug delivery to the colon. It degrades in the human colon due to enzymes like *β-mannanase*, influenced by bacteria such as *Bacteroides* and *Ruminococci*.

4.2. Application in Medicine and Pharmacy

Carob seed peels and endosperm have valuable pharmaceutical and medicinal applications due to the bioactive components and good functionality. Research indicates that carob seed peels have a significant antioxidant effect against mood disorders, abdominal obesity, anxiety and depression, and mental disorders such as schizophrenia. The endosperm showed promise for use in pharmaceuticals due to its favorable characteristics of biocompatibility, biodegradability, and mucoadhesive properties in forming various dosage forms, including tablets, gels, and nanoparticles. Locust bean gum (LBG) is derived from carob and can have an array of health advantages (i.e., it can help gastrointestinal support, have hypolipidemic benefits, help manage diabetes) as well as the capacity to create various drug delivery forms (including microcapsules, microparticles, and nanoparticles) since it has the capacity to gel and control drug release.

5. CONCLUSION

The carob (*Ceratonia siliqua* L.) is a prominent Mediterranean species, not just because of its environmental and economic significance, but due to its diverse phytochemical profile. It is rich in secondary metabolites that can deliver a wide range of biological activities, in particular, polyphenols, flavonoids and tannins. These bioactive components manifest potent biological activities in terms of antioxidant and antimicrobial, inflammatory, antidiabetic, and anticancer activities, demonstrating the potential of carob to be used for prevention and treatments of human diseases. Within the food and drug industries, the use of a variety of carob-derived secondary metabolites, provides consumers and pharmaceutical companies natural options as an alternative to their synthetic counterparts, and following current trends for functional foods and plant-based medicines. Further, exploiting various aspects of the plant, such as the pods, seeds leaves and bark, promotes a sustainable approach to the utilization of the plant holistically.

REFERENCES

Abidar, S., Boiangiu, R. S., Dumitru, G., Todirascu-Ciornea, E., Amakran, A., Cioanca, O., Hritcu, L., & Nhiri, M. (2020). The Aqueous Extract from *Ceratonia siliqua* Leaves Protects against 6-Hydroxydopamine in Zebrafish: Understanding the Underlying Mechanism. *Antioxidants*, *9*(4), 304. DOI: 10.3390/antiox9040304 PMID: 32276477

Aboura, I., Nani, A., Belarbi, M., Murtaza, B., Fluckiger, A., Dumont, A., Benammar, C., Tounsi, M. S., Ghiringhelli, F., Rialland, M., Khan, N. K., & Hichami, A. (2017). Protective effects of polyphenol-rich infusions from carob (*Ceratonia siliqua*) leaves and cladodes of Opuntia ficus-indica against inflammation associated with diet-induced obesity and DSS-induced colitis in Swiss mice. *Biomedicine and Pharmacotherapy*, *96*, 1022–1035. DOI: 10.1016/j.biopha.2017.11.125 PMID: 29221725

Abu Hafsa, S. H., Ibrahim, S. A., & Hassan, A. A. (2017). Carob pods (*Ceratonia siliqua* L.) improve growth performance, antioxidant status and caecal characteristics in growing rabbits. *Journal of Animal Physiology and Animal Nutrition*, *101*(6), 1307–1315. DOI: 10.1111/jpn.12651 PMID: 28133861

Abulyazid, I., Elhalim, S. A. A., Sharada, H. M., Aboulthana, W. M., & Elhalim, S. T. A. A. (2017). Hepatoprotective effect of carob pods extract (*Ceratonia siliqua* L.) against cyclophosphamide induced alterations in rats. *International Journal of Current Pharmaceutical Review and Research.*, *8*(2), 149–162. DOI: 10.25258/ijcprr.v8i02.9199

Ahanger, M. A., Bhat, J. A., Siddiqui, M. H., Rinklebe, J., & Ahmad, P. (2020). Integration of silicon and secondary metabolites in plants: A significant association in stress tolerance. *Journal of Experimental Botany*, *71*(21), 6758–6774. DOI: 10.1093/jxb/eraa291 PMID: 32585681

Atta, A. H., Atta, S. A., Khattab, M. S., El-Aziz, T. H. A., Mouneir, S. M., Ibrahim, M. A., Nasr, S. M., & Emam, S. R. (2023). *Ceratonia siliqua* pods (Carob) methanol extract alleviates doxorubicin-induced nephrotoxicity via antioxidant, anti-inflammatory and anti-apoptotic pathways in rats. *Environmental Science and Pollution Research International*, *30*(35), 83421–83438. DOI: 10.1007/s11356-023-28146-z PMID: 37341944

Azab, A. (2022). D-Pinitol—Active natural product from carob with notable insulin regulation. *Nutrients*, *14*(7), 1453. DOI: 10.3390/nu14071453 PMID: 35406064

Batlle, I., & Tous, J. (1997). *Carob tree. Ceratonia siliqua L. Promoting the conservation and use of under-utilised and neglected crops Institute of Plant Genetics and Crop Plant Research*. Gatersleben/International Plant Genetic Resources Institute.

Ben Ayache, S., Behija Saafi, E., Emhemmed, F., Flamini, G., Achour, L., & Muller, C. D. (2020). Biological activities of aqueous extracts from carob plant (*Ceratonia siliqua* L.) by antioxidant, analgesic and proapoptotic properties evaluation. *Molecules (Basel, Switzerland)*, *25*(14), 3120. DOI: 10.3390/molecules25143120 PMID: 32650498

Ben Tahar, S., Diane, A., Amalich, S., Chiki, Z., Hajji Nabih, M., Boulika, H., & Idrissi Kandri, N. (2024). Optimization of ultrasound-assisted extraction of bioactive compounds from carob pulp using response surface methodology. *Journal of Food Measurement and Characterization*, *18*(9), 7942–7952. DOI: 10.1007/s11694-024-02776-4

Boublenza, I., Lazouni, H. A., Ghaffari, L., Ruiz, K., Fabiano-Tixier, A. S., & Chemat, F. (2017). Influence of roasting on sensory, antioxidant, aromas, and physicochemical properties of carob pod powder (*Ceratonia siliqua* L.). *Journal of Food Quality*, *4193672*(1), 1–10. DOI: 10.1155/2017/4193672

Brassesco, M. E., Brandão, T. R., Silva, C. L., & Pintado, M. (2021). Carob bean (*Ceratonia siliqua* L.): A new perspective for functional food. *Trends in Food Science & Technology*, *114*, 310–322. DOI: 10.1016/j.tifs.2021.05.037

Cegledi, E., Dobroslavić, D., Zorić, Z., Repajić, M., & Garofulić, I. E. (2024). Antioxidant Activity of Carob Tree (*Ceratonia siliqua* L.) Leaf Extracts Obtained by Advanced Extraction Techniques. *Processes (Basel, Switzerland)*, *12*(4), 658. DOI: 10.3390/pr12040658

Čepo, D. V., Mornar, A., Nigović, B., Kremer, D., Radanović, D., & Dragojević, I. V. (2014). Optimization of roasting conditions as an useful approach for increasing antioxidant activity of carob powder. *Lebensmittel-Wissenschaft + Technologie*, *58*(2), 578–586. DOI: 10.1016/j.lwt.2014.04.004

Chaalal, M., Ydjedd, S., Chemache, L., López-Nicolás, R., Sánchez-Moya, T., Frontela-Saseta, C., Ros-Berruezo, G., & Kati, D. E. (2023). Evaluation of the antimicrobial potential of digested and undigested carob phenolic extracts: Impact on selected gut microbiota. *Acta Alimentaria*, *52*(4), 612–622. DOI: 10.1556/066.2023.00172

Chan, S. P., & Colagiuri, S. (2015). Systematic review and meta-analysis of the efficacy and hypoglycemic safety of gliclazide versus other insulinotropic agents. *Diabetes Research and Clinical Practice*, *110*(1), 75–81. DOI: 10.1016/j.diabres.2015.07.002 PMID: 26361859

Christou, C., Poulli, E., Yiannopoulos, S., & Agapiou, A. (2019). GC-MS analysis of D-pinitol in carob: Syrup and fruit (flesh and seed). *Journal of Chromatography. B, Analytical Technologies in the Biomedical and Life Sciences, 1116*, 60–64. DOI: 10.1016/j.jchromb.2019.04.008 PMID: 30986609

Custódio, L., Fernandes, E., & Romano, A. (2007). Quantification of polyphenols in carob tree (*Ceratonia siliqua* L.) fruits and leaves in Portuguese cultivars. In II International Symposium on Human Health Effects of Fruits and Vegetables. *Acta Horticulturae*, (841), 503–506. DOI: 10.17660/ActaHortic.2009.841.69

Dahmani, W., Elaouni, N., Abousalim, A., Akissi, Z. L. E., Legssyer, A., Ziyyat, A., & Sahpaz, S. (2023). Exploring Carob (*Ceratonia siliqua* L.): A Comprehensive Assessment of Its Characteristics, Ethnomedicinal Uses, Phytochemical Aspects, and Pharmacological Activities. *Plants, 12*(18), 3303. DOI: 10.3390/plants12183303 PMID: 37765467

Dallali, S., Aloui, F., Selmi, H., & Sebei, H. (2018). Comparison of the chemical composition and the antioxidant activity of the leaves of Carob tree (*Ceratonia siliqua* L.) collected in three sites of Djebel Zaghouan (Tunisia). *Journal of New Sciences Agriculture and Biotechnology CIRS.*, (21), 3429–3438.

Darwish, W. S., Khadr, A. E. S., Kamel, M. A. E. N., Abd Eldaim, M. A., El Sayed, I. E. T., Abdel-Bary, H. M., Ullah, S., & Ghareeb, D. A. (2021). Phytochemical characterization and evaluation of biological activities of egyptian carob pods (*Ceratonia siliqua* L.) aqueous extract: *In vitro* study. *Plants, 10*(12), 2626. DOI: 10.3390/plants10122626 PMID: 34961100

De la Fuente-Fernández, M., de la Fuente-Muñoz, M., Román-Carmena, M., Amor, S., García-Redondo, A. B., Blanco-Rivero, J., González-Hedström, D., Espinel, A. E., García-Villalón, A. L., & Granado, M. (2022). Carob Extract Supplementation Together with Caloric Restriction and Aerobic Training Accelerates the Recovery of Cardiometabolic Health in Mice with Metabolic Syndrome. *Antioxidants, 11*(9), 1803. DOI: 10.3390/antiox11091803 PMID: 36139877

Elaoufi, M. M., Bouterfas, K., Djebbar, A. A., Meziani, S., Rezki, H., Kermas, F., Benali, M., & Yasmina, B. M. (2022). Chemical composition, anti-ulcer and anti-inflammatory effects of carob pods (*Ceratonia siliqua* L.) polyphenols from ain temouchent. *Journal of Microbiology, Biotechnology and Food Sciences, 12*(2). Advance online publication. DOI: 10.55251/jmbfs.5427

Elbouzidi, A., Taibi, M., Ouassou, H., Ouahhoud, S., Ou-Yahia, D., Loukili, E. H., Aherkou, M., Mansouri, F., Bencheikh, N., Laaraj, S., Bellaouchi, R., Saalaoui, E., Elfazazi, K., Berrichi, A., Abid, M., & Addi, M. (2023). Exploring the multi-faceted potential of carob (*Ceratonia siliqua* var. Rahma) leaves from Morocco: A comprehensive analysis of polyphenols profile, antimicrobial activity, cytotoxicity against breast cancer cell lines, and genotoxicity. *Pharmaceuticals (Basel, Switzerland)*, *16*(6), 840. DOI: 10.3390/ph16060840 PMID: 37375787

Fogarasi, M., Neme , S. A., Fărca , A., Socaciu, C., Semeniuc, C. A., Socaciu, M. I., & Socaci, S. (2024). Bioactive secondary metabolites in mushrooms: A focus on polyphenols, their health benefits and applications. *Food Bioscience*, *62*, 105166. DOI: 10.1016/j.fbio.2024.105166

Furman, B. L. (2015). Streptozotocin-induced diabetic models in mice and rats. *Current Protocols in Pharmacology*, *70*(1), 5–47. DOI: 10.1002/0471141755.ph0547s70 PMID: 26331889

García-Díez, E., López-Oliva, M. E., Caro-Vadillo, A., Pérez-Vizcaíno, F., Pérez-Jiménez, J., Ramos, S., & Martín, M. Á. (2022). Supplementation with a Cocoa–Carob blend, alone or in combination with metformin, attenuates diabetic cardiomyopathy, cardiac oxidative stress and inflammation in Zucker diabetic rats. *Antioxidants*, *11*(2), 432. DOI: 10.3390/antiox11020432 PMID: 35204314

Ghanemi, F. Z., & Belarbi, M.Fatima Zohra GHANEMIMeriem BELARBI. (2021). Phytochemistry and Pharmacology of *Ceratonia siliqua* L. leaves. *Journal of Natural Product Research and Applications.*, *1*(1), 69–82. DOI: 10.46325/jnpra.v1i01.7

Ghanemi, F. Z., Belarbi, M., Fluckiger, A., Nani, A., Dumont, A., De Rosny, C., Aboura, I., Khan, A. S., Murtaza, B., Benammar, C., Lahfa, B. F., Patoli, D., Delmas, D., Rébé, C., Apétoh, L., Khan, N. A., Ghringhelli, F., Rialland, M., & Hichami, A. (2017). Carob leaf polyphenols trigger intrinsic apoptotic pathway and induce cell cycle arrest in colon cancer cells. *Journal of Functional Foods*, *33*, 112–121. DOI: 10.1016/j.jff.2017.03.032

Gregoriou, G., Neophytou, C. M., Vasincu, A., Gregoriou, Y., Hadjipakkou, H., Pinakoulaki, E., Christodoulou, M. C., Ioannou, G. D., Stavrou, I. J., Christou, A., Kapnissi-Christodoulou, C. P., Aigner, S., Stuppner, H., Kakas, A., & Constantinou, A. I. (2021). Anti-cancer activity and phenolic content of extracts derived from cypriot carob (*Ceratonia siliqua* L.) pods using different solvents. *Molecules (Basel, Switzerland)*, *26*(16), 5017. DOI: 10.3390/molecules26165017 PMID: 34443605

Gruendel, S., Otto, B., Garcia, A. L., Wagner, K., Mueller, C., Weickert, M. O., Heldwein, W., & Koebnick, C. (2007). Carob pulp preparation rich in insoluble dietary fibre and polyphenols increases plasma glucose and serum insulin responses in combination with a glucose load in humans. *British Journal of Nutrition*, *98*(1), 101–105. DOI: 10.1017/S0007114507701642 PMID: 17381962

Hussein, W. A., Salem, A. A. E., Fahmy, H. A., Mouneir, S. M., Soliman, A. S., & Abbas, M. S. (2022). Effect of carob, doum, and cinnamon powder on blood lipid profile in diabetic rats. *Egyptian Journal of Chemistry*, *65*(9), 317–328. DOI: 10.21608/ejchem.2022.114446.5202

Ikram, A., Khalid, W., Wajeeha Zafar, K.-U., Ali, A., Afzal, M. F., Aziz, A., Faiz ul Rasool, I., Al-Farga, A., Aqlan, F., & Koraqi, H. (2023). Nutritional, biochemical, and clinical applications of carob: A review. *Food Science & Nutrition*, *11*(7), 3641–3654. DOI: 10.1002/fsn3.3367 PMID: 37457186

Ioannou, G. D., Savva, I. K., Christou, A., Stavrou, I. J., & Kapnissi-Christodoulou, C. P. (2023). Phenolic Profile, Antioxidant Activity, and Chemometric Classification of Carob Pulp and Products. *Molecules (Basel, Switzerland)*, *28*(5), 2269. DOI: 10.3390/molecules28052269 PMID: 36903513

Karmous, I., Taheur, F. B., Zuverza-Mena, N., Jebahi, S., Vaidya, S., Tlahig, S., Mhadhbi, M., Gorai, M., Raouafi, M., Debara, M., Bouhamda, T., & Dimkpa, C. O. (2022). Phytosynthesis of zinc oxide nanoparticles using *Ceratonia siliqua* L. and evidence of antimicrobial activity. *Plants*, *11*(22), 3079. DOI: 10.3390/plants11223079 PMID: 36432809

Khazaei, F., Bozorgi, M., & Khazaei, M. (2023). Anticancer effect of carob bean extract on human prostate cancer cell lines: Apoptosis induction and Bax/Bcl-2 ratio improvement. *Middle East Journal of Cancer*, *14*(3), 363–369. DOI: 10.30476/mejc.2022.93823.1704

Khelouf, I., Jabri Karoui, I., & Abderrabba, M. (2023). Chemical composition, *in vitro* antioxidant and antimicrobial activities of carob pulp (*Ceratonia siliqua* L.) from Tunisia. *Chemicke Zvesti*, *77*(10), 6125–6134. DOI: 10.1007/s11696-023-02926-w

Kim, I. S., Kim, C. H., & Yang, W. S. (2021). Physiologically active molecules and functional properties of soybeans in human health—A current perspective. *International Journal of Molecular Sciences*, *22*(8), 4054. DOI: 10.3390/ijms22084054 PMID: 33920015

Kim, J. I., Kim, J. C., Joo, H. J., Jung, S. H., & Kim, J. J. (2005). Determination of total chiro-inositol content in selected natural materials and evaluation of the antihyperglycemic effect of pinitol isolated from soybean and carob. *Food Science and Biotechnology*, *14*(4), 441–445.

Lv, J., Yang, S., Zhou, W., Liu, Z., Tan, J., & Wei, M. (2024). Microbial regulation of plant secondary metabolites: Impact, mechanisms and prospects. *Microbiological Research*, *283*, 127688. DOI: 10.1016/j.micres.2024.127688 PMID: 38479233

Macho-González, A., Garcimartín, A., López-Oliva, M. E., Celada, P., Bastida, S., Benedí, J., & Sánchez-Muniz, F. J. (2020b). Carob-fruit-extract-enriched meat modulates lipoprotein metabolism and insulin signaling in diabetic rats induced by high-saturated-fat diet. *Journal of Functional Foods*, *64*, 103600. DOI: 10.1016/j.jff.2019.103600

Macho-González, A., López-Oliva, M. E., Merino, J. J., García-Fernández, R. A., Garcimartín, A., Redondo-Castillejo, R., Bastida, S., Sánchez-Muniz, F. J., & Benedí, J. (2020a). Carob fruit extract-enriched meat improves pancreatic beta-cell dysfunction, hepatic insulin signaling and lipogenesis in late-stage type 2 diabetes mellitus model. *The Journal of Nutritional Biochemistry*, *84*, 108461. DOI: 10.1016/j.jnutbio.2020.108461 PMID: 32739787

Meziani, S., Oomah, B. D., Zaidi, F., Simon-Levert, A., Bertrand, C., & Zaidi-Yahiaoui, R. (2015). Antibacterial activity of carob (*Ceratonia siliqua* L.) extracts against phytopathogenic bacteria *Pectobacterium atrosepticum.Microbial Pathogenesis*, *78*, 95–102. DOI: 10.1016/j.micpath.2014.12.001 PMID: 25489722

Mouniane, Y. Chriqui, A., El-Khadir, I., Bensaid, A., Arabi, R., Zoubir, M.H., Mabrouki, J., Hmouni. (2024). Investigation on the Phytosociology and Soil Characteristics of Carob Tree (*Ceratonia siliqua* L.) in Northeast Morocco: Implications for Biodiversity Conservation and Ecosystem Restoration. In: Mabrouki, J., Azrour, M. (eds) Integrated Solutions for Smart and Sustainable Environmental Conservation. Studies in Systems, Decision and Control, vol 527. Springer, Cham. https://doi.org/DOI: 10.1007/978-3-031-55787-3_10

Nadhem, A., Valentina, C., Sami, F., Pierluigi, C. (2012). Inhibitory Effect of Carob (*Ceratonia siliqua*) Leaves Methanolic Extract on Listeria monocytogenes.

Ortega, N., Macia, A., Romero, M. P., Trullols, E., Morello, J. R., Anglès, N., & Motilva, M. J. (2009). Rapid Determination of Phenolic Compounds and Alkaloids of Carob Flour by Improved Liquid Chromatography Tandem Mass Spectrometry. *Journal of Agricultural and Food Chemistry*, *57*(16), 7239–7244. DOI: 10.1021/jf901635s PMID: 19624131

Othmen, K. B., Elfalleh, W., Beltrán, J. M. G., Esteban, M. Á., & Haddad, M. (2020). An *in vitro* study of the effect of carob (*Ceratonia siliqua* L.) leaf extracts on gilt-head seabream (*Sparus aurata* L.) leucocyte activities. Antioxidant, cytotoxic and bactericidal properties. *Fish & Shellfish Immunology, 99*, 35–43. DOI: 10.1016/j.fsi.2020.02.005 PMID: 32032761

Owen, R. W., Haubner, R., Hull, W. E., Erben, G., Spiegelhalder, B., Bartsch, H., & Haber, B. (2003). Isolation and structure elucidation of the major individual polyphenols in carob fibre. *Food and Chemical Toxicology, 41*(12), 1727–1738. DOI: 10.1016/S0278-6915(03)00200-X PMID: 14563398

Papaefstathiou, E., Agapiou, A., Giannopoulos, S., & Kokkinofta, R. (2018). Nutritional characterization of carobs and traditional carob products. *Food Science & Nutrition, 6*(8), 2151–2161. DOI: 10.1002/fsn3.776 PMID: 30510716

Papagiannopoulos, M., Wollseifen, H. R., Mellenthin, A., Haber, B., & Galensa, R. (2004). Identification and Quantification of Polyphenols in Carob Fruits (*Ceratonia siliqua* L.) and Derived Products by HPLC-UV-ESI/MS^n. *Journal of Agricultural and Food Chemistry, 52*(12), 3784–3791. DOI: 10.1021/jf030660y PMID: 15186098

Papakonstantinou, E., Orfanakos, N., Farajian, P., Kapetanakou, A. E., Makariti, I. P., Grivokostopoulos, N., Ha, M. A., & Skandamis, P. N. (2017). Short-term effects of a low glycemic index carob-containing snack on energy intake, satiety, and glycemic response in normal-weight, healthy adults: Results from two randomized trials. *Nutrition (Burbank, Los Angeles County, Calif.), 42*, 12–19. DOI: 10.1016/j.nut.2017.05.011 PMID: 28870473

Qasem, M. A., Noordin, M. I., Arya, A., Alsalahi, A., & Jayash, S. N. (2018). Evaluation of the glycemic effect of *Ceratonia siliqua* pods (Carob) on a streptozotocinnicotinamide induced diabetic rat model. *PeerJ, 6*, e4788. Advance online publication. DOI: 10.7717/peerj.4788 PMID: 29844959

Rašković, A., Martić, N., Tomas, A., Andrejić-Višnjić, B., Bosanac, M., Atanasković, M., Nemet, M., Popović, R., Krstić, M., Vukmirović, S., & Stilinović, N. (2023). Carob Extract (*Ceratonia siliqua* L.): Effects on Dyslipidemia and Obesity in a High-Fat Diet-Fed Rat Model. *Pharmaceutics, 15*(11), 2611. DOI: 10.3390/pharmaceutics15112611 PMID: 38004588

Reuter, S., Gupta, S. C., Chaturvedi, M. M., & Aggarwal, B. B. (2010). Oxidative stress, inflammation, and cancer: How are they linked? *Free Radical Biology & Medicine, 49*(11), 1603–1616. DOI: 10.1016/j.freeradbiomed.2010.09.006 PMID: 20840865

Rico, D., Martín-Diana, A.B., Martínez-Villaluenga, C., Aguirre, L., Silván, J. M., Dueñas, M., De Luisf, D.A., Lasa, A. (2019). *In vitro* approach for evaluation of carob by-products as source bioactive ingredients with potential to attenuate metabolic syndrome (MetS). Heliyon. 5(1), e01175. https://doi.org/ iyon.2019. e01175DOI: 10.1016/j.hel

Rodríguez-Solana, R., Coelho, N., Santos-Rufo, A., Gonçalves, S., Pérez-Santín, E., & Romano, A. (2019a). The influence of *in vitro* gastrointestinal digestion on the chemical composition and antioxidant and enzyme inhibitory capacities of carob liqueurs obtained with different elaboration techniques. *Antioxidants*, *8*(11), 563. DOI: 10.3390/antiox8110563 PMID: 31744100

Rodríguez-Solana, R., Salgado, J. M., Pérez-Santín, E., & Romano, A. (2019b). Effect of carob variety and roasting on the antioxidant capacity, and the phenolic and furanic contents of carob liquors. *Journal of the Science of Food and Agriculture*, *99*(6), 2697–2707. DOI: 10.1002/jsfa.9437 PMID: 30350333

Roseiro, L. B., Duarte, L. C., Oliveira, D. L., Roque, R., Bernardo-Gil, M. G., Martins, A. I., Sepúlveda, C., Almeida, J., Meireles, M., Gírio, F. M., & Rauter, A. P. (2013). Supercritical, ultrasound and conventional extracts from carob (*Ceratonia siliqua* L.) biomass: Effect on the phenolic profile and antiproliferative activity. *Industrial Crops and Products*, *47*, 132–138. DOI: 10.1016/j.indcrop.2013.02.026

Rtibi, K., Selmi, S., Grami, D., Amri, M., Eto, B., El-Benna, J., Sebai, H., & Marzouki, L. (2017). Chemical constituents and pharmacological actions of carob pods and leaves (*Ceratonia siliqua* L.) on the gastrointestinal tract: A review. *Biomedicine and Pharmacotherapy*, *93*, 522–528. DOI: 10.1016/j.biopha.2017.06.088 PMID: 28686965

Şahin, H., Topuz, A., Pischetsrieder, M., & Özdemir, F. (2009). Effect of roasting process on phenolic, antioxidant and browning properties of carob powder. *European Food Research and Technology*, *230*(1), 155–161. DOI: 10.1007/s00217-009-1152-7

Sęczyk, L., Świeca, M., & Gawlik-Dziki, U. (2016). Effect of carob (*Ceratonia siliqua* L.) flour on the antioxidant potential, nutritional quality, and sensory characteristics of fortified durum wheat pasta. *Food Chemistry*, *194*, 637–642. DOI: 10.1016/j.foodchem.2015.08.086 PMID: 26471602

Sigge, G. O., Iipumbu, L., & Britz, T. J. (2011). Proximate composition of carob cultivars growing in South Africa. *South African Journal of Plant and Soil*, *28*(1), 17–22. DOI: 10.1080/02571862.2011.10640008

Stavrou, I. J., Christou, A., & Kapnissi-Christodoulou, C. P. (2018). Polyphenols in Carobs: A Review on Their Composition, Antioxidant Capacity and Cytotoxic Effects, and Health Impact. *Food Chemistry, 269*, 355–374. DOI: 10.1016/j.foodchem.2018.06.152 PMID: 30100447

Tetik, N., Turhan, I., Oziyci, H. R., & Karhan, M. (2011). Determination of D-pinitol in carob syrup. *International Journal of Food Sciences and Nutrition, 62*(6), 572–576. DOI: 10.3109/09637486.2011.560564 PMID: 21466274

Tewari, R., Gupta, M., Ahmad, F., Rout, P. K., Misra, L., Patwardhan, A., & Vasudeva, R. (2017). Extraction, quantification and antioxidant activities of flavonoids, polyphenols and pinitol from wild and cultivated Saraca asoca bark using RP-HPLC-PDA-RI method. *Industrial Crops and Products, 103*, 73–80. DOI: 10.1016/j.indcrop.2017.03.036

Ullah, A., Munir, S., Badshah, S. L., Khan, N., Ghani, L., Poulson, B. G., Emwas, A. H., & Jaremko, M. (2020). Important flavonoids and their role as a therapeutic agent. *Molecules (Basel, Switzerland), 25*(22), 5243. DOI: 10.3390/molecules25225243 PMID: 33187049

Xie, J., Wang, Z., Cui, H., Nie, H., Zhang, T., Gao, X., & Qiao, Y. (2020). Effects of enzymatic hydrolysate of locust bean gum on digestibility, intestinal morphology and microflora of broilers. *Journal of Animal Physiology and Animal Nutrition, 104*(1), 230–236. DOI: 10.1111/jpn.13245 PMID: 31762097

Ydjedd, S., Bouriche, S., López-Nicolás, R., Sánchez-Moya, T., Frontela-Saseta, C., Ros-Berruezo, G., Rezgui, F., Louaileche, H., & Kati, D. E. (2017). Effect of *in vitro* gastrointestinal digestion on encapsulated and nonencapsulated phenolic compounds of carob (*Ceratonia siliqua* L.) pulp extracts and their antioxidant capacity. *Journal of Agricultural and Food Chemistry, 65*(4), 827–835. DOI: 10.1021/acs.jafc.6b05103 PMID: 28094929

Zahorec, J., Šoronja-Simović, D., Petrović, J., Šereš, Z., Pavlić, B., Sterniša, M., Možina, S. S., Ačkar, Đ., Šubarić, D., & Jozinović, A. (2024). The Effect of Carob Extract on Antioxidant, Antimicrobial and Sensory Properties of Bread. *Applied Sciences (Basel, Switzerland), 14*(9), 3603. DOI: 10.3390/app14093603

Zhu, B. J., Zayed, M. Z., Zhu, H. X., Zhao, J., & Li, S. P. (2019). Functional polysaccharides of carob fruit: A review. *Chinese Medicine, 14*(1), 40. DOI: 10.1186/s13020-019-0261-x PMID: 31583011

Chapter 12

The Genus Origanum: Secondary Metabolites, Therapeutic Properties, and Traditional Uses

Mustafa Eray Bozyel
https://orcid.org/0000-0001-5556-4880
Dokuz Eylül University, Turkey

Elif Merdamert-Bozyel
https://orcid.org/0000-0001-5470-2372
Health Institutes of Türkiye, Turkey

Cenker Yaman
https://orcid.org/0000-0002-3559-9098
Graduate School of Natural and Applied Sciences, Dokuz Eylül University, Turkey

Gizem Gül
https://orcid.org/0000-0003-3928-2917
Dokuz Eylül University, Turkey

Selime Deniz Bozkurt
https://orcid.org/0009-0003-4782-8884
Dokuz Eylül University, Turkey

Kerem Canlı
https://orcid.org/0000-0001-6061-6948
Dokuz Eylül University, Turkey

ABSTRACT

The genus Origanum (Lamiaceae) encompasses a variety of species recognized for their medicinal properties. It has a wide distribution in the Northern Hemisphere, particularly in the Mediterranean Basin. The term "oregano" is used to refer to several species within the genus Origanum. Origanum species have been used in traditional medicinal practices since ancient times to treat various ailments. Secondary metabolites produced by this genus are important as they take an active role in numerous therapeutic properties and biological activities, including antibacterial, antifungal, antiviral, antioxidant, anti-inflammatory, and antitumor effects. The most prevalent secondary metabolites in this genus are carvacrol, thymol, gamma-terpinene, p-cymene, and linalool. These secondary metabolites

DOI: 10.4018/979-8-3693-9112-9.ch012

play an important role in the therapeutic properties and biological activities of the genus. This study aims to present a comprehensive review of the traditional uses of the genus Origanum, its secondary metabolites, and their therapeutic properties.

1. INTRODUCTION

The utilization of plants for medicinal and therapeutic purposes has historical roots that extend back to the earliest periods of human civilization. In their quest for sustenance, early humans experimented with a diverse array of plant species. Edible plants were consumed as food, while those deemed toxic or possessing adverse effects were either avoided or utilized as instruments of defense. Additionally, plants that elicited physiological responses—such as perspiration, defecation, healing, or hallucination—were designated for medicinal applications and practices of divination. Over millennia, humans have honed their ability to harness a wide range of plants as potential remedies for various ailments. Approximately four thousand years ago, the Chinese emperor Qien Nong (Chi'en Nung) compiled a seminal guide to medicinal plants, titled Ben Zao (Pen Tsao). This foundational text offers comprehensive information regarding the properties and applications of over three hundred plant species, several of which retain significance in contemporary medicine. Simultaneously and subsequently, the Sumerians documented prescriptions on clay tablets, while the Egyptians chronicled their medical knowledge on rolls of papyrus. The earliest known medical document, the Papyrus Kahun, dates back to the reign of King Amenemhet III (1840-1792 BCE) and addresses women's health issues and various medical conditions. Among the most notable of these medical papyri is the Ebers Papyrus, which provides an extensive account of the pharmaceutical practices prevalent during that era. It includes detailed instructions on the preparation and administration of various plant-based remedies, specifically those aimed at treating parasitic infections and gastrointestinal disorders. Many of these plants continue to be utilized in both traditional and modern medical practices.

The Greeks and Romans owe a significant debt to earlier civilizations for their extensive herbal knowledge, a body of work meticulously documented in Dioscorides' "De Materia Medica" and the comprehensive 37-volume natural history authored by Pliny the Elder. These foundational texts have been preserved through translations into Arabic by notable figures such as Rhazes and Avicenna. The understanding and application of medicinal plants were further advanced by monastic communities in Europe, who not only cultivated various medicinal species but also translated these pivotal Arabic manuscripts. The establishment of the first recognized apothecaries in Baghdad during the 9th century marked a significant development in the field. By the thirteenth century, London emerged as a critical center for the trade of herbs and spices, highlighting the growing importance of herbal commerce. However, the progression of medical science encountered considerable obstacles during the Dark Ages, primarily due to the prevailing Christian doctrine that regarded disease as a divine punishment for sin. This belief influenced some women, who viewed the pain of childbirth as an opportunity for penance. Within the confines of monastic life, the diligent translation of herbals and other sources of natural medicine continued, enabling the preservation of this knowledge. The Renaissance period ushered in a new context for the evolution of herbal traditions; William Caxton played a pivotal role by printing numerous medical treatises, while Nicholas Culpeper translated the complete "Physicians' Pharmacopoeia" which was published in 1653 under the title "The English Physician and Complete Herbals" and continues to be in print to the present day. Moreover, the rise of alchemy and the resulting dichotomy between the "new philosophy" of reason and empirical investigation and the established traditions encompassing ancient medical doctrines, herbalism, astrology, and the occult signified the end of the golden age of herbals. The witch hunts of this era precipitated the decline of village "healing women," as women were systematically barred from pursuing scholarly activities in this domain. Non-professional healers were often labeled as heretics, further stigmatizing their practices. Consequently, the use of herbs became increasingly associated with magic and the occult, forming a complex and problematic association that has proven difficult to dismantle. Despite this, the knowledge and practices of folk herbalism continued, particularly in economically disadvantaged regions, despite herbalism's exclusion from mainstream medical education.

The growing awareness regarding the potential adverse effects of pharmaceuticals, exemplified by the tragic outcomes associated with substances such as thalidomide, has sparked renewed interest in the investigation of herbal remedies as viable sources of natural medicines. This interest is particularly pronounced among vulnerable populations, including pregnant women, children, individuals with chronic conditions (notably chronic stress) who have not achieved satisfactory responses to conventional treatments, and those with immunosuppressed states. These groups have benefitted significantly from safe and effective treatments that eschew the use of toxic pharmacological agents. The impact of environmental pollution, food additives, and contaminated water, among myriad other factors, on human health and immune function is profound. In response to these challenges, there is an imperative to transition away from chemically based interventions and to explore therapeutic strategies that enhance the body's resilience amidst the demands of contemporary living. As the research into the bioactive constituents of herbs progresses, an increasing number of ancient treatments and tonics are being rediscovered, recognized, and reintegrated into modern therapeutic practices. The global transport network has facilitated unprecedented access to a diverse array of medicinal plants from various regions, including ginseng, guarana, tea tree oil, aloe vera, and ginkgo biloba. Notably, a considerable proportion of the pharmacopeia used in academic medicine, such as aspirin derived from the white willow, can be traced back to folk remedies, notwithstanding the historical marginalization of these traditional practices by mainstream medical science. Until recently, the exploration of folk and tribal medicines has been largely serendipitous. However, since the conclusion of the Second World War, there has been a marked increase in systematic investigations of traditional medical systems aimed at the identification of novel pharmaceutical preparations. Current estimates suggest that over 120 prescription drugs are derived from plants, with approximately 25 percent of all prescriptions containing one or more active ingredients sourced from botanicals. There exists a substantial evidence base supporting the integration of herbal remedies into conventional medical frameworks. For instance, extracts from the yew tree have demonstrated significant efficacy in inhibiting malignant cell proliferation in humans, particularly in the treatment of pediatric leukemia. Similarly, the rosy periwinkle has shown promise in the management of specific forms of leukemia. Conducting a comparative and evaluative analysis of folk and academic medical systems presents inherent challenges. On one hand, the indiscriminate dismissal of folk medicine may lead to the inappropriate rejection of established and proven methodologies, including essential immunizations and pharmaceuticals required for the treatment of chronic and serious illnesses that were previously nonexistent. Conversely, the potential hazards associated with folk medicine are often emphasized without a balanced acknowledgment of its contributions to conventional medicine and the commonalities that exist between the two approaches. Presently, there is an increasing recognition of the effectiveness of natural remedies, with their use gradually gaining acceptance and endorsement, particularly for minor ailments that can be appropriately managed at home, such as headaches, mild digestive disturbances, and sore throats. However, it remains inadvisable to treat severe conditions, particularly those affecting the liver, heart, or kidneys, or serious illnesses in young children, without professional intervention; such cases warrant referral to qualified practitioners, (Shealy, 1998).

According to estimates from the World Health Organization (WHO), approximately 88% of countries worldwide incorporate traditional medicine into their healthcare practices. This broad category encompasses various modalities, including herbal remedies, yoga, acupuncture, and indigenous healing therapies. In the realm of pharmaceutical formulations, it is estimated that over 40% are derived from natural products, with several breakthrough medications originating from traditional medicinal practices; notable examples include aspirin and artemisinin, (Mansinhos, Gonçalves, & Romano, 2024).

The historical use of herbal medicines in medical treatment is well-documented, as these remedies are often employed to manage a wide range of diseases owing to the diverse array of active compounds they contain and their relatively benign side effect profiles. Conversely, synthetic pharmaceuticals tend to demonstrate greater efficacy in targeting specific diseases but are frequently associated with a higher incidence of adverse effects. A significant limitation of herbal medicines is their delayed onset of action, which necessitates extended use to achieve optimal therapeutic outcomes, (Özata, 2019).

Despite advancements in pharmacological research and recent therapeutic developments, bacterial, fungal, and viral infections continue to represent substantial public health challenges, particularly in developing nations, (Cos *et al.,* 2006).

The Lamiaceae family, characterized by aromatic herbage, quadrangular stems, and verticillate inflorescences, is widely distributed across the globe, exhibiting a pronounced presence in both tropical and temperate regions, including the Mediterranean and tropical upland savannas, (Dorman *et al.,* 2004).

The Lamiaceae family holds considerable significance in the realm of medicinal and aromatic plants, serving as a primary source of essential oils and phenolic compounds. These compounds are valued for their diverse medicinal properties and various commercial applications, underscoring the family's importance in both pharmaceutical and economic contexts.

The aerial parts of numerous aromatic plants within this family, particularly those from the genera *Origanum*, *Satureja*, and *Thymus*, are frequently incorporated into food products due to their organoleptic properties. In Türkiye, these plants are commonly consumed in the form of herbal teas. Furthermore, members of the Lamiaceae family have been utilized in traditional medicine to address a variety of ailments, including asthma, muscle pain, indigestion, diarrhea, nausea, rheumatism, and infectious diseases. A comprehensive review of the literature indicates that species within thc Lamiaccac family exhibit a range of biological activities, including anti-inflammatory, antioxidant, antibacterial, antifungal, and antiviral properties, (Dorman *et al.,* 2004).

In culinary contexts, several species from the Lamiaceae family are predominantly employed, including oregano and marjoram (*Origanum*), thyme (*Thymus*), sage (*Salvia*), mint (*Mentha*), rosemary (*Rosmarinus*), basil (*Ocimum*), and lavender (*Lavandula*). Moreover, various genera within the Lamiaceae family, such as Salvia, *Lavandula*, *Teucrium*, and *Phlomis*, have gained popularity as ornamental plants for gardens and indoor settings, owing to their aromatic qualities and ease of cultivation. Notably, these species are among the most effectively propagated through stem cuttings.

From an industrial and economic perspective, these medicinal and aromatic plants play a significant role in the development of the cosmetics, agro-food, pharmaceutical, and fragrance industries. The genera *Mentha* and *Lavandula* are particularly valuable within the cosmetics sector, featuring a diverse array of species utilized therein. Commonly recognized species for flavoring in the food industry include *Rosmarinus officinalis* L., *Origanum majorana* L., and *Ocimum basilicum* L. Likewise, *Satureja montana* L., *Mentha* x *piperita* L., *Salvia officinalis* L., and *Sideritis scardica* Griseb. are routinely harnessed in beverage formulations and teas. Collectively, these species are acknowledged as rich sources of bioactive compounds, particularly phenolic compounds and terpenes, contributing to their widespread application and importance in various industries, (Mansinhos, Gonçalves, & Romano, 2024).

As the sixth largest family among angiosperms, Lamiaceae comprises over 245 genera and approximately 7,886 species distributed worldwide, featuring numerous economically and medicinally important species. The largest genera within the family include *Salvia* L. (945 species), *Scutellaria* L. (360 species), and *Stachys* L. (300 species), along with *Plectranthus* L'Hér. Additionally, significant genera, such as *Hyptis* Jacq. (280 species), *Teucrium* (250 species), *Vitex* L. (250 species), *Thymus* L. (220 species), and *Nepeta* L. (200 species), are also part of this family. Twelve distinct subfamilies have been identified within Lamiaceae, namely *Ajugoideae*, *Callicarpoideae*, *Cymarioideae*, *Lamioideae*, *Nepetoideae*, *Peronematoideae*, *Premnoideae*, *Prostantheroideae*, *Scutellarioideae*, *Symphorematoideae*, *Tectonoideae*, and *Viticoideae*.

In Türkiye, the Lamiaceae family ranks as the third largest in terms of taxonomic diversity and the fourth largest concerning species richness, encompassing 48 genera and 782 taxa. Of these, 603 are species, 179 are subspecies, and 190 are varieties. Notably, 346 taxa are endemic to Türkiye, constituting approximately 44% of the total. Moreover, 23 hybrid species have been identified, of which 19 are endemic (82%). These findings underscore Türkiye's significance as a center of Lamiaceae diversity within the Old World, hosting approximately 10% of all known species of this family globally. The five largest genera in Türkiye, based on the number of taxa, are *Stachys* (118 taxa), *Salvia* L. (107 taxa), *Sideritis* (53 taxa), *Phlomis* L. (53 taxa), and *Teucrium* (48 taxa), (Güner *et al.,* 2012) (Celep & Dirmenci, 2017) (Selvi *et al.,* 2022).

Türkiye is strategically located at the intersection of three distinct phytogeographic regions, which exhibit notable climatic and ecological diversity. The distribution of Lamiaceae taxa within Türkiye is as follows: 293 taxa are documented in the Mediterranean region (37.4%), 287 in the Irano-Turanian region (36.7%), 90 in the Euro-Siberian (Circumboreal) region (11.5%), and 112 taxa fall under unknown or multiregional phytogeographic elements (14.3%). Within the Mediterranean phytogeographic region, 61% of the taxa are endemic, alongside 50% in the Irano-Turanian region and 13% in the Euro-Siberian region. Some endemic taxa display wide distributions across Türkiye, resulting in ambiguities related to their phytogeographic classification. Notably, these taxa account for 13% of the total number of endemic species identified. Over time, various Lamiaceae genera have migrated between phytogeographic regions, adapting to specific habitats across the country. The genera Stachys, *Salvia*, *Sideritis*, *Phlomis*, *Teucrium*, *Nepeta*, *Thymus*, *Scutellaria*, *Origanum*, and *Clinopodium* are particularly distinguished for their species richness in Türkiye, and they also demonstrate a relatively high endemism ratio. Considering the substantial number of taxa and the notable endemism ratios, coupled with the country's diverse habitats, climates, soil types, extensive altitudinal range, and a variety of pollinators, it becomes apparent that Türkiye serves as an exceptional model for studying the evolution and speciation of the Lamiaceae family within the Old World, (Celep & Dirmenci, 2017).

The genus *Origanum* is classified within the Lamiaceae family, and its etymology reveals a rich heritage; the name *Origanum* is derived from the Greek term όριγανον (origanon), which itself is rooted in the words ρος (oros, meaning "mountain") and γάνος (ganos, meaning "brightness"). This nomenclature reflects the plant's natural habitat, typically found at altitudes ranging from 400 to 1800 meters in sunny locations, (Sakkas & Papadopoulou, 2017).

The genus *Origanum* (subfamily *Nepetoideae*, tribe *Mentheae*, subtribe *Menthineae*) encompasses 43 species, including 51 taxa and 15 hybrids distributed globally, (Ietswaart, 1980) (Ietswaart, 1982). Its species are predominantly located in the Mediterranean region and are native to tropical and temperate areas of Asia, Africa, and Europe. Additionally, *Origanum* has been introduced to diverse regions, including India, the western and eastern coasts of North America, and Mexico, (Marrelli, Statti, & Conforti, 2018). Türkiye is notable for hosting the highest diversity within this genus, with 23 recorded species (26 taxa), 8 hybrids, and one suspected species, of which 20 are endemic, (Ietswaart, 1980) (Davis, Mill, & Tan, 1988) (Duman, 2000).

Species within the *Origanum* genus are characterized by their strong aromatic properties and are typically perennial herbs or subshrubs. They exhibit significant morphological and chemical diversity, with key chemical constituents including carvacrol, thymol, linalool, and p-cymene. The therapeutic potential of *Origanum* species is well-documented in folk medicine, where they are commonly utilized as teas and culinary herbs. Empirical studies have highlighted their various pharmacological effects, such as antispasmodic, antimicrobial, expectorant, antioxidant, anticholinesterase, and carminative activities, (Başer & Kirimer, 2006) (Yilmaz et al., 2017). Consequently, the applications of *Origanum* plants are extensive, being used not only as tea and in food products but also in traditional medicinal practices for managing infectious diseases and in cancer prevention and treatment of gastrointestinal disorders, (Marrelli *et al.*, 2016).

2. CHEMICAL COMPOSITION OF THE GENUS ORIGANUM

The genus *Origanum* comprises a diverse array of species characterized by their distinct chemical compositions. Predominantly, these chemicals consist of secondary metabolites, which encompass a wide variety of structures. Notable among these are terpenes—including monocyclic monoterpenes, bicyclic monoterpenes, acyclic monoterpenes, sesquiterpenes, diterpenoids, and triterpenoids—as well as an array of phenolic compounds, including phenols, phenolic acids, and flavonoids. Collectively, these secondary metabolites play significant roles in the therapeutic properties and potential applications of *Origanum* species.

2.1. Secondary Metabolites of the Genus Origanum

2.1.1. Terpenes in the Genus Origanum

The genus *Origanum* is notable for its rich composition of terpenes, particularly the monocyclic monoterpenes carvacrol, and thymol, which are central to its commercial appeal, (Skoula & Harborne, 2002) (Khoury *et al.*, 2016). In addition to these primary compounds, various chemically related substances have been identified, including α-terpinene, γ-terpinene, p-cymene, p-cymenene, p-cymen-7-ol, p-cymen-8-ol, as well as carvacrol and thymol methyl ethers, carvacrol and thymol acetates, terpinen-4-ol, thymoquinone, and thymohydroquinone (Figure 1), (Skoula & Harborne, 2002) (Ozkan, Baydar, & Erbas, 2010).

Moreover, species within the *Origanum* genus are characterized by a diversity of bicyclic monoterpenes. Prominent among these are α-pinene, β-pinene, borneol, camphene, camphor, isoborneol, sabinene, thujene, and various forms of sabinene hydrate—namely, cis-sabinene hydrate, trans-sabinene hydrate, cis-sabinene hydrate acetate, and trans-sabinene hydrate acetate—as well as cis-sabinol and trans-sabinol (Figure 2), (Skoula & Harborne, 2002) (Han *et al.*, 2017).

Additionally, several acyclic monoterpenes such as β-myrcene, geraniol, linalool, and linalyl acetate have been recognized in *Origanum* species (Figure 3), (Skula *et al.*, 1999).

The most frequently isolated sesquiterpenes exhibit notable variety, including α-cadinol, α-copaene, α-humulene, α-muurolene, β-bisabolene, β-bourbonene, β-caryophyllene, β-caryophyllene oxide, β-cubebene, γ-cadinene, γ-muurolene, aromandrene, germacrene, germacrene-D-ol, and bicyclogermacrene (Figure 4), Skoula & Harborne, 2002) (Bisht *et al.*, 2009) (Pirigharnaei *et al.*, 2011).

Diterpenoids have been isolated from only two species of *Origanum: Origanum pampaninii* and *Origanum akhdarense*. Specific compounds identified include akhdarenol, akhdardiol, akhdartriol, and isoakhdartriol (Figure 5), (Skoula & Harborne, 2002) (Passannanti *et al.*, 1984) (Piozzi, Paternostro, & Passannanti, 1985).

Furthermore, the major triterpenoids identified in *Origanum* species are ursolic and oleanolic acids, along with β-amyrin, uvaol, betulin, and betulic acid (Figure 6), Skoula & Harborne, 2002).

2.1.2. Phenolic Compounds in the Genus Origanum

The *Origanum* genus is characterized by a diverse array of phenolic compounds, with hydroquinone being the most frequently isolated phenolic compound in various *Origanum* species. Additionally, previous studies have identified hydroquinone monomethyl ether and the glucoside arbutin (hydroquinone-O-glucoside) as significant constituents (Figure 7), (Assaf *et al.*, 1987) (Ifantis, Solujić, & Skaltsa, 2012) (Lukas *et al.*, 2010).

Within the realm of phenolic acids, several compounds have been documented in *Origanum* species, including p-hydroxybenzoic acid, vanillic acid, syringic acid, and protocatechuic acid. Hydroxycinnamic acids such as caffeic and cinnamic acids, along with their esterified derivatives, notably rosmarinic acid and chlorogenic acid, have also been identified (Figure 7), (Skoula & Harborne, 2002)

Moreover, an extensive range of flavonoids has been reported across various species within the *Origanum* genus. Identified flavonoids include acacetin, apigenin, aromadendrin, axillarin, apigenin-7-O-glucuronide, and apigenin-7,4′-dimethylether, along with chrysin, chrysoeriol, cinaroside, and cirsimaritin. Further investigations have revealed additional flavonoids, including chrysoeriol-7-O-glucuronide, chrysosplenol-D, desmethylnobiletin, eriodictyol, and eriodictiol-7-O-glucoside. Noteworthy compounds such as galangin, genkwanin, isoorientin, isovitexin, kaempferol, luteolin, luteolin-7-O-glucuronide, luteolin-7-O-rutinoside, mosloflavone, naringenin, neglectein, quercetin, and penduletin have also been documented. Furthermore, compounds like retusin, taxifolin, thymonin, thymusin, 6-hydroxyluteolin-7,3′-dimethylether, and 6-hydroxyluteolin-7,3′,4′-trimethylether have been identified (Figure 8), (Skoula & Harborne, 2002) (Ifantis, Solujić, & Skaltsa, 2012) (Cavero *et al.*, 2006) (Nagy *et al.*, 2011) (Radušienė *et al.*, 2008) (Skoula *et al.*, 2008).

These findings underline the rich phytochemical diversity present in the *Origanum* genus, highlighting its potential applications in various fields, including pharmacology and nutrition.

Figure 1. The most frequently occurring monocyclic monoterpenes in the Origanum species (Marrelli, Statti, & Conforti, 2018)

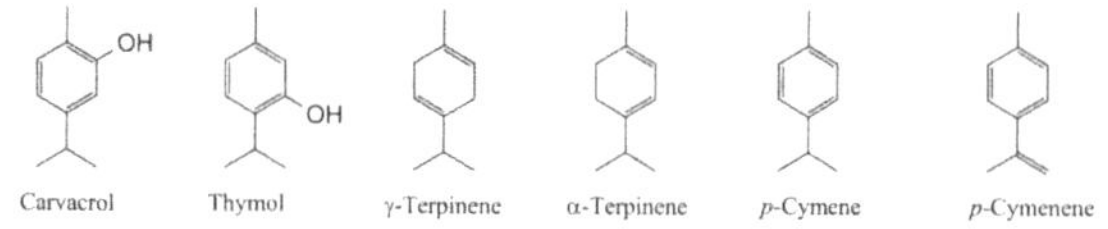

Figure 2. The most frequently occurring bicyclic monoterpenes in the Origanum species Marrelli, Statti, & Conforti, 2018)

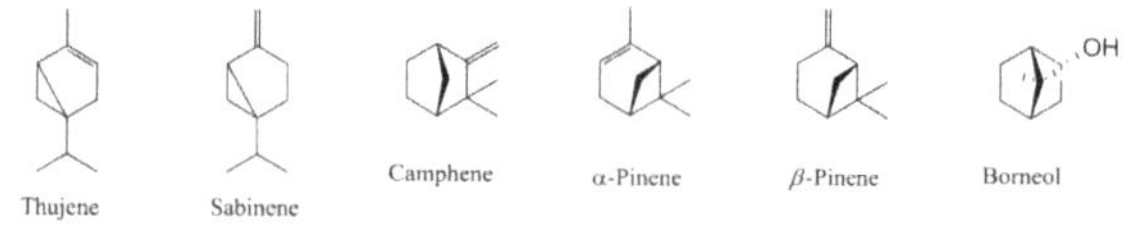

Figure 3. The most frequently occurring acyclic monoterpenes in the Origanum species Marrelli, Statti, & Conforti, 2018)

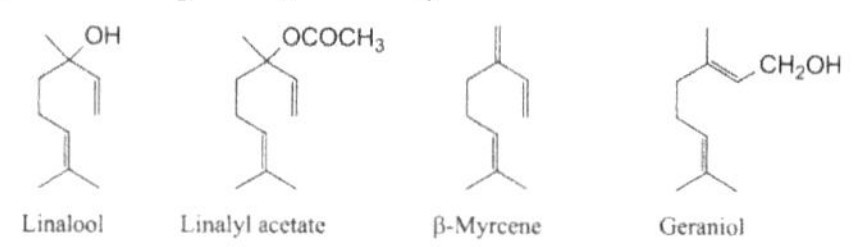

Figure 4. The most frequently occurring sesquiterpenes in the Origanum species Marrelli, Statti, & Conforti, 2018)

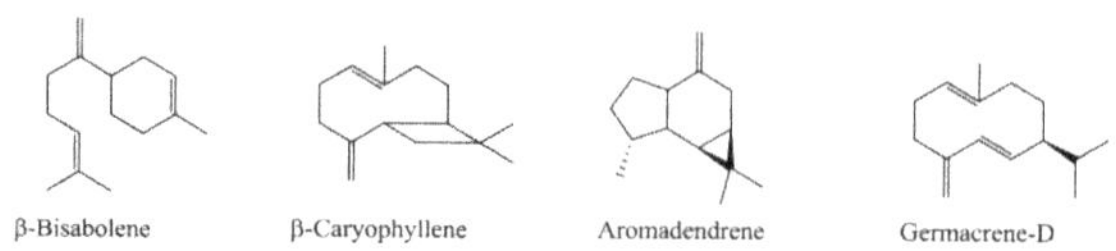

Figure 5. The most frequently occurring diterpenes in the Origanum species Marrelli, Statti, & Conforti, 2018)

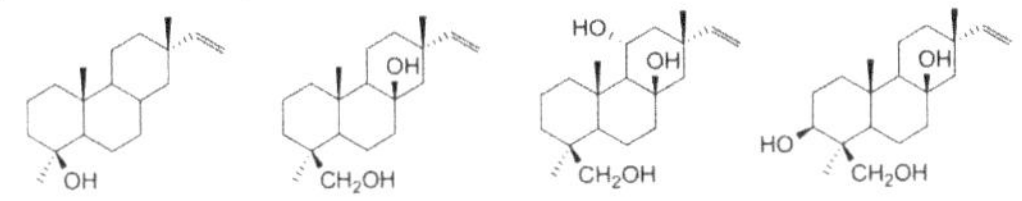

Akhdarenol Akhdardiol Akhdartriol Isoakhdartriol

Figure 6. The most frequently occurring triterpenes in the Origanum species Marrelli, Statti, & Conforti, 2018)

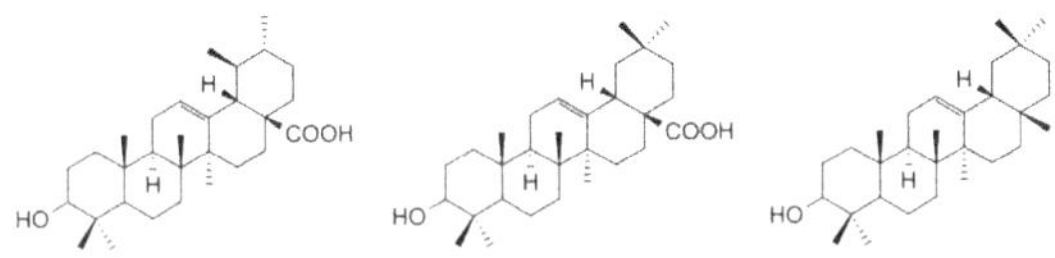

Ursolic acid Oleanoic acid β-Amyrin

Figure 7. The most frequently occurring phenols in the Origanum species Marrelli, Statti, & Conforti, 2018)

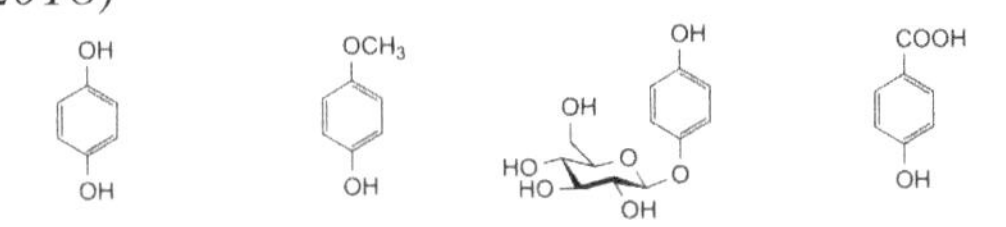

Hydroquinone Hydroquinone monomethyl ether Arbutin *p*-Hydroxybenzoic acid

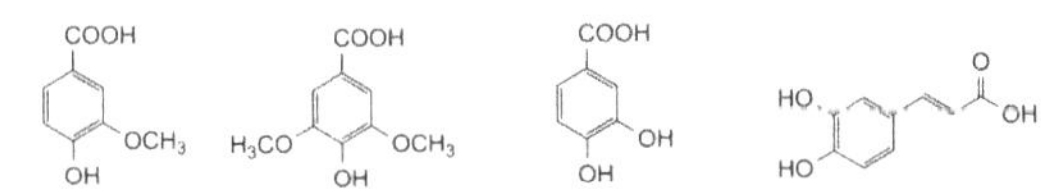

Vanillic acid Syringic acid Protocatechuic acid Caffeic acid

Figure 8. The most frequently occurring flavonoids in the Origanum species Marrelli, Statti, & Conforti, 2018)

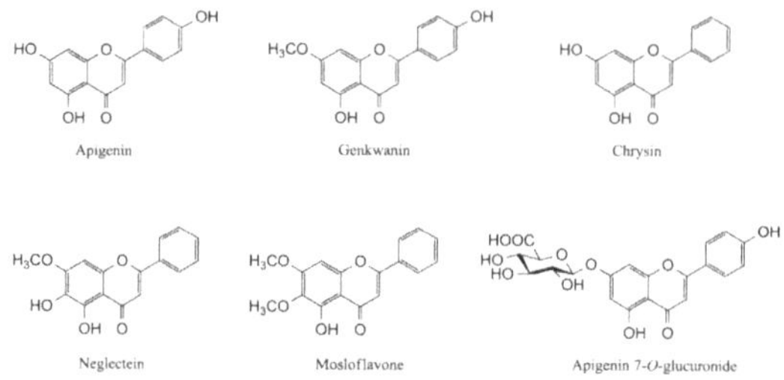

3. BIOLOGICAL ACTIVITIES AND THERAPEUTIC PROPERTIES OF THE GENUS ORIGANUM

3.1. Antimicrobial Activities

Origanum, a genus of plants renowned for its culinary and medicinal applications across various cultures, is recognized as an important aromatic and medicinal species. Numerous studies have investigated the chemical composition of essential oils extracted from *Origanum* species, which are widely utilized as flavoring agents in a variety of culinary contexts, including sauces, soups, as well as meat and fish dishes. Traditionally, *Origanum* has been employed in folk medicine for the treatment of various ailments, such as diarrhea, rheumatism, indigestion, headaches, muscle pain, and asthma, (Erenler *et al.*, 2017). Moreover, this genus has been shown to exhibit significant antimicrobial activity against foodborne bacteria and fungi, (Busatta *et al.*, 2008).

3.1.1. Antibacterial Activity

In a recent study conducted by Canli *et al.* (2023), the antimicrobial efficacy of the ethanol extract of *Origanum onites* was investigated. The researchers employed both disk diffusion and minimum inhibitory concentration (MIC) tests to evaluate the extract's activity against a diverse range of microbial strains, including 30 distinct bacterial strains representing 28 unique species, among which several demonstrated multidrug resistance, as well as two fungal strains. The findings revealed that the ethanol extract of *Origanum onites* exhibited significant antimicrobial activity across the tested microbial strains. Notably, the highest level of efficacy was observed against *Enterococcus faecium*, a Gram-positive bacterium, where a concentration of 100 μL resulted in an inhibition zone measuring 52 mm. Additionally, the Gram-negative bacteria *Pseudomonas aeruginosa* DSMZ 50071 and *Pseudomonas fluorescens* P1 displayed considerable sensitivity, with an inhibition zone of 24 mm observed with the 100 μL application of the ethanol extract. The results for *Acinetobacter baumannii*, a multidrug-resistant strain, were particularly remarkable, indicating a level of activity that surpassed that of all positive controls. Furthermore, all tested fungal strains exhibited greater efficacy than the positive controls. The authors attributed the strong antimicrobial effects observed in the study to the presence of bioactive compounds within the ethanol extract of *Origanum onites*, particularly carvacrol, which comprised 82.34% of the extract and was identified as a key contributor to its potent antimicrobial properties.

In their study, Harmati *et al.* (2017) evaluated the in vivo efficacy of a combination of essential oils derived from *Satureja hortensis* and *Origanum vulgare* subsp. *hirtum* against *Helicobacter pylori*. This research aimed to develop novel therapeutic agents for *H. pylori* infections, which are known to contribute to various gastrointestinal and extra-gastrointestinal disorders, as well as serving as significant risk factors for gastric carcinoma and MALT lymphoma. The findings from this investigation demonstrated that the synergistic effect of the essential oil mixture surpassed the efficacy of the individual oils in the treatment of *H. pylori* infections.

This study investigated the antimicrobial properties of essential oils derived from the aerial parts of three *Origanum* species: *O. libanoticum*, *O. ehrenbergii*, and *O. syriacum*. The oils were tested against *Candida albicans* and six pathogenic bacteria, specifically *Escherichia coli*, *Pseudomonas aeruginosa*, *Enterococcus faecalis*, *Salmonella enteritidis*, *Staphylococcus aureus*, and *Bacillus subtilis* subsp. *spizizenii*. The essential oils of *O. syriacum* and *O. ehrenbergii* exhibited significant antimicrobial activity, particularly against *Bacillus spizizenii*, *Escherichia coli*, and *Enterococcus faecalis*, with minimum inhibitory concentration (MIC) values of 0.4 mg/ml. Additionally, these oils demonstrated effects against *Staphylococcus aureus*, with MIC values of 0.4 and 0.6 mg/ml, respectively. However, both essential oils showed no efficacy against the remaining three bacterial species, with MIC values exceeding 2 mg/ml. A comparative analysis of the chemical composition of the essential oils indicated that the antimicrobial activity of *O. syriacum* and *O. ehrenbergii* is primarily attributed to the presence of phenolic monoterpenes, specifically thymol and carvacrol, (Al Hafi *et al.*, 2016).

De Martino *et al.* (2009) conducted a comprehensive investigation into the chemical composition and antimicrobial properties of essential oils extracted from three distinct populations of *Origanum vulgare* L. subsp. *hirtum*, which were naturally occurring in the Campania region of southern Italy. The study assessed the antibacterial efficacy of these essential oils against a range of bacterial species, including *Bacillus cereus*, *Bacillus subtilis*, *Staphylococcus aureus*, *Staphylococcus epidermidis*, *Streptococcus faecalis*, *Escherichia coli*, *Proteus mirabilis*, *Proteus vulgaris*, *Pseudomonas aeruginosa*, and *Salmonella typhi* Ty2. The results indicated notable antimicrobial activity against Gram-positive bacteria, with a particular emphasis on *S. epidermidis*. Among the Gram-negative bacteria tested, only *E. coli* demonstrated sensitivity to the essential oils. The variability in antimicrobial activity observed across the three populations was primarily ascribed to the concentrations of phenolic compounds, specifically thymol, carvacrol, and carvacrol methyl ether. Furthermore, the synergistic effects of trace active constituents, such as γ-terpinene and p-cymene, were also found to contribute significantly to the overall antimicrobial effectiveness of the essential oils.

Furthermore, the essential oils extracted from three species of *Origanum*—specifically *O. dictamnus*, *O. libanoticum*, and *O. microphyllum*—were evaluated for their potential antimicrobial properties. The findings revealed significant antimicrobial activity, particularly against Gram-positive pathogens. Notably, among the Gram-negative bacteria tested, only *Escherichia coli* exhibited sensitivity to the essential oils of *O. dictamnus* and *O. microphyllum*, (Marrelli *et al.,* 2016).

3.1.2. Antifungal Activity

Císarová *et al.* (2016) conducted a comprehensive evaluation of the antifungal efficacy of 15 essential oils against three species of *Aspergillus*. The study revealed that *Origanum vulgare* demonstrated the most significant antifungal activity, characterized by a minimum inhibitory dosage (MID) of 31.5 µl/l of air. This remarkable effectiveness was consistently observed across all tested strains, particularly when *O. vulgare* was utilized in conjunction with other essential oils.

Waller *et al.* (2016) evaluated the anti-Sporothrix spp. activity of the essential oil of *O. majorana* Linn. (marjoram) against 18 fungal isolates of *Sporothrix brasiliensis* from humans, dogs, and cats, as well as a standard strain of *Sporothrix chenckii*. The recent evidence of resistance to itraconazole among *Sporothrix* spp. represents a significant public health concern. No significant difference was observed between the minimum inhibitory concentrations (MIC), while *Origanum majorana* demonstrated superior minimum fungicidal concentrations (MFC) compared to itraconazole. All tested strains demonstrated susceptibility to the essential oil, exhibiting fungistatic activity at concentrations of ≤ 2.25–9 mg/ml, while fungicidal activity was observed at concentrations between 2.25 and 18 mg/ml.

In a study conducted by Sharifzadeh and Shokri (2016), the antifungal properties of essential oils derived from Iranian flora were evaluated against *Candida albicans*, with a focus on assessing their efficacy against fluconazole-resistant and susceptible strains of this pathogen. Among the essential oils tested, *Origanum vulgare* was identified as one of the most potent, exhibiting the lowest minimum inhibitory concentration (MIC) against *C. albicans*. The essential oil of *O. vulgare*, sourced from Iran, is notably rich in monoterpene phenols, with thymol being a prominent component. While the exact antifungal mechanism of thymol remains inadequately understood, it is hypothesized to disrupt the integrity of the fungal cell membrane and cell wall, ultimately contributing to the deterioration of the yeast. Additionally, substantial antifungal activity against *Candida albicans* has also been documented by Miller *et al.* (2015) for an essential oil derived from *O. vulgare*.

The essential oils derived from *Origanum majorana* and *Origanum vulgare* were assessed for their efficacy against clinically isolated strains of *Microsporum canis*, *Trichophyton mentagrophytes*, *T. erinacei*, *T. terrestre*, and *Microsporum gypseum*. These fungi are recognized as primary causative agents of zoonotic and environmental dermatophytoses in humans, (Nardoni *et al.*, 2015). Among the tested essential oils, *Origanum vulgare* exhibited the highest effectiveness, with a minimum inhibitory concentration (MIC) ranging from 0.025% to 0.5%.

3.2. Antioxidant Activity

Reactive oxygen species (ROS), which include the hydroxyl radical, superoxide, and singlet oxygen, are free radicals that have the potential to induce cellular damage. This oxidative stress is implicated in the pathogenesis of various diseases, including cancer, cardiovascular disorders, and neurodegenerative conditions such as Parkinson's and Alzheimer's diseases, (Valko *et al.*, 2007). While synthetic antioxidants such as butylated hydroxytoluene (BHT), propyl gallate (PG), butylated hydroxyanisole (BHA), and tert-butylhydroquinone (TBHQ) are widely utilized to mitigate oxidative damage, their associated toxicity has led to a growing demand for natural antioxidants. Research has demonstrated that compounds found in fruits and vegetables can effectively scavenge ROS. Thus, it is evident that plant extracts rich in antioxidant compounds hold considerable significance in both pharmacological applications and the food industry, (Balasundram, Sundram, & Samman, 2006) (Miguel, 2010).

Gonçalves *et al.* (2017) conducted an evaluation of the antioxidant properties of methanolic extracts derived from *Origanum vulgare* subsp. *virens*. The study revealed that the extract exhibited significant scavenging activity against DPPH and ABTS radicals, as well as pronounced ferric-reducing power. Additionally, a noteworthy total phenolic content was quantified in the extract. High-Performance Liquid Chromatography with Diode Array Detection (HPLC-DAD) analysis identified rosmarinic acid as the predominant compound; however, other chemical constituents may also play a role in the observed antioxidant activity.

Aras *et al.* (2017) conducted a comprehensive evaluation of the antioxidant activity of *O. acutidens* leaves, employing the DPPH, FRAP, and CUPRAC methodologies. Their findings elucidated that the water extract of this species demonstrated significant efficacy in scavenging DPPH radicals.

The hydroalcoholic extract of *Oregano vulgare* L. subsp. *viridulum* (Martin-Donos) Nyman, a plant with traditional culinary significance among the Calabrian population in Southern Italy, has been shown to exhibit strong antioxidant activity against the DPPH radical, as reported by Conforti *et al.* (2011a). However, this extract demonstrated only weak antioxidant activity when evaluated using the β-carotene bleaching method (Marrelli *et al.*, 2015) and exhibited minimal inhibitory effects on nitric oxide (NO) production in the LPS-stimulated RAW 264.7 mouse macrophage cell line, (Conforti *et al.*, 2011a). In contrast, the ethanolic extract of the aerial parts of *Oregano heracleoticum* L. displayed significant radical scavenging capacity as assessed through the 1,1-Diphenyl-2-picrylhydrazil (DPPH) assay, as well as pronounced antioxidant activity in the β-carotene bleaching test. Furthermore, the assay for NO production inhibition, conducted using the murine monocytic macrophage RAW 264.7 cell line, indicated that this extract demonstrated noteworthy activity, (Conforti *et al.*, 2011b).

The essential oils extracted from three species of *Origanum*—namely, *O. dictamnus*, *O. libanoticum*, and *O. microphyllum*—were assessed for their potential antioxidant activity using two spectrophotometric methods: the DPPH (2,2-diphenyl-1-picrylhydrazyl) assay and the FRAP (Ferric Reducing Antioxidant Power) test. The evaluation revealed that these essential oils exhibited limited antiradical activity. Notably, the oil derived from *O. dictamnus* demonstrated a modest capacity for free radical scavenging, (Marrelli *et al.*, 2016).

Furthermore, Özbek *et al.* (2017) provided evidence supporting the antioxidant potential of the essential oil derived from *O. rotundifolium*, highlighting its effectiveness in scavenging ABTS, hydrogen peroxide (H_2O_2), and superoxide radicals.

3.3. Antiproliferative Activity

Natural products serve as a fundamental source of inspiration for drug discovery and development aimed at addressing human diseases. Numerous studies have substantiated the anticancer properties associated with various traditional medicines and natural products. Additionally, these natural products, characterized by their complex mixtures of chemical compounds, possess the potential to target multiple vulnerabilities within cancer cells while sparing non-cancerous cells from toxicity, (Ovadje *et al.,* 2015).

The cytotoxic properties of the essential oil derived from *Origanum vulgare* subsp. *hirtum,* along with its principal constituents—carvacrol, thymol, citral, and limonene—have been systematically assessed in hepatocarcinoma HepG2 cells. The essential oil exhibited a significant capacity to inhibit cell viability in a dose-dependent manner. Importantly, it demonstrated reduced cytotoxicity towards the non-tumor cell line HEK293, as reported by Elshafie *et al.* (2017).

The extract of *O. rotundifolium,* along with several isolated compounds, was evaluated for its antiproliferative effects against a variety of cell lines, including C6, HeLa, and Vero cells. Among these, vitexin exhibited the most significant antiproliferative activity across all tested cell lines. Notably, the extract demonstrated enhanced activity compared to the isolated compounds, which may be attributed to the synergistic interactions among the diverse phytochemical constituents, (Erenler *et al.,* 2017).

The essential oils extracted from *Origanum dictamnus, Origanum libanoticum,* and *Origanum microphyllum* were evaluated for their anti-cancer properties against two human cancer cell lines: the colon carcinoma cell line LoVo and the hepatocarcinoma cell line HepG2. All tested samples demonstrated a reduction in cell viability in a dose-dependent manner. Notably, the essential oil of *O. dictamnus* exhibited the most pronounced inhibitory effect on both cell lines at the highest concentration tested (100 mg/ml), achieving an inhibition rate of 58.39% after 24 hours of incubation, particularly against the colon carcinoma cell line. In comparison, at the same concentration, the essential oils of *O. microphyllum* and *O. libanoticum* induced inhibition rates of 47.12% and 48.15%, respectively, (Marrelli *et al.,* 2016).

The essential oil derived from *O. onites* has been the focus of extensive investigation concerning its antiproliferative, antiangiogenic, and cytoprotective effects across various cell lines, including H-ras transformed rat embryonic fibroblasts (5RP7) and hepatoma cells (HepG2). Research findings indicate that this oil possesses the ability to inhibit cell viability and induce apoptosis in 5RP7 cells. Notably, comparative analyses demonstrate that the oil exhibits a lower cytotoxicity towards HepG2 cells in comparison to carvacrol and thymol, while also providing protection against H2O2-induced cytotoxicity, (Tepe, Cakir, & Sihoglu Tepe, 2016).

3.4. Antidiabetic Activity

Diabetes mellitus is a metabolic disorder characterized by impairment in insulin action or secretion. There exists a robust correlation between diabetes and an elevated risk of various cardiovascular and metabolic complications, including stroke, coronary heart disease, hypertension, renal failure, and dyslipidemia, (Olokoba, Obateru, &

Olokoba, 2012). In recent years, plant extracts have emerged as promising candidates for the management and treatment of diabetes, owing to their high concentrations of antioxidants and their potential health-promoting properties, (Kooti *et al.*, 2016).

The investigation conducted by Soliman, Nassan, and Ismail (2016) explored the effects of an aqueous extract derived from the leaves of *Oregano majoranum* on dyslipidemia, hypoglycemia, and hyperinsulinemia in a rat model of type 2 diabetes. The results indicated that the administration of the *O. majoranum* extract resulted in significant improvements in dyslipidemia, with normalized biochemical parameters observed in the type 2 diabetic rats. Additionally, there was a notable reduction in both glucose and insulin levels. The extract was found to up-regulate the expression of key genes associated with carbohydrate and lipid metabolism, such as adiponectin, glucose transporter-2 (GLUT-2), and lipoprotein lipase (LPL). Moreover, the extract effectively reversed the histopathological alterations identified in the livers and kidneys of the diabetic rats, suggesting its potential therapeutic role in managing the complications associated with type 2 diabetes.

The antioxidant and anti-inflammatory properties of *Origanum* species have prompted Vujicic *et al.* (2016) to explore the potential of *O. vulgare* L. subsp. *hirtum* as a therapeutic intervention for Type 1 diabetes. Their investigation revealed that the ethyl acetate extract significantly impedes the onset of Type 1 diabetes by attenuating the pro-inflammatory M1/Th1/Th17 response and facilitating a shift in the macrophage population towards the protective M2 phenotype. Additionally, the methanolic extract of oregano demonstrated specific regulatory effects on IL-17-producing T lymphocytes, (Vujicic *et al.*, 2015). In contrast, the ethyl acetate extract displayed a broad range of immunomodulatory effects, suggesting its potential utility in mitigating islet-directed inflammation, (Vujicic *et al.*, 2016).

Furthermore, existing literature indicates that the extended application of *O. onites* L. essential oil may be beneficial in preventing or at least delaying the onset of specific complications related to diabetes mellitus. This intervention has been associated with significant reductions in levels of aspartate aminotransferase (AST), urea, and cholesterol, (Tepe, Cakir, & Sihoglu Tepe, 2016) (Lermioglu *et al.*, 1997).

4. TRADITIONAL USES OF THE GENUS ORIGANUM

The genus *Origanum* has been utilized in traditional medicine for the treatment of various health conditions. Notably, it has been employed to address respiratory ailments, including asthma and bronchitis, as well as coughs. Additionally, its applications extend to gastrointestinal disorders such as diarrhea, indigestion, and abdominal pain. Furthermore, *Origanum* is recognized for its antibacterial and anti-inflammatory properties and has been utilized in managing menstrual disorders and diabetes. This study presents a comprehensive overview of the ethnobotanical applications of *Origanum* taxa, along with their ethnopharmacological uses within the context of Turkish traditional medicine, as detailed in Table 1. Furthermore, Table 2 outlines various multi-herbal formulas that incorporate Origanum species in conjunction with other plants.

Table 1. Traditional uses of the genus origanum

Botanical names*	**Turkish names**	**Common names**	**Used parts**	**Usage forms**	**Uses**	**References**
Origanum sp.	Mercanköşk, Güveti otu, Kekik, Oğlan çiçeği	Marjoram, Oregano	Aerial parts	Infusion	Stomach ache, intestinal diseases, cold	(Tuzlaci, 2016)
			Branches	Infusion	Cold, flu	(Polat *et al.*, 2012)
			Flowering branches	Infusion	Cold, flu	(Polat, Satil, & Çakılcıoğlu, 2011)
			Flowering parts	Infusion	Abdominal pain	(Tuzlaci, 2016)
			Whole plant	Oil	Nausea	(Tuzlaci, 2016)
			Flowers, Leaves, Branches	Tea	Cough, cold	(Deniz, Serteser, & Kargıoğlu, 2010)
Origanum acutidens (Hand.-Mazz.) Ietsw. ****(End.)**	Zemul, Anıh, Anık, Dağ kekiği, Koç anığı, Sarı adaçayı,	Oregano	Aerial parts	Infusion	Anti-influenza	(Sargin, 2021)
			Aerial parts	Infusion	Cough, sedative, stomach ailments	(Karakaya *et al.*, 2019)
			Aerial parts	Infusion	Urinary tract diseases	(Tuzlaci, 2016)
			Aerial parts	Unspecified	Abdominal pain	(Terzioğlu & Coşkunçelebi, 2021)
			Flowers	Decoction	Cough, flu, stomach ailments	(Karakaya *et al.*, 2019)
			Flowers	Tea, infusion	Abdominal pain	(Kadıoğlu, Kadıoğlu, & Karagöz Sezer, 2021)
			Flowers		Hemorrhoid	(Kadıoğlu, Kadıoğlu, & Karagöz Sezer, 2021)
			Leaves	Infusion	Cold, flu, sedative	(Polat, 2019)

continued on following page

Table 1. Continued

Botanical names*	Turkish names	Common names	Used parts	Usage forms	Uses	References
			Leaves	Infusion	Sedative, kidney stone, circulatory system disorders	(Akbulut & Zengin, 2023)
			Leaves	Spice	Unspecified	(Kadıoğlu, Kadıoğlu, & Karagöz Sezer, 2021)
			Young aerial parts	Spice	Unspecified	(Doğan & Tuzlacı, 2015)
			Aerial parts, Flowering branches	Decoction	Abdominal pain	(Ozturk & Altay, 2017)
			Flowers, Leaves	Decoction	Abdominal pain	(Kadıoğlu, Kadıoğlu, & Karagöz Sezer, 2021)
			Flowers, Leaves	Spice	Unspecified	(Kadıoğlu, Kadıoğlu, & Karagöz Sezer, 2021)
Origanum bilgeri P.H.Davis ****(End.)**	Tüylümercan, Kekik	Noname	Aerial parts	Infusion	Cold	(Tuzlaci, 2016) (Ozturk & Altay, 2017) (Senkardes & Tuzlaci, 2014)
Origanum hypericifolium O.Schwarz & P.H.Davis ****(End.)**	Delikmercan, Acımık, Çökelek kekiği, Kekik, Kozalı kekik, Mercan köşkü	Noname	Aerial parts	Infusion	Abdominal pain, cold	(Tuzlaci, 2016)
			Aerial parts	Infusion	Abdominal pain, cold	(Bulut *et al.*, 2017)
			Aerial parts	Infusion	Anti-influenza	(Sargin, 2021)
			Aerial parts	Infusion	Diabetes, Prostate diseases	(Ozturk & Altay, 2017)
			Flowering parts, Leaves	Infusion	Breast cancer	(Tuzlaci, 2016) (Bozyel *et al.*, 2019)
			Flowers, Leaves	Decoction	Breast cancer	(Sağıroğlu, Dalgıç, & Toksoy, 2013)

continued on following page

Table 1. Continued

Botanical names*	Turkish names	Common names	Used parts	Usage forms	Uses	References
Origanum majorana L. (syn.: *Origanum dubium* Boiss.)	Mercanköşk, nane kekiği, Çorba kekiği, yağ kekiği, Daş kekik, Kekik, Macur otu, Farekulağı, Kanarya otu, püren kekiği, Guyotu, Ak kekik, Kekik çay, Eşekkekiği, Sakarkekik	Sweet marjoram, Pot marjoram, marjoram	Aerial parts	Boiled	Indigestion, stomach ache	(Doğan & Ugulu, 2013)
			Aerial parts	Infusion	Asthma	(Melikoğlu, Kurtoğlu, & Kültür, 2015)
			Aerial parts	Infusion	Cold, catarrh	(Bulut et al., 2017)
			Aerial parts	Infusion	Cough, sedative	Yeşilada et al. (1993)
			Aerial parts	Infusion	Diabetes	Arıtuluk & Ezer (2012); Karaman & Elgin Cebe (2016)
			Aerial parts	Infusion	Sore throat, cold	(Şenkardeş & Tuzlacı, 2014).
			Aerial parts	Infusion	Stomach ulcer	(Kültür *et al.*, 2018)
			Aerial parts	Infusion	Stomach ache	(Erbay, Anıl, & Melikoğlu, 2017)
			Aerial parts	Infusion	Urinary tract diseases	(Tuzlaci, 2016)
			Aerial parts	Tea, aromatic water, oil	Stomach ache, cold, wound healing, sedative, diaphoretic, skin problems	(Cinbilgel & Kurt, 2019)
			Aerial parts	Unspecified	Expectorant, diaphoretic, muscle pain, wound healing	(Akan & Bakir Sade, 2015)
			Flowers	Decoction	Sedative, stomach upset, diuretic, constipation	(Çömlekçioğlu & Karaman, 2008)
			Flowering branches	Infusion	Anti-influenza	(Sargin, 2021)

continued on following page

Table 1. Continued

Botanical names*	Turkish names	Common names	Used parts	Usage forms	Uses	References
			Flowering branches	Infusion	Cold, flu, stomach ache	(Sargin & Büyükcengiz, 2019)
			Flowering branches	Infusion, powdered	Sedative, stomachic, diuretic, carminative, diaphoretic, constipation	(Ozturk, Altay, & Gönenç, 2017)
			Flowering branches	Infusion, Aerial part juice, Leaf powder, Spice	Cold, flu, stomach ache, pharyngitis, pleasure and medicinal tea	(Sargin, 2015)
			Fresh shoots	Raw eaten	Sedative	(Tuzlaci, 2016)
			Leaves	Boiled in water + honey	Bronchital calmative	(Uysal *et al.*, 2012)
			Leaves	Infusion, crushed	Respiratory tract diseases, flu, asthma	(Sargin, Akçicek, & Selvi, 2013)
			Leaves	Infusion, Poultice	Cold, flu, asthma, pleasure and medicinal tea	(Sargin, Selvi, & López, 2015)
			Flowers, Leaves	Decoction	Stomach ache	(Bulut & Tuzlaci, 2015)
			Flowers, Leaves	Infusion	Cold	(Bulut & Tuzlaci, 2015)
			Flowers, Leaves	Unspecified	Spice	(Tutenocakli, 2023)
			Flowering branches, Leaves	Decoction	Insomnia, whooping cough, migraine	(Korkmaz & Karakurt, 2014)
			Flowering branches, Leaves	Decoction	Stomach ache	(Erbay, Anıl, & Melikoğlu, 2017)
			Flowering branches, Leaves	Infusion	Sedative	(Tuzlaci, 2016)
			Flowering parts, Leaves	Infusion	Diuretic	(Tuzlaci, 2016)
			Leaves, Seeds	Unspecified	Stomach ache, atherosclerosis	(Uysal *et al.*, 2010)
			Leaves, Shoots	Decoction	Stomach ache	(Sağıroğlu, Dalgıç, & Toksoy, 2013)

continued on following page

Table 1. Continued

Botanical names*	Turkish names	Common names	Used parts	Usage forms	Uses	References
			Unspecified	Infusion, spice	Hypotension, pleasure tea	(Sargin, Selvi, & Büyükcengiz, 2015)
			Unspecified	Unspecified	Abdominal pain, inguinal pain, menstrual regulator, vasoconstrictor, cold, pharyngitis, stomachic, medicinal tea	(Kayiran, 2019)
			Unspecified	Unspecified	Common cold	(Başer *et al.*, 2006)
			Unspecified	Unspecified	Stomach ache, cold	(Bulut & Tuzlaci, 2009)
Origanum minutiflorum O.Schwarz & P.H.Davis *(End.)	Tokakekik, Sütçüler kekiği, Kekik, eşekkekiği	Spartan oregano	Aerial parts	Decoction	Stomach ache	(Yeşilada *et al.*, 1993)
			Aerial parts	Infusion	Stomach ache	(Tuzlaci, 2016)
			Aerial parts	Poultice	Stomach ache, rheumatism	(Tuzlaci, 2016)
			Aerial parts	Poultice	Toothache, stomach ache, rheumatism	(Yeşilada *et al.*, 1993)
			Aerial parts	Tea	Cold, stomach ache	(Cinbilgel & Kurt, 2019)
			Flowers, Leaves	Infusion, essential oil	Abdominal pain, waist pain	(Fakir, Korkmaz, & Güller, 2009)
			Leaves, Stems	Infusion	Pain reliever, digestive, antimicrobial	(Aksoy, Çelik, & Tunay, 2016)
			Flowers, Leaves, Shoots	Infusion	Cold, flu, throat infection	(Ozturk, Altay, & Gönenc, 2017) (Fakir, Korkmaz, & Icel, 2016)
			Flowers, Leaves, Shoots	Infusion	Spices, Cold, flu, throat infection	(Korkmaz, Fakir, & Güller, 2011)
			Flowers, Leaves, Shoots	Decoction, Infusion	Cold, flu, throat infection, stomach ache, toothache, rheumatism, abdominal pain	(Ozturk & Altay, 2017)
			Unspecified	Unspecified	Food, beverage, spice, medicine, apiculture	(Demirel & Dutkuner, 2021)

continued on following page

Table 1. Continued

Botanical names*	Turkish names	Common names	Used parts	Usage forms	Uses	References
			Unspecified	Unspecified	General health, cold, stomach ache, skin cleanser, flu, pain reliever, spice	(Korkmaz & Fakir, 2009)
Origanum onites L.	Bilyalı kekik, Eşek kekiği, Eşekkekiği, Güve kekiği, Karakekik, Taş kekiği, Kekik, Dağ kekiği, Akbaş kekik, Kırkbaş kekik, koca Lealı kekik, tokalı kekik, bilya kekik, arı kekiği, Mercanköşk, Ak kekik, Deli kekik, Beyaz kekik, Toklu baş kekiği, güve otu, topbaş kekik, akbaşlı, akbaşlı kekik, kaya kekiği, koca kekik, İzmir kekiği	Pot marjoram, Oregano, Turkish oregano, Cretan oregano	Aerial parts	Boiled	Stomach ache	(Doğan & Ugulu, 2013)
			Aerial parts	Decoction	Cold, stomach ache	(Yeşilada *et al.*, 1993)
			Aerial parts	Decoction	Cough, flu	(Uysal *et al.*, 2012)
			Aerial parts	Decoction	Diabetes	(Sarikaya, Öner, & Harput, 2010)
			Aerial parts	Decoction	Digestive regulatory	(Akyol & Altan, 2013)
			Aerial parts	Decoction	Eczema	(Erarslan, Ecevit Genç, & Kültür, 2020)
			Aerial parts	Decoction	Ithching	(Polat & Satil, 2012) (Tuzlaci, 2016)

continued on following page

Table 1. Continued

Botanical names*	Turkish names	Common names	Used parts	Usage forms	Uses	References
			Aerial parts	Decoction	Stomach ache, bronchitis, anti-inflamatory, immunogenic, antiemetic, carminative, expectorant, cough, antihypertensive	(Sağıroğlu, Dalgıç, & Toksoy, 2013)
			Aerial parts	Essential oil	Head ache	(Erbay, Anil, & Melikoğlu, 2018)
			Aerial parts	İnfusion	Abdominal ailments, cold, high cholesterol, sedative, cardiovascular disease, antiparasitic	(Arican, Yeşil, & Ecevit Genç, 2013)
			Aerial parts	Infusion	Abdominal pain, cough, stomach ailments	(Bulut *et al.*, 2017)
			Aerial parts	Infusion	Cold, stomach disorders, dyspepsia	(Kalankan, Özkan, & Akbulut, 2015)
			Aerial parts	Infusion	Covid-19	(Akbulut & Özkan, 2023)
			Aerial parts	Infusion	Eczema, grayout, immune-boosting, vertigo	(Tuzlaci, 2016)
			Aerial parts	Infusion	Head ache, abdominal pain, cold, the sniffles, flu, bronchitis	(Erucar, Tan, & Miski, 2023)
			Aerial parts	Infusion	Hyperglycaemia, diabetes	(Erucar, Tan, & Miski, 2023)
			Aerial parts	Infusion	Hypertension, tachycardia	(Erucar, Tan, & Miski, 2023)
			Aerial parts	Infusion	Muscle development in children/teenager	(Erucar, Tan, & Miski, 2023)
			Aerial parts	Infusion	Stomach ailments, antiseptic, cholesterol	(Güner & Selvi, 2016)
			Aerial parts	Infusion	Stomach ache, stomachic	(Erucar, Tan, & Miski, 2023)
			Aerial parts	Infusion	Stomach ache	(Erbay, Anıl, & Melikoğlu, 2017)

continued on following page

Table 1. Continued

Botanical names*	Turkish names	Common names	Used parts	Usage forms	Uses	References
			Aerial parts	Infusion	Stomach ache	(Bulut & Tuzlaci, 2015)
			Aerial parts	Infusion	Stomachic, diuretic	(Selvi, Dağdelen, & Kara, 2013)
			Aerial parts	Infusion	Tachycardia	(Gulec, Erarslan, & Kültür, 2023)
			Aerial parts	Infusion	Weak nails strengthening	(Erucar, Tan, & Miski, 2023)
			Aerial Parts	Oil	Diabetes	(Polat & Satil, 2012)
			Aerial parts	Oil	Nausea	(Erucar, Tan, & Miski, 2023)
			Aerial parts	Oil	Toothache	(Sağıroğlu, Dalgıç, & Toksoy, 2013)
			Aerial parts	Decoction, Salve	Eczema	(Sağıroğlu, Dalgıç, & Toksoy, 2013)
			Aerial parts	Infusion, Crushed	Gastrointestinal diseases, bronchitis, respiratory tract diesases & flu, hypertension & tachycardia	(Sargin, Akçicek, & Selvi, 2013)
			Aerial parts	Infusion, Crushed	Hypertension	(Olcay & Kültür, 2020)
			Aerial parts	Infusion, Essential oil	Upper back pain	Bozyel, Merdamert Bozyel, & Canli, 2020
			Aerial parts	Infusion, essential oil, Paste, Aerial part juice, Oil extracted, Drop	Angina, bronchitis, pharyngitis, laryngitis, cold, flu, haircare, carminative, costiveness, intestinal spasm, dyspepsia, head ache, nail care, hypertension, tachycardia, diabetes, pleasure, medicinal tea	(Sargin, Selvi, & López, 2015)
			Aerial Parts	Tea, Medicinal	Cold	(Nacakci & Dutkuner, 2018)

continued on following page

Table 1. Continued

Botanical names*	Turkish names	Common names	Used parts	Usage forms	Uses	References
			Aerial parts	Unspecified	Abdominal pain, stomach flu, sprain	(Kincal, Ceylan, & Görk, 2021)
			Flowering branches	Decoction	Toothache	(Uzun & Kaya, 2019)
			Flowering branches	Infusion	Abdominal pain	Polat & Satil, 2012
			Leaves	Dried	Spice	Akyol & Altan, 2013
			Leaves	Fresh	Toothache, head ache	Polat & Satil, 2012
			Aerial parts, Flowers	Infusion	Body strengthening	Erucar, Tan, & Miski, 2023
			Aerial parts, Flowering branches	Infusion	Diabetes	Arituluk & Ezer, 2012
			Aerial parts, Leaves	Aromatic water	Diarrhea	(Karahüseyin & Sari, 2019)
			Aerial parts, Leaves	Infusion	Diarrhea	(Karahüseyin & Sari, 2019)
			Aerial parts, Leaves	Infusion/ Decoction	Diarrhea	(Karahüseyin & Sari, 2019)
			Flowering parts, Leaves	Dried	Tetter, diuretic	(Tuzlaci, 2016)
			Flowering parts, Leaves	Infusion	Eczema, hemorrhoid	(Tuzlaci, 2016)
			Flowers, Leaves	Decoction	Abdominal pain, nausea, bronchitis	(Akan & Pekmez, 2018)
			Flowers, Leaves	Decoction	Cold, stomach ache, indigestion	(Akbaş, Çıtakoğlu, & Davran, 2024)
			Flowers, Leaves	Infusion	Asthma	(Melikoğlu, Kurtoğlu, & Kültür, 2015)
			Flowers, Leaves	Infusion	Cold, flu, hyperglycaemia	(Akbulut, Karakose, & Özkan, 2019)
			Flowers, Leaves	infusion	Diabetes	(Karaman & Elgin Cebe, 2016)
			Flowers, Leaves	Infusion, Essential oil	Abdominal pain, toothache, head ache	(Fakir, Korkmaz, & Icel, 2016)

continued on following page

Table 1. Continued

Botanical names*	Turkish names	Common names	Used parts	Usage forms	Uses	References
			Flowers, Leaves	Unspecified	Spice	(Akan & Pekmez, 2018)
			Flowers, Leaves	Unspecified	Tea	(Tutenocakli, 2023)
			Leaves, Stems	Tea, Spice	Unspecified	(Tanaydin, Satil, & Çakılcıoğlu, 2022)
			Aerial parts, Flowers, Flowering branches	Foot bath	Immune-boosting	(Sargin & Dogan, 2023)
			Flowers, Leaves, Shoots	Infusion	Spices, cold, flu, throat infection	(Korkmaz, Fakir, & Güller, 2011)
			Flowers, Leaves, Shoots	Volatile oil	Throat infection	(Korkmaz, Fakir, & Güller, 2009)
			Flowers, Leaves, Stems	Decoction	Spice, cold	(Çömlekçioğlu & Karaman, 2008)
			Flowers, Leaves, Stem barks	Infusion	Diabetes, cough	(Güler, Erkan, & Uğurlu, 2020)
			Flowering branches, Fresh shoots, Leaves	Tea, Water, Oil, Spice	Cholesterol, vasodilating, cold, cough, diabetes, burn insecticidal	(Cinbilgel & Kurt, 2019)
			Aerial parts, Flowers, Leaves, Oil, Shoots	Infusion	Antiseptic, abdominal ailments, cold, high cholesterol, sedative, cardiovascular disease, antiparasitic, throat infection, moth repellent	(Ozturk, Altay, & Gönenç, 2017)
			Unspecified	Oil	Abdominal pain	(Kincal, Ceylan, & Görk, 2021)
			Unspecified	Oil	Burn	(Tuzlaci, 2016)
			Unspecified	Oil	Hemorrhoid	(Polat & Satil, 2012)
			Unspecified	Medicinal, Spice	Stomach ache, head ache, toothache, diabetes, protection for lice	(Öz Aydın *et al.*, 2006)

continued on following page

Table 1. Continued

Botanical names*	Turkish names	Common names	Used parts	Usage forms	Uses	References
			Unspecified	Unspecified	Cold	(Başer *et al.*, 2006)
			Unspecified	Unspecified	Food, beverage, spice, medicine	(Demirel & Dutkuner, 2021)
			Unspecified	Unspecified	General health, cold, stomach ache, skin cleanser, flu, pain reliever, spice	(Korkmaz & Fakir, 2009)
			Unspecified	Unspecified	Stomach ache	(Bulut & Tuzlaci, 2009) (Ersen Bak & Cifci, 2020)
Origanum rotundifolium Boiss.	Yuvarlak mercan, Anıh, Aylık otu,	Round-leaved oregano	Aerial parts	Decoction (bath)	Infant gas pains	(Bozyel, Merdamert Bozyel, & Canli, 2020)
			Aerial parts	Infusion	Cough, sedative, stomach ailments	(Karakaya *et al.*, 2019)
Origanum saccatum P.H.Davis **(End.)**	Tahtacı kekiği, Bayır çayı, Çay otu, Cıngıllı kekik, Kekik, Cıngıllı Ot	Noname	Aerial parts	Infusion	Herniated thoracic/lumbar disc	(Albayrak & Daskin, 2018)
			Aerial parts, Flowering branches	Infusion	Anti-influenza	(Sargin, 2021)
			Aerial parts, Flowering branches	Infusion	Cold, flu	(Sargin & Büyükcengiz, 2019)
			Aerial parts, Flowering branches	Infusion, Aerial part juice, Oil extracted, Leaf powder, Spice	Cold, flu, stomach ache, herniated disc, Pharyngitis, pleasure & medicinal tea	(Sargin, 2015)
			Flowering branches, Leaves	Tea	Relaxing tea, stomach ache	(Cinbilgel & Kurt, 2019)
			Flowers, Leaves, Shoots	Distilled water	Cholesterol, blood sugar, digestive, respiratory system disease, ulcer, intestines disease, arthrosis, waist pain	(Fakir, Korkmaz, & Güller, 2009)

continued on following page

Table 1. Continued

Botanical names*	Turkish names	Common names	Used parts	Usage forms	Uses	References
			Aerial parts, Flowers, Juice, Leaves, Shoots,	Infusion, Distilled Water, Powdered	Cholesterol, diabetes, digestive and respiratory system diseases, stomach ulcer, gastro-intestinal diseases, arthritis, waist pain, cold, flu, stomach ache, pharyngitis, herniated disc	(Ozturk & Altay, 2017)
Origanum sipyleum L. **(End.)	Mor mercan, Kekik, Bayır kekiği, Mor çay, Ak kekik, Mercan köşk	Showy pink oregano, Sipyle Marjoram	Aerial parts	Decoction	Stomach ache	(Akıllıgöz & Başaran, 2021)
			Flowers	Decoction	Respiratory tract diseases, covid-19	(Koyuncu *et al.*, 2010)
			Flowers	Unspecified	Insomnia, shortness of breath	(Erucar, Tan, & Miski, 2023)
			Flowering parts	Dried	Moth repellent	(Tuzlaci, 2016)
			Leaves	Infusion	Stomach ulcer, carminative, antihypertensive, diuretic	(Tuzlaci, 2016)
			Flowers, Leaves	Dried	Spice	(Altay *et al.*, 2015)
			Flowers, Leaves	Infusion	Medicinal tea	(Altay *et al.*, 2015)
			Flowering branches, Leaves	Infusion	Cold	(Tuzlaci, 2016)
			Flowering branches, Leaves	Tea, spice	Hemorrhoid, diabetes	(Cinbilgel & Kurt, 2019)
			Flowers, Leaves, Shoots	Distilled water	Cholesterol, blood sugar, digestive, respiratory system disease, ulcer, intestines disease, arthrosis, waist pain	(Fakir, Korkmaz, & Güller, 2009)

continued on following page

Table 1. Continued

Botanical names*	Turkish names	Common names	Used parts	Usage forms	Uses	References
			Flowers, Leaves, Shoots	Oil	Cholesterol, blood sugar	(Korkmaz, Fakir, & Güller, 2011)
			Flowers, Leaves, Shoots	Tea, Distilled Water, Infusion	Cholesterol, diabetes, respiratory system diseases, ulcer, gastro-intestinal diseases, arthritis, waist pain, digestive system disorders, diuretic, antiseptic, stomach ache, carminative, indigestion, back pain, pharyngitis, asthma, expectorant, rheumatism, appetizing, cardiac diseases, cough, head ache, sore throat, abdominal pain, sprain pain, injury pain, cold, flu, tension, flatulence	(Ozturk & Altay, 2017)
			Flowers, Leaves, Shoots	Unspecified	Stomach ulcer	(Kültür *et al.*, 2018)
			Unspecified	Spice, medicinal	Unspecified	(Demirel & Dutkuner, 2021)
			Unspecified	Unspecified	General health, cold, stomach ache, skın cleanser, flu, pain reliever, spice	(Korkmaz & Fakir, 2009)
Origanum syriacum L.	Hababa, kekik, Atkekiği, Dağ nanesi	Syrian oregano, Biblical-hyssop, Lebanese oregano	Leaves	Unspecified	common cold, diabetes	(Güzel & Güzelşemme, 2018)
			Stems	Decoction	Stomach ache	(Erbay, Anil, & Melikoğlu, 2017)
			Flowers, Leaves, Oil, Seeds	Maceration	Rheumatism, eye ailment, burns, stomach troubles, sedative	(Ozturk, Altay, & Gönenç, 2017)

continued on following page

Table 1. Continued

Botanical names*	Turkish names	Common names	Used parts	Usage forms	Uses	References
			Unspecified	Unspecified	Pneumonia, asthma, cough, anthelminthic, toothache, intestinal cleanser, cold, flu, abdominal pain, hernia, pharyngitis, medicinal tea	(Demirci Kayiran, 2019)
Origanum syriacum subsp. *bevanii* (Holmes) Greuter & Burdet	Hababa, Göğ otu, At kekiği, Dağ kekiği, Kekik, Eşek kekiği, eşşek kekiği, güve kekiği, boz kekik, sihilin kekiği, sahilin kekiği, Halil İbrahim kekiği	Noname	Aerial parts	Infusion	Medicinal tea, cold, flu, cough, colic spasms, menstrual pains, spice	(Kerar & Akan, 2019)
			Aerial parts	Chew, Tea	Mouth sore	(Demirci & Özhatay, 2012)
			Leaves	Infusion	Cold	(Tuzlaci, 2016) (Güzel & Kayıkçı, 2023)
			Aerial parts, Flowering branches	Infusion	Anti-influenza	(Sargin, 2021)
			Aerial parts, Flowering branches	Infusion	Cold, flu, pharyngitis, stomach ache	(Sargin & Büyükcengiz, 2019)
			Aerial parts, Flowering branches	Infusion, Aerial part juice, Oil extracted, Leaf powder, Spice	Cold, flu, pharyngitis, stomach ache, pyrosis, indigestion pains seen in the riding animals like horses & donkeys, pleasure & medicinal tea	(Sargin, 2015)
			Branches, Flowers, Leaves	Unspecified	Spice	(Boz, İldeniz, & Cabi, 2022)
			Unspecified	Infusion, Spice	Cold, flu, pharyngitis, stomach ache, pleasure tea	(Sargin, Selvi, & Büyükcengiz, 2015)

continued on following page

Table 1. Continued

Botanical names*	Turkish names	Common names	Used parts	Usage forms	Uses	References
Origanum vulgare L.	Karakınık, Kekik otu, Keklik otu, Anuk, Anık, Kekik, Kaya kekiği, taş kekik, kokulu kekik, sarı kekik, tapan kekiği, yayla kekiği, Gevey otu, Dağ kekiği, Deli kekik, Karakekik, Güve kekiği, kaba topağı, Boylu kekik, Güvelik otu, Güve otu, Dost otu	Wild marjoram, Ornamental oregano, Oregano	Aerial parts	Aromatic water	Stomachic, intestinal pain	(Yeşilada *et al.*, 1993)
			Aerial parts	Decoction	Dyspepsia, stomach ache	(Kültür *et al.*, 2021)
			Aerial parts	Decoction	Intestinal pain	(Yeşilada *et al.*, 1993
			Aerial parts	Decoction	Kidney stone	(Sağıroğlu & Aydin, 2024)
			Aerial parts	Decoction	Menstrual pains	(Unal & Altundağ Çakır, 2024)
			Aerial parts	Infusion	Anti-influenza	(Sargin, 2021)
			Aerial parts	Infusion	Tachycardia, vasodilator	(Gulec, Erarslan, & Kültür, 2023)
			Aerial parts	Mordanting	Yellow dye, green dye	(Badem *et al.*, 2019)
			Aerial parts	Tea	Food	(Hayta, Polat, & Selvi, 2014)
			Aerial parts	Unspecified	Lower back pain	(Boyzel, Merdamert Bozyel, & Canli, 2020)
			Aerial parts	Unspecified	Spice	(Kültür *et al.*, 2021)
			Flowering branches	Infusion	Cold, flu	(Polat & Satil, 2012)
			Fruits	Spice	Food, dyspepsia	(Hayta, Polat, & Selvi, 2014)
			Leaves	Chew	Toothache	(Uzun & Kaya, 2019)

continued on following page

Table 1. Continued

Botanical names*	Turkish names	Common names	Used parts	Usage forms	Uses	References
			Leaves	Decoction	Antihypertensive, high cholesterol	(Polat *et al.*, 2015)
			Leaves	Decoction	High cholesterol, cold, flu	(Şahin & Kılıç, 2022)
			Leaves	Decoction	Hypertension	(Olcay & Kültür, 2020)
			Leaves	Fresh	Toothache, head ache	(Polat & Satil, 2012)
			Leaves	Infusion	Sedative	(Tuzlaci, 2016)
			Leaves	Infusion, Decoction	Hemorrhoid	(Sari & Erarslan, 2023)
			Aerial parts, Flowering branches	Lotion, mash, gargle, infusion	Acne vulgaris	(Korkmaz & Karakurt, 2015)
			Aerial parts, Flowering branches	Lotion, Mash, Infusion, Hair bath, Gargle	Baldness, carminative, costiveness, intestinal spasm, dyspepsia, diet, weight loss, haircare, acne treatment, toothache, tachycardia, intestinal worms, pleasure and medicinal tea	(Sargin, Selvi, & López, 2013)
			Aerial parts with/ without flowers, Flowering branches	Foot bath	Immune-boosting	(Sargin & Dogan, 2023)
			Flowers, Leaves	Spice	Unspecified	(Korkmaz & Karakurt, 2014) (Uzun & Palabas Uzun, 2011)
			Flowering branches, Leaves	Infusion	Diuretic, carminative, sedative, diaphoretic	(Yeşil & İnal, 2021)
			Flowers, Leaves, Shoots	Distilled water	Cholesterol, blood sugar, digestive, respiratory system disease, ulcer, intestines disease, arthrosis, waist pain	(Fakir, Korkmaz, & Güller, 2009)

continued on following page

Table 1. Continued

Botanical names*	Turkish names	Common names	Used parts	Usage forms	Uses	References
			Flowers, Leaves, Shoots	Oil	Cholesterol, blood sugar	(Korkmaz, Fakir, & Güller, 2011)
Origanum vulgare subsp. *gracile* (K.Koch) Ietsw.	Kuşzemulu, Kekik, Dağ kekiği, Karakınık, Eşek kekiği, Kır kekiği,	Russian oregano	Aerial parts	Infusion	Antitussives	(Demir, 2020)
			Aerial parts	Infusion	Diabetes	(Aritukul & Ezer, 2012)
			Aerial parts	Infusion	Shortness of breath, enuresis	(Altundağ Çakır, 2017)
			Aerial parts	Decoction, Infusion	hypertension	(Olcay & Kültür, 2020)
			Aerial parts	Unspecified	Spice	(Yeşil & İnal, 2019)
			Fresh aerial parts	boiled	Preparation of pastry and pancake	(Kılıç & Bağcı, 2013)
			Fresh aerial parts	spice	Unspecified	(Doğan & Tuzlacı, 2015) (Kılıç & Bağcı, 2013)
			Flowers	Tea	Unspecified	(Doğan & Tuzlacı, 2015)
			Flowers	Unspecified	Vulnerary, stomach ache, hypertension, epilepsy, head ache, asthma, digestive	(Terzioğlu & Coşkunçelebi, 2021)
			Flowering branches	Infusion	Asthma	(Melikoğlu, Kurtoğlu, & Kültür, 2015)
			Leaves	Decoction	Cold, flu, urinary inflammations	(Özdemir Nath & Kültür, 2022)
			Aerial parts, Flowering branches, Leaves	Infusion	Anti-influenza	(Sargin, 2021)

continued on following page

Table 1. Continued

Botanical names*	Turkish names	Common names	Used parts	Usage forms	Uses	References
Origanum vulgare subsp. *hirtum* (Link) Ietsw.	Karamercan, Nuz otu, Nuzlu ot, Kekik, Güve otu, Kak otu, Uzun kekik, Kekikotu, Köfteotu, Ayaklı kekik, Kekik otu, Keklik otu, Kara kekik, Taş kekiği, Yayla kekiği, Istanbul kekiği, deli kekik, Karakekik, Güve kekiği, Yer kekiği, Keklik, Ak kekik, Mercan köşk, Düğümlü kekik, Güce kekiği, Baharat otu, Güveci, Koru çayı, Uzun kekik, Yaban kekiği, Güvey kekiği	Greek oregano	Aerial parts	Decoction	Kidney stone	(Sağıroğlu & Aydin, 2024)
			Aerial parts	Decoction	Stomach ache	(Uysal *et al.*, 2012)
			Aerial parts	Infusion	Abdominal pain, cold, cholesterol, nausea, inflamation, cancer	(Baykan *et al.*, 2023)
			Aerial parts	Infusion	Anti-influenza	(Bulut *et al.*, 2017)
			Aerial parts	Infusion	Cold, flu	(Kızılarslan Hançer *et al.*, 2020)
			Aerial parts	Infusion	Stomach ailments	(Bulut *et al.*, 2017)
			Aerial parts	Infusion	Stomach ailments, diabetes	(Bulut & Tuzlaci, 2015)
			Aerial parts	Infusion	Stomach ailments, hemorrhoid, appetite stimulant	(Güner & Selvi, 2016)

continued on following page

Table 1. Continued

Botanical names*	Turkish names	Common names	Used parts	Usage forms	Uses	References
			Aerial parts	Oil	Gingivitis	(Bulut & Tuzlaci, 2015)
			Aerial parts	Decoction, Infusion, Oil	Gingival diseases	(Uzun & Kaya, 2019)
			Aerial parts	Unspecified	Spice added to "tarhana"	(Kızılarslan & Özhatay, 2012)
			Aerial parts	Unspecified	Preservative for dried fruit "kak"	(Kızılarslan & Özhatay, 2012)
			Aerial parts	Unspecified	Tea	(Kızılarslan & Özhatay, 2012)
			Branches with leaves	Tea, Spice	Unspecified	(Satil, Akcicek, & Selvi, 2008)
			Leaves	Chew	Head ache	(Erbay, Anil, & Melikoğlu, 2018)
			Leaves	Infusion	Diabetes	(Arituluk & Ezer, 2012) (Karaman & Elgin Cebe, 2016) (Ecevit Genç & Özhatay, 2006)
			Leaves	Tea	Asthma	(Melikoğlu, Kurtoğlu, & Kültür, 2015)
			Aerial parts, Leaves	Infusion	Diabetes	(Karaman & Elgin Cebe, 2016)
			Flowers, Leaves	Decoction	Stomach ache, rheumatism	(Sağıroğlu, Dalgıç, & Toksoy, 2013)
			Flowers, Leaves	Infusion	Diabetes, hemorrhoid	(Altay *et al.*, 2015)
			Flowers, Leaves	Tea, Spice	Unspecified	(Tanaydin, Satil, & Çakılcıoğlu, 2022)
			Flowers, Leaves, Shoots	Unspecified	Cholesterol, blood sugar, digestive, respiratory system diseases, stomach ulcer, intestinal diseases, arthrosis, waist pain	(Ozturk, Altay, & Gönenç, 2017)
			Unspecified	Medical, spice	Toothache, cold	(Öz Aydın *et al.*, 2006)
			Unspecified	Oil	Low back pain	(Tuzlaci, 2016)

continued on following page

Table 1. Continued

Botanical names*	Turkish names	Common names	Used parts	Usage forms	Uses	References
			Unspecified	Unspecified	Cold	(Başer et al., 2006)
			Unspecified	Unspecified	Diabetes, stomach diseases, gingivitis	(Bulut & Tuzlaci, 2009)
			Unspecified	Unspecified	Medicinal	(Aydin & Yeşil, 2018)
			Unspecified	Unspecified	Rheumatic pain	(Ersen Bak & Cifci, 2020)
Origanum vulgare subsp. *viridulum* (Martrin-Donos) Nyman (syn.: *O. vulgare* subsp. *viride* (Boiss.) Hayek)	İstanbul kekiği, Mercanköşk, Çay otu, domurcak çayı, Çay çiçeği, Dağ çiçeği, Adaçayı, Dağ anığı, Kekik, Çay kekiği, Güvey otu, Hoş otu, Kaya kekiği, Taş kekik, Sarı kekik, Tapan kekiği, Yayla kekiği, Dağ kekiği, kokulu kekik, şabla kekiği, tuzlu kekik	Italian oregano, Winter marjoram	Aerial parts	Decoction	Cold	(Saraç, Özkan, & Akbulut, 2013)
			Aerial parts	Infusion	Cold, sore throat, diaphoretic, diuretic	(Akıllıgöz & Başaran, 2021)
			Aerial parts	Infusion	Stomach ache	(Erbay, Anil, & Melikoğlu, 2018)
			Aerial parts	Spice	Unspecified	(Çalışkan, Yıldırım, & Şenkardeş, 2020) (Polat *et al.*, 2015)
			Aerial parts	Unspecified	Cold	(Çalışkan, Yıldırım, & Şenkardeş, 2020)
			Aerial parts	Decoction, Spice, Herbal Tea	Cold, flu	(Bağcı & Keskin, 2022)
			Flowering branches	Infusion	Anti-influenza	Sargin, 2021
			Aerial parts, Leaves	Decoction, Dried eaten	Cancer cure, spice	(Akbulut & Zengin, 2023)

continued on following page

Table 1. Continued

Botanical names*	Turkish names	Common names	Used parts	Usage forms	Uses	References
			Flowering plant, Leaves	Infusion	Stomach ulcer	(Kültür *et al.*, 2018)
			Flowers, Leaves, Stems	Food, Tea	Unspecified	(Ecevit Genç & Özhatay, 2006)
Origanum vulgare subsp. *vulgare* L.	Dağ kekiği, uzun kekik, kırçayı, Grip otu, adaçayı, Mercan köşk, Karakınık, dağ çayı	European Oregano	Aerial parts	Decoction	Diabetes	(Arituluk & Exer, 2012) (Karaman & Elgin Cebe, 2016)
			Aerial parts	Decoction	Relaxing, bronchodilator in influenza	(Karcı et al., 2017)
			Aerial parts	Decoction	Kidney stone	(Tuzlaci, 2016)
			Aerial parts	Infusion	Stomach disorders, abdominal pain, cold, flu, diabetes, bone strengthening	(Tuzlaci, 2016)
			Aerial parts	Dried, powdered and mixed with honey	Wound healing	(Tuzlaci, 2016)
			Flowers, Leaves	Decoction	Diabetes, flu	Kayabaşı, Tümen, & Polat, 2023
			Fruits, Whole plant	Decoction	Cold, Infection, asthma	Eminağaoğlu, Göktürk, & Akyıldırım Beğen, 2017
			Flowers, Leaves, Stem barks	Infusion	Pharyngitis	(Güler, Erkan, & Uğurlu, 2020)
Origanum x *majoricum* L.	Mercanköşk	Italian Oregano, Hardy sweet marjoram	Aerial parts	Infusion	Urenary diseases, nausea, stomach ache, cold, flu	(Polat & Satil, 2012)

"*" (6); "**(End.)" Endemic taxon

Table 2. Multi-herbal formulas of the genus origanum

Botanical names	Turkish names	Common names	Used parts	Usage forms	Uses	References
Origanum onites Juglans regia	Bilyalı kekik Ceviz	Turkish oregano +Persian walnut	Aerial parts +Leaves	Henna	Hair strengthening	(Erucar, Tan, & Miski, 2023)
Origanum onites Matricaria chamomilla	Bilyalı kekik Alman papatyası	Turkish oregano +Scented mayweed	Aerial parts +Aerial parts	Infusion	Bronchitis	(Erucar, Tan, & Miski, 2023)
Origanum onites Salvia sp.	Bilyalı kekik Adaçayı	Turkish oregano +Sage	Aerial parts +Leaves	Infusion	Anti-influenza	(Sargin, 2021)
Origanum onites Salvia sp.	Bilyalı kekik Adaçayı	Turkish oregano +Sage	Aerial parts with flowers, flowering branches +Leaves	Infusion	Immune-boosting	(Sargin & Dogan, 2023)
Origanum onites Salvia sp.	Bilyalı kekik Adaçayı	Turkish oregano +Sage	Aerial parts +Aerial parts	Infusion	Severe flu	(Erucar, Tan, & Miski, 2023)
Origanum onites Vitis vinifera	Bilyalı kekik Asma	Turkish oregano + Grape vine	Aerial parts +Vinegar	Infusion mixed with vinegar	Blood cancer	(Tuzlaci, 2016)
Origanum onites Pimpinella anisum Mentha sp.	Bilyalı kekik Anason Nane	Turkish oregano +Anise +Mint	Aerial parts with flowers, flowering branches +Leaves +Leaves	Infusion	Immune-boosting	(Sargin & Dogan, 2023)
Origanum onites Vitex agnus-castus Thymus sp.	Bilyalı kekik Hayıt Kekik	Turkish oregano + Lilac chaste tree +Thyme	Aerial parts, leaves +Aerial parts +Aerial parts	Cooked with flour and water	Diarrhea	(Karahüseyin & Sarı, 2019)
Origanum onites Salvia sp. *Thymus* sp. *Mentha* sp.	Bilyalı kekik Adaçayı Kekik Nane	Turkish oregano +Sage +Tyhme +Mint	Aerial parts +Aerial parts +Aerial parts +Aerial parts	Infusion + salt (Foot bath)	Foot pain	(Erucar, Tan, & Miski, 2023)

continued on following page

Table 2. Continued

Botanical names	Turkish names	Common names	Used parts	Usage forms	Uses	References
Origanum onites *Petroselinum crispum* *Allium cepa* *Olea europaea*	Bilyalı kekik Maydanoz Soğan Zeytin	Turkish oregano +Garden parsley +Common onion +Olive	Aerial parts +Aerial parts +Tubers +Oil	Boiled and applied as poultice	Infertility in women	(Erucar, Tan, & Miski, 2024)
Origanum vulgare *Salvia* sp.	Karakınık Adaçayı	Wild marjoram +Sage	Aerial parts with/ without flowers, flowering branches +Leaves	Infusion	Immune-boosting	(Sargin & Dogan, 2023)
Origanum vulgare *Pimpinella anisum* *Mentha* sp.	Karakınık Anason Nane	Wild marjoram +Anise +Mint	Aerial parts with/ without flowers, flowering branches +Leaves +Leaves	Infusion	Immune-boosting	(Sargin & Dogan, 2023)
Origanum vulgare *Petroselinum crispum* *Mentha pulegium*	Karakınık Maydanoz Yarpuz	Wild marjoram + Garden parsley + Pennyroyal	Leaves +Leaves +Leaves	Infusion	Immune-boosting	(Sargin & Dogan, 2023)
Origanum vulgare *Petroselinum crispum* *Mentha x piperita*	Karakınık Maydanoz Nane	Wild marjoram + Garden parsley + Peppermint	Leaves +Leaves +Leaves	Infusion	Immune-boosting	(Sargin & Dogan, 2023)
Origanum vulgare *Cistus laurifolius* *Populus alba* *Reseda lutea* *Salvia tomentosa*	Karakınık Karağan Ak kavak Muhabbetçiçeği Şalba	Wild marjoram +Laurel-leaved cistus +White poplar +Wild mignonette +Balsamic sage	Aerial parts +Aerial parts + Sprouts + Aerial parts + Aerial parts	Mordanting	Yellow dye	(Badem *et al.*, 2019)

continued on following page

Table 2. Continued

Botanical names	Turkish names	Common names	Used parts	Usage forms	Uses	References
Origanum vulgare subsp. *hirtum* *Melissa officinalis*	Karamercan Oğulotu	Greek oregano +Lemon balm	Aerial parts +Aerial parts	Infusion	Nausea	(Bulut & Tuzlaci, 2009)
Origanum vulgare subsp. *hirtum* *Tilia tomentosa*	Karamercan Gümüşi ıhlamur	Greek oregano +Silver lime	Aerial parts +Flowers	Infusion	Cold	(Bulut & Tuzlaci, 2009)
Origanum vulgare subsp. *hirtum* *Petroselinum crispum* *Mentha pulegium*	Karamercan Maydanoz Yarpuz	Greek oregano + Garden parsley + Pennyroyal	Leaves +Leaves +Leaves	Infusion	Immune-boosting	(Tuzlaci, 2016)

"*" (6); "**(End.)" Endemic taxon

5. CONCLUSION

The relationship between plants and humans is a complex and enduring phenomenon that has traversed the entirety of human history. The utilization of plant resources has facilitated the satisfaction of diverse human needs, encompassing food, medicine, shelter, fuel, clothing, perfumes, and cosmetics. The transmission of knowledge regarding these botanical applications has occurred through both oral traditions and written texts across generations.

In contemporary society, there has been a marked increase in interest surrounding plant-derived pharmaceuticals, particularly in response to the rising awareness of the adverse effects associated with synthetic drugs. This burgeoning field, known as ethnopharmacology, focuses on the exploration of plants as a source of medicinal compounds and has led to the introduction of numerous novel pharmaceuticals into the market.

The therapeutic efficacy of these herbal remedies is significantly influenced by the presence of secondary metabolites. This study provides an in-depth examination of the Origanum genus, emphasizing its secondary metabolites, biological activities, and traditional applications. The findings robustly support the hypothesis that various species within the Origanum genus may possess valuable therapeutic properties in the management of a range of pathological conditions, including bacterial and fungal infections, diabetes, and cancer.

REFERENCES

Akan, H., & Bakır Sade, Y. (2015). Investigation of the ethnobotanical aspects of Kâhta town and Narince village. *BEU Journal of Science*, *4*(2), 219–248.

Akan, H., Öz, A., & Pekmez, H. (2018). Some of the plant species used among the local people in Ortaca (Muğla). *Turkish Journal of Agriculture-Food Science and Technology, 6*(9), 1168-1174.

Akbaş, K., Çıtakoğlu, M., & Davran, S. (2024). Natural plants of the Sandras Mountain (Köyceğiz-Muğla) traditionally employed for therapeutic purposes. *Turkish Journal of Forestry, 25*(1), 32-40.

Akbulut, S., Karakose, M., & Özkan, Z. C. (2019). Traditional uses of some wild plants in Kale and Acıpayam provinces in Denizli. *Kastamonu University Journal of Forestry Faculty, 19*(1), 72-81.

Akbulut, S., & Özkan, Z. (2023). Medicinal and aromatic plants use preference against COVID-19 symptoms in Northern Anatolia. *Artvin Çoruh University Journal of Forestry Faculty*, *24*(1), 87–95.

Akbulut, S., & Zengin, Z. (2023). Ethnobotanical survey of wild plants used in Gümüşhane province (Turkey). *Boletín Latinoamericano y del Caribe de Plantas Medicinales y Aromáticas*, *22*(2), 237–254. DOI: 10.37360/blacpma.23.22.2.18

Akıllıgöz, Y., & Başaran, A. (2021). Evaluation of ethnobotanical studies conducted in Ankara Province on the COVID-19 pandemic. *Journal of Integrative Anatolian Medicine, 2*(3), 20-55.

Aksoy, A., Çelik, J., & Tunay, H. (2016). Some plants which are used and sold by the folk in the Bazaar at Gazipaşa (Antalya) district and intended use of them. *Research Journal of Biological Sciences*, *9*(2), 55–61.

Akyol, Y., & Altan, Y. (2013). Ethnobotanical studies in the Maldan Village (Province Manisa, Turkey). *Marmara Pharmaceutical Journal*, *17*(1), 21–25. DOI: 10.12991/201317388

Al Hafi, M., El Beyrouthy, M., Ouaini, N., Stien, D., Rutledge, D., & Chaillou, S. (2016). Chemical composition and antimicrobial activity of *Origanum libanoticum, Origanum ehrenbergii*, and *Origanum syriacum* growing wild in Lebanon. *Chemistry & Biodiversity*, *13*(5), 555–560. DOI: 10.1002/cbdv.201500178

Albayrak, N. B., & Daşkın, R. (2018). Medicinal plants used in Orhaneli and Büyükorhan Districts (Bursa–Northwest Anatolia). *Phytologia Balcanica, 24*(3), 381-388.

Altay, V., Karahan, F., Sarcan, Y. B., & İlçim, A. (2015). An ethnobotanical research on wild plants sold in Kırıkhan district Hatay/Turkey herbalists and local markets. *Biological Diversity and Conservation, 8*(2), 81-91.

Altundağ Çakır, E. (2017). Traditional knowledge of wild edible plants of Iğdır Province (East Anatolia, Turkey). *Acta Societatis Botanicae Poloniae, 86*(4), 3568. https://doi.org/DOI: 10.5586/asbp.2017.3568

Aras, A., Silinsin, M., Bingöl, M. N., & Bursal, E. (2017). Identification of bioactive polyphenolic compounds and assessment of antioxidant activity of *Origanum acutidens.International Letters of Natural Sciences*, *66*, 1–8. . DOI: 10.56431/p-b670qx

Arican, Y. E., Yeşil, Y., & Ecevit Genç, G. (2013). A preliminary ethnobotanical survey of Kumluca (Antalya). *Journal of the Faculty of Pharmacy Istanbul University*, *43*(2), 95–102.

Arıtuluk, Z. C., & Ezer, N. (2012). Plants used for diabetes in Turkey-II. *Hacettepe University Journal of Faculty of Pharmacy*, *2*, 179–208.

Assaf, M. H., Ali, A. A., Makboul, M. A., Beck, J. P., & Anton, R. (1987). Preliminary study of phenolic glycosides from *Origanum majorana*, quantitative estimation of arbutin; cytotoxic activity of hydroquinone. *Planta Medica*, *53*(4), 343–345. DOI: 10.1055/s-2006-962734

Aydın, A., & Yeşil, Y. (2018). An ethnobotanical preliminary study in İkizce (Ordu-Turkey) district. *Bağbahçe Scientific Journal, 5*(3), 25-43. https://doi.org/DOI: 10.1234/bsj.2018.0053

Badem, M., Korkmaz, N., Sener, S. O., Kanbolat, S., Ozgen, U., Sevgi, S., et al. (2019). Biological screening of traditional medicinal plants from villages of Akkuş (Ordu) in Turkey on the effects of tyrosinase. *Journal of Pharmaceutical Research International, 25*(6), 1-10. https://doi.org/DOI: 10.2345/jpri.2019.0472

Bağcı, Y., & Keskin, L. (2022). An ethnobotanical field survey in the Kadınhanı district of Konya in Turkey. *KSU Journal of Agricultural and Natural Sciences, 25*(2), 312-336. https://doi.org/DOI: 10.5556/ksujans.2022.4569

Balasundram, N., Sundram, K., & Samman, S. (2006). Phenolic compounds in plants and agri-industrial by-products: Antioxidant activity, occurrence, and potential uses. *Food Chemistry*, *99*(1), 191–203. DOI: 10.1016/j.foodchem.2005.07.042

Başer, K. H. C., & Kirimer, N. (2006). Essential oils of Lamiaceae plants of Turkey. *Acta Horticulturae*, (723), 163–172. DOI: 10.17660/ActaHortic.2006.723.18

Başer, K. H. C., Tümen, G., Malyer, H., & Kirimer, N. (2006). Plants used for common cold in Turkey. In *Proceedings of the IVth International Congress of Ethnobotany (ICEB 2005)* (pp. 133–137).

Baykan, S., Ozturk, B., Sahin, B., & Senol, S. G. (2023). Ethnobotanical study of medicinal plants in Nemrut Mountain, Adiyaman-Türkiye. *Journal of Research in Pharmacy, 27*(6), 2250-2269. https://doi.org/DOI: 10.5337/jrp.2023.2403

Bisht, D., Chanotiya, C. S., Rana, M., & Semwal, M. (2009). Variability in essential oil and bioactive chiral monoterpenoid compositions of Indian oregano (*Origanum vulgare* L.) populations from northwestern Himalaya and their chemotaxonomy. *Industrial Crops and Products, 30*(3), 422–426. DOI: 10.1016/j.indcrop.2009.07.014

Boz, E., İldeniz, H. K., & Cabi, E. (2022). Some ethnobotanical information from Gönen (Balıkesir) District. *Acta Biologica Turcica, 35*(4), 1-17. https://doi.org/DOI: 10.9876/actabiol.2022.38497

Bozyel, M. E., Merdamert Bozyel, E., Canlı, E., & Altuner, E. M. (2019). Anticancer uses of medicinal plants in Turkish traditional medicine. *Kahramanmaras Sütçü Imam Üniversitesi Tarim ve Doga Dergisi, 22*(Suppl 2), 465–484. DOI: 10.18016/ksutarimdoga.vi.550334

Bozyel, M. E., Merdamert Bozyel, E., & Canli, K. (2020). Turkish herbal medicine in the treatment of back pain. In *Ethnomedicinal Plant Use and Practice in Traditional Medicine* (pp. 235–251). IGI Global. DOI: 10.4018/978-1-7998-1320-0.ch012

Bozyel, M. E., Merdamert Bozyel, E., & Canli, K. (2020). Ethnobotanical uses of medicinal plants for the treatment of herniated disc in Turkish traditional medicine. In *Ethnomedicinal Plant Use and Practice in Traditional Medicine* (pp. 221–234). IGI Global. DOI: 10.4018/978-1-7998-1320-0.ch011

Bulut, G., Haznedaroğlu, M. Z., Doğan, A., Koyu, H., & Tuzlacı, E. (2017). An ethnobotanical study of medicinal plants in Acipayam (Denizli-Turkey). *Journal of Herbal Medicine, 10*, 64–81. DOI: 10.1016/j.hermed.2017.08.001

Bulut, G., & Tuzlacı, E. (2009). Folk medicinal plants of Bayramiç (Çanakkale-Turkey). *Journal of the Faculty of Pharmacy Istanbul University, 40*, 87–99.

Bulut, G., & Tuzlacı, E. (2015). An ethnobotanical study of medicinal plants in Bayramiç. *Marmara Pharmaceutical Journal, 19*(3), 268–282. DOI: 10.12991/mpj.201519392830

Busatta, C., Vidal, R. S., Popiolski, A. S., Mossi, A. J., Dariva, C., Rodrigues, M. R. A., Corazza, F. C., Corazza, M. L., Vladimir Oliveira, J., & Cansian, R. L. (2008). Application of *Origanum majorana* L. essential oil as an antimicrobial agent in sausage. *Food Microbiology, 25*(1), 207–211. DOI: 10.1016/j.fm.2007.07.003

Çalışkan, G., Yıldırım, G., & Şenkardeş, İ. (2020). A study on herbs used in food in Rize province within the context of gastronomy tourism. *Journal of Social and Humanities Research, 7*(51), 573-583. https://doi.org/DOI: 10.1305/jshr.2020.0034

Canli, K., Bozyel, M. E., Turu, D., Benek, A., Şimşek, O., & Altuner, E. M. (2023). Biochemical, antioxidant properties and antimicrobial activity of steno-endemic *Origanum onites.Microorganisms, 11*(8), 1987. DOI: 10.3390/microorganisms11081987

Cavero, S., García-Risco, M. R., Marín, F. R., Jaime, L., Santoyo, S., Señoráns, F. J., Reglero, G., & Ibañez, E. (2006). Supercritical fluid extraction of antioxidant compounds from oregano: Chemical and functional characterization via LC–MS and in vitro assays. *The Journal of Supercritical Fluids, 38*(1), 62–69. DOI: 10.1016/j.supflu.2005.01.003

Celep, F., & Dirmenci, T. (2017). Systematic and biogeographic overview of Lamiaceae in Turkey. *Natural Volatiles & Essential Oils, 4*(4), 14–27.

Çinbilgel, İ., & Kurt, Y. (2019). A research on species diversity and ethnobotanical utilization of Lamiaceae family in Southern Turkey. *Süleyman Demirel University Journal of Science and Technology Institute, 23*(1), 90–107.

Císarová, M., Tančinová, D., Medo, J., & Kačániová, M. (2016). The in vitro effect of selected essential oils on the growth and mycotoxin production of *Aspergillus* species. *Journal of Environmental Science and Health. Part B, Pesticides, Food Contaminants, and Agricultural Wastes, 51*(10), 668–674. DOI: 10.1080/03601234.2016.1191887

Çömlekçioğlu, N., & Karaman, Ş. (2008). The medicinal plants found in the local herbal markets in the city of Kahramanmaras in Turkey. *KSU Journal of Science and Engineering, 11*(1), 23–32.

Conforti, F., Marrelli, M., Carmela, C., Menichini, F., Valentina, P., Uzunov, D., Statti, G. A., Duez, P., & Menichini, F. (2011). Bioactive phytonutrients (omega fatty acids, tocopherols, polyphenols), in vitro inhibition of nitric oxide production and free radical scavenging activity of non-cultivated Mediterranean vegetables. *Food Chemistry, 129*(4), 1413–1419. DOI: 10.1016/j.foodchem.2011.05.085

Conforti, F., Marrelli, M., Menichini, F., Tundis, R., Statti, G. A., Solimene, U., & Menichini, F. (2011). Chemical composition and protective effect of oregano (Origanum heracleoticum L.) ethanolic extract on oxidative damage and on inhibition of NO in LPS-stimulated RAW 264.7 macrophages. *Journal of Enzyme Inhibition and Medicinal Chemistry*, *26*(3), 404–411. DOI: 10.3109/14756366.2010.519336

Cos, P., Vlietinck, A. J., Berghe, D. V., & Maes, L. (2006). Anti-infective potential of natural products: How to develop a stronger in vitro 'proof-of-concept'. *Journal of Ethnopharmacology*, *106*(3), 290–302. DOI: 10.1016/j.jep.2006.04.003

Davis, P. H., Mill, R. R., & Tan, K. (1988). *Flora of Turkey and the East Aegean Islands* (Suppl. 1, Vol. 10). Edinburgh University Press.

De Martino, L., De Feo, V., Formisano, C., Mignola, E., & Senatore, F. (2009). Chemical composition and antimicrobial activity of the essential oils from three chemotypes of *Origanum vulgare* L. ssp. *hirtum* (Link) Ietswaart growing wild in Campania (Southern Italy). *Molecules (Basel, Switzerland)*, *14*(8), 2735–2746. DOI: 10.3390/molecules14082735

Demir, İ. (2020). An ethnobotanical study of medicinal plants used in Hizan District (Bitlis-Turkey). *Yuzuncu Yil University Journal of Agricultural Sciences, 30*(4), 732-741. https://doi.org/DOI: 10.29129/yuzujag.2020.4319

Demirci, S., & Özhatay, N. (2012). An ethnobotanical study in Kahramanmaraş (Turkey); wild plants used for medicinal purpose in Andirin, Kahramanmaraş. *Turkish Journal of Pharmaceutical Sciences, 9*(1), 75-92.

Demirci Kayıran, S. (2019). Dioskorides'in *De Materia Medica* adlı eserindeki tıbbi bitkilerin Doğu Akdeniz'de günümüzdeki kullanımlarının araştırılması. *Lokman Hekim Dergisi*, *9*(2), 189–202. DOI: 10.31020/mutftd.519382

Demirel, O., & Dutkuner, İ. (2021). A study of ethnobotany in Sütçüler (Isparta). In *International Aegean Symposiums on Innovation Technologies & Engineering-IV (September 11-12, 2021)Proceedings Book* (pp. 19–37).

Deniz, L., Serteser, A., & Kargıoğlu, M. (2010). Local names and ethnobotanical features of some plants in Usak University (Usak) and its near vicinity. *Afyon Kocatepe University Journal of Science and Engineering*, *1*, 57–72.

Doğan, A., & Tuzlacı, E. (2015). Wild edible plants of Pertek (Tunceli-Turkey). *Marmara Pharmaceutical Journal*, *19*(2), 126–135. DOI: 10.12991/mpj.20151910459

Doğan, Y., & Ugulu, I. (2013). Medicinal plants used for gastrointestinal disorders in some districts of Izmir province, Turkey. *Studies on Ethno-Medicine*, *7*(3), 149–161. DOI: 10.1080/09735070.2013.11886456

Dorman, H. D., Bachmayer, O., Kosar, M., & Hiltunen, R. (2004). Antioxidant properties of aqueous extracts from selected Lamiaceae species grown in Turkey. *Journal of Agricultural and Food Chemistry*, *52*(4), 762–770. DOI: 10.1021/jf034908v

Duman, H. (2000). Origanum L. In A. Güner, N. Özhatay, T. Ekim, & K. H. C. Başer (Eds.), *Flora of Turkey and the East Aegean Islands* (Suppl. 2, Vol. 11, pp. 297–313). Edinburgh University Press.

Ecevit Genç, G. & Özhatay, N. (2006). An ethnobotanical study in Çatalca (European part of Istanbul) II. Turkish Journal of Pharmaceutical Sciences, 3(2), 73-89.

Elshafie, H. S., Armentano, M. F., Carmosino, M., Bufo, S. A., De Feo, V., & Camele, I. (2017). Cytotoxic activity of *Origanum vulgare* L. on hepatocellular carcinoma cell line HepG2 and evaluation of its biological activity. *Molecules (Basel, Switzerland)*, *22*(9), 1435. DOI: 10.3390/molecules22091435

Eminağaoğlu, Ö., Göktürk, T., & Beğen, H. A. (2017). Traditional uses of medicinal plants and animals of Hatila Valley National Park, Artvin. *Biological Diversity and Conservation*, *10*(3), 33–42.

Erarslan, Z. B., Ecevit Genç, G., & Kültür, Ş. (2020). Medicinal plants traditionally used to treat skin diseases in Turkey—Eczema, psoriasis, vitiligo. *Journal of the Faculty of Pharmacy Ankara University*, *44*(1), 137–166.

Erbay, M. Ş., Anıl, S., & Melikoğlu, G. (2017). Plants used as painkillers in folk medicine in Turkey-I: Stomachache. *Marmara Pharmaceutical Journal*, *21*(4), 741–755. DOI: 10.12991/mpj.2017.0

Erbay, M. Ş., Anıl, S., & Melikoğlu, G. (2018). Plants used as painkillers in traditional treatment in Turkey-II: Headache. *Marmara Pharmaceutical Journal*, *22*(1), 29–36. DOI: 10.12991/mpj.2018.37

Erenler, R., Meral, B., Sen, O., Elmastaş, M., Aydin, A., Eminagaoğlu, O., & Topcu, G. (2017). Bioassay-guided isolation, identification of compounds from *Origanum rotundifolium* and investigation of their antiproliferative and antioxidant activities. *Pharmaceutical Biology*, *55*(1), 1646–1653. DOI: 10.1080/13880209.2017.1310906

Erşen Bak, F., & Çifci, K. (2020). Traditional uses of some medicinal plants in the central villages of Artvin. *Artvin Coruh University Journal of Forestry Faculty, 21*(2), 318-329.

Erucar, F. M., Tan, N., & Miski, M. (2023). Ethnobotanical records of medicinal plants of Turkey effective on stress management compiled with the literature survey in their chemical content and activities. *Records of Natural Products*, *17*(1), 1–92. DOI: 10.25135/rnp.324.2203.2372

Fakir, H., Korkmaz, M., & Güller, B. (2009). Medicinal plant diversity of western Mediterranean region in Turkey. *Journal of Applied Biological Sciences, 3*(2), 33–43.

Fakir, H., Korkmaz, M., & Icel, B. (2016). Medicinal plants traditionally used for pain alleviation in Antalya province, Turkey. *Studies on Ethno-Medicine, 10*(3), 314–324. DOI: 10.1080/09735070.2016.11905503

Gonçalves, S., Moreira, E., Grosso, C., Andrade, P. B., Valentão, P., & Romano, A. (2017). Phenolic profile, antioxidant activity and enzyme inhibitory activities of extracts from aromatic plants used in Mediterranean diet. *Journal of Food Science and Technology, 54*(1), 219–227. DOI: 10.1007/s13197-016-2453-z

Gulec, M., Erarslan, Z. B., & Kültür, Ş. (2023). The medicinal plants traditionally used against cardiovascular diseases in Turkey. *International Journal of Traditional Complementary Medicine Research, 4*(2), 81–96. DOI: 10.53811/ijtcmr.1232190

Güler, B., Erkan, Y., & Uğurlu, E. (2020). Traditional uses and ecological resemblance of medicinal plants in two districts of the Western Aegean Region (Turkey). *Environmental Development and Sustainability, 22*, 2099-2120. 134.

Erbay, M. Ş., & Sarı, A. (2018). Plants used in traditional treatment against hemorrhoids in Turkey. *Marmara Pharmaceutical Journal, 22*(2), 110-132.

Güner, A., Aslan, S., Ekim, T., Vural, M., & Babaç, M. T. (Eds.). (2012). *Türkiye bitkileri listesi (damarlı bitkiler).* Nezahat Gökyiğit Botanik Bahçesi ve Flora Araştırmaları Derneği Yayını.

Güner, Ö., & Selvi, S. (2016). Wild medicinal plants sold in Balıkesir/Turkey herbal markets and their using properties. *Biological Diversity and Conservation, 9*(2), 96–101.

Güzel, Y., & Güzelşemme, M. (2018). Wild plants used as herbal tea in Antakya and Defne provinces of Hatay. *ANADOLU Journal of Aegean Agricultural Research Institute, 28*(1), 1-5.

Güzel, Y., & Kayıkçı, S. (2023). Traditional foraged spice, sauce, and egg-painting plants of Hatay, Türkiye: Bringing the traditional into commerce. *Anadolu Journal of Aegean Agricultural Research Institute, 33*(2), 237-258. https://doi.org/DOI: 10.1234/ajaari.2023.33452

Han, F., Ma, G. Q., Yang, M., Yan, L., Xiong, W., Shu, J. C., Zhao, Z., & Xu, H. (2017). Chemical composition and antioxidant activities of essential oils from different parts of the oregano. *Journal of Zhejiang University. Science. B., 18*(1), 79–84. DOI: 10.1631/jzus.B1600377

Harmati, M., Gyukity-Sebestyén, E., Dobra, G., Terhes, G., Urbán, E., Decsi, G., Mimica-Dukić, N., Lesjak, M., Simin, N., Pap, B., Nemeth, I. B., & Buzas, K. (2017). Binary mixture of *Satureja hortensis* and *Origanum vulgare* subsp. *hirtum* essential oils: In vivo therapeutic efficiency against *Helicobacter pylori* infection. *Helicobacter*, *22*(2), e12350. DOI: 10.1111/hel.12350

Hayta, S., Polat, R., & Selvi, S. (2014). Traditional uses of medicinal plants in Elazığ (Turkey). *Journal of Ethnopharmacology, 154*(3), 613-623. https://doi.org/DOI: 10.1016/j.jep.2014.04.025

Ietswaart, J. H. (1980). Leiden Botanical Series: Vol. 4. *A taxonomic revision of the genus Origanum (Labiatae)*. Brill. DOI: 10.1007/978-94-009-9156-9

Ietswaart, J. H. (1982). Origanum L. In Davis, P. H. (Ed.), *Flora of Turkey and the East Aegean Islands* (Vol. 7, pp. 297–313). Edinburgh University Press.

Ifantis, T. M., Solujić, S., & Skaltsa, H. (2012). Secondary metabolites from the aerial parts of *Origanum scabrum* Boiss. & Heldr. *Biochemical Systematics and Ecology*, *44*, 289–294. DOI: 10.1016/j.bse.2012.06.014

Kadıoğlu, S., Kadıoğlu, B., & Karagöz Sezer, K. (2021). Ethnobotanical properties of natural plants in Kop Mountain Pass (Bayburt/Turkey). *Biological Diversity and Conservation*, *14*(2), 264–276. DOI: 10.46309/biodicon.2021.925769

Kadıoğlu, S., Kadıoğlu, B., & Karagöz Sezer, K. (2024). Usage of shrub and tree-form plants in traditional folk medicine. *Muş Alparslan University Journal of Agricultural and Natural Sciences*, *4*(1), 9–22.

Kalankan, G., Özkan, Z. C., & Akbulut, S. (2015). Medicinal and aromatic wild plants and traditional usage of them in Mount Ida (Balıkesir/Turkey). *Journal of Applied Biological Sciences*, *9*(3), 25–33.

Karahüseyin, S., & Sarı, A. (2019). Plants used in traditional treatment against diarrhea in Turkey. *Istanbul Journal of Pharmacy, 49*(1), 33-44.

Karakaya, S., Polat, A., Aksakal, Ö., Sümbüllü, Y. Z., & İncekara, Ü. (2019). Plants used in traditional medicine and other uses in South of Erzurum (Turkey): An ethnobotanical study. *Ethnobotany Research and Applications*, *18*, 1–18. DOI: 10.32859/era.18.13.1-18

Karaman, Ö., & Elgin Cebe, G. (2016). Diabetes and antidiabetic plants used in Turkey. *Journal of Faculty of Pharmacy Ankara University*, *40*(3), 47–61.

Kayabaşı, N. P., Tümen, G., & Polat, R. (2023). Ethnobotanical study on the medicinal plants in the Manyas province (Balıkesir, Turkey). [IJTK]. *Indian Journal of Traditional Knowledge*, *22*(1), 83–91.

Kerar, B. A., & Akan, H. (2019). Aktepe ve Zeytinoba köyleri (Hassa/Hatay-Türkiye) arasında kalan bölgenin florası ve etnobotaniği üzerine bir araştırma. *Bağbahçe Bilim Dergisi, 6*(3), 76-96.

Khoury, M., Stien, D., Eparvier, V., Ouaini, N., & El Beyrouthy, M. (2016). Report on the medicinal use of eleven Lamiaceae species in Lebanon and rationalization of their antimicrobial potential by examination of the chemical composition and antimicrobial activity of their essential oils. *Evidence-Based Complementary and Alternative Medicine : eCAM*, *2547169*(1), 2547169. Advance online publication. DOI: 10.1155/2016/2547169

Kılıç, Ö., & Bağcı, E. (2013). An ethnobotanical survey of some medicinal plants in Keban (Elazığ-Turkey). *Journal of Medicinal Plants Research, 7*(23), 1675-1684. https://doi.org/DOI: 10.5897/JMPR2013.4205

Kıncal, S., Ceylan, O., & Görk, G. (2021). Ethnobotanical features of Ula (Muğla/ Turkey) district. *Biological Diversity and Conservation*, *14*(1), 69–81. DOI: 10.46309/ biodicon.2021.768665

Kızılarslan, Ç., & Özhatay, N. (2012). An ethnobotanical study of the useful and edible plants of İzmit. *Marmara Pharmaceutical Journal, 16*(3), 194-200. https:// doi.org/DOI: 10.12991/mpj.2012.234

Kızılarslan Hançer, Ç., Sevgi, E., Altınbaşak, B. B., Altundağ Çakır, E., & Akkaya, M. (2020). Traditional knowledge of wild edible plants of Biga (Çanakkale), Turkey. *Acta Societatis Botanicae Poloniae, 89*(1), 8914. https://doi.org/DOI: 10.5586/ asbp.2020.8914

Kooti, W., Farokhipour, M., Asadzadeh, Z., Ashtary-Larky, D., & Asadi-Samani, M. (2016). The role of medicinal plants in the treatment of diabetes: A systematic review. *Electronic Physician*, *8*(1), 1832–1842. DOI: 10.19082/1832

Korkmaz, M., & Fakir, H. (2009). Determination of final consumer characteristics of non-wood forest products (A case study for Isparta City). *Süleyman Demirel University Faculty of Forestry Journal*, *10*(2), 10–20.

Korkmaz, M., Fakir, H., & Güller, B. (2011). Consumer preferences for medicinal and aromatic plant products: Surveys of urban consumers and sellers in western Mediterranean region of Turkey. *Journal of Medicinal Plants Research*, *5*(10), 2054–2063.

Korkmaz, M., & Karakurt, E. (2014). Medicinal plants sold in the herbal markets in Kelkit (Gümüşhane). *Suleyman Demirel University Journal of Natural and Applied Sciences*, *18*(3), 60–80.

Korkmaz, M., & Karakurt, E. (2015). Traditional uses of wild edible plants in Kelkit (Gümüşhane) district. *Research Journal of Biological Sciences, 8*(2), 31-39. https://doi.org/DOI: 10.3923/rjbs.2015.03139

Koyuncu, O., Yaylaci, O., Öztürk, D., Potoglu Erkara, I., Savaroglu, F., Akcoskun, O., et al. (2010). Risk categories and ethnobotanical features of the Lamiaceae taxa growing naturally in Osmaneli (Bilecik/Turkey) and environs. *Biological Diversity and Conservation, 3*(3), 31-45.

Kültür, Ş., Altınbaşak, O., Anıl, S., & Melikoğlu, G. (2018). Medicinal plants used in the treatment of stomach ulcers in Turkey. *Marmara Pharmaceutical Journal*, *22*(1), 1–14.

Kültür, Ş., Gürdal, B., Sari, A., & Melikoğlu, G. (2021). Traditional herbal remedies used in kidney diseases in Turkey: An overview. *Turkish Journal of Botany, 45*(4), 269-287. https://doi.org/DOI: 10.1063/tjb.2021.0589

Lermioglu, F., Bagci, S., Onderoglu, S., Ortac, R., & Tugrul, L. (1997). Evaluation of the long-term effects of oleum origani on the toxicity induced by administration of streptozotocin in rats. *Journal of Pharmacy & Pharmaceutical Sciences*, *49*(11), 1157–1161.

Lukas, B., Schmiderer, C., Mitteregger, U., & Novak, J. (2010). Arbutin in marjoram and oregano. *Food Chemistry*, *121*(1), 185–190. DOI: 10.1016/j.foodchem.2009.12.028

Mansinhos, I., Gonçalves, S., & Romano, A. (2024). How climate change-related abiotic factors affect the production of industrial valuable compounds in Lamiaceae plant species: A review. *Frontiers in Plant Science*, *15*, 1370810. DOI: 10.3389/fpls.2024.1370810

Marrelli, M., Conforti, F., Formisano, C., Rigano, D., Arnold, N. A., Menichini, F., & Senatore, F. (2016). Composition, antibacterial, antioxidant and antiproliferative activities of essential oils from three *Origanum* species growing wild in Lebanon and Greece. *Natural Product Research*, *30*(6), 735–739. DOI: 10.1080/14786419.2015.1040993

Marrelli, M., Cristaldi, B., Menichini, F., & Conforti, F. (2015). Inhibitory effects of wild dietary plants on lipid peroxidation and on the proliferation of human cancer cells. *Food and Chemical Toxicology*, *86*, 16–24. DOI: 10.1016/j.fct.2015.09.011

Marrelli, M., Statti, G. A., & Conforti, F. (2018). *Origanum* spp.: An update of their chemical and biological profiles. *Phytochemistry Reviews*, *17*(4), 873–888. DOI: 10.1007/s11101-018-9566-0

Melikoğlu, G., Kurtoğlu, S., & Kültür, Ş. (2015). Traditional medicinal plants used in asthma treatment in Turkey. *Marmara Pharmaceutical Journal*, *19*(1), 1–11.

Miguel, M. G. (2010). Antioxidant activity of medicinal and aromatic plants. A review. *Flavour and Fragrance Journal*, *25*(5), 291–312. DOI: 10.1002/ffj.1961

Miller, A. B., Cates, R. G., Lawrence, M., Soria, J. A. F., Espinoza, L. V., Martinez, J. V., & Arbizú, D. A. (2015). The antibacterial and antifungal activity of essential oils extracted from Guatemalan medicinal plants. *Pharmaceutical Biology*, *53*(4), 548–554. DOI: 10.3109/13880209.2014.932391

Nacakcı, F. M., & Dutkuner, İ. (2018). A study of ethnobotany in Kumluca (Antalya). *Turkish Journal of Forestry*, *19*(2), 113–119. DOI: 10.18182/tjf.421970

Nagy, T. O., Solar, S., Sontag, G., & Koenig, J. (2011). Identification of phenolic components in dried spices and influence of irradiation. *Food Chemistry*, *128*(2), 530–534. DOI: 10.1016/j.foodchem.2011.03.037

Nardoni, S., Giovanelli, S., Pistelli, L., Mugnaini, L., Profili, G., Pisseri, F., et al. (2015). In vitro activity of twenty commercially available, plant-derived essential oils against selected dermatophyte species. *Natural Product Communications*, *10*(8), 1934578X1501000840.

Olcay, B., & Kültür, Ş. (2020). Medicinal plants used in traditional treatment of hypertension in Turkey. *International Journal of Science and Technology Research*, *6*(3), 80–95.

Olokoba, A. B., Obateru, O. A., & Olokoba, L. B. (2012). Type 2 diabetes mellitus: A review of current trends. *Oman Medical Journal*, *27*(4), 269–273. DOI: 10.5001/omj.2012.68

Ovadje, P., Roma, A., Steckle, M., Nicoletti, L., Arnason, J. T., & Pandey, S. (2015). Advances in the research and development of natural health products as mainstream cancer therapeutics. *Evidence-Based Complementary and Alternative Medicine : eCAM*, *751348*, 1–12. Advance online publication. DOI: 10.1155/2015/751348

Öz Aydın, S., Dirmenci, T., Tümen, G., & Başer, K. H. C. (2006). Plants used as analgesic in the folk medicine of Turkey. In *Proceedings of the IVth International Congress of Ethnobotany (ICEB 2005)* (pp. 167-171). Ege Yayinlari.

Özata, N. (2019). *Fitoterapi ve aromaterapi*. Istanbul Tıp Kitabevleri.

Özbek, H., Güvenalp, Z., Özek, T., Sevindik, H. G., Yuca, H., Yerdelen, K. Ö., & Demirezer, L. Ö. (2017). Chemical composition, antioxidant and anticholinesterase activities of the essential oil of *Origanum rotundifolium* Boiss. from Turkey. *Records of Natural Products, 11*(5), 485–490. DOI: 10.25135/rnp.62.16.05.040

Özdemir Nath, E., & Kültür, Ş. (2022). An ethnobotanical study of medicinal plants in Savaştepe (Balikesir-Turkey). *Clinical and Experimental Health Sciences, 12*(4), 954-980. https://doi.org/DOI: 10.5532/cehs.2022.1405

Ozkan, G., Baydar, H., & Erbas, S. (2010). The influence of harvest time on essential oil composition, phenolic constituents and antioxidant properties of Turkish oregano (*Origanum onites* L.). *Journal of the Science of Food and Agriculture, 90*(2), 205–209. DOI: 10.1002/jsfa.3788

Ozturk, M., & Altay, V. (2017). An overview of the endemic medicinal and aromatic plants of Turkey—conservation and sustainable use. In *International Congress on Medicinal and Aromatic Plants Full Text Proceedings Book* (pp. 11-39).

Ozturk, M., Altay, V., & Gönenç, T. M. (2017). Herbal medicine from high mountains in the East Mediterranean. In *Drug discovery from herbs: Approaches and applications* (pp. 327–367). DAYA Publishing House.

Passannanti, S., Paternostro, M., Piozzi, F., & Barbagallo, C. (1984). Diterpenes from the genus *Amaracus.Journal of Natural Products, 47*(5), 885–889. DOI: 10.1021/np50035a027

Piozzi, F., Paternostro, M., & Passannanti, S. (1985). A minor diterpene from *Amaracus akhdarensis.Phytochemistry, 24*(5), 1113–1114. DOI: 10.1016/S0031-9422(00)83201-X

Pirigharnaei, M., Zare, S., Heidary, R., & Khara, J., EmamaliSabzi, R., & Kheiry, F. (2011). The essential oils compositions of Iranian oregano (*Origanum vulgare* L.) populations in field and provenance from Piranshahr district, West Azarbaijan province, Iran. *Avicenna Journal of Phytomedicine, 1*(2), 106–114.

Polat, R. (2019). Ethnobotanical study on medicinal plants in Bingöl (City center), Turkey. *Journal of Herbal Medicine, 16*, 100211. DOI: 10.1016/j.hermed.2018.01.007

Polat, R., Cakilcioglu, U., Kaltalioğlu, K., Ulusan, M. D., & Türkmen, Z. (2015). An ethnobotanical study on medicinal plants in Espiye and its surrounding (Giresun-Turkey). *Journal of Ethnopharmacology, 163*, 1-11. https://doi.org/DOI: 10.1016/j.jep.2014.12.019

Polat, R., Çakılcıoğlu, U., Ulusan, M. D., Gür, F., & Türkmen, Z. (2015). Investigations of ethnobotanical aspect of wild plants sold in Espiye Giresun/Turkey local markets. *Biological Diversity and Conservation, 8*(3), 114-119. https://doi.org/DOI: 10.1305/bdc.2015.0915

Polat, R., & Satıl, F. (2012). An ethnobotanical survey of medicinal plants in Edremit Gulf (Balıkesir–Turkey). *Journal of Ethnopharmacology*, *139*(2), 626–641. DOI: 10.1016/j.jep.2011.12.004

Polat, R., & Satıl, F. (2012). Research on some medicinal plants commercially sold in the Havran and Burhaniye region (Balıkesir-Turkey). *Bocconea, 24*, 311-317.

Polat, R., Satıl, F., & Çakılcıoğlu, U. (2011). Medicinal plants and their use properties of plants sold in the herbal market in Bingöl, Turkey district. *Biological Diversity and Conservation*, *4*(3), 25–35. DOI: 10.17515/bio.dc.2011.4.3.03

Polat, R., Selvi, S., Çakılcıoğlu, U., & Açar, M. (2012). Investigations of ethnobotanical aspects of wild plants sold in Bingöl (Turkey) local markets. *Biological Diversity and Conservation*, *5*(3), 155–161. DOI: 10.17515/bio.dc.2012.5.3.12

Radušienė, J., Ivanauskas, L., Janulis, V., & Jakštas, V. (2008). Composition and variability of phenolic compounds in *Origanum vulgare* from Lithuania. *Biologija (Vilnius, Lithuania)*, *54*(1), 45–49. DOI: 10.2478/v10054-008-0009-5

Sağıroğlu, M., & Aydın, D. (2024). An ethnobotanical research in Cumalıkızık and its surroundings (Bursa). *Afyon Kocatepe University Journal of Science and Engineering, 24*(4), 758-772. https://doi.org/DOI: 10.5432/afkose.2024.1569

Sağıroğlu, M., Dalgıç, S., & Toksoy, S. (2013). Medicinal plants used in Dalaman (Muğla), Turkey. *Journal of Medicinal Plants Research*, *7*(28), 2053–2066. DOI: 10.5897/JMPR2013.2590

Şahin, T., & Kılıç, Ö. (2022). A review: Some plants used for hemorrhoids in Turkey traditional medicine. *Russian Journal of Biological Research, 9*(1), 8-29. https://doi.org/DOI: 10.3905/rjbiolres.2022.0097

Sakkas, H., & Papadopoulou, C. (2017). Antimicrobial activity of basil, oregano, and thyme essential oils. *Journal of Microbiology and Biotechnology*, *27*(3), 429–438. DOI: 10.4014/jmb.1608.08024

Saraç, D. U., Özkan, Z. C., & Akbulut, S. (2013). Ethnobotanic features of Rize/Turkey province. *Biological Diversity and Conservation, 6*(3), 57-66. https://doi.org/DOI: 10.2195/bdc.2013.0566

Sargin, S. A. (2015). Ethnobotanical survey of medicinal plants in Bozyazı district of Mersin, Turkey. *Journal of Ethnopharmacology*, *173*, 105–126. DOI: 10.1016/j.jep.2015.07.009

Sargin, S. A. (2021). Potential anti-influenza effective plants used in Turkish folk medicine: A review. *Journal of Ethnopharmacology*, *265*, 113319. DOI: 10.1016/j.jep.2020.113319

Sargın, S. A., Akçicek, E., & Selvi, S. (2013). An ethnobotanical study of medicinal plants used by the local people of Alaşehir (Manisa) in Turkey. *Journal of Ethnopharmacology*, *150*(3), 860–874. DOI: 10.1016/j.jep.2013.09.040

Sargin, S. A., & Büyükcengiz, M. (2019). Plants used in ethnomedicinal practices in Gulnar district of Mersin, Turkey. *Journal of Herbal Medicine*, *15*, 100224. DOI: 10.1016/j.hermed.2018.06.003

Sargin, S. A., & Dogan, Y. (2023). Immune-boosting plants used in Turkish folk medicine and their potential against COVID-19. In *Ethnopharmacology and Drug Discovery for COVID-19: Anti-SARS-CoV-2 agents from herbal medicines and natural products* (pp. 479–548). Springer Nature Singapore. DOI: 10.1007/978-981-99-3664-9_18

Sargin, S. A., Selvi, S., & Büyükcengiz, M. (2015). Ethnomedicinal plants of Aydıncık district of Mersin, Turkey. *Journal of Ethnopharmacology*, *174*, 200–216. DOI: 10.1016/j.jep.2015.08.008

Sargin, S. A., Selvi, S., & López, V. (2015). Ethnomedicinal plants of Sarıgöl district (Manisa), Turkey. *Journal of Ethnopharmacology*, *171*, 64–84. DOI: 10.1016/j.jep.2015.05.031

Sarı, F., & Erarslan, Z. B. (2023). A scoping review of traditional medicinal plants used to treat acne vulgaris in Türkiye. *European Journal of Integrative Medicine, 64*, 102305. https://doi.org/DOI: 10.1016/j.eujim.2023.102305

Sarıkaya, S., Öner, H., & Harput, Ş. (2010). Medicinal plants used for the treatment of diabetes in Turkey. *Journal of the Faculty of Pharmacy Ankara University*, *39*(4), 317–342.

Satıl, F., Akçiçek, E., & Selvi, S. (2008). An ethnobotanical study in Madra Mountain (Balıkesir—İzmir) and vicinity. *Research Journal of Biological Sciences, 1*(1), 31-36. https://doi.org/DOI: 10.3923/rjbs.2008.03136

Selvi, S., Dağdelen, A., & Kara, S. (2013). Medicinal and aromatic plants consumed as herbal tea and collected from Ida Mountains (Balıkesir-Edremit). *Tekirdag Ziraat Fakültesi Dergisi*, *10*(2), 26–33.

Selvi, S., Polat, R., Çakilcioğlu, U., Celep, F., Dirmenci, T., & Ertuğ, Z. F. (2022). An ethnobotanical review on medicinal plants of the Lamiaceae family in Turkey. *Turkish Journal of Botany*, *46*(4), 283–332. DOI: 10.55730/1300-008X.2712

Şenkardeş, İ., & Tuzlacı, E. (2014). Some ethnobotanical notes from Gündoğmuş District (Antalya/Turkey). *Journal of Marmara University Institute of Health Sciences*, *4*(2), 63–75. DOI: 10.5455/musbed.20140303070652

Sharifzadeh, A., & Shokri, H. (2016). Antifungal activity of essential oils from Iranian plants against fluconazole-resistant and fluconazole-susceptible *Candida albicans.Avicenna Journal of Phytomedicine*, *6*(2), 215–226.

Shealy, C. N. (1998). *The illustrated encyclopedia of healing remedies*. Element Books.

Skoula, M., Gotsiou, P., Naxakis, G., & Johnson, C. B. (1999). A chemosystematic investigation on the mono- and sesquiterpenoids in the genus *Origanum* (Labiatae). *Phytochemistry*, *52*(4), 649–657. DOI: 10.1016/S0031-9422(99)00268-X

Skoula, M., Grayer, R. J., Kite, G. C., & Veitch, N. C. (2008). Exudate flavones and flavanones in *Origanum* species and their interspecific variation. *Biochemical Systematics and Ecology*, *36*(8), 646–654. DOI: 10.1016/j.bse.2008.05.003

Skoula, M., & Harborne, J. B. (2002). The taxonomy and chemistry of *Origanum*. In Kintzios, S. E. (Ed.), *Oregano: The genera Origanum and Lippia* (pp. 67–108). Taylor & Francis.

Soliman, M. M., Nassan, M. A., & Ismail, T. A. (2016). *Origanum majoranum* extract modulates gene expression, hepatic and renal changes in a rat model of type 2 diabetes. *Iranian Journal of Pharmaceutical Research : IJPR*, *15*(Suppl), 45–54. DOI: 10.22037/ijpr.2016.5595

Tanaydın, G., Satıl, F., & Çakılcıoğlu, U. (2022). An ethnobotanical research on plants used for food purposes in Bigadiç (Balıkesir-Turkey). *Turkish Journal of Natural Sciences, 11*(4), 142-147.

Tepe, B., Cakir, A., & Sihoglu Tepe, A. (2016). Medicinal uses, phytochemistry, and pharmacology of *Origanum onites* (L.): A review. *Chemistry & Biodiversity*, *13*(5), 504–520. DOI: 10.1002/cbdv.201500069

Terzioğlu, S., & Coşkunçelebi, K. (2021). Medicinal plants of northeast Anatolia. In *Biodiversity, Conservation and Sustainability in Asia: Volume 1: Prospects and Challenges in West Asia and Caucasus* (pp. 275-337). Cham: Springer International Publishing. DOI: 10.1007/978-3-030-59928-7_11

Tutenocakli, T. (2023). Plants consumed as food in an ethnobotanical perspective: The case study of Yenice-Canakkale-Turkey. *Current Trends in Natural Sciences, 12*(23), 224–233. DOI: 10.47068/ctns.2023.v12i23.025

Tuzlacı, E. (2016). *Türkiye Bitkileri Geleneksel İlaç Rehberi.* Istanbul Tıp Kitabevleri.

Ünal, S., & Altundağ Çakır, E. (2024). Natural dye plants in Sındırgı Yağcıbedir Carpets (Balıkesir, Turkey). *Eurasian Journal of Forestry Science, 12*(2), 66-72. https://doi.org/DOI: 10.3059/ejfs.2024.0715

Uysal, İ., Gücel, S., Tütenocakli, T., & Öztürk, M. (2012). Studies on the medicinal plants of Ayvacik-Çanakkale in Turkey. *Pakistan Journal of Botany, 44*(Suppl 1), 239–244.

Uysal, İ., Onar, S., Karabacak, E., & Çelik, S. (2010). Ethnobotanical aspects of Kapıdağ peninsula (Turkey). *Biological Diversity and Conservation, 3*(3), 15–22.

Uzun, A., & Palabas Uzun, S. (2011). Medicinal and aromatic plant taxa of Altındere Valley (Maçka/Trabzon). In *Proceedings of the 2nd International Non-Wood Products Symposium* (pp. 269-282). https://doi.org/DOI: 10.1234/inwp.2011.0298

Uzun, M., & Kaya, A. (2019). Traditional medicinal plants used for oral and dental diseases in Turkey. *Biological Diversity and Conservation, 12*(1), 138-148.

Valko, M., Leibfritz, D., Moncol, J., Cronin, M. T., Mazur, M., & Telser, J. (2007). Free radicals and antioxidants in normal physiological functions and human disease. *The International Journal of Biochemistry & Cell Biology, 39*(1), 44–84. DOI: 10.1016/j.biocel.2006.07.001

Vujicic, M., Nikolic, I., Kontogianni, V. G., Saksida, T., Charisiadis, P., Orescanin-Dusic, Z., Blagojevic, D., Stosic-Grujicic, S., Tzakos, A. G., & Stojanovic, I. (2015). Methanolic extract of *Origanum vulgare* ameliorates type 1 diabetes through anti-oxidant, anti-inflammatory and anti-apoptotic activity. *British Journal of Nutrition, 113*(5), 770–782. DOI: 10.1017/S0007114514004048

Vujicic, M., Nikolic, I., Kontogianni, V. G., Saksida, T., Charisiadis, P., Vasic, B., Stosic-Grujicic, S., Gerothanassis, I. P., Tzakos, A. G., & Stojanovic, I. (2016). Ethyl acetate extract of *Origanum vulgare* L. ssp. hirtum prevents streptozotocin-induced diabetes in C57BL/6 mice. *Journal of Food Science, 81*(7), H1846–H1853. DOI: 10.1111/1750-3841.13333

Waller, S. B., Madrid, I. M., Ferraz, V., Picoli, T., Cleff, M. B., de Faria, R. O., Meireles, M. C. A., & de Mello, J. R. B. (2016). Cytotoxicity and anti-*Sporothrix brasiliensis* activity of the *Origanum majorana* Linn. oil. *Brazilian Journal of Microbiology : Publication of the Brazilian Society for Microbiology*, *47*(4), 896–901. DOI: 10.1016/j.bjm.2016.07.017

Yeşil, Y., & İnal, İ. (2019). Traditional knowledge of wild edible plants in Hasankeyf (Batman Province, Turkey). *Acta Societatis Botanicae Poloniae, 88*(3), 3633. https://doi.org/DOI: 10.5586/asbp.2019.3633

Yeşil, Y., & İnal, İ. (2021). Ethnomedicinal plants of Hasankeyf (Batman-Turkey). *Frontiers in Pharmacology, 11*, 624710. https://doi.org/DOI: 10.3389/fphar.2021.624710

Yeşilada, E., Honda, G., Sezik, E., Tabata, M., Goto, K., & Ikeshiro, Y. (1993). Traditional medicine in Turkey IV: Folk medicine in the Mediterranean subdivision. *Journal of Ethnopharmacology*, *39*(1), 31–38. DOI: 10.1016/0378-8741(93)90048-A

Yılmaz, H., Çarıkçı, S., Kılıç, T., Dirmenci, T., Arabacı, T., & Gören, A. C. (2017). Screening of chemical composition, antioxidant and anticholinesterase activity of section *Brevifilamentum* of *Origanum* (L.) species. *Records of Natural Products*, *11*(5), 439–455. DOI: 10.25135/rnp.56.17.04.029

Chapter 13
Medicinal Uses of Secondary Metabolites in the Genus Salvia

Elif Merdamert-Bozyel
https://orcid.org/0000-0001-5470-2372
Health Institutes of Türkiye, Turkey

Mustafa Eray Bozyel
https://orcid.org/0000-0001-5556-4880
Dokuz Eylül University, Turkey

Dilay Turu
https://orcid.org/0000-0002-8485-0488
Graduate School of Natural and Applied Sciences, Dokuz Eylül University, Turkey

Atakan Benek
https://orcid.org/0000-0001-6726-5968
Dokuz Eylül University, Turkey

Kerem Canlı
https://orcid.org/0000-0001-6061-6948
Dokuz Eylül University, Turkey

ABSTRACT

The Salvia genus, commonly referred to as "sage", represents the largest genus within the family Lamiaceae. Approximately 1,000 species of the Salvia genus are known to grow naturally, primarily in southern Europe but also in other regions worldwide. A significant proportion of the species are utilized in traditional medi-

DOI: 10.4018/979-8-3693-9112-9.ch013

cine. In vitro and in vivo studies with Salvia species have confirmed the presence of numerous secondary metabolites with various biological activities and therapeutic properties. The Salvia genus contains a variety of secondary metabolites, including sterols, flavonoids, sesquiterpenoids, sesterpenoids, diterpenoids, triterpenoids, and essential oils. This study aims to present a comprehensive analysis of the use of the genus Salvia in traditional medicine and the therapeutic effects of its secondary metabolites.

1. INTRODUCTION

The findings regarding the medicinal applications of plants substantiate their utilization since ancient times. The employment of plant-derived medicines constitutes a vital component of the cultural practices within rural societies, even in developed nations. In eras when the advancement of medical practices lagged behind contemporary standards, communities relied on plants in their natural forms for therapeutic purposes. The applications of plants span diverse domains, including but not limited to spices, teas, ornamental uses, medicinal preparations, dyes, the flavoring industry, culinary practices, and the cosmetics sector. Furthermore, technological advancements over time have broadened these applications, enhancing the roles that plants play in various industries, (Berber et al., 2013) (Baytop, 1999).

Phytochemicals, often referred to as plant chemicals, are biologically active compounds synthesized by plants, (Liu, 2004).

Among the various plant families, the Lamiaceae family exhibits the highest diversity in terms of phytochemical composition. The most significant biologically active compounds within this family are secondary metabolites, which have garnered increasing scholarly attention due to their diverse applications and effects, (IARC, 1980).

Notably, phenolic compounds stand out as the most crucial group of secondary metabolites, particularly due to their decongestant properties. Phenolic substances are recognized as paramount natural antioxidants and are classified as polyphenolic compounds, which are ubiquitous across all plant parts. Among these polyphenolic compounds, flavonoids, coumarins, cinnamic acid derivatives, tocopherols, and phenolic acids are particularly prevalent in decongestant formulations. The extensive array of secondary metabolites present in the Lamiaceae family underscores the importance of continued research into their potential health benefits and therapeutic applications, (IARC, 1980).

1.1 General Characteristics of the Lamiaceae Family

The Lamiaceae family, commonly known as the mint family, exhibits a global distribution, with the notable exception of the frigid Polar Regions. The economic and medicinal significance of this family is extensively documented in the scientific literature. Species within the Lamiaceae family are predominantly herbaceous perennials or shrubs, typically characterized by their aromatic properties and diverse uses in various cultural, culinary, and therapeutic applications. The Lamiaceae family, renowned for its extensive diversity, encompasses a wide array of flowering plants with a cosmopolitan distribution. Among its largest genera are *Salvia*, comprising approximately 900 species; *Scutellaria*, with around 360 species; *Stachys* and *Plectranthus*, each containing 300 species; *Hyptis*, totaling 280 species; *Thymus*, which includes 220 species; and *Nepeta*, with 200 species. A significant number of these taxa are utilized in culinary applications as spices and vegetables. Overall, the Lamiaceae family consists of approximately 250 genera and 7,900 species globally, highlighting its ecological and agricultural importance, (Kaya, 2024).

The Lamiaceae family holds considerable significance due to its rich biodiversity and notable economic value. The chemical composition within this family is both diverse and complex. A substantial body of scholarly research has focused on the essential oils derived from various genera within Lamiaceae. In addition, investigations have explored a range of other bioactive compounds, including diterpenes, triterpenes, and phenolic compounds. Notably, the *Salvia* genus is critical within this family, distinguished by its unique taxonomic characteristics and an array of active compounds that may play essential roles in ecological processes, (Rahmanifar, Livadariu, & Cornea, 2023).

1.2 General Characteristics of the Salvia Genus

The *Salvia* genus, commonly referred to as sage, represents the largest aggregation of plant species within the Lamiaceae family, encompassing over 900 distinct species globally. This genus is particularly diverse, with a significant representation of species across the Americas, South America, as well as East and Southeast Asia. The term "*Salvia*" is etymologically derived from the Latin word "salvere," which implies meanings such as "to heal," "to do good," and "to be healthy".

Historically, the anxiolytic and fatigue-relieving properties of various species within this genus have been recognized for centuries. Contemporary scientific research has corroborated these claims, revealing that *Salvia* species may confer numerous benefits, including enhancements in memory function, along with exhibiting antioxidant, antibacterial, antidiabetic, and antitumor properties.

Moreover, *Salvia* has diverse applications across the fields of alternative medicine, pharmacology, perfumery, and cosmetics. Its significance extends into apiculture, as the intricate and aromatic flowers of *Salvia* are valuable to beekeeping practices, (Rahmanifar, Livadariu, & Cornea, 2023).

2. BIOCHEMICAL CONTENTS OF THE SALVIA GENUS

The *Salvia* genus encompasses a notable group of utilitarian plants that have maintained their significance throughout history. Numerous wild-growing *Salvia* species are utilized in traditional medicine across diverse cultural contexts, often serving as a form of sage or a tobacco substitute, attributable to the similarities in leaf texture and morphology. Extensive research has identified a variety of secondary metabolites within these species. The phytochemical profile of *Salvia* is characterized by the production of monoterpenoids, particularly those bearing abietan or clerodane skeletons, in addition to triterpenoids and flavonoids. Investigations into the secondary metabolites of *Salvia* species have revealed their potential to exhibit properties such as antioxidant, antibacterial, antimutagenic, anti-inflammatory, and cytotoxic activities, (Er *et al.,* 2013).

3. SECONDARY METABOLITES AND BIOLOGICAL ACTIVITIES OF THE SALVIA GENUS

Secondary metabolites are organic compounds that do not directly contribute to the growth, development, or reproduction of living organisms. Throughout history, the beneficial properties of medicinal plants have been exploited by various industries, including food, pharmaceuticals, and cosmetics. Unlike primary metabolites, the absence of secondary metabolites does not result in immediate mortality; however, it can lead to long-term disruptions in an organism's survival, fertility, or phenotypic characteristics, and in some cases, may not produce any discernible effects.

These compounds frequently play crucial roles in the plant defense mechanism. As previously noted, secondary metabolites are not essential to the fundamental molecular architecture of cells. They typically exist in limited quantities and may have negligible direct influence on growth and development. When present, they are often localized to specific tissues, organs, or developmental stages. Additionally, secondary metabolites may be restricted to particular genera or species and often arise under specific conditions, such as environmental stress or specialized nutritional inputs.

In recent years, a substantial body of research has emerged underscoring the significance and medicinal value of secondary metabolites found in the *Salvia* genus. As a result, considerable efforts have been directed toward the development of alternative methods for the production of key plant compounds, with a particular emphasis on secondary metabolites.

These secondary metabolites play a crucial role in various industrial applications, including the formulation of medicinal agents, cleansing products (such as soaps), essential oils, adhesives, chewing gum, resins, rubber, spices for food and beverages, and a range of other materials.

The compounds in question play a crucial role in various essential functions within plants, including the regulation of hormones, promotion of growth, mitigation of microbial contamination, attraction of pollinators, and deterrence of herbivores and insects. These processes enable plants to not only survive but also thrive within their ecological niches while minimizing damage from herbivorous animals and insects. The diverse chemical families to which these compounds belong, including alkaloids and flavonoids, equip plants with sophisticated defense mechanisms against microbial threats, herbivory, and ultraviolet radiation. Furthermore, secondary metabolites are instrumental in attracting pollinating insects to flowers, thus facilitating reproductive success.

Prior research has established that the genus *Salvia* is a rich source of valuable secondary metabolites, particularly terpenoids and flavonoids, which are present in its roots, leaves, and flowers. Notably, the concentration of these metabolites is maximized during the flowering stage. Among these compounds, rosmarinic acid and salvianolic acid, both belonging to the flavonoid group, are formed through the dimerization and tetramerization of caffeic acid, respectively. These secondary metabolites have been shown to exhibit a diverse array of biological activities, including antioxidant, antiplatelet, antitumor, and antiviral properties. It is hypothesized that the observed antimicrobial, antioxidant, and anticancer effects of *Salvia* are attributable to the presence of specific compounds within its essential oil, (Rahmanifar, Livadariu, & Cornea, 2023).

As a result, despite the relatively low concentrations of these metabolites found in plants, they continue to serve as the only economically viable source for a significant number of these valuable compounds. Furthermore, research has demonstrated that these plants exhibit notable hypoglycaemic properties.

The medicinal metabolites found in *Salvia* plants are primarily categorized into three main groups: monoterpenes, triterpenes, and diterpenes, along with phenolic acids. Monoterpenes such as cineole, thujone, and camphor, as well as triterpenes including ursolic acid and oleanolic acid, are predominantly observed in the essential oils of these plants. Together with flavonoids, these compounds are more abundant in the above-ground parts of Salvia than in other plant structures. Conversely, diterpenoids and phenolic acids are the principal constituents found in the root system, (Abu-Izneid *et al.,* 2020).

Among the phenolic acids present in *Salvia* species, caffeic acid and its derivatives are noteworthy. Notably, caffeic acid often exists in a dimeric form as rosmarinic acid (RA), which stands out as the most significant phenolic acid within the genus. Furthermore, caffeic acid trimers and tetramers are of particular interest regarding their therapeutic potential. The key phenolic acids identified in *Salvia* include caffeic acid, dihydroxyphenyl lactic acid, chlorogenic acid, and danshensu (caffeic acid monomers), alongside RA (caffeic acid dimer), salvianolic acid A (caffeic acid trimer), and salvianolic acid B, (Rahmanifar, Livadariu, & Cornea, 2023).

3.1 Secondary Metabolites of the *Salvia* Genus

3.1.1 Sesquiterponoids

Sesquiterpenes constitute the most extensive category of plant secondary metabolites, characterized by the presence of three isoprene units. These compounds exhibit a widespread distribution across various angiosperms, as well as among several gymnosperms and bryophytes. Sesquiterpenes and their derivatives are biosynthesized in diverse plant structures, which include leaves, fruits, and roots. A defining attribute of sesquiterpenes and their related derivatives is their role in plant defense mechanisms, attributed to their antifungal, antibacterial, and antiviral properties, (Abu-Izneid *et al.,* 2020).

In recent decades, an expanding body of literature has highlighted the beneficial effects of sesquiterpenes on a plethora of metabolic disorders, such as hyperglycemia, hyperlipidemia, cardiovascular complications, neural disorders, diabetes, and cancer. This compound class can be categorized into six distinct subgroups: aliphatic sesquiterpenes, germacrane sesquiterpenes, carotenoid sesquiterpenes, caryophyllane sesquiterpenes, guaiane sesquiterpenes, and various other sesquiterpenes, (Wu *et al.,* 2012).

3.1.1.1 Germacrane Sesquiterpenoids

Germacrane sesquiterpenoids represent a distinct class of sesquiterpenes characterized by a unique 10-membered ring system and varying arrangements of functional groups. Salviadienol A and B are notable as the first germacrane sesquiterpenes isolated from *Salvia chinensis*, (Wu *et al.,* 2012).

3.1.1.2 Aliphatic Sesquiterpene

The chemical composition of *Salvia* encompasses a range of aliphatic sesquiterpenes, notably including salvinine, which is specifically derived from *Salvia divaricate*, (Wu *et al.*, 2012).

3.1.1.3 Carotenes

Carotene sesquiterpenes, commonly known as daucane sesquiterpenes, represent a subclass of terpenoid compounds characterized by their unique structural properties. Notably, the chemical compound 1,5-epoxysalvial-4(14)-ene has been identified in the plant species *Salvia sclarea*, highlighting the phytochemical diversity within this genus, (Wu *et al.*, 2012).

3.1.1.4 Caryophyllanes

Caryophyllane sesquiterpenes represent a distinctive class of natural bicyclic sesquiterpenes that are characterized by a specific 4/9-ring system, (Wu *et al.*, 2012).

3.1.1.5 Guaiane Sesquiterpene

Among the nine identified guaiane sesquiterpenes, nubiol has been found in several specific compounds, namely nubenolide, nubenolide acetate, bisnubidiol, and bisnubenolide. These compounds are derived from the plant *Salvia nubicola*, (Wu *et al.*, 2012).

3.1.1.6 Other Sesquiterpenes

The predominant sesquiterpenes identified in *Salvia palaefolia* belong to this category, (Wu *et al.*, 2012).

3.1.2 Diterpenes

Diterpenes are a class of natural compounds characterized by a skeletal structure comprised of 20 carbon atoms. The biosynthesis of these compounds can be elucidated by examining the various cyclization processes of geranylgeranyl diphosphate (GGPP). Diterpenes are prevalent across a multitude of plant families and some animal species. They are biosynthesized through two primary pathways: the mevalonic acid pathway (MVA) and the deoxylulose phosphate pathway (DOXP). The cyclization process plays a pivotal role in the generation of diverse diterpene carbon skeletons, forming a major branch of the biosynthetic pathway for cyclic diterpenes.

The biological significance of diterpenes is noteworthy, as numerous members of this class have been shown to exhibit significant biological activities. For example, compounds such as taxol, cafestol, and kahweol have been identified to possess anticancer properties. Moreover, diterpenes derived from the *Salvia* genus constitute the largest group of secondary metabolites within this class. This broad grouping can be further classified based on their structural characteristics into five subgroups: Tibetan diterpenoids, clerodane diterpenoids, pimarane diterpenoids, labdane diterpenoids, and various other diterpenoids, (Wu *et al.,* 2012).

3.1.2.1 Abietan Diterpenoid Derivatives

The compounds within this genus have been shown to possess a variety of intriguing biological activities, garnering considerable interest from the pharmacological community. The predominant component group of the *Salvia* genus is comprised of abietans and their rearranged derivatives, (Wu *et al.,* 2012).

3.1.2.2 Clerodanes

Clerodin, a class of bitter diterpenoids, was initially extracted from *Clerodendron infortunatum* (Family Verbenaceae). Its structure and stereochemistry, excluding the absolute configuration, were elucidated through X-ray crystallographic analysis of a bromolactone derivative. The fundamental hydrocarbon framework has since been designated as clerodane. Clerodanes are prevalent across a diverse range of plant families and are characterized by four adjacent stereocenters, which exist in either a cis or trans decalin configuration. Additionally, clerodane diterpenoids exhibit a wide array of biological properties, highlighting their potential significance in various fields of research, (Wu *et al.,* 2012).

3.1.2.3 Pimaranes

Pimaran diterpenes represent a distinct class of tricyclic hydrophenanthrene-nucleated diterpenoids that exhibit close biosynthetic affinities with labdane. These compounds are prevalent across a diverse array of plant families. Within the scope of *Salvia* species, pimaran diterpenes are recognized as a relatively minor group of constituents. Notably, among the various members of the *Salvia* genus, particularly within the subgenus P. Dec., *Salvia parryi* has been hypothesized to exhibit a significant abundance of pimaran diterpenes. To date, a total of twenty distinct pimaran diterpenes have been successfully isolated from various *Salvia* species, (Wu *et al.,* 2012).

3.1.2.4 Labdanes

Labdan, a compound belonging to the bicyclic diterpenoid family, is characterized by its decaline system and a C-6 ring that can exist in either an open or closed configuration, as exemplified by manoyl oxide and its derivatives. Labdan-type diterpenes are extensively distributed across various natural sources and have been shown to exhibit a wide range of significant biological activities. Numerous labdane diterpenoids have been successfully isolated from the *Salvia* genus, highlighting their ecological and pharmacological relevance, (Wu *et al.,* 2012).

3.1.3 Sesterterpenoids

3.1.3.1 C-23 Terpenoids

A novel class of terpenes featuring unique skeletal structures has been identified within the *Salvia* genus. These compounds exhibit 6/6/7-, 6/6/8-, or 6/6/5/5-ring configurations, characterized by the presence of a lactone linkage between carbon atoms C-6 and C-22. Additionally, the structures are denoted as C-6-, C-6-, or C-6-, C-6-, C-6-, C-6-, and C-6-decalin, reflecting their intricate molecular architecture, (Wu *et al.,* 2012).

3.1.3.2 C-25 Terpenoids

C-25 sesterpenes are generally synthesized from the aerial parts of plant species within the *Salvia genus*, (Wu *et al.,* 2012).

3.1.4 Triterpenoids and Steroids

The group is categorized into subgroups based on their structural characteristics, encompassing the following categories: ursane-type triterpenoids, oleanane-type triterpenoids, lupane-type triterpenoids, dammarane-type triterpenoids, steroids, and various other triterpenoids, (Wu *et al.,* 2012).

3.1.4.1 Ursanes

The compounds oleanolic acid and salvistamineol were successfully isolated from the respective species *Salvia officinalis* and *Salvia staminea*, (Horiuchi *et al.,* 2007) (Topçu, *et al.,* 2003). Six novel ursane-type triterpenoids were isolated from the roots of *Salvia kronenburgii*, (Topçu, *et al.,* 2003) (Topçu, *et al.,* 2004). Four novel ursane triterpenoids were successfully isolated from the aerial parts of *Salvia argentea.* The subgroup consisted of four distinct examples: 3-Oxours-12-ene-1β,11α-diol derived from *Salvia haenkei*; 3-epiursolic acid obtained from

Salvia lanata; santolinoic acid extracted from *Salvia santolinifolia*; and salvin A, also sourced from *S. santolinifolia*, (Wu *et al.,* 2012).

3.1.4.2 Oleananes

2α,3β-Dihydroxyolean-28-oic acid has been identified as an oleanane-type triterpenoid extracted from *Salvia hierosolymitana*. In the present study, several chemical compounds were identified, specifically: 1β,2α,3β,11α-tetrahydroxyolean-12-ene, 3β-acetoxyolean-12-ene-lβ,2α,11α-triol, and 3β-hydroxy-l-oxoolean-12-en-28-oic acid, commonly referred to as virgatic acid. Additionally, three oleanane-type triterpenoids, each characterized by a double bond between carbon atoms C-12 and C-13, were isolated from four different species of the genus *Salvia*. These species include *Salvia kronenburgii*, *Salvia argentea*, *Salvia virgata*, and *Salvia santolinifolia*. One of the notable compounds identified is 3α,6α,24-trihydroxyolean-12-en-28-oic acid, also known as salvin B, (Wu *et al.,* 2012).

The triterpenoids Przewanoic acids A and B, derived from *Salvia przewalskii*, are characterized by the presence of a 12,13-cyclo group. Furthermore, an examination of *Salvia lanigera* has led to the identification of an oleanane-type triterpene featuring a lactone bridge between the C-28 and C-13 positions. Reglin is characterized as an ester that consists of an abietane quinone diterpene structure, combined with a triterpenoid acyl moiety, (Ortega *et al.,* 1995).

3.1.4.3 Lupanes

The roots of *Salvia palaestina* were extracted using acetone, resulting in the isolation of four lupane-type triterpenes characterized by a double bond between C-20 and C-29. Additionally, seven lupane-type triterpenes from four distinct *Salvia* species were identified, specifically: 1β,11α,20-trihydroxy-lupan-3-one; lupane-3β,11α,20-triol; 3β-acetoxylupane-11α,20-diol; 3-oxolupane-11α,20-diol; monogynol A; 3β-O-trans-p-coumaroylmonogynol A; and 3β-O-cis-p-coumaroylmonogynol A. Further analysis revealed that four additional lupane-type triterpenes were detected in the species *Salvia deserta*, *Salvia phlomoides*, *Salvia macrochlamys*, and *Salvia montbretii*, all of which contained a hydroxy group at C-20, (Wu *et al.,* 2012).

3.1.4.4 Dammaranes

Three novel 20,24-epoxydammarane triterpenes, referred to as santolins A, B, and C, were isolated from the acetone-soluble fraction of the methanol extract of *Salvia santolinifolia* Salvilymitone. Furthermore, two new triterpenoids, designated salvilymitone and salvilymitol, were obtained from *Salvia hierosolymitana,* (Wu *et al.,* 2012).

3.1.4.5 Other Triterpenoids

In 1999, Ahmad and his colleagues published two pivotal papers addressing *Salvia bucharica*. In these studies, they reported the successful isolation and identification of salvadiol as well as salvadiones A and B. Notably, salvadiol features a novel carbon skeleton derived from the precursor icetexone, which is hypothesized to form via the autoxidation of myrcene, (Wu *et al.*, 2012).

3.1.4.6 Steroids

The steroids brassicasterone, 1-oxo-7α-hydroxysitosterol, and stigmast-4-en-3-one were successfully isolated from the plant species *Salvia multicaulis*, *Salvia glutinosa*, and *Salvia amplexicaulis*, respectively, (Wu *et al.*, 2012).

3.1.5 Polyphenols

Salvia spp. is distinguished by the presence of two principal categories of active constituents. In addition to the previously noted lipophilic terpenoids, a second category of metabolites has been identified, primarily comprising water-soluble polyphenolics. Notable examples of these polyphenolic compounds include salvianolic acid B, danshensu, and protocatechuic aldehyde, among others. Moreover, the polyphenols can be classified into two subgroups on the basis of their structural characteristics: phenolic acids and flavonoids, (Wu *et al.*, 2012).

3.1.5.1 Phenolic Acids

Beginning in the 1980s, researchers from China and Japan have extensively investigated the water-soluble constituents of Danshen (*Salvia miltiorrhiza*), resulting in the isolation of over twenty phenolic acids from this medicinal plant. Notably, these phenolic acids encompass caffeic acid monomers as well as oligomers, which are commonly known as depsides or salvianolic acids. This ongoing research underscores the significance of Danshen in phytochemistry and its potential therapeutic applications. Phenolic acids have been shown to play a significant role in the prevention of various human diseases. Notably, the primary effects of phenolic acids in Tanshen include their antioxidant, anticoagulant, and cytoprotective properties, (Wang, Morris-Natschke, & Lee, 2007).

Przewalskinone B is a novel anthraquinone that has been successfully isolated from *Salvia przewalskii*. Within the *Salvia* genus, the predominant class of water-soluble compounds consists of polar phenolic acids. Additionally, from *Salvia moorcroftiana*, researchers have isolated nonyl 4-hydroxybenzoate and 4-hydroxy-2-isopropyl-5-methylphenyl O-α-L-rhamnopyranosyl-(1→2)-β-D-glucopyranoside, both of which are derivatives of benzene Two phenolic esters were characterized in the acetone extract of *Salvia microphylla*: eicosaheptanoic acid 2-(p-hydroxyphenyl)ethyl ester and hexacosylferulate. Additionally, a novel cyclic phenyl acetamide was isolated from the rhizome of *Salvia miltiorrhiza,* (Wang, Morris-Natschke, & Lee, 2007).

The compound 4-(1-hydroxy-5-methylnaphthalen-2-yl)-2-methyl-4-oxobutyl acetate, also known as salvianonol, was isolated from the same plant species, (Don *et al.,* 2006).

3.1.5.2 Flavonoids

A novel flavanone, designated as nubatin, has been successfully extracted from the specimen of *Salvia nubicola*, which was collected in Quetta, Pakistan, (Wu *et al.,* 2012). In the course of this study, several flavonoids were identified and characterized. The identified flavonoids include 6,8-di-C-glucosylapigenin (commonly known as vicenin-2), luteolin 7-O-β-D-glucoside, luteolin 7-O-glucuronide, luteolin 3′-O-glucuronide, and 6-hydroxyluteolin 7-O-glucoside. Additionally, six distinct flavonoids were isolated and characterized from *Salvia officinalis*. Furthermore, three additional flavonoids were extracted and characterized from the same plant species: 6-methoxyluteolin 7-O-glucoside, 6-hydroxyluteolin 5-O-glucoside, and 6-hydroxyluteolin 7-O-glucuronide. This comprehensive analysis contributes to the understanding of the flavonoid profile present in *S. officinalis* and its potential applications, (Wu *et al.,* 2012).

Two novel flavone glycosides, namely apigenin 7-O-β-D-glucopyranosyl-(1‴→4″)-β-D-glucopyranoside (referred to as apigenin 7-O-cellobioside) and apigenin 7,4′-O,O-di-β-D-glucopyranoside (designated apigenin 7,4′-O,O-diglucoside), have been successfully isolated from the petals of *Salvia uliginosa,* (Veitch *et al.,* 1998).

The novel anthocyanin identified in the plant species associated with the blue coloration of its flowers is delphinidin 3-O-[6-O-(p-coumaroyl)-β-D-glucopyranoside]-5-O-[4-O-acetyl-6-O-malonyl-β-D-glucopyranoside]. In a series of three publications, Zahid and colleagues extensively explored this topic. Between 2001 and 2003, the species *Salvia moorcroftiana* was both isolated and characterized, leading to the discovery of four new flavonoid glycosides: genkwanin 4′-O-α-L-arabinopyranosyl-(1→6)-β-D-galactopyranoside, genkwanin 4′-[O-α-L-rhamnopyranosyl-(1→2)-β-D-galactopyranoside], genkwanin 4′-[O-α-L-arabinopyranosyl-(1→3)-α-L-rhamnopyranoside] and genkwanin 4′-O-{α-L-rhamnopyranosyl-(1→2)-[α-L-rhamnopyranosyl-(1→6)]-β-D-galactopyranoside}, (Wu *et al.,* 2012).

Additionally, 8-methoxygenistein 7-O-α-L-rhamnoside 4′-O-β-D-glucoside was also successfully isolated from *Salvia moorcroftiana*, contributing to the understanding of the phytochemical diversity within this species, (Wu *et al.,* 2012).

3.1.5.3 Others

The aerial components of *Salvia nemorosa* underwent comprehensive chemical analysis, leading to the isolation of three novel megastigmane glycosides, designated as salvionosides A, B, and C. In a separate investigation of *Salvia miltiorrhiza*, two notable compounds were identified: a 2,5-disubstituted furan and a nitrogen-containing compound. Furthermore, the ethanol extract of Dalmatian sage (*Salvia officinalis*) was found to yield three glycosidically bound flavor precursors, (Don *et al.*, 2006) (Don *et al.*, 2005).

Among the compounds examined, salvianolic acid N demonstrated significant inhibitory effects on HIV-1 integrase (IN) in vitro, along with a notable reduction of HIV-1 p24 antigen levels in MT-4 cell lines, (Zhang *et al.*, 2008a) (Zhang *et al.*, 2008b). Furthermore, two lignan diesters, namely secoisolariciresinol diester and secoisolariciresinol branched fatty diester, were successfully isolated from the seeds of *S. plebeia* (20,21). The subsequent tables provide a comprehensive enumeration of the secondary metabolites that have been identified within the *Salvia* genus (Table 1-4).

Table 1. Sesquiterponoids of the Salvia genus

1	salvinine	*S. divaricata*	24	(1R,5R)-1,5-epoxysalvial-4(14)-ene	*S. sclarea*
2	salviadienol A	*S. chinensis*	25	(2R,5E)-2,12-epoxycaryophyll-5- ene	*S. sclarea*
3	3β,6β,8a-triacetoxy-4β,5α-epoxy-1-oxogermacr-10(14)-ene	*S. roborowskii*	26	(2R,5E)-caryophyll-5-en-12-al	*S. sclarea*
4	3β,6β,8a-triacetoxy-4β,5α-epoxygermacr-1(10)E-Ene	*S. roborowskii*	27	(2S,5E)-caryophyll-5-en-12-al	*S. sclarea*
5	3β,6β,8a-triacetoxy-4β,5α:1α,10β-diepoxygermacrane	*S. roborowskii*	28	caryophyllene oxide	*S. sclarea* *S. palaefolia*
6	salviadienol B	*S. chinensis*	29	4,10-epoxy-6α-hydroxyguaiane (= buchariol)	*S. bucharica*
7	trijugin A	*S. trijuga*	30	isospathulenol	*S. sclarea*
8	trijugin B	*S. trijuga*	31	(1β,3β,4α,5α,6α,8α)-guai-10(14)- ene-3,4,6,8-tetrol 3,6,8-triacetate	*S.roborowskii*
9	trijugin C	*S. trijuga*	32	spathulenol	*S. eupatorium* *S. sclarea*
10	trijugin D	*S. trijuga*	33	nubiol	*S. nubicola*
11	trijugin E	*S. trijuga*	34	nubenolide	*S. nubicola*
12	trijugin F	*S. trijuga*	35	nubenolideacetate	*S. nubicola*

continued on following page

Table 1. Continued

13	trijugin G	*S. trijuga*	36	bisnubidiol	*S. nubicola*
14	trijugin H	*S. trijuga*	37	bisnubenolide	*S. nubicola*
15	trijugin I	*S. trijuga*	38	1α,9β-dibenzoyloxy-2β,3β,4β-trihydroxydihydro-β-agarofuran	*S. palaefolia*
16	(1aS*,6R*,6aS*,7aR*,9aR*)-1a,2,6,6a,7a,8,9,9a-octahydro-1a,5,7atrimethylbisoxireno[4,5:8,9] cyclodeca[1,2-b]furan-6-yl acetate (=castanin B)6-acetoxyglechomafuran	*S. castanea* *S. roborowskii*	39	lα-acetoxy-11-hydroxy-2,8-dioxoeudesman-3-en-12-oic acid methyl ester	*S. palaefolia*
17	glechomafuran	*S. palaefolia*	40	11-hydroxy-3,8-dioxo-eudesman-1,4-dien-12-oic acid methyl ester	*S. palaefolia*
18	castanin C	*S. castanea*	41	β-eudesmol	*S. microphylla*
19	castanin D	*S. castanea*	42	8α-hydroxy-β-eudesmol	*S. microphylla*
20	castanin E	*S. castanea*	43	1α-acetoxy-2-oxoeudesman-3,7(11)-dien-8β,12-olide	*S. palaefolia*
21	castanin F	*S. castanea*	44	1α-hydroxy-2-oxoeudesman-3,7(11)-dien-8β,12-olide	*S. palaefolia*
22	(4R*,5R*,5aS*,8S*,8aR*,8bR*)-8-formyl-4,5,5a,6,7,8,8a,8b-octahydro- 5,8b-dihydroxy-3,5a,8-trimethyl-2-oxo-2H-indeno[4,5-b]furan-4-yl acetate (= castanin A)	*S. castanea*	45	1α,8α-dihydroxy-2-oxoeudesman-3,7(11)-dien-8β,12-olide	*S. palaefolia*
23	(3β,4α,6α,8β,9β,10α)-8-(acetyloxy)-3,4:9,10-diepoxygermacr-7(11)-eno- 12,6-lactone	*S. roborowskii*	46	1α-acetoxy-8α-hydroxy-2-oxoeudesman-3,7(11)-dien-8,12- olide	*S. palaefolia*

(Wu *et al.*, 2012)

Table 2. Diterpenoids of the Salvia genus

1	O-methylpisiferic acid methyl ester	*S.blepharochlaena*	273	salvilimbinol	*S. limbata*
2	pisiferic acid	*S.blepharochlaena*	274	4-dehydrosalvilimbinol	*S. limbata*
3	O-methylpisiferic acid	*S.blepharochlaena*	275	sclareapinone	*S. sclarea* *S. prionitis*
4	candelabrone	*S. palaestina* *S. candelabrum*	276	4,14-dihydroxysaprorthoquinone	*S. eriophora*
5	12-O-methylcandelabrone	*S. palaestina*	277	salvisyrianone	*S. syriaca*
6	forskalinone	*S. forskahlei*	278	prionoid D	*S. prionitis*

continued on following page

Table 2. Continued

7	20-norinuroyleanol	*S. semiatrata*	279	4-hydroxysaprorthoquinone	*S. prionitis*
8	1-isopropyl-4b,8,8-trimethyl-9-oxo-4b,5,6,7,8,8a,9,10-octahydrophenanthrene-2,3,10-triyl triacetate	*S. melissodora*	280	prionoid E	*S. prionitis*
9	14-hydroxy-12-methoxy-abieta-8,11,13-trien-3-one	*S. multicaulis*	281	2-hydroxysaprorthoquinone	*S. limbata*
10	12-peroxyabieta-8,11,13-trien-6-one	*S. multicaulis*	282	saprorthoquinone	*S. prionitis*
11	1-oxoferruginol	*S. napifolia*	283	4.5-seoo-5,10-friedo-abieta-4(18),5(10),6,8,13-pentaene-1,11,12-trione (= 1-oxoaethiopinone)	*S. argentea*
12	6-oxoferruginol	*S. napifolia*	284	4,5-seco-5,10-friedo-abieta-4(18),5,6,8,13-pentaene-11,12-dione	*S. aethiopis*
13	1-oxo-5-hydroxyabieta-8,11,13-trien-18-oic acid	*S. candidissima*	285	prionoid F	*S. prionitis*
14	euphraticol	*S. euphratica*	286	sahandinone	*S. sahendica*
15	euphracal	*S. euphratica*	287	12-hydroxy-sapriparaquinone	*S. limbata* *S. prionitis*
16	2α-hydroxyferruginyl-2,12-dimethyl ether	*S. pachystachys*	288	limbinal	*S. limbata*
17	14-hydroxyferruginol	*S. montbretii*	289	3,12-dihydroxysapriparaquinon-1-ene	*S. limbata*
18	(3S,4aS,10aS)-1,2,3,4,4a,9,10,10aoctahydro-6-hydroxy-7-isopropyl-1,1,4a-trimethyl-9-oxophenanthren-3-yl acetate (= 2α-acetoxysugiol)	*S. miltiorrhiza*	290	prineoparaquinone	*S. prionitis*
19	16-hydroxycarnosic acid	*S. mellifera* *S. apiana* *S. chinopeplica*	291	2,3-dehydrosalvipisone	*S. sclarea*
20	sugiol	*S. miltiorrhiza* *S. tomentosa* *S. broussonetii* *S. canariensis* *S. pachystachys* *S. przewalskii*	292	acetylsalvipisone	*S. sclarea*

continued on following page

Table 2. Continued

21	ferruginol	*S.blepharochlaena* *S. candidissima* *S. apiana* *S. argentea* *S. broussonetii* *S. cilicica* *S. miltiorrhiza* *S. montbretii* *S. przewalskii* *S. sclarea* *S. tiliaefolia* *S. wiedemannii* *S. potentillifolia* *S. mellifera* *S. syriaca* *S. cyanescens* *S. napifolia* *S. microstegia* *S. candidissima* *S. eriophora* *S. hypargeia* *S. bracteata* *S. viridis* *S. multicaulis*	293	12-isopentenyl-3-oxosalvipisone	*S. cyanescens*
22	hypargenin A (= 6β,12-dihydroxyabieta-8,11,13-triene-1,7-dione)	*S. hypargeia*	294	1,4-dihydro-6-methyl-2-(1-methylethyl)-5-(4-methylpent-4-enyl)naphthalene-1,4-dione	*S. sahendica*
23	hypargenin B (= 12,15-dihydroxyabieta-8,11,13-trien-7-one)	*S. hypargeia*	295	1-oxosalvipisone	*S.candidissima*
24	hypargenin C (= 12-hydroxyabieta-8,11,13-triene-6,7-dione)	*S. hypargeia*	296	12-hydroxy-4,5-seco-5,10-friedo-4(18),5(10),6,8,12-abietapentaene-11,14-dione	*S. aethiopis*
25	hypargenin E (= 6β,14-dihydroxyabieta-8,11,13-trien-1-one)	*S. hypargeia*	297	saprionide	*S. prionitis*
26	iguestol	*S. broussonetii*	298	saprirearine	*S. prionitis*
27	salviviridinol	*S. viridis*	299	prionoid A	*S. prionitis*
28	abieta-9,12,14-trien-7-one	*S. amplexicaulis*	300	salvonitin	*S. prionitis*
29	16-acetoxycarnosic acid	*S. mellifera*	301	sapriolactone	*S. prionitis*
30	abieta-8,11,13-triene-11,12,16,20-tetraol	*S. mellifera*	302	de-O-ethylsalvonitin	*S. prionitis*
31	12-methoxyabieta-8,11,13-trien-11-ol	*S. candidissima*	303	prionoid B	*S. prionitis*
32	pomiferin A	*S. pomifera*	304	salvibretol	*S. montbretii*
33	pomiferin B	*S. pomifera*	305	sahandone	*S. sahendica*
34	pomiferin C	*S. pomifera*	306	prionoid C	*S. prionitis*
35	pomiferin D	*S. pomifera*	307	cariocal	*S. anastomosans*
36	pomiferin E	*S. pomifera*	308	16-hydroxyrosmadial	*S. mellifera*
37	10-acetylferruginol	*S. microstegia*	309	7,8-seco-para-ferruginone	*S. prionitis*
38	abieta-8,11,13-triene-5,11,12-triol	*S. microstegia*	310	rosmanoyl carnosate	*S. canariensis*
39	abieta-8,11,13-trien-3-one	*S. wiedemannii*	311	7,7′-bistaxodione	*S. montbretii*

continued on following page

Table 2. Continued

40	2α-hydroxysugiol diacetate	*S. cardiophylla*	312	11,11′-didehydroxy-7,7′-dihydroxytaxodione	*S. montbretii*
41	2α-hydroxysugiol	*S. cardiophylla*	313	microstegiol	*S. microstegia* *S. prionitis*
42	salviol	*S. cardiophylla* *S. tomentosa*	314	1-oxosalvibretol	*S. montbretii*
43	7-oxocarnosic acid diacetate	*S. canariensis*	315	candidissiol	*S. condidissima* *S. sclarea*
44	6-oxo-7β-hydroxycarnosic acid diacetate	*S. canariensis*	316	3-oxo-tilifolidione	*S. thymoides*
45	6-oxo-7α-hydroxycarnosic acid diacetate	*S. canariensis*	317	3-hydroxytilifolidione	*S. thymoides*
46	12-methoxycarnosic acid	*S. lanigera* *S. tomentosa* *S. officinalis*	318	dichroanal B	*S. dichroantha*
47	abietatriene-7β,15-diol	*S. sapinae*	319	dichroanal A	*S. dichroantha*
48	methyl carnosoate	*S. lanigera* *S. officinalis*	320	derivatives of 353	*S. dichroantha*
49	12-methoxy-11,7-dihydroxy-dehydroabietane	*S. bicolor*	321	salvicanaric acid	*S. canariensis* *S. munzii*
50	20-oxoinuroyleanol	*S. coulteri*	322	hongencaotone	*S. prionitis*
51	3β-hydroxydehydroabietic acid	*S. oxyodon*	323	bisprioterone B	*S. prionitis*
52	pomiferin F	*S. pomifera*	324	bisprioterone A	*S. prionitis*
53	pomiferin G	*S. pomifera*	325	bisprioterone C	*S. prionitis*
54	7-oxoferruginol-18-al	*S. sclarea*	326	salvicanol	*S. apiana* *S. canariensis* *S. przewalskii* *S. coulteri*
55	methyl 12-O-methylcarnosoate	*S. africana-lutea*	327	aegyptinone B	*S. aegyptiaca*
56	cryptojaponol	*S. barrelieri*	328	icetexone	*S. gilliessi* *S. ballotaeflora* *S. candicans*
57	inuroyleanol	*S. barrelieri*	329	paramiltioic acid	*S.paramiltiorrhiza*
58	carnosic acid	*S. mellifera*	330	epi-danshenspiroketallactone	*S. glutinosa* *S. przewalskii*
59	demethylcryptojaponol	*S. phlomoides*	331	10,11,14-trihydroxy-12-methoxy-9(10→20)abeoabieta-8,11,13-trien-7-one	*S. coulteri*
60	3β-hydroxydemethylcryptojaponol	*S. pubescens*	332	demethylsalvicanol	*S. broussonetii*
61	15-hydroxyabieta-8,11,13-trien-7-one	*S. albocaerulea*	333	przewalskin C	*S. przewalskii*
62	trilobinone	*S. triloba*	334	przewalskin D	*S. przewalskii*
63	safficinolide	*S. officinalis*	335	fruticulin A	*S. fruticulosa*
64	salvidorol	*S. dorrii*	336	1(10)-seco-2(10)-cycloicetexane (= salvimultine)	*S. multicaulis*
65	salvirecognone	*S. recognita*	337	19-deoxyicetexone	*S. ballotaeflora*
66	salvirecognine	*S. recognita*	338	5-epi-icetexone	*S. gilliessi*

continued on following page

Table 2. Continued

67	16-hydroxy-6,7-didehydroferruginol	*S. apiana*	339	19-deoxyisoicetexone	*S. ballotaeflora*
68	6,7-dehydrosempervirol	*S. apiana*	340	5,6-dihydro-6α-hydroxysalviasperanol	*S. aspera*
69	abieta-6,8,11,13-tetraene-6,12,14-triol	*S. napifolia*	341	brussonol	*S. broussonetii*
70	hypargenin D (= 12-hydroxyabieta-6,8,11,13-tetraen-3-one)	*S. hypargeia*	342	salviasperanol	*S. aspera*
71	6,7-didehydroferruginol	*S. apiana*	343	3,11,11a,11b-tetrahydro-8,11-dihydroxy-2a-methyl-9-(1-methylethyl)benzo[5,6] cyclohept[1,2,3-cd]isobenzofuran-	*S. candicans*
72	11,12-dimethoxyabieta-6,8,11,13-tetraen-20-oic acid methyl ester	*S. canariensis*	344	2,7,10(2aH)-trione	*S. ballotaeflora*
73	cryptanol	*S. cryptantha* *S. cilicica* *S. euphratica* *S. pachystachys* *S. wiedemannii*	345	7,20-dihydroanastomosine	*S. anastomosans*
74	trilobinol	*S. triloba*	346	anastomosine	*S. przewalskii*
75	20(10→5)abeoabieta-1(10),6,8,11,13-pentaene-11,12,16-triol	*S. apiana*	347	przewalskin E	*S. semiatrata* *S. tiliaefolia* *S. thymoides*
76	19(4→3)abeo-O-demethylcryptojaponol	*S. pubescens*	348	5-nor-3-oxo-tilifolidione	*S. thymoides*
77	12-O-methylcandesalvone A	*S. palaestina*	349	danshenspiroketallactone	*S. glutinosa* *S. miltiorrhiza* *S. przewalskii*
78	12-O-methyl-2-oxocandesalvone A	*S. palaestina*	350	aegyptinone A	*S. aegyptiaca*
79	candesalvone A	*S. candelabrum*	351	dichroanal B	*S. dichroantha*
80	blephaein	*S.blepharochlaena*	352	2α-hydroxysalvicanaric acid	*S. texana*
81	salvitchihatine	*S. tchihatcheffii*	353	salvicanaraldehyde	*S. munzii*
82	7-oxo-11,12,14-trihydroxy-20-methoxyabieta-5,8,11,13-tetraene	*S. candidissima*	354	4,8-dimethyl-8,9-dihydro-10,12-dioxa-benzo[a]anthracene-7,11-dione (= salviamone)	*S. miltiorrhiza*
83	salvinolone	*S. prionitis*	355	salprionin	*S. prionitis*
84	montbretyl 12-methyl ether (= 6-hydroxy-12-methoxyabieta-5,8,11,13-tetraen-7-one)	*S. montbretii*	356	przewalskin B	*S.przewalskii*
85	6-hydroxysalvinolone	*S. montbretii*	357	12-methoxy-8,11,13-abietatrien-20,11-olide	*S. officinalis*
86	14-deoxycoleon U	*S. phlomoides*	358	9-isopropyl-2,2,5-trimethyl-8H-phenaleno[1,9bc]furan-8-one (= salvilenone)	*S.miltiorrhiza*
87	6,11-dihydroxy-12-methoxyabieta-5,8,11,13-tetraen-7-one	*S. phlomoides*	359	3-hydroxysalvilenone	*S. prionitis*
88	multicaulin	*S.blepharochlaena* *S. multicaulis*	360	wiedemannic acid	*S.wiedemannii*
89	7,8-dimethyl-2-(1-methylethy) phenanthren-3-ol	*S. hydrangea* *S. multicaulis*	361	heldrichinic acid	*S.heldrichiana*

continued on following page

Table 2. Continued

90	11,12-dihydroxy-20-nor-5(10),6,8,11,13-abietapentaen-1-one (= arucadiol)	*S. anastomosans* *S. prionitis* *S. argentea*	362	lanigerone	*S. lanigera*
91	1,2,3,4-tetrahydro-5-hydroxy-7-isopropyl-1,1-dimethyl-4-oxophenanthren-6-yl palmitate	*S. miltiorrhiza*	363	salvinolactone	*S. prionitis*
92	3β-hydroxy-8,11,13(14),15-abietatetraen-18-oic acid	*S.tomentosa*	364	miltipolone	*S. castanea*
93	nemorosin	*S. nemorosa*	365	castanolide	*S. castanea*
94	abieta-8,11,13-triene-11,12,20-triol	*S. mellifera*	366	epi-castanolide	*S. castanea*
95	11,12,16-trihydroxyabieta-8,11,13-trien-20-al	*S. mellifera*	367	salvigreside A	*S. greggii*
96	2-oxocandesalvone A	*S. palaestina*	368	salvigreside B	*S. greggii*
97	12-O-methyl-2-oxocandesalvone A	*S. palaestina*	369	salvigreside C	*S. greggii*
98	sageone	*S. officinalis* *S. mellifera*	370	19-O-acetoxy-15,16-epoxy-ent-cleroda-3,13(16),14-triene-6,18-diol	*S. fulgens*
99	11,12,16-trihydroxy-20-norabieta-5(10),8,11,13-tetraen-1-one	*S. mellifera*	371	19-acetoxy-15,16-epoxy-6-hydroxy-ent-cleroda-3,13(16),14trien-18-al	*S. fulgens*
100	9,10-dihydro-7,8-dimethyl-2-(1-methylethyl)phenanthren-3-ol	*S. hydrangea*	372	hardwickiic acid	*S. regla*
101	maytenoquinone	*S. melissodora*	373	divinatorin A	*S. divinorum*
102	viridinol	*S. viridis*	374	divinatorin B	*S. divinorum*
103	2α,7,11-trihydroxy-7,9(11),13-abietatrien-12-one	*S. texana*	375	divinatorin C	*S. divinorum*
104	6,12-dihydroxyabieta-5,8,11,13-tetraen-7-one (= montbretol	*S. miltiorrhiza* *S. montbretii*	376	divinorin F	*S. divinorum*
105	2-oxotaxodione	*S. texana*	377	divinatorin D	*S. divinorum*
106	7-hydroxytaxodione	*S. montbretii*	378	divinatorin E	*S. divinorum*
107	2α-hydroxytaxodione	*S. texana*	379	kerlinic acid	*S. keerlii*
108	2α-hydroxytaxodone	*S. texana*	380	thymonin	*S. thymoides*
109	2α,7-dihydroxytaxodone	*S. texana*	381	derivative of 392	*S. thymoides*
110	fruticulin B	*S. fruticulosa*	382	derivative of 392	*S. thymoides*
111	2α,10β-dihydroxy-12-oxo-norabieta-9(11),13-dien (= salvipiliferol)	*S. pilifera*	383	7β-hydroxythymonin	*S. thymoides*
112	viridone	*S. viridis*	384	derivative of 395	*S. thymoides*
113	2α,11-dihydroxy-5,7,9(11),13-abietatetraen-12-one	*S. texana*	385	derivative of 395	*S. thymoides*
114	5,6-dehydro-2α,7-dihydroxytaxodone	*S. texana*	386	clerodermic acids	*S. regla*
115	5,6-didehydro-7-hydroxytaxodone	*S. munzii*	387	7β-18,19-trihydroxy-ent-cleroda-3,13-dien-16,15-olide	*S. melissodora*
116	15-deoxyfuerstione (= 11-hydroxy-5,7,9(11),13-abietatetraen-12-one)	*S.moorcraftiana*	388	lasianthin	*S. lasiantha*

continued on following page

Table 2. Continued

117	7-hydroxy-12-methoxy-20-norabieta-1,5(10),7,9,12-pentaene-6,14-dione	*S. cilicica*	389	salvidivin D	*S. divinorum*
118	horminone	*S.blepharochlaena* *S. anastomosans* *S. barrelieri* *S. tomentosa* *S. candidissima* *S. cryptantha.* *S. pachystachys* *S. sahendica* *S. wiedemannii* *S. lanata* *S. verbenaca*	390	salvigreside D	*S. greggii*
119	7-acetylhorminone	*S.blepharochlaena*	391	salvidivin C	*S. divinorum*
120	19-hydroxyroyleanone	*S. chinopeplica*	392	brevifloralactone	*S. melissodora* *S. breviflora*
121	abieta-8,12-diene-11,14-dione	*S. cilicica*	393	1-deacetoxy-8-epi-salvinorin G	*S. divinorum*
122	deacetylnemorone	*S. anastomosans*	394	salvidivin A	*S. divinorum*
123	deacetoxynemorone	*S. anastomosans*	395	salvidivin B	*S. divinorum*
124	royleanonic acid	*S. plebeia*	396	prionitin	*S. sahendica*
125	trilobic acid	*S. triloba*	397	pachystazone (abiet-5-en-7-one)	*S.pachystachys* *S.condidissima*
126	candelabroquinone	*S.candelabrum*	398	brevifloralactone acetate	*S. breviflora*
127	6-oxoroyleanone-18-oic acid	*S. divaricata*	399	salvimadrensinone	*S. madrensis*
128	6-oxo-12-methylroyleanone-18-oic acid	*S. divaricata*	400	salvimadrensinol	*S. madrensis*
129	horminone-18-oic acid	*S. divaricata*	401	salvimadrensin	*S. madrensis*
130	12-deoxy-7,7-dimethoxy-6-oxoroyleanone	*S. nutans*	402	portulide C	*S. melissodora*
131	16-hydroxyroyleanone	*S. apiana*	403	7α-hydroxyneoclerodane-3,13-diene-18,19:15,16-diolide	*S. microphylla* *S. melissodora* *S. thymoides*
132	2β-hydroxyroyleanone	*S. cryptantha*	404	semiatrin	*S. semiatratha*
133	19-hydroxy-7α-acetoxyroyleanone	*S. regla*	405	7-acetoxy-12(R)-hydroxyneocleroda-3,13-diene-18,19:15,16-diolide (= kerlinolide)	*S. keerlii*
134	7α-ethoxyroyleanone	*S.lavandulaefolia*	406	7α-oxo-neocleroda-3,13-diene-18,19:15,16 diolide	*S. thymoides*
135	7α-ethoxy-12-O-methyl-royleanone	*S.lavandulaefolia*	407	salvigresin	*S. greggii*
136	7,12-diacetylhorminon-18-al	*S. candicans*	408	1(10)-dehydrosalviarin	*S. sousae*
137	20-hydroxy-7α-acetoxyroyleanone	*S. lanata*	409	15,16-epoxy-2β-O-β-D-glucopyranosylneocleroda-3,13(16),14-trien-18,19-olide	*S. amarissima*
138	7-oxoroyleanone-12-methyl ether	*S. barrelieri*	410	15,16-epoxy-2β-O-tetraacetyl-β-D-glucopyranosylneocleroda-3,13(16),14-trien-18,19-olide	*S. amarissima*
139	virgatol (= 12,16,17-trihydroxy-8,12-abietadiene-11,14-dione)	*S. virgata*	411	neocleroda-3,13(16),14-trien-15,16-epoxy-18,19-olide	*S. amarissima*
140	bractealine	*S. bracteata*	412	salvisplendin C	*S. splendens*

continued on following page

Table 2. Continued

141	12-methyl-5-dehydrohorminone	*S. multicaulis*	413	(5R,9R,10S)-7S-acetoxy-15,16-epoxy-1S,2S,12-trihydroxy-ent-cleroda-3,13(16),14-trien-18,19-olide	*S. haenkei*
142	12-methyl-5-dehydroacetylhorminone	*S. multicaulis*	414	7α-acetoxy-2β-hydroxy-ent-cleroda-3,13-diene-18,19:16,15-diolide	*S. melissodora*
143	neocryptotanshinone II	*S. miltiorrhiza*	415	7β-hydroxy-ent-cleroda-3,13-diene-18,19:16,15-diolide	*S. melissodora*
144	kronenquinone	*S. kronenburgii*	416	7α-acetoxy-ent-cleroda-3,13-diene-18,19:16,15-diolide	*S. melissodora*
145	12-deoxydanshenxinkun B	*S. glutinosa*	417	2β,7α-dihydroxy-ent-cleroda-3,13-diene-18,19:16,15-diolide	*S. melissodora*
146	danshenxinkun B	*S. glutinosa* *S. miltiorrhiza*	418	2β-acetoxy-7α-hydroxy-ent-cleroda-3,13-diene-18,19:16,15-diolide	*S. melissodora*
147	(-)-danshexinkun A	*S. miltiorrhiza* *S. trijuga*	419	7-oxo-ent-cleroda-3,13-dien-18,19:16,15-diolide	*S. melissodora*
148	trilobiol	S. triloba	420	2β-hydroxy-ent-cleroda-3,13-diene-18,19:16,15-diolide	*S. melissodora*
149	oleoyl neocryptotanshinone	*S. miltiorrhiza*	421	2β-hydroxy-7-oxo-ent-cleroda-3,13-diene-18,19:16,15-diolide	*S. melissodora*
150	miltionone I	*S. miltiorrhiza*	422	7α-hydroxy-ent-cleroda-3,13-diene-18,19:16,15-diolide	*S. melissodora*
151	royleanone	*S. anastomosans* *S. fruticulosa* *S. nutans* *S. pachystachys* *S. tomentosa* *S. pratensis* *S. ringens*	423	salvinicin A	*S. divinorum*
152	oleoyl danshenxinkun A	*S. miltiorrhiza*	424	salvinicin B	*S. divinorum*
153	12-deoxy-6,7-dehydroroyleanone	*S. nutans*	425	salvinorin A	*S. divinorum*
154	ambreinolide-18-oic acid	*S. palaestina*	426	divinorin B	*S. divinorum*
155	13-epi-manoyloxide-15,18-dioic acid	*S. palaestina*	427	salvinorin C	*S. divinorum*
156	15-normanoyloxide-14,18-dioic acid	*S. palaestina*	428	salvinorin D	*S. divinorum*
157	8α-acetoxy-14,15,16-trinorlabdan-13-oic acid	*S. palaestina*	429	salvinorin E	*S. divinorum*
158	6α-hydroxy-8α-acetoxy-13,14,15,16-tetranorlabdan-12-oic acid	*S. yosgadensis*	430	salvinorin F	*S. divinorum*
159	hypargenin F (= 5,12-dihydroxyabieta-6,8,12-triene-11,14-dione)	*S. hypargeia* *S. montbretii*	431	salvinorin G	*S. divinorum*
160	12-deoxy-6-hydroxy-6,7-dehydroroyleanone	*S. nutans*	432	salvinorin H	*S. divinorum*
161	6,7-dehydroroyleanone	*S. aegyptiaca* *S. moorcraftiana*	433	salvinorin I	*S.divinorum*
162	6α-hydroxy-11,12-dioxo-8,13-abieta-diene	*S. recognita*	434	17β-salvinorin J	*S.divinorum*
163	11,12,-dioxoabieta-8,13-dien (= miltirone)	*S. napifolia* *S. miltiorrhiza*	435	17α-salvinorin J	*S.divinorum*

continued on following page

Table 2. Continued

164	7β-hydroxy-8,13-abietadiene-11,12-dione	*S. miltiorrhiza*	436	linearolactone (= linearifoline)	*S.polystachya* *S. lineata*
165	salviphlomone	*S. phlomoides*	437	(5R,9R)-15,16-epoxy-10S-hydroxy-ent-cleroda-3,13(16),14-triene-17,12S:18,19-diolide	*S. haenkei*
166	1R-hydroxy-20-nor-5(10),6,8,13-abietatetraene-11,12-dione (= 1R-hydroxymiltirone)	*S. argentea*	438	(5R,9R)-15,16-epoxy-ent-cleroda-3,7,13(16),14-tetraene-17,12S:18,19-diolide	*S.wagneriana*
167	4-methylenemiltirone	*S. miltiorrhiza*	439	(5R,9R)-15,16-epoxy-10S-hydroxy-ent-cleroda-3,7,13(16),14-tetraene-17,12S:18,19-diolide	*S. haenkei*
168	multiorthoquinone	*S.blepharochlaena* *S. multicaulis*	440	15,16-epoxy-4β, 8α,10β-trihydroxyneocleroda-1,13(16),14-triene-17,12R:18,19-diolide	*S. infuscata*
169	demethylmultiorthoquinone	*S.blepharochlaena* *S. multicaulis*	441	splendidin	*S. splendens*
170	18,20-dinor-1,3,5(10),6,8,13-abietahexaene-11,12-dione	*S. glutinosa*	442	salviarin	*S. greggii* *S. splendens* *S.rhyacophila*
171	salvibracteone	*S. bracteata*	443	splenolide B	*S. splendens*
172	12-O-methylcarnosol	*S. officinalis*	444	splenolide A	*S. splendens*
173	16-hydroxyisorosmanol	*S. mellifera*	445	1-O-acetylspenolide A	*S. splendens*
174	16-hydroxy-20-deoxocarnosol	*S. mellifera*	446	salvisplendin A	*S. splendens*
175	16-acetoxycarnosol	*S. canariensis*	447	15,16-epoxy-8α-hydroxyneocleroda-2,13(16),14-triene-17,12R:18,19-diolide	*S. reflexa*
176	isogaldosol	*S. mellifera*	448	6β-hydroxy salviarin	*S.rhyacophila*
177	przewalskin	*S. przewalskii*	449	6β-acetoxy salviarin	*S.rhyacophila*
178	deoxocarnosol 12-methyl ether	*S. canariensis*	450	10β-acetoxy salviarin	*S.rhyacophila*
179	isocarnosol	*S. lanigera*	451	7,8β-dihydrosalviacoccin	*S. greggii*
180	przewalskin F	*S. przewalskii*	452	salvisplendin B	*S. splendens*
181	6α,12,19-trihydroxy-11,14-dioxo-8,12-abietadien-20,7β-olide	*S. gilliessi*	453	salviacoccin	*S. coccinea*
182	przewalskin G	*S. przewalskii*	454	splenolide C	*S. splendens*
183	yunnannin A	*S. yunnanensis*	455	(4S,5R,9S,10R)-15,16-epoxy-ent-cleroda-1,13 (16),14-triene-17,12S:18,19-diolide	*S. haenkei*
184	7,20-epoxyroyleanone	*S. napifolia*	456	polystachyne D	*S.polystachya*
185	12-hydroxyabieta-11,14-quinone-(20→7)-lactone	*S. columbariae*	457	polystachyne E	*S.polystachya*
186	rosmanol	*S. rubescens* *S. tomentosa* *S. canariensis* *S. officinalis* *S. pachyphylla*	458	1α,2α-epoxy-3,4α-dihydrolinearolactone	*S. reptans*
187	6,7-dimethoxy-7-epi-rosmanol	*S. officinalis*	459	1α,10α-epoxysalviarin	*S. lineata*
188	16-hydroxyrosmanol	*S. mellifera*	460	2β,3β:15,16-diepoxy-10β-hydroxyneocleroda-7,13(16),14-triene-17,12R:18,19-diolide (= epoxysalviacoccin)	*S. plebeia*

continued on following page

Table 2. Continued

189	16-hydroxy-epi-rosmanol	*S. mellifera*	461	1,2-dihydro-6α,7α-epoxylinearifoline	*S. sousae*
190	7α,11,12-trihydroxyabieta-8,11,13-trien-20-oic acid-20,6-lactone	*S. canariensis*	462	8,12(R)-epoxyneocleroda-3,13(14)-diene-18,19:15,16-diolide (= kerlin)	*S. keerlii*
191	16-hydroxicarnosol	*S. rubescens* *S. chinopeplica* *S. mellifera*	463	splenolide B	*S. splendens*
192	11,12-di-O-methylcarnosol	*S. rubescens*	464	dehydrokerlin	*S.polystachya* *S.rhyacophila*
193	6-epi-demethylesquirolin D	*S.anastomosans* *S. aspera*	465	salvisplendin D	*S. splendens*
194	7β-methoxyrosmanol	*S. dorrii*	466	salvifolin	*S. tiliaefolia* *S. dugesii*
195	16-hydroxy-7-methoxyrosmanol	*S. rubescens* *S. munzii*	467	polystachyne A	*S. polystachya*
196	deacetylsessein	*S. regla*	468	polystachyne B	*S. polystachya*
197	7α-hydroxy-12,19-dihydroxyabieta-8,12-diene-11,14-dione-19,20-δ-lactone	*S. candicans*	469	polystachyne C	*S. polystachya*
198	sessein	*S. regla* *S. sessei*	470	salvifarin	*S. farinacea*
199	7α-hydroxy-12-dihydroxy-19-methylabieta-8,12-diene-11,14-dione-19,20-δ-lactone	*S. candicans*	471	trans-1,2-dihydrosalvifaricin	*S. fulgens*
200	conacytone	*S.ballotaeflora* *S. candicans*	472	salvixalapoxide	*S. xalapensis*
201	methylenedihydrotanshinquinone	*S. miltiorrhiza* *S. trijuga*	473	2α-hydroxy-7-epi-8β,17-dihydrolanguiduline	*S. tonalensis* *S. miltiorrhiza* *S. sousae*
202	galdosol	*S. mellifera*	474	tonalenin	*S. tonalensis*
203	sagequinone methide A	*S. officinalis*	475	isosalvisousolide	*S. sousae*
204	12-hydroxy-11,14-dioxo-6,8,12-abietatrien-19,20-olide	*S. gilliessi*	476	7-epi-languiduline	*S. tonalensis*
205	12-acetoxy-11,14-dioxo-6,8,12-abietatrien-19,20-olide	*S. gilliessi*	477	salvilanguiduline A	*S. languidula*
206	8-hydroxy-12-oxoabieta-9(11),13-dien-20-oic acid 8,20-lactone	*S.wiedemannii*	478	salvilanguiduline B	*S. languidula*
207	2α,8-dihydroxy-12-oxoabieta-9(11),13-dien-20-oic acid-8,20-lactone (= piliferalactone)	*S. pilifera*	479	salvilanguiduline C	*S. languidula*
208	2α,20-dihydroxy-12-oxoabieta-9(11),13-dien-8,20-ether (= piliferol)	*S. pilifera*	480	salvilanguiduline D	*S. languidula*
209	pachyphyllone	*S. pachyphylla*	481	salvifulgenolide	*S. fulgens*
210	3β-acetoxyabiet-8(14)-en-18-oic acid 9α,13α-endoperoxide	*S. oxyodon*	482	salvixalapadiene	*S. xalapensis*
211	3β-hydroxyabiet-8(14)-en-18-oic acid 9α,13α-endoperoxide	*S. oxyodon*	483	isosalvixalapadiene	*S. xalapensis*
212	1,2,5,6-tetrahydrotanshinone I	*S.miltiorrhiza*	484	salvianduline C	*S.lavanduloides*
213	trijuganone B	*S. trijuga*	485	salvireptanolide	*S. reptans*

continued on following page

Table 2. Continued

214	methylenetanshiquinone	*S.miltiorrhiza* *S. trijuga*	486	rhyacophiline	*S. rhyacophila*
215	3α,17-dihydroxytanshinone II	*S. hians*	487	7-epi-rhyacophiline	*S. rhyacophila*
216	tanshindiol A	*S. miltiorrhiza*	488	7,8-didehydrorhyacophiline	*S. reflexa*
217	tanshindiol B	*S. miltiorrhiza*	489	cardiophyllidin	*S. cardiophylla*
218	carnosol	*S. canariensis* *S.chinopeplica* *S. officinalis* *S. rubescens*	490	polystachyne F	*S. polystachya*
219	tanshindiol C	*S. miltiorrhiza*	491	salvianduline A	*S.lavanduloides*
220	3(-hydroxytanshinone IIA	*S. miltiorrhiza*	492	salvianduline B	*S.lavanduloides*
221	tanshinone IIB	*S.miltiorrhiza*	493	derivative of 535	*S.lavanduloides*
222	nortanshinone	*S. miltiorrhiza*	494	bisditerpenoid derivative	*S. wagneriana*
223	7α-methoxyrosmanol	*S. dorrii* *S.chinopeplica*	495	bisditerpenoid derivative	*S. wagneriana*
224	15,16-dihydrotanshinone I	*S. glutinosa* *S. miltiorrhiza* *S. trijuga* *S. nipponica*	496	blepharolide A	*S.blepharophylla*
225	tanshinone I	*S. glutinosa* *S. miltiorrhiza* *S. przewalskii* *S. trijuga*	497	salvianduline D	*S. lavanduloides*
226	danshenol C	*S.yunnanensis* *S. trijuga*	498	spiroleucantholide	*S. leucantha*
227	6-methylcryptotanshinone	*S. aegyptiaca*	499	salvileucalin B	*S. leucantha*
228	17-hydroxycryptotanshinone	*S. munzii*	500	salvigenolide	*S. fulgens*
229	6-deoxo-5,6-didehydrolanugon Q	*S. apiana*	501	salvifaricin	*S. farinacea* *S. dugesii* *S. leucantha*
230	miltionone II	*S. miltiorrhiza*	502	2β-hydroxysalvigenolide	*S. xalapensis*
231	danshenol A	*S. glutinosa*	503	blepharolide B	*S. blepharophylla*
232	neotanshinlactone	*S. miltiorrhiza*	504	dugesin B	*S. dugesii*
233	trijuganone A	*S. trijuga*	505	salvileucantholide	*S. leucantha*
234	isotanshinone I	*S. glutinosa*	506	salviandulin E	*S. leucantha*
235	isotanshinone II	*S. glutinosa*	507	dugesin A	*S. dugesii*
236	dihydroisotanshinone II	*S. glutinosa*	508	(-)-isopimara-8(14),15-diene	*S. parryi*
237	derivative of tanshinone IIA	*S. miltiorrhiza*	509	7α-hydroxyisopimara-8(14),15-diene	*S. parryi*
238	derivative of tanshinone IIA	*S. miltiorrhiza*	510	isopimara-8(14),15-dien-7-one	*S. parryi*
239	derivative of tanshinone IIA	*S. miltiorrhiza*	511	sandaracopimaric acid	*S. fulgens*
240	salviamine E	*S. yunnanensis*	512	7α-hydroxysandaracopimaric acid	*S. microphylla*
241	salviamine F	*S. yunnanensis*	513	methyl 7α-hydroxysandaracopimarate	*S. microphylla*
242	salviamine B	*S. yunnanensis*	514	7-oxo-sandaracopimarate	*S. microphylla*
243	salviamine C	*S. yunnanensis*	515	7-oxo-sandaracopimaric acid	*S. microphylla*
244	salviamine D	*S. yunnanensis*	516	salvipimarone	*S. multicaulis*

continued on following page

Table 2. Continued

245	isosalviamine E	*S. yunnanensis*	517	7α-acetoxyisopimara-8(14),15-diene-18-oic acid	*S. microphylla*
246	salvianan	*S. miltiorrhiza*	518	isopimaric acid	*S. greggii* *S. wiedemannii*
247	neosalvianen	*S. miltiorrhiza*	519	14α-hydroxy-7,15-isopimaradien-18-oic acid	*S. greggii*
248	salvianen	*S. miltiorrhiza*	520	14α-hydroxyisopimara-7,15-diene	*S. parryi*
249	salviamine A	*S. yunnanensis*	521	14α,18-dihydroxy-7,15-isopimaradiene	*S. greggii*
250	isosalviamine C	*S. yunnanensis*	522	3β-hydroxy-7,15-isopimaradien-18-oic acid methyl ester	*S. greggii*
251	isosalviamine D	*S. yunnanensis*	523	14-oxo-pimaric acid	*S. wiedemannii*
252	isosalviamine A	*S. trijuga*	524	11β-hydroxymanoyl oxide	*S. candidissima*
253	isosalviamine B	*S. trijuga*	525	isopimara-8,15-dien-7-one	*S. parryi*
254	3-oxosapriparaquinone	*S. prionitis*	526	isopimara-6,8(14),15-triene	*S. parryi*
255	tanshinone IIA	*S. glutinosa* *S.miltiorrhiza* *S.przewalskii*	527	parryin	*S. parryi*
256	cryptotanshinone	*S.ballotaeflora* *S. apiana* *S. glutinosa* *S. mellifera* *S. miltiorrhiza* *S. munzii* *S. przewalskii* *S. trijuga*	528	7α-hydroxy-labd-8(17)-en-15-oic (= salvic acid)	*S. eupatorium*
257	15-epi-danshenol A	*S. glutinosa* *S. glutinosa*	529	8(17)-labdene-3α,7β-diacetoxy-15-oic acid	*S. eupatorium*
258	dihydroisotanshinone I	*S. glutinosa* *S. miltiorrhiza*	530	7α-hydroxy-14,15-dinor-13-oxo-8(17)-labdene	*S. eupatorium*
259	formyltanshinone	*S. miltiorrhiza*	531	sclareol	*S. sclarea*
260	salviadione	*S. miltiorrhiza*	532	manool	*S. sclarea* *S. officinalis*
261	prioline	*S. prionitis*	533	salvitrijudin A	*S. digitaloides*
262	salvigerone	*S. lanigera*	534	methyl 3α-hydroxy-8α-acetoxy-13,14,15,16-tetranorlabdan-12-oate	*S. aethiopis*
263	salvipalestinoic acid	*S. palaestina*	535	6α-hydroxynorambreinolide	*S. yosgadensis*
264	methyl 12-O-methylsalvipalestinoate	*S. palaestina*	536	3α-hydroxynorambreinolide	*S. aethiopis*
265	candesalvolactone	*S.candelabrum*	537	6α-hydroxyambreinolide	*S. yosgadensis*
266	3,4-secoisopimara-4(18),7,15-triene-3-oic acid	*S. cinnabarina*	538	norambreinolide-18,6α-olide	*S. sahendica*
267	candesalvoquinone	*S.candelabrum*	539	8-acetoxy-13,14,15,16-tetranorlabdan-12-oic acid-18,6α-olide	*S. sahendica*
268	12-O-methylcandesalvone B	*S.candelabrum*	540	2,6-dimethyl-10-(p-tolyl)undeca-2,6-diene	*S. dorisiana*
269	candesalvones B	*S.candelabrum*	541	salviolone	*S. miltiorrhiza*
270	candesalvone B methyl ester	*S.candelabrum*	542	salviatalin A	*S. digitaloides*

continued on following page

Table 2. Continued

271	limbinol	*S. limbata*	543	8(17),12E,14-labdatrien-6,19-olide	*S. leriaefolia*
272	acetyllimbinol	*S. limbata*	544	2α-hydroxyambreinolide	*S. palaestina*

(Wu *et al.*, 2012).

Table 3. Sesterterpenes of the Salvia genus

1	przewalskin A	*S.przewalskii*
2	13,14-dioxo-11-hydroxy-7-methoxy-hassane- 8,11,15-trien-22,6-olide	*S. apiana*
3	rel-(5S,6S,7S,10R,12S,13R)-7-hydroxy-11,16- dioxoapiana-8,14-dien-22,6-olide	*S. officinalis*
4	rel-(5S,6S,7R,10R,12S,13R)-7-hydroxy-11,16- dioxoapiana-8,14-dien-22,6-olide	*S. officinalis*
5	rel-(5S,6S,7S,10R,12R,13S)-7-hydroxy-11,16- dioxoapiana-8,14-dien-22,6-olide	*S. officinalis*
6	14-hydroxy-7-methoxy-11,16-dioxoapian-8- en-22,6-olide	*S. apiana*
7	7-methoxy-11,16-dioxoapian-8,14-dien-22,6- olide	*S. apiana*
8	yosgadensonol	*S.yosgadensis*
9	13-epi-yosgadensonol	*S.yosgadensis*
10	6-dehydroxyyosgadensonol	*S. limbata*
11	6-dehydroxy-13-epi-yosgadensonol	*S. limbata*
12	6α,14-dihydroxymanoyloxide-15,17-dien-16,19-olide (=yosgadensolide A)	*S.yosgadensis*
13	6α,14-dihydroxy-13-epi-manoyloxide-15,17- dien-16,19-olide	*S.yosgadensis*
14	salvileucolide methyl ester derivative	*S. hypoleuca*
15	salvimirzacolide	*S.mirzayanii*
16	salvisyriacolide	*S. syriaca*
17	8α,13,14-threo-trihydroxylabd-15,17-dien- 16,19-olide-23-oic acid	*S. palaestina*
18	8α,13,14-erythro-trihydroxylabd-15,17-dien- 16,19-olide-23-oic aci	*S. palaestina*
19	3α,8α,13,14-erythro-tetrahydroxylabd-15,17- dien-16,19-olide	*S. palaestina*
20	cyclic peroxide	*S. hypoleuca*
21	6α,16-dihydroxymanoyloxide-14,17-dien- 16,19-olide (= yosgadensolide B)	*S.yosgadensis*
22	3-epi-salviaethiopisolide	*S. aethiopis*
23	salviaethiopisolide	*S. aethiopis*
24	14-hydroperoxy-13(21)-dehydro-13,14-dihydrosalvileucolide-6,23-lactone	*S. hypoleuca*
25	15,16-dehydrosalvileucolide-6,23-lactonetrans-epoxide	*S. hypoleuca*
26	15,16-dehydrosalvileucolide-6,23-lactone-cisepoxide	*S. hypoleuca*
27	13,14-bis-epi-trans-epoxide	*S. hypoleuca*
28	salvileucolidone	*S. hypoleuca*
29	salvileucolide-6,23-lactone	*S. hypoleuca*

continued on following page

Table 3. Continued

30	8-hydroxy-13-hydroperoxylabd-14,17-dien- 19,16:23,6α-diolide	*S. sahendica*
31	17,18,19,20-tetranor-13-epi-manoyloxide-14- en-16-oic acid-23,6α-olide	*S. sahendica*

(Wu *et al.*, 2012)

Table 4. Triterpenoids of the Salvia genus

1	maslinic acid (= 2α-hydroxyoleanolic acid)	*S. canariensis*	76	yunnaneic acid A	*S. yunnanensis*
2	oleanolic acid	*S. officinalis* *S. amplexicaulis* *S. ballotaeflora* *S. longystyla*	77	yunnaneic acid B	*S. yunnanensis*
3	3β,11α,21α-trihydroxyurs-12-ene (=salvistamineol)	*S. staminea*	78	yunnaneic acid D	*S. yunnanensis*
4	1β,2α-dihydroxy-3β-acetoxy-11-oxours-12-ene	*S. kronenburgii*	79	yunnaneic acid C	*S. yunnanensis*
5	1β,2α,3β,11α-tetrahydroxyurs-12-ene	*S. kronenburgii*	80	sagerinic acid	*S. officinalis*
6	3α-acetoxyurs-12-ene-1β,11α-diol	*S. kronenburgii*	81	luteolin 7-O-glucuronide	*S. officinalis*
7	1β,3α,11α-trihydroxyurs-12-ene	*S. kronenburgii*	82	luteolin 3′-O-glucuronide	*S. officinalis*
8	2α,3β,11α-trihydroxyurs-12-ene	*S. kronenburgii*	83	6-hydroxyluteolin 7-O-glucoside	*S. officinalis*
9	3β-acetoxy-urs-12-ene-2α,11α-dial	*S. argentea*	84	6-methoxyluteolin 7-O-glucoside	*S. tomentosa*
10	3β acetoxy urs-12-ene-1β,2α,11α-triol	*S. argentea*	85	6-hydroxyluteolin 5-O-glucoside	*S. verticillata* *S. tomentosa*
11	3β-acetoxy-urs-12-ene-1β,2α,11α,20β-tetraol	*S. argentea*	86	4-{4-O-[6-(4-hydroxybenzoyl)-O-β-D-glucopyranosyl]-3-hydroxyphenyl} butan-2-one (= salviaplebeiaside)	*S. plebeia*
12	3β-acetoxy-urs-12-ene-2α,11α,20β-triol	*S. argentea*	87	salvionoside B	*S. nemorosa*
13	3-oxours-12-ene-1β,11α-diol	*S. haenkei*	88	salvionoside C	*S. nemorosa*
14	3-epi-ursolic acid	*S. lanata*	89	4-hydroxyacetophenone 4-O-(6′-O-β-D-apiofuranosyl)-β-D-glucopyranoside	*S. officinalis*
15	santolinoic acid	*S. santolinifolia*	90	6-O-caffeoyl-β-D-fructofuranosyl-(2→1)-α-D-glucopyranoside	*S. officinalis*
16	2α,3β,5α-trihydroxyurs-12-en-28-oic acid (= salvin A)	*S. santolinifolia*	91	1-O-caffeoyl-β-D-apiofuranosyl-(1→6)-β-D-glucopyranoside	*S. officinalis*

continued on following page

Table 4. Continued

17	3,11-dioxoursun-12-ene	*S. mellifera*	92	1-O-p-hydroxybenzoyl-β-D-apiofuranosyl-(1→6)-β-D-glucopyranoside	*S. officinalis*
18	urs-12-ene-3α,11α-diol S. willeana	*S. willeana*	93	1-O-(2,3,4-trihydroxy-3-methyl) butyl-6-O-feruloyl-β-D-glucopyranoside	*S. officinalis*
19	3α,24-dihydroxyolean-12-en-28-oic acid	*S. nicolsoniana*	94	octanol ester of cis-O-methyl caffeic acid dimer	*S. forskahlei*
20	3α,24-dihydroxyolean-12-en-28,30-dioic acid	*S. nicolsoniana*	95	7,8-dihydroxy-2-(3,4-dihydroxyphenyl)-1,2-dihydronaphthalene-1,3-dicarboxylic acid di(1-carboxy-2-(3,4-dihydroxyphenyl))ethyl ester (= salvianolic acid L)	*S. officinalis*
21	2α-acetoxyurs-5,12-diene-3β,11α-diol	*S. kronenburgii*	96	4,4′-bisbenzoic acid heptyl ester	*S. multicaulis*
22	3-oxo-13(28)-epoxyursan-11-ene	*S. mellifera*	97	di(4,4′-hexyloxycarbonylphenyl) ether	*S. heldrichiana*
23	3β,6α,23-trihydroxyurs-12,19(29)-dien-28- oic acid	*S.hierosolymitana*	98	melitric acid A	*S. officinalis*
24	2α,3β,20β,23-tetrahydroxyurs-12,19 (29)- dien-28-oic acid	*S. chinensis*	99	salvianolic acid I	*S. cavaleriei*
25	23-(trans-p-coumaroyloxy)-3β,6α,30-trihydroxyurs-12-en-28-oic acid	*S.hierosolymitana*	100	methyl melitrate A	*S. officinalis*
26	2α,3β-dihydroxyolean-28-oic acid	*S.hierosolymitana*	101	salvianolic acid D	*S.miltiorrhiza*
27	1β,2α,3β,11α-tetrahydroxyolean-12-ene	*S. kronenburgii*	102	salvianolic acid E	*S.miltiorrhiza*
28	3β-acetoxyolean-l2-ene-2α,11α-dial	*S. argentea*	103	prionitiside A	*S. prionitis*
29	3β-acetoxyolean-12-ene-lβ,2α,11α-triol	*S. argentea*	104	prionitiside B	*S. prionitis*
30	3β-hydroxy-l-oxoolean-12-en-28-oic acid (= virgatic acid)	*S. virgata*	105	salvianolic acid J	*S. flava*
31	3α,6α,24-trihydroxyolean-12-en-28-oic acid (= salvin B)	*S. santolinifolia*	106	lithospermate B	*S. miltiorrhiza*
32	salvinemorol	*S. nemorosa*	107	salvianolic acid B	*S. miltiorrhiza*
33	24-nor-2α,3β-dihydroxyolean-4(23),12-ene	*S.hierosolymitana*	108	dimethyl heptamethylsalvianolate B	*S. miltiorrhiza*
34	2R,3R-dihydroxy-24-nor-4(23),12- oleanadien-28-oic acid	*S. carduacea*	109	nubatin	*S. nubicola*

continued on following page

Table 4. Continued

35	2α,3α,16α-trihydroxy-24-nor-4(23),12- oleandien-28-oic acid	*S. palaestina*	110	delphinidin 3-O-[6-O-(p-coumaroyl)-β-D-glucopyranoside]-5-O-[4-O-acetyl-6-O-malonyl-β-D-glucopyranoside]	*S. uliginosa*
36	przewanoic acid B	*S. przewalskii*	111	luteolin 7-O-β-D-glucoside	*S. officinalis*
37	santolin B	*S. santolinifolia*	112	6-hydroxyluteolin 7-O-glucuronide	*S. officinalis*
38	santolin A	*S. santolinifolia*	113	apigenin 7-O-β-D-glucopyranosyl-(1‴→4″)-β-D-glucopyranoside(apiyenin 7-O-cellobioside)	*S. uliginosa*
39	santolin C	*S. santolinifolia*	114	(1S,2R,4R)-1,8-epoxy-p-menthan-2-yl-O-β-D-glucopyranoside	*S. officinalis*
40	salvadione A	*S. bucharica*	115	loliolide	*S. divinorum*
41	przewanoic acid A	*S. przewalskii*	116	genkwanin 4′-O-α-L-arabinopyranosyl-(1→6)-β-D-galactopyranoside	*S. moorcroftiana*
42	1β,11α-dihydroxyolean-18-en-3-one	*S. deserta*	117	genkwanin 4′-[O-α-L-rhamnopyranosyl-(1→2)-β-D-galactopyranoside]	*S. moorcroftiana*
43	23-hydroxygermanicone	*S. pomifera*	118	genkwanin 4′-[O-α-L-arabinopyranosyl-(1→3)-α-L-rhamnopyranoside]	*S. moorcroftiana*
44	olean-13(18)-ene-2α,3β,11α-triol	*S. pinnata*	119	8-methoxygenistein 7-O-α-L-rhamnoside 4′-O-β-D-glucoside	*S. triloba*
45	olean-(13)18-ene-2β,3β-diol	*S. horminum*	120	genkwanin 4′-O-{α-L-rhamnopyranosyl-(1→2)-[α-L-rhamnopyranosyl-(1→ 6)]-β-D-galactopyranoside}	*S. moorcroftiana*
46	3β-hydroxyoleanan-13β→28 lactone	*S. lanigera*	121	4-hydroxy-2-isopropyl-5-methylphenyl O-α-L-rhamnopyranosyl-(1→2)-β-D-glucopyranoside	*S. moorcroftiana*
47	2α,20β-dihydroxy-3β-acetoxyurs-9(11),12-diene	*S. kronenburgii*	122	przewalskinone B	*S. przewalskii*
48	1β,2α-dihydroxy-3β-acetoxyurs-9(11),12-diene	*S. kronenburgii*	123	nonyl 4-hydroxybenzoate	*S. moorcroftiana*
49	deacetyloxysessein-7α-(3β-hydroxyolean-12- en-28-oate) (= reglin	*S. regla*	124	eicosaheptanoic acid 2-(p-hydroxyphenyl)ethyl ester	*S. microphylla*
50	lupeol	*S. palaestina*	125	hexacosylferulate	*S. microphylla*
51	lup-20(29)-ene-2α,3β-diol	*S. palaestina*	126	eugenylglucoside	*S. officinalis*
52	lup-20(29)-ene-3β,23-diol	*S. palaestina*	127	trans-p-coumaric acid 4-O-(2′-O-β-D-apiofuranosyl)-β-D-glucopyranoside	*S. officinalis*

continued on following page

Table 4. Continued

53	2α-methoxylup-20(29)-en-3β-ol	*S. palaestina*	128	4-(1-hydroxy-5-methylnaphthalen-2-yl)-2-methyl-4-oxobutyl acetate (= salvianonol)	*S. miltiorrhiza*
54	palestinol	*S. triloba*	129	cis-p-coumaric acid 4-O-(2′-O-β-D-apiofuranosyl)-β-D-glucopyranosid	*S. officinalis*
55	7β-hydroxylup-20(29)-en-3-one	*S. pratensis*	130	salvianolic acid N	*S. yunnanensis* *S. chinensis* *S. prionitis*
56	1β,11α-dihydroxylup-20(29)-en-3-one	*S. deserta*	131	salvionoside A	*S. nemorosa*
57	(1β,3β)-lup-20(29)-ene-1,3,30-triol	*S. sclareoides*	132	methyl salvianolate A	*S. yunnanensis*
58	3α-O-acetyl-20(29)-lupen-2α-ol	*S. trijuga*	133	ethyl salvianolate A	*S. yunnanensis*
59	1β,11α,20-trihydroxylupan-3-one	*S. deserta*	134	lithospermic acid	*S. yunnanensis*
60	lupane-3β,11α,20-triol	*S. phlomoides*	135	cis-lithospermic acid	*S. yunnanensis*
61	3β-acetoxylupane-11α,20-diol	*S. phlomoides*	136	lignan secoisolariciresinol diester	*S. plebeia*
62	3-oxolupane-11α,20-diol	*S. phlomoides*	137	secoisolariciresinol branched fatty diester	*S. plebeia*
63	monogynol A	*S. macrochlamys*	138	sagecoumarin	*S. miltiorrhiza* *S. officinalis*
64	3α-hydroxy-20-oxo-30-norlupane	*S. nubicola*	139	(6R,9R)-3-oxo-α-ionol β-D-glucopyranoside	
65	3β-O-trans-p-coumaroylmonogynol A	*S. montbretii*	140	(6R,9S)-3-oxo-α-ionol β-D-glucopyranoside	
66	3β-O-cis-p-coumaroylmonogynol A	*S. montbretii*	141	(E)-4-[5-(hydroxymethyl)furan-2-yl] but-3-en-2-one	
67	20S,24R-epoxydammar-12β,25-diol-3-one	*S. bicolor*	142	5-(methoxymethyl)-1H-pyrrole-2-carbaldehyde	
68	7β,25-dihydroxy-(20S,24R)-epoxydammaran- 3-one (= salvilymitone)	*S.hierosolymitana*	143	5-(3-hydroxypropyl)-7-methoxy-2-(3′-methoxy-4′-hydroxyphenyl)-3-benzo[b]furancarbaldehyde	*S. miltiorrhiza*
69	(20S,24R)-epoxydammarane-3β,7α,25-triol (= salvilymitol)	*S.hierosolymitana*	144	apigenin 7,4′-O,O-di-β-D-glucopyranoside (apigenin 7,4′-O,O-diglucoside)	*S. uliginosa*
70	salvadiol	*S. bucharica*	145	salvianolic acid A	*S. yunnanensis* *S. miltiorrhiza* *S. flava* *S. prionitis*
71	salvadione B	*S. bucharica*	146	6,8-di-C-glucosylapigenin (= vicenin-2)	*S. officinalis*
72	brassicasterone	*S. multicaulis*	147	octanol ester of trans-O-methyl caffeic acid dimer	*S. forskahlei*

continued on following page

Table 4. Continued

73	1-oxo-7α-hydroxysitostero	*S. glutinosa*	148	2,10,11-trihydroxy-8-methoxy-1,6,7,8-tetrahydro-2H-benzo[e] azecine-3,5-dione	*S. miltiorrhiza*
74	stigmast-4-en-3-one	*S. amplexicaulis*	149	ethyl O-β-D-glucopyranosyl tuberonate	*S. officinalis*
75	salvianolic acid C	*S. miltiorrhiza*			

(Wu *et al.*, 2012)

3.2 Biological Activities

The genus *Salvia* is distinguished by its extensive geographic distribution and diverse ethnobotanical applications. Numerous species within this genus have been utilized for centuries, notably in traditional Chinese medicine, to promote longevity. A prominent example is Danshen (*Salvia miltiorrhiza*), which has garnered significant attention for its medicinal properties. Tanshinones, a class of natural products first isolated from *S. miltiorrhiza* and other *Salvia* species in 1934, are of particular interest. The principal constituents of this group include tanshinone IIA, 3-hydroxytanshinone, tanshinone IIB, and cryptotanshinone. These compounds possess a broad spectrum of pharmacological activities, encompassing antibacterial, antifungal, antioxidant, anti-inflammatory, antineoplastic, and antiplatelet aggregation effects. In recent decades, there has been a marked increase in interest among medicinal chemists and clinicians regarding the therapeutic potential of *Salvia* constituents as antimicrobial, antioxidant, antitumor, and antifeeding agents. Various natural compounds derived from different *Salvia* species, as well as their hemisynthetic derivatives, have been extensively investigated by numerous research teams. A select number of these constituents have demonstrated particularly promising activity against bacterial and tumor cell lines, highlighting their potential as valuable agents in the pharmaceutical landscape, (Wu *et al.*, 2012).

3.2.1 Antioxidant Activity

In recent years, the application of synthetic antioxidant compounds in food products has faced increasing restrictions due to the potential adverse effects associated with these substances. As a result, there has been a growing emphasis on identifying natural sources of food antioxidants that offer effective and safer alternatives. Among these, *Salvia* species emerge as a promising natural source, renowned for their favorable culinary attributes and traditional use in extending the shelf life of various food products, (Wu *et al.,* 2012).

Research indicates that phenolic acids possess significant antioxidant properties, including the ability to inhibit lipid peroxidation and scavenge free radicals. This study investigates the antioxidant activities of methanol extracts obtained from six *Salvia* species native to Turkey: *S. caespitosa*, *S. hypargeia*, *S. euphratica*, *S. sclarea*, *S. candidissima*, and *S. aethiopis*. Utilizing the DPPH free radical-scavenging assay, the results revealed that *S. euphratica* exhibited the highest antioxidant activity, with an IC_{50} value of 20.7 ± 1.22 µg/mL, followed closely by *S. sclarea* with an IC_{50} of 23.4 ± 0.97 µg/mL among the polar subfractions. In the β-carotene/linoleic acid test system, the polar extract of *S. hypargeia* demonstrated superior antioxidant activity compared to the polar extracts of the other *Salvia* species examined, achieving a remarkable inhibition rate of 69.2% ± 1.90%, (Sharma, Fagan, & Schaefer, 2019).

Additionally, *S. sclarea* displayed an inhibition rate of 63.5% ± 4.24%. For comparative purposes, the inhibition rate of the synthetic antioxidant butylated hydroxytoluene (BHT) was determined to be 96%. These findings underscore the potential of *Salvia* species as viable natural alternatives for synthetic antioxidants in food preservation. The antioxidant activities exhibited by the polar extracts of various *Salvia* species, in comparison to butylated hydroxytoluene (BHT), indicate that the incorporation of sage extract may serve as an effective strategy for enhancing the shelf life of perishable food products that contain fats, (Tepe *et al.,* 2006).

The antioxidant activity of candesalvone, candelabroquinone, 12-O-methylcandesalvone, candesalvone B methyl ester, and candelabrone was systematically evaluated in both enzyme-dependent and enzyme-independent assays of lipid peroxidation. The results indicated that the enzyme-dependent system produced IC_{50} values ranging from 3.49 to 10.42 µg, whereas the enzyme-independent system demonstrated IC_{50} values between 1.40 and 13.40 µg. These findings highlight the differential potency of these compounds as antioxidants in various biochemical contexts, (Janicsák *et al.,* 2003).

The antioxidant activities of sage polyphenols, which include flavone glycosides and various derivatives of rosmarinic acid, were evaluated for their efficacy in scavenging DPPH and superoxide anion radicals. The assessment revealed variability in the antioxidant activity among the flavonoids under investigation. Notably, flavonoids possessing a catechol B-ring, such as luteolin glycosides, demonstrated significantly greater antioxidant capacity compared to those lacking this structural feature, such as apigenin glycosides, (Lu & Foo, 2001).

The compounds extracted from *Salvia miltiorrhiza* include rosmarinquinone, dehydrorosmarinquinone, miltirone I, tanshinone IIA, cryptotanshinone, and dihydrotanshinone. The antioxidant activity of these quinones in lard at 100 °C was evaluated using a Rancimat apparatus. The following structural features have been identified as correlating with enhanced antioxidant activity: (a) the presence of additional conjugated double bonds within the A ring; (b) the substitution of a furan ring with a dihydrofuran ring; and (c) the presence of an isopropyl substituent positioned ortho to a quinone carbonyl, as opposed to the alternative of a dihydrofuran ring, (Weng & Gordon, 1992).

The antioxidant activity of the compounds isolated from *Salvia officinalis* was assessed using the oil stability index method. Among the compounds evaluated, carnosol, rosmanol, epi-rosmanol, isorosmanol, galdosol, and carnosic acid displayed significantly strong antioxidant activity, comparable to that of α-tocopherol, (Miura, Kikuzaki, & Nakatanni, 2002). The primary compounds identified in the antioxidant phenolic extracts derived from *Salvia officinalis* include rosmarinic acid and carnosol, (Santos-Gomes *et al.*, 2002).

Within the class of abietane diterpenes, inuroyleanol has been identified as exhibiting the highest scavenging activity against DPPH (1,1-diphenyl-2-picrylhydrazyl) as well as the most significant inhibition of lipid peroxidation in the β-carotene-linoleic acid system. Conversely, inuroyleanol displayed the lowest scavenging activity for superoxide anions, while abietane 7-oxoroyleanone-12-methyl ether demonstrated the highest superoxide anion scavenging capacity, exhibiting antioxidant potential comparable to that of the well-established antioxidant L-ascorbic acid. Notably, abietane 7-oxoroyleanone-12-methyl ether proved to be more active than both BHT (butylated hydroxytoluene) and α-tocopherol. Additionally, the antioxidant activity of Royleanone was found to be superior in both systems compared to that of horminone and 7-acetylhorminone. These findings suggest that quinonoids or fully substituted C-ring phenolic abietane diterpenoids, which are devoid of any substituents other than a keto group at C-7, are likely to exhibit reduced antioxidant activity. In the DPPH free radical scavenging assay, 7-acetoxyroyleanone-12-methyl ether, a methyl derivative of 7-acetylhorminone at the C-12 position, exhibited a markedly enhanced activity, with efficacy up to four to five times greater than that of the control, (Wu *et al.*, 2012).

This notable effect can be ascribed to the increased scavenging capacity imparted by the methoxy group at the C-12 position, which likely contributes to its superior antioxidant properties. The enhanced efficacy of carnosic acid, characterized by the presence of ortho-dihydroxy groups on the aromatic ring C, has been extensively documented in contrast to royleanonic acid, which features a hydroxy-p-benzoquinone moiety. This disparity in antioxidant activity has been ascribed to the capacity of carnosic acid to inhibit oxidative processes through the donation of hydrogen atoms, thereby effectively scavenging free radicals in both the DPPH and β-carotene–linoleic acid systems, (Wu *et al.*, 2012).

Research has established that orthodihydroxy phenols, as well as compounds featuring a hydroxy and a methoxy group, are capable of forming more stable radicals through the donation of hydrogen atoms. This phenomenon has been observed in the case of inuroyleanol. It can therefore be hypothesized that these types of abietanes will exhibit enhanced antioxidant activity in comparison to abietanes that contain monohydroxy phenol or p-quinoid C ring structures. The generation of reactive oxygen species (ROS) has been implicated as a critical contributor to the pathogenesis of neurodegenerative diseases, including stroke, Alzheimer's disease (AD), and Parkinson's disease (PD), all of which are characterized by neuronal death. These conditions predominantly affect the elderly population and are responsible for approximately 60% of all dementia cases in individuals aged 65 and older. Furthermore, it is estimated that about 60% of all dementia cases occur within this demographic. The *Salvia* genus of plants has a long-standing history in the treatment of various neurodegenerative diseases. Compounds such as caffeic acid, danshensu, rosmarinic acid, prolithospermic acid, salvianolic acid A, and salvianolic acid B have exhibited inhibitory effects against lipid peroxidation induced by iron-cysteine and hemolysis of erythrocytes provoked by hydrogen peroxide. Within these investigations, salvianolic acid A has been identified as the most potent compound. Moreover, caffeic acid and its derivatives have demonstrated significant free radical scavenging activity, (Wu *et al.,* 2012).

The tetrameric form of lithospermic acid B and its magnesium salt exhibit the most pronounced bioactivity, in contrast to the trimeric lithospermic acid and dimeric rosmarinic acid, which display comparatively lower yet notable efficacy. Furthermore, the monomeric caffeic acid is characterized by the least activity among the compounds studied. Notably, rosmarinic acid, salvianolic acid A, and salvianolic acid B have demonstrated significant antioxidant properties, primarily through their capacity to scavenge superoxide anion radicals (O_2-). A structural-activity relationship (SAR) analysis indicates that the presence of hydroxy groups and a saturated linkage between aromatic rings are critical determinants of free radical scavenging activity, (Wang, Morris-Natschke, & Lee, 2007).

3.2.2 Cytotoxicity Activity

Plants have significantly contributed to the discovery and development of effective anticancer agents. Notably, more than 60% of the anticancer agents currently in use are derived from natural sources, which include plants, marine organisms, and microorganisms. This underscores the importance of natural products in the ongoing quest for novel therapeutic agents in oncology, (Kabouche *et al.,* 2007) (Valeriote *et al.,* 2002).

In a study conducted in 2000, Liu demonstrated that the aqueous extract of *Salvia miltiorrhiza* exerted significant effects on HepG2 hepatoma cells *in vitro*. The findings indicated that the extract suppressed cellular proliferation, induced notable morphological changes, and initiated apoptotic pathways, (Liu, Shen, & Ong, 2000).

The hypoxia-inducible factor-1 (HIF-1) has emerged as a crucial target in the development of novel anticancer therapeutics. Recent investigations have identified several isolated compounds, including sibiriquinone A, sibiriquinone B, cryptotanshinone, and dihydrotanshinone I, sourced from *Salvia miltiorrhiza,* which exhibit significant inhibitory effects on hypoxia-induced luciferase expression. The half-maximal inhibitory concentration (IC_{50}) values for these compounds were determined to be 0 for the inhibition of luciferase expression. Notably, the IC_{50} values in AGS cells, a human gastric cancer cell line, were recorded at 34 μM, 3.36 μM, 1.58 μM, and 2.05 μM, while for Hep3B cells, a human hepatocarcinoma cell line, the corresponding values were 0.28 μM, 3.18 μM, 1.36 μM, and 2.29 μM, respectively. These findings underscore the potential of these compounds as promising candidates in the targeting of HIF-1 for anticancer therapies, (Dat *et al.,* 2007).

The compound Danshenol A exhibited significant inhibitory effects on the proliferation of various cancer cell lines, including K562 (IC_{50} = 0.53 μg/mL), T-24 (IC_{50} = 7.94 μg/mL), QGY (IC_{50} = 4.65 μg/mL), and Me180 (IC_{50} = 6.89 μg/mL). In a related investigation, Yunnanin A demonstrated moderate inhibitory activity against the QGY cell line (IC_{50} = 16.75 μg/mL) and the Me180 cell line (IC_{50} = 5.84 μg/mL), (Xu *et al.,* 2006).

Furthermore, an *in vitro* evaluation of the cytotoxicity of carnosol and its derivatives, 20-deoxocarnosol and 16-hydroxycarnosol, was conducted against a spectrum of cancer cell lines, including A2780 (ovarian cancer), SW1573 (nonsmall-cell lung cancer), WiDr (colon cancer), T-47D (breast cancer), and HBL-100 (breast cancer). All tested compounds manifested GI_{50} values ranging from 3.6 to 35 μM across the five cancer cell lines. Notably, the A2780 and HBL-100 cell lines exhibited heightened sensitivity, with GI_{50} values between 3.6 and 5.4 μM, (Wu *et al.,* 2012).

Moreover, the isolation of taxodione from *S. staminea* demonstrated pronounced cytotoxicity across several cell lines. The recorded IC_{50} values for BC1, LU1, COL2, KB, KB-VI, LNCaP, P388, and A2780 were 1.2, 5.1, 0.7, 3.4, 4.1, and 0 μg/mL, respectively. Additional IC_{50} values measured were 7, 0.3, and 9.0 μg/mL, respectively. Salvileucalin B also exhibited notable cytotoxic activity against the A549 and HT-29 cell lines, with IC_{50} values of 5.23 and 1.88 μg/mL, respectively, (Wu *et al.,* 2012).

3.2.3 Anti-HIV Activity

In the three decades following the initial identification of the human immunodeficiency virus (HIV) as the causative agent of acquired immune deficiency syndrome (AIDS), more than 40 million individuals have become infected. A significant number of secondary metabolites extracted from plant sources have undergone rigorous screening to evaluate their in vitro anti-HIV efficacy, (Wu *et al.,* 2012).

A novel polyphenol, salvianolic acid N, extracted from the aqueous roots of *Salvia yunnanensis*, has demonstrated the capacity to inhibit both HIV-1 reverse transcriptase (RT) and integrase (IN). The inhibitory concentration (IC_{50}) values were determined to range between 67.10 and 193.39 μg/mL for RT and between 1.78 and 18.5 μg/mL for IN. Additionally, it was observed that salvianolic acid N, at non-toxic concentrations, exerts an inhibitory effect on HIV-1 p24 antigen expression in MT-4 cell lines, with a toxicity concentration (TC_{50}) value ranging from 3.7 to 24. Notably, at a concentration of 10 μg/mL, the IC_{50} for the inhibition of p24 in MT-4 cell cultures was calculated to be between 0.649 and 4.28 μg/mL, yielding a selective index (SI) of 5.63 to 5.70, (Wu *et al.,* 2012).

Furthermore, Przewalskin A and B displayed modest anti-HIV-1 activity, with effective concentration (EC_{50}) values of 41 and 30 μg/mL, respectively. The anti-HIV-1 activities of salvianolic acid A, methyl salvianolate A, ethyl salvianolate A, lithospermic acid, and cis-lithospermic acid were also assessed for their ability to inhibit p24 antigen expression in HIV-1-infected MT-4 cell cultures. The resulting EC_{50} values for these compounds were found to be 2.07, 1.62, 1.44, 3.99, and 6.11 μg/mL, respectively, (Wu *et al.,* 2012).

3.2.4 Antimicrobial Activity

The compound methyl 12-O-methylcarnosoate, isolated from *Salvia africana-lutea*, demonstrated a minimum inhibitory concentration (MIC) of 28 micromoles per liter against *Mycobacterium tuberculosis*, (Hussein *et al.,* 2007). Furthermore, the antibacterial properties of horminone and 7-acetylhorminone were found to be significant across various bacterial strains. Specifically, against *Staphylococcus aureus* ATCC 6538 P, the MICs were reported at 6.5 μg/mL and 10 μg/mL, respectively. For *Staphylococcus epidermidis* ATCC 12226, the observed MICs were 1.5 μg/mL and 6 μg/mL. Additionally, *Bacillus subtilis* ATCC 6633 displayed MIC values of 1.5 μg/mL and 3 μg/mL for these compounds, (Wu *et al.,* 2012).

In recent studies, the compound horminone was shown to exhibit antimicrobial activity against *Enterococcus faecalis* ATCC 29212, with a minimum inhibitory concentration (MIC) of 14 μg/mL. Additionally, O-Methylpisiferic acid demonstrated selectivity in its activity, being effective only against *Bacillus subtilis* ATCC

6633, with MIC values of 30, 25, 32, 25, and 20 μg/mL. For *Bacillus subtilis*, the MICs ranged from 25 to 35 μg/mL, with values exceeding 45 μg/mL recorded at higher concentrations, including 60 μg/mL and values between 15 and 20 μg/mL. *Staphylococcus aureus* showed MIC values of 6 to 4 μg/mL, values exceeding 45 μg/mL, and additional measurements of 10 to 8 μg/mL, with multiple readings of 6 to 4 μg/mL, (Wu *et al.*, 2012).

Furthermore, 1-Oxoferruginol demonstrated effective antimicrobial activity against *Bacillus subtilis*, *Staphylococcus aureus*, and *Staphylococcus epidermidis*, each exhibiting an MIC of 15.6 μg/mL, while showing modest activity against *Proteus mirabilis* (>250 μg/mL). On the other hand, Microstegiol displayed minimal activity against *Bacillus subtilis*, with an MIC of >250 μg/mL. Notably, Sclareol exhibited significant antimicrobial efficacy against a range of bacteria, including *Staphylococcus aureus*, *Staphylococcus epidermidis*, *Escherichia coli*, *Proteus vulgaris*, and *Pseudomonas aeruginosa*, with MIC values of 15.6 μg/mL, 15.6 μg/mL, 62.5 μg/mL, 62.5 μg/mL, and 31.3 μg/mL, respectively. The antibacterial properties of 8(17),12E,14-labdatrien-6,19-olide have been demonstrated against *Staphylococcus aureus*. In addition, the compounds salvipisone and aethiopinone displayed significant antibacterial activity against *Staphylococcus aureus*, with minimum inhibitory concentration (MIC) values ranging from 18.75 to 37.5 μg/mL, and against *Staphylococcus epidermidis*, with MIC values between 9.37 and 75.0 μg/mL. Compound 350 also exhibited antimicrobial efficacy against two Gram-positive organisms, specifically *Staphylococcus aureus* and *Micrococcus luteus*, with MIC values of 20.0 μM and 15.0 μM, respectively. Moreover, oleanolic acid and ursolic acid demonstrated MICs of 8 μg/mL and 4 μg/mL, respectively, while also exhibiting antimicrobial activity against *Streptococcus pneumoniae* and methicillin-resistant *Staphylococcus aureus* (MRSA), (Wu *et al.*, 2012) (Norouzi, Babalar, & Mirmasoumi, 2017).

The antimicrobial activity of *Salvia fruticosa* ethanol extract (SFEt) was evaluated using the disk diffusion method against 39 bacterial strains, including 11 multidrug-resistant (MDR) bacteria, and 2 fungal strains. The extract exhibited a broad-spectrum antimicrobial activity, particularly against *Staphylococcus epidermidis* DSMZ 20044 (21 mm inhibition zone) and *Proteus vulgaris* (MDR) (13 mm inhibition zone), indicating significant efficacy against Gram-positive and Gram-negative bacteria. Of particular note was the finding that *Streptococcus pneumoniae* (MDR) demonstrated a higher degree of susceptibility to SFEt than several conventional antibiotics, thus underlining its potential in combating antibiotic resistance. The biochemical composition of SFEt, analyzed via GC-MS, revealed 23 chemical constituents, with D-camphor (20.27%) as the dominant compound, followed by (+)-borneol (9.59%), caryophyllene (8.11%), and lupeol acetate (6.28%). These bioactive compounds are recognized for their antimicrobial and antioxidant properties, suggesting that the observed biological activity of *S. fruticosa* is likely due to their combined or synergistic effects. The presence of several unidentified components in the extract further suggests the potential discovery of novel bioactive molecules. The antimicrobial potency of *S. fruticosa* and its biochemical profile supports its potential use as a natural alternative to synthetic antimicrobial agents. Further studies are warranted to isolate and characterize its active compounds, (Bozyel *et al.,* 2023).

3.2.5 Others Biological Activities

Acetylcholinesterase (AChE) inhibitors represent the sole class of pharmacological agents that has received regulatory approval for the treatment of Alzheimer's disease (AD). Recent studies have demonstrated that the compounds dihydrotanshinone, cryptotanshinone, tanshinone, and tanshinone A exhibit significant inhibitory activity against AChE. Their respective c log P values, measured at 2.4, 3.4, 4.8, and 5.8, indicate a potential for these compounds to effectively traverse the blood-brain barrier, thereby enhancing their therapeutic applicability in the context of AD, (Ren *et al.,* 2004).

The crude extract of *Salvia eriophora* and five isolated compounds—namely, 4,14-dihydroxysaprorthoquinone, aethiopinone, ferruginol, 4,12-dihydroxysapriparaquinone, and 6,7-dehydroroyleanone—were subjected to evaluation for their cardiovascular activities utilizing Wistar Albino rats. The findings revealed significant cardiovascular effects, characterized by a notable reduction in direct blood pressure, alongside a modest increase in heart rate; however, the latter did not reach statistical significance. Additionally, the comparative cytotoxic effects of demethylsalvicanol, 14-deoxycoleon U, and demethylcryptojaponol were assessed on insect Sf9 and mammalian CHO cells. The results indicated that demethylsalvicanol exhibited moderate antifeedant activity against *Leptinotarsa decemlineata*, whereas 14-deoxycoleon U demonstrated the highest potency as an antifeedant. In contrast, demethylcryptojaponol displayed considerable toxicity towards this insect, (Wu *et al.,* 2012).

The clerodane diterpenoid salvinorin A, recognized as the principal active constituent of the psychotropic plant *Salvia divinorum*, has been identified as a potent agonist at the κ-opioid receptor. Additionally, safficinolide has been shown to reduce the yield of vesicular stomatitis virus (VSV), while sageone exhibits notable antiviral activity, demonstrating inactivation effects against both VSV and herpes simplex virus type 1 (HSV-1), (Wu *et al.,* 2012).

4. TRADITIONAL USES OF SALVIA GENUS

The *Salvia* genus has a significant historical presence in traditional medicine, employed for the treatment of a variety of health conditions. Notably, *Salvia* species have been utilized to address respiratory ailments, including asthma and bronchitis, as well as persistent coughs. In addition, these plants have been recognized for their efficacy in treating gastrointestinal disorders, such as diarrhea, indigestion, and abdominal pain. Moreover, Salvia exhibits pronounced antibacterial and anti-inflammatory properties, which contribute to its application in managing menstrual disorders and diabetes. This study aims to provide a comprehensive overview of the ethnobotanical applications of *Salvia* taxa, particularly within the framework of Turkish traditional medicine, as summarized in Table 5. Furthermore, Table 6 delineates various multi-herbal formulas that incorporate *Salvia* species alongside other botanical constituents.

Table 5. Traditional uses of the Salvia genus

Botanical names*	**Turkish names**	**Common names**	**Used parts**	**Usage forms**	**Uses**	**References**
Salvia sp.	Adaçayı	Sage	Unspecified	Unspecified	Kidney diseases	(Kültür *et al.*, 2021)
			Aerial parts	Infusion	Abdominal pain, bronchitis, cough	((Tuzlaci, 2016))
			Leaves	Infusion	Cold, antifungal	((Tuzlaci, 2016))
Salvia absconditiflora (Montbret & Aucher ex Benth.) Greuter & Burdet (syn.: *S. cryptantha* Montbret & Aucher ex Benth.) **(End.)**	Kara şalba, Öksürük otu, Kara ot, garaot, garaod, Adaçayı, Yabani Adaçayı, Ada çayı, Ballık otu, Kokulu ot, Sarı şabla, Çalba, Kayışkıran, Şabla, Yakıs ablası,	Sage, Turkish black sage	Aerial parts	Infusion	Asthma	(Melikoğlu, Kurtoğlu, & Kültürr, 2015)
			Aerial parts	Infusion	Cardiovascular diseases	(Gulec, Erarslan, & Kultur, 2023)
			Aerial parts	Infusion	Cough, bronchitis	(Demirci & Özhatay, 2012)

continued on following page

Table 5. Continued

Botanical names*	Turkish names	Common names	Used parts	Usage forms	Uses	References
			Aerial parts	Infusion	Hemorrhoid	Erbay & Sari, 2018) (Şahin, T., & Kılıç, 2022)
			Aerial parts	Infusion	Immune-Boosting	(Sargin & Dogan, 2023)
			Aerial parts	Infusion	Stomach diseases, cold, bronchitis, cough, flu, sore throat, hemorrhoid, heart diseases, wound healing, antiseptic	((Tuzlaci, 2016))
			Aerial parts	Infusion	Stomach diseases, diuretic, heart diseases, hemorrhoid	(Tuzlacı & Şenkardeş, 2011)
			Aerial parts	Infusion	Tea	(Şenkardeş & Tuzlacı, 2016)
			Flowering parts	Infusion	Abdominal pain, shortness of breath, cough, fatigue	((Tuzlaci, 2016))
			Flowering parts	Infusion	Asthma, cough, expectorant	(Tuzlacı & Şenkardeş, 2011)
			Leaves	Decoction	Stomach ache	(Erbay, Anil, & Melikoğlu, 2017)
			Leaves	Decoction	Stomach ache, cold	(Doğan & Bağcı, 2011)
			Leaves	Infusion	Stomach ache, cold	((Tuzlaci, 2016))
			Leaves	Infusion	Sore throat, shortness of breath	(Akbulut, 2021)
			Whole plant	Infusion	Kidney stone	(Kültür *et al.*, 2021)
			Whole plant	Infusion, gargle	Fatigue, cough, stomach pain, antibiotics, flu, kidney stones, body resistance, throat inflammation, pharyngitis, bronchitis	(Korkmaz & Karakurt, 2015)

continued on following page

Table 5. Continued

Botanical names*	Turkish names	Common names	Used parts	Usage forms	Uses	References
			Aerial parts, Flowers, Leaves	Poultice with dough	Anti-influenza	(Sargin, 2021)
			Aerial parts, Flowers, Leaves	Infusion, Leaves are eaten by chewing, Mixture, Cataplasm	Stomach ache, cold and flu, bronchitis, asthma, pleasure and medicinal tea	(Sargin, Selvi, & López, 2015)
			Aerial parts, Flowers, Leaves, Whole plant	Decoction, Infusion	Cough, bronchitis, sore throat, stomach disorders, stomach ache, antiseptic, asthma, expectorant, diuretic, hemorrhoid, heart diseases, insomnia, gynoecological disorders, cold and flu, emollient, abdominal pain, fatigue	(Ozturk & Altay, 2017)
Salvia adenocaulon P.H.Davis **(End.)**	Kızlaryülmesi	Taseli sage	Aerial parts	Tea	Anti-stress, calming nerves, sedative and fatigue, throat inflammation, cold, and blood cleaner	(Erucar, Tan, & Miski, 2023)
Salvia adenophylla Hedge & Hub.-Mor. **(End.)**	Poruk, Dağ çayı	Unspecified	Aerial parts	Infusion	Abdominal pain	((Tuzlaci, 2016)) Bulut et al. (2017)
Salvia aethiopis L.	Habeş adaçayı, Adaçayı, Karakoyun Teği, Maldili, Tüylü Adaçayı	Mediterranean sage, African sage	Aerial parts	Infusion	Cold	(Koyuncu *et al.*, 2010)
			Aerial parts	Infusion	Stomach ache, cold, shortness of breath, heart diseases	((Tuzlaci, 2016))
			Aerial parts	Infusion, Decoction	Heart diseases	(Gulec, Erarslan, & Kultur, 2023)

continued on following page

Table 5. Continued

Botanical names*	Turkish names	Common names	Used parts	Usage forms	Uses	References
			Leaves	Cooked with yogurt	Unspecified	(Altundağ Çakır, 2017)
			Leaves	Infusion	Cold	((Tuzlaci, 2016))
			Stems	Eaten raw after bark is peeled	Unspecified	(Altundağ Çakır, 2017)
			Unripe fruits	Eaten	Food	(Şenkardeş & Tuzlacı, 2016)
			Leaves, flowers	Decoction	Stomach ailments	(Doğan & Bağcı, 2011)
Salvia aramiensis Rech.f.	Pohur, Adaçayı, Buhur ağacı, Yara otu	Amanos Mountain sage, Aramenian salve	Leaves	Decoction	Bronchitis	(Altay & Çelik, 2017)
			Leaves	Infusion	Anti-influenza	(Sargin, 2021)
			Leaves	Infusion	Medicinal tea for cough, cold and flu and diabetes	(Güzel & Güzelşemme, 2018)
			Leaves	Unspecified	Cold, diabetes, cough, bronchitis	(Altay *et al.*, 2015)
			Flowers, Leaves	Infusion	Bronchitis	((Tuzlaci, 2016))
			Flowers, Leaves	Unspecified	Spice, flavouring	(Güzel & Kayıkçı, 2023)
Salvia argentea L.	Gümüş şalba, Adaçayı	Silver sage	Aerial parts	Infusion	Cold	((Tuzlaci, 2016)) (Koyuncu *et al.*, 2010)
Salvia aucheri subsp. *canescens* (Boiss. & Heldr.) Celep, Kahraman & Doğan **(End.)	Koramaz	Lilac waving sage	Leaves	Infusion	Abdominal pain, cold, sedative	((Tuzlaci, 2016))
Salvia brachyantha (Bordz.) Pobed.	Kazan şalbası, Gazangulpu	Unspecified	Aerial parts	Infusion	Cold	((Tuzlaci, 2016))
			Leaves	Stuffed	Food	(Altundağ Çakır, 2017)
Salvia bracteata Banks & Sol.	Çoban şalbası, Adaçayı	Shepherd's sage	Aerial parts	Infusion	Cold	((Tuzlaci, 2016))

continued on following page

Table 5. Continued

Botanical names*	Turkish names	Common names	Used parts	Usage forms	Uses	References
			Aerial parts	Infusion	Cold, medicinal tea	(Koyuncu *et al.*, 2010)
			Fresh aerial parts	Tea	Unspecified	(Doğan & Tuzlacı, 2015)
			Leaves	Infusion	Abdominal pain, cold	((Tuzlaci, 2016))
Salvia cadmica Boiss.	Kaya şalbası, Adaçayı	Anatolian wand sage	Aerial parts	Crushed	Hemostatic	((Tuzlaci, 2016))
			Aerial parts	Infusion	Abdominal pain	(56)
			Aerial parts	Infusion	Abdominal pain, cold	((Tuzlaci, 2016))
			Aerial parts	Infusion	Cold, medicinal tea	(Koyuncu *et al.*, 2010)
			Aerial parts	Infusion, crushed	Cold, flu	(Ozturk & Altay, 2017)
			Unspecified	Unspecified	Cold, sore throat	(Erzurumlu, 2021)
Salvia cadmica var. *cadmica* Boiss. ****(End.)**	Kaya şalbası, Ada çayı	Anatolian wand sage	Aerial parts	Tea	Cold, flu	(Cinbilgel & Kurt, 2019)
Salvia candidissima Vahl	Galabor, Adaçayı	Blazing white sage, Silver sage	Leaves	Infusion	Anti-influenza	(Sargin, 2021)
			Whole plant	Infusion	Kidney stone	(Kültür *et al.*, 2021)
Salvia candidissima subsp. *candidissima* Vahl	Galabor, Adaçayı, Öküzgötü	Eastern blazing white sage	Aerial parts	Infusion	Cold	((Tuzlaci, 2016))
			Aerial parts	Infusion	Cold, medicinal tea	(Koyuncu *et al.*, 2010)
			Leaves	Infusion	Cold, flu	((Tuzlaci, 2016))
			Stems	Unspecified	Young stems are eaten by peeling the bark	(Yapar, 2024)
			Whole plant	Infusion, gargle	Fatigue, cough, stomach pain, antibiotics, flu, kidney stones, body resistance, throat inflammation, pharyngitis, bronchitis	(Korkmaz & Karakurt, 2015)

continued on following page

Table 5. Continued

Botanical names*	Turkish names	Common names	Used parts	Usage forms	Uses	References
Salvia ceratophylla L.	Tarak şalba, Adaçayı, Öküz Pöçüğü	Comb sage	Stems	Fresh	Food	(Güneş & Özhatay, 2011)
			Whole plant	Decoction	Fatigue, cough, antibiotic, flu, sweat odour	(Korkmaz & Karakurt, 2014)
			Whole plant	Gargle	throat inflammation	(Korkmaz & Karakurt, 2014)
Salvia chrysophylla Stapf **(End.)	Boz şalba, Bozçavla	Goldleaf Sage	Aerial parts	Decoction	Rheumatism	(Ozturk & Altay, 2017)
			Aerial parts	Infusion	Rheumatism	((Tuzlaci, 2016))
			Aerial parts	Poultice	Rheumatism	((Tuzlaci, 2016))
			Aerial parts	Poultice, decoction	Rheumatism	(Yeşilada *et al.*, 1993)
Salvia cyanescens Boiss. & Balansa **(End.)	Mor galabor, Kazankarası	Turkish lilac sage	Aerial parts	Decoction	Diabetes	(Ozturk & Altay, 2017) (Han & Bulut, 2015)
			Aerial parts	Infusion	Diabetes	((Tuzlaci, 2016))
Salvia dichroantha Stapf **(End.)	Kutnu	West Anatolian sage	Flowers	Food	Its nectar sucked	(Celik & Yesil, 2020)
			Leaves	Infusion	Stomach ache, wound healing, abscess	((Tuzlaci, 2016))
			Leaves	Infusion	Abdominal pain, stomach ache	(Ozturk & Altay, 2017)
Salvia divaricata Montbret & Aucher ex Benth. **(End.)	Saplı şalba	Unspecified	Leaves	Infusion	Constipation, stomach, sedative	(Ozturk & Altay, 2017)
			Leaves	Unspecified	Constipation, stomachic, calmatine	(Terzioğlu & Coşkunçelebi, 2021)
Salvia forskahlei L.	Dolma yaprağı, Karadeniz adaçayı, Ağbandık	Sarma sage	Aerial parts	Decoction	Influenza, expectorant	(Karci *et al.*, 2017)

continued on following page

Table 5. Continued

Botanical names*	Turkish names	Common names	Used parts	Usage forms	Uses	References
			Leaves	Compress	Wound healing	(Karaköse, 2022)
			Leaves	Infusion	Constipation, Stomach, Sedative	(Akbulut & Bayramoglu, 2013)
			Leaves	Unspecified	Influenza, constipant, stomach, calmative	(Terzioğlu & Coşkunçelebi, 2021)
Salvia fruticosa Mill.	Adaçayı, Ada çayı, Moşapla, Moşaplı, Boşotu, Muşapla, Puşapla, Yakıotu, Elma Ada çayı, çalba, geyik elması, Elma çayı, Elmalı adaçayı, Anadolu adaçayı, Almageyik, Şapla, Yakı otu, Moşaplı, dağ çayı, Boş, Boşapla,	Turkish sage, Greek sage	Aerial parts	Boiled with textile	Red dye	(Ozdemir Nath & Kültürr, 2015)
			Aerial parts	Infusion	Cold, abdominal pain, throat pain, eczema, stomach disease, cough, kidney problems, inflammation, wound healing	(Ozdemir Nath & Kultur, 2022)
			Aerial parts	Infusion	Head ache	(Erbay, Anil, & Melikoğlu, 2018)
			Aerial parts	Infusion	Head ache, sore throat, stomach ailments (before breakfast)	(Bulut & Tuzlaci, 2015)
			Aerial parts	Unspecified	Antipyretic, sore throat	(Uysal *et al.*, 2010)
			Aerial parts	Unspecified	Cold and flu, abdominal pain	(Kincal, Ceylan, & Görk, 2021)
			Aerial parts	Unspecified	Gingival diseases	(Uzun & Kaya, 2019)
			Fruits	Unspecified	Food	(Akan & Pekmez, 2018)

continued on following page

Table 5. Continued

Botanical names*	Turkish names	Common names	Used parts	Usage forms	Uses	References
			Leafy branches	Infusion	Stomach ache	(Erbay, Anil, & Melikoğlu, 2017)
			Leaves	Boiled in water+ sugar	Antiseptic, dyspepsia, cold, tonsilitis	(Uzun & Kaya, 2019)
			Leaves	Decoction	Asthma, bronchitis	(Boz, İldeniz, & Cabi, 2022)
			Leaves	Decoction	Stomach ache, tonsillits, antisudofiric, catarrh, flu, sinusitis	Sağıroğlu, Dalgıç, & Toksoy, 2013)
			Leaves	Infusion	Constipation, Stomach, Sedative	(Akbulut & Bayramoglu, 2013)
			Leaves	Infusion	Tea	(Yalçın, Akan, & Çakılcıoğlu, 2022)
			Leaves	Infusion	Wound healing	(Ozdemir Nath & Kultur, 2022)
			Leaves	Kept in vinegar	Calcification	(Ozdemir Nath & Kultur, 2022)
			Leaves	Oil	Asthma, bronchitis, diuretic, menstruation regulating	Sağıroğlu, Dalgıç, & Toksoy, 2013)
			Leaves	Salve	Carminative	Sağıroğlu, Dalgıç, & Toksoy, 2013)
			Leaves	Tea	Stomach ache, cold, tonsilitis, sinusitis, antiseptic	(Akan & Pekmez, 2018)
			Leaves	Decoction, gargle	Cold, toothache	(Boz, İldeniz, & Cabi, 2022)
			Aerial parts, Essential oil	Infusion, Lotion	anti-influenza	(Sargin, 2021)
			Aerial parts, Leaves	Decoction	Respiratory disorders and kidney diseases	(Ötnü & Akan, 2020)

continued on following page

Table 5. Continued

Botanical names*	Turkish names	Common names	Used parts	Usage forms	Uses	References
			Flowers, Leaves	Decoction	Cold, Stomach ache	(Akbaş, Çıtakoğlu, & Davran, 2024)
			Flowers, Leaves	Decoction, Infusion	Urinary tract infection, carminative, Constipation, Stress-induced insomnia, Sedative	(Palasoglu & Eminagaoglu, 2022)
			Flowers, Leaves	Infusion, oil	Stomach ache	(Fakir, Korkmaz, & Icel, 2016)
			Flowers, Leaves, Shoots	Oil	Carminative	(Korkmaz, Fakir, & Guller, 2011)
			Flowers, Leaves, Shoots	Oil	Carminative, diuretic, antiseptic	(Fakir, Korkmaz, & Güller, 2009)
			Unspecified	Fresh Oil	Asthma	(Melikoğlu, Kurtoğlu, & Kültürr, 2015)
			Unspecified	Oil	Scorpion sting	((Tuzlaci, 2016))
			Unspecified	Unspecified	Cold	(Başer *et al.*, 2006)
			Unspecified	Unspecified	Sore throat, stomach ache	(Öz Aydın *et al.*, 2006)
			Unspecified	Unspecified	Sore throat, head ache, stomach diseases	(Bulut & Tuzlaci, 2009)
Salvia glutinosa L.	Oklu şalba, Purçuma	Sticky sage	Leaves	Unspecified	Wound healing, burn	((Tuzlaci, 2016)) (Saraç, Özkan, & Akbulut, 2013)
			Leaves	Unspecified	Wound healing, antimicrobial, immunostimulant, anti-inflammatory, astringent, vermifuge, cicatrising, mouth disease	(Terzioğlu & Coşkunçelebi, 2021)
			Flowering parts, Leaves	Infusion	Heart diseases, arteriosclerosis	((Tuzlaci, 2016))

continued on following page

Table 5. Continued

Botanical names*	Turkish names	Common names	Used parts	Usage forms	Uses	References
Salvia hispanica L.	Chia tohumu	Chia	Seeds	Infusion	Weight loss	(Alkış, Parmaksiz, & Akan, 2021)
			Seeds	Unspecified	Brain diseases, heart diseases, weight loss	(Ötnü & Akan, 2020)
Salvia huberi Hedge **(End.)	Meryemiye	Unspecified	Leaves	Infusion	Constipation, stomach, sedative	(Ozturk & Altay, 2017)
Salvia hydrangea DC. ex Benth.	Koç şalba, Koçotu	Unspecified	Aerial parts	Infusion	Diabetes	(Sarikaya, Öner, & Harput, 2010)
			Flowering branches	Infusion	Stomach diseases, cold, diabetes, antipyretic	((Tuzlaci, 2016))
Salvia hypargeia Fisch. & C.A.Mey. **(End.)	Siyahot, Ada çayı, Iccak otu	Turkish mountain sage	Aerial parts	Infusion	Tea	(Şenkardeş & Tuzlacı, 2016)
			Roots	Decoction	Cold	((Tuzlaci, 2016))
			Aerial parts, Sap	Infusion	Heartstroke	(Gulec, Erarslan, & Kultur, 2023)
			Flowering branches, roots	Boiled, infusion	Stomach ache, cough, cold	(Ozturk & Altay, 2017)
Salvia limbata C.A.Mey.	Maldili, Kedi kuyruğu	Lulling sage	Aerial parts	Boiled	Toothache	((Tuzlaci, 2016))
			Aerial parts	Infusion	Toothache	((Tuzlaci, 2016))
			Aerial parts	Decoction	Stomach ache	(Bozkurt, 2024)
			Stems	Eaten raw after bark is peeled	Unspecified	(Altundağ Çakır, 2017)
Salvia macrochlamys Boiss. & Kotschy	Gevrek şalba	Pinklip sage	Aerial parts	Infusion	Shortness of breath, cardiovascular diseases	((Tuzlaci, 2016))
Salvia multicaulis Vahl	Adaçayı, Çobandöşeği, Çay otu, Dağ çayı, Süt otu, Dağ Reyhanı, kürtreyhanı	Many-stemmed sage, Kurdish basil	Aerial parts	Crushed	Oedema	((Tuzlaci, 2016))

continued on following page

Table 5. Continued

Botanical names*	Turkish names	Common names	Used parts	Usage forms	Uses	References
			Aerial parts	Decoction	Cold, flu	(Hayta, Polat, & Selvi, 2014)
			Aerial parts	Decoction	Diabetes	(Sarikaya, Öner, & Harput, 2010) (Arituluk & Ezer, 2012) (Karaman & Elgin Cebe, 2016)
			Aerial parts	Infusion	Appetite stimulant, respiratory diseases, urinary tract diseases, asthma, bronchitis	(Sirri, Özaslan, & Fidan, 2021)
			Aerial parts	Infusion	Cold, flu	(Baykan *et al.*, 2023)
			Aerial parts	Infusion	Tea	(Yalçın, Akan, & Çakılcıoğlu, 2022)
			Aerial parts	Infusion	Wound healing, flu, cough, labor pain, anti-inflammatory, antidote	(Akgul *et al.*, 2018)
			Aerial parts	Infusion, Decoction	Anti-influenza	(Sargin, 2021)
			Aerial parts	Dried, boiled and poultice	Oedema	((Tuzlaci, 2016))
			Aerial parts	Unspecified	Stomach ache	(Akan *et al.*, 2013)
			Fresh aerial parts	Tea		(Doğan & Tuzlacı, 2015)
			Fruits	Infusion	Urinary problems, abdominal pain, menstrual pain, bronchitis	(Yeşil & İnal, 2021)
			Leaves	Infusion	Head ache, skin diseases, appetite suppressant	(Akbulut & Karaköse, 2023)
			Leaves	Tea	Unspecified	(Yeşil & İnal, 2021)

continued on following page

Table 5. Continued

Botanical names*	Turkish names	Common names	Used parts	Usage forms	Uses	References
			Leaves	Unspecified	Wound healing	(Terzioğlu & Coşkunçelebi, 2021) (Ozturk, Altay, & Gönenç, 2017)
			Leaves	Unspecified	Wound healing, tea	(Cakilcioglu, Turkoglu, & Kürşat, 2007)
			Whole plant	Decoction	Fatigue, cough, antibiotic, flu, sweat odour	(Korkmaz & Karakurt, 2014)
			Whole plant	Gargle	throat inflammation	(Korkmaz & Karakurt, 2014)
			Whole plant	Infusion	Kidney stone	(Kültür *et al.*, 2021)
			Whole plant	Tea	Several disorders	(Kaya, Dağlı, & Tosyagülü Çelik, 2020)
			Whole plant	Infusion, gargle	Fatigue, cough, stomach pain, antibiotics, flu, kidney stones, body resistance, throat inflammation, pharyngitis, bronchitis	(Korkmaz & Karakurt, 2015)
			Whole plant	Unspecified	Anorexia, respiratory and urinary tract disorders, weakness, cough, stomach diseases, kidney stones, asthma, throat inflammation, pharyngitis, bronchitis, diabetes, tonsil infection, indigestion, pain, cold, natural antibiotic, sedative	(Karahan *et al.*, 2023)
			Flowers, Leaves	Tea	Unspecified	(Demir & Ayaz, 2022)
			Aerial parts, Flowers, Leaves	Decoction	Heart attack risk	(Gulec, Erarslan, & Kultur, 2023)

continued on following page

Table 5. Continued

Botanical names*	Turkish names	Common names	Used parts	Usage forms	Uses	References
Salvia napifolia Jacq.	Ters şalba, Çay otu	Turkish whorled clary	Aerial parts	Unspecified	Tea	(Özdemir & Kültürr, 2017)
			Leaves	Infusion	Cold	((Tuzlaci, 2016))
Salvia nemorosa L.	Gehareş, Adaçayı, Hanımana otu	Purple wood sage	Aerial parts	Crushed	Hemostatic, wound healing	((Tuzlaci, 2016))
			Aerial parts	Decoction	Urinary disorders, stomach ache	(Bozkurt, 2024)
			Aerial parts	Infusion	Cold	((Tuzlaci, 2016))
			Aerial parts	Unspecified	Hemostatic, cold, catarrh	(Terzioğlu & Coşkunçelebi, 2021)
			Flowering branches	Infusion	Cold	((Tuzlaci, 2016))
			Leaves	Dried eaten	Spice	(Akbulut & Zengin, 2023)
Salvia officinalis L.	Tıbbi adaçayı, Adaçayı, Deve dili, Acı elma otu	Garden sage, Culinary sage, golden sage, Common sage, sage, Sage tea	Aerial parts	Infusion	Anti-influenza	(Sargin, 2021)
			Aerial parts	Infusion	Appetizer, blood purifier, carminative, antimicrobial, cold, fatigue reliever, stress reliever, hand and foot tremor, throat infections	(Akan & Bakir Sade, 2015)
			Aerial parts	Infusion	Kidney diseases	(Kültür *et al.*, 2021)
			Aerial parts	Infusion after drying	Immune-boosting	(Sargin & Dogan, 2023)
			Aerial parts	Poultice	Rheumatism	(Akan & Bakir Sade, 2015)
			Aerial parts	Infusion, gargle	Gingivitis	(Uzun & Kaya, 2019)
			Leaves	Boiled and drunk	Stomach ache	(Doğan & Ugulu, 2013)

continued on following page

Table 5. Continued

Botanical names*	Turkish names	Common names	Used parts	Usage forms	Uses	References
			Leaves	Decoction	Cholesterol, mouth sores, hepatoprotective, sedative	(Kavakli, Kaya, & Ugurlu, 2020)
			Leaves	Decoction	Sedative, memory booster, immune-boosting, antiseptic, antistress, digestive, sore throat, gynaecological disorders, weight loss, liver cleanser	(Kayakli, Yaylaci, & Ugurlu, 2015)
			Leaves	Infusion	Abdominal pain, cough	(Güler, Manav, & Uğurlu, 2015)
			Leaves	Infusion	Constipation, stomach, sedative	(Akbulut & Bayramoglu, 2013)
			Leaves	Infusion	Kidney stone	(Kültür *et al.*, 2021)
			Leaves	Infusion	Severe acute respiratory syndrome coronavirus 2 (SARS-CoV-2)-COVID-19	(Akbulut & Özkan, 2023)
			Leaves	Infusion	Sore throat, tonsilitis, pyorrhoea, carminative, antinausea, diuretic, sweat off	(Akbulut, Karaköse, & Özkan, 2019)
			Leaves	Tea	İnflammation, fatigue	(Yaşar *et al.*, 2019)
			Leaves	İnfusion, gargle	Sore throat, shortness of breath	(Akbulut, 2021)
			Leaves	Unspecified	Food, Respriatory diseases	(Sari, Kültürr, & Koçyiğit, 2023)
			Leaves	Unspecified	Flu, colds, throat infections	(Tütenocaklı & Uysal, 2014)
			Leaves	Unspecified	Gynecological diseases, painful menstrual	(Cakir & Akan, 2023)

continued on following page

Table 5. Continued

Botanical names*	Turkish names	Common names	Used parts	Usage forms	Uses	References
			Flowers, Leaves	Decoction	Cold, diuretic and respiratory disorders	(Çömlekçioğlu & Karaman, 2008)
			Flowers, Leaves	Decoction	Digestive, diuretic, carminative, insomnia, gingivitis, tonsillitis, cold, flu, throat diseases, skin wounds	(Bağcı, Dural, & Savran, 2006)
			Flowers, Leaves	Decoction	Stomach ache	(Güler, Erkan, & Uğurlu, 2020) (184)
			Flowers, Leaves	Infusion	Cough, flu, throat inflammation	(Aslan, 2018)
			Flowers, Leaves	Tea	Cold, flu	(Sarikaya & Karabay, 2021)
			Flowers, Leaves	Unspecified	Bronchitis, ulcer, gout, rheumatism, inflammation, dizziness, tremor, paralysis, diarrhoea	(Ekren & Corbaci, 2021)
			Flowering branches, leaves	Infusion	Kidney diseases	(Kültür *et al.*, 2021)
			Flowers, Leaves, Stems	Unspecified	Tea	(Tütenocaklı, 2023)
			Unspecified	Unspecified	Cold	(Başer *et al.*, 2006)
			Unspecified	Unspecified	Diuretic, menstrual problems, wound healing, vaginal fungus, digestive, diuretic, carminative, stimulant, anti-inflammatory, anti-cold	(Demirci Kayiran, 2019)
Salvia palaestina Benth.	Sürmeli şalba, Adaçayı, Dağ çayı	Palestinian sage	Aerial parts	Crushed	Hemostatic, wound healing	((Tuzlaci, 2016))
			Aerial parts	Infusion	Abdominal pain, menstrual pain	(Yeşil & İnal, 2021)

continued on following page

Table 5. Continued

Botanical names*	Turkish names	Common names	Used parts	Usage forms	Uses	References
			Aerial parts	Infusion	Anti-influenza	(Sargin, 2021)
			Aerial parts	Infusion	Cold, cough, diabetes	((Tuzlaci, 2016))
			Aerial parts	Infusion	Immune-boosting	(Sargin & Dogan, 2023)
			Aerial parts	Unspecified	Fragrance	(Eksik & Akan, 2021)
			Leaves	Infusion	Cold	(Şahin Fidan & Akan, 2019)
			Leaves	Unspecified	Cold	(Kocabas, Erol, & Aktolun, 2017)
			Leaves	Unspecified	Wound healing	(Cakilcioglu, Turkoglu, & Kürşat, 2007)
			Whole plant	Infusion	Insomnia	(Erucar, Tan, & Miski, 2023)
			Whole plant	Poultice	Burns, scars	(Erucar, Tan, & Miski, 2023)
			Whole plant	Tea	Several disorders	(Kaya, Dağlı, & Tosyagülü Çelik, 2020)
Salvia pilifera Montbret & Aucher ex Benth. **(End.)**	Etekli şalba, Mor Adaçayı	Sage	Aerial parts	Unspecified	Alzheimer's disease, nerve damage, antibacterial, antioxidant	(Karahan *et al.*, 2023)
Salvia pinnata L.	Çanak şalbası, Ellik otu	Featherleaf sage	Aerial parts	Infusion	Cold	((Tuzlaci, 2016))
			Aerial parts	Infusion	Cold, medicinal tea	(Koyuncu *et al.*, 2010)
Salvia pisidica Boiss. & Heldr. ex Benth. **(End.)**	Benli şalba	Unspecified	Aerial parts, flowering branches	Infusion	Cold	(Ozturk & Altay, 2017)
Salvia poculata Náb.	Küllü şalba, Öküzpörçüğü	Ashen sage	Leaves	Unspecified	In making "sarma" dish	(Sirri & Sirri, 2020)

continued on following page

Table 5. Continued

Botanical names*	Turkish names	Common names	Used parts	Usage forms	Uses	References
Salvia potentillifolia Boiss. & Heldr. ex Benth. **(End.)**	Sarıporuk, Adaçayı		Unspecified	Unspecified	Cold	(Başer *et al.*, 2006)
Salvia recognita Fisch. & C.A.Mey. **(End.)**	Puslu şalba, Yaygın Adaçayı	Turkish cliff sage	Aerial parts	Unspecified	Cold, antibacterial, antifungal, antioxidant, antiseptic, carminative, diuretic, spasmolytic, stomachic, diaphoretic	(Karahan *et al.*, 2023)
Salvia rosifolia Sm. **(End.)**	Gülmeryemiye, Adaçayı	Unspecified	Leaves	Infusion	Constipation, stomach, sedative	(Ozturk & Altay, 2017)
			Whole plant	Infusion	Kidney stone	(Kültür *et al.*, 2021)
			Whole plant	Infusion, gargle	Fatigue, cough, stomach pain, antibiotics, flu, kidney stones, body resistance, throat inflammation, pharyngitis, bronchitis	(Korkmaz & Karakurt, 2015)
Salvia russellii Benth.	Kurdeşk, Yabani küncü	Blue whorled clary	Aerial parts	Infusion	Abdominal pain, cold	((Tuzlaci, 2016))
			Stems	Fresh stems are peeled and eaten	Food	(Akan, Korkut, & Balos, 2008)
Salvia sclarea L.	Paskulak, Şalba, Dağ çayı, Misk adaçayı, Kıtırak otu, Adaçayı, Arı otu, yalancı çay, Yağlıkara	Clary, Clary sage, Clary wort	Aerial parts	Dried	Spice	(Koyuncu *et al.*, 2010)
			Aerial parts	Infusion	Hemorrhoid	(Koyuncu *et al.*, 2010)
			Flowers	Aromatic water	Stomach ache	(Erucar, Tan, & Miski, 2023)
			Flowers	Fresh	Wart	(Yeşilada *et al.*, 1993)

continued on following page

Table 5. Continued

Botanical names*	Turkish names	Common names	Used parts	Usage forms	Uses	References
			Flowering branches	Aromatic water	Nervousness, tension situation, sedative	(Erucar, Tan, & Miski, 2023)
			Flowering branches	Decoction	Hypertension	(Olcay & Kültürr, 2020)
			Flowering branches	Decoction	Stomach ache	(Erbay, Anil, & Melikoğlu, 2017)
			Leaves	Crushed	Rheumatism	(Han & Bulut, 2015)
			Leaves	Decoction	Cold, cardiovascular diseases	(Eminağaoğlu, Göktürk, & Akyıldırım Beğen, 2017)
			Leaves	Fresh	Sedative	(Akbulut & Zengin, 2023)
			Leaves	Infusion	Colds and flu, gastric pain	(Görhan & Öztürk, 2021)
			Leaves	Tea	Cold	(Cinbilgel & Kurt, 2019)
			Leaves	Tea	Unspecified	(Doğan & Tuzlacı, 2015)
			Leaves	Unspecified	Cold, stomachic, constipant, treatment of sunstroke, sore throat	(Terzioğlu & Coşkunçelebi, 2021)
			Leaves		Sunburn	(Altay & Karahan, 2017)
			Whole plant	Infusion	Kidney stone	(Kültür *et al.*, 2021)
			Whole plant	Infusion, gargle	Fatigue, cough, stomach pain, antibiotics, flu, kidney stones, body resistance, throat inflammation, pharyngitis, bronchitis	(Korkmaz & Karakurt, 2015)
			Flowers, Leaves	Infusion	Sore throat	(Fakir, Korkmaz, & Icel, 2016)
			Flowering branches, Leaves	Infusion	Anti-influenza	(Sargin, 2021)

continued on following page

Table 5. Continued

Botanical names*	Turkish names	Common names	Used parts	Usage forms	Uses	References
			Flowers, Leaves, Shoots	Infusion	Sore throat, throat inflammation, antitussive, stomach cold, depression, gynaecological disease, ulcer and intestines spasm, cold, exhaustion, antitussive	(Fakir, Korkmaz, & Güller, 2009)
			Unspecified	Apiculture	Unspecified	(Demirel & Dutkuner, 2021)
			Unspecified	Unspecified	Aphrodisiac, eye problems, oedema, stomachic, antitussive	(Demirci Kayiran, 2019)
			Unspecified	Unspecified	Stomach ache, kidney pain	(Erzurumlu, 2021)
Salvia staminea Montbret & Aucher ex Benth.	Erkek şalba, Adaçayı, Gazankulpu	Iranian sage	Aerial parts	Dried	Wound healing	((Tuzlaci, 2016))
			Leaves	Cooked with bulgur	Food	(Altundağ Çakır, 2017)
			Whole plant	Decoction	Fatigue, cough, antibiotic, flu, sweat odour	(Korkmaz & Karakurt, 2014)
			Whole plant	Dried	Newborn wounds	(Güneş & Özhatay, 2011)
			Whole plant	Gargle	Throat inflammation	(Korkmaz & Karakurt, 2014)
Salvia suffruticosa Montbret & Aucher ex Benth.	Kalın şalba, Çay otu		Aerial parts	Tea	Unspecified	(Doğan & Tuzlacı, 2015)
			Leaves	Decoction	Wound healing	((Tuzlaci, 2016))
			Leaves	Infusion	Cold	((Tuzlaci, 2016))

continued on following page

Table 5. Continued

Botanical names*	Turkish names	Common names	Used parts	Usage forms	Uses	References
Salvia syriaca L.	Çevlikotu, Sıvsıvok, Kılkırk, Melvent, Adaçayı, Almaşık	Syrian sage	Aerial parts	Raw eaten	Gastric antacid	((Tuzlaci, 2016))
			Aerial parts	Unspecified	Child's toy	(Akan *et al.*, 2013)
			Aerial parts	Unspecified	Tea	(Akan & Balos, 2023)
			Flowers	Decoction	Infertility in women	(Karakaya *et al.*, 2019)
			Fruits	Dried	Spice	(Akgul *et al.*, 2018)
			Galls	Raw eaten	Snack	(Yeşil, Çelik, & Yılmaz, 2019)
			Roots	Cleaned and eaten or roasted and added to pilaf.	Unspecified	(Aslan, Akan, & Pekmez, 2020)
			Seeds	Unspecified	Food	(Akan & Balos, 2023)
			Whole plant	Infusion	Kidney stone	(Kültür *et al.*, 2021)
			Whole plant	Infusion, gargle	Fatigue, cough, stomach pain, antibiotics, flu, kidney stones, body resistance, throat inflammation, pharyngitis, bronchitis	(Korkmaz & Karakurt, 2015)
			Flowers, Leaves	Infusion	Anti-influenza	(Sargin, 2021)
			Flowers, Leaves	Infusion	Carminative, expectorant	(Karakaya *et al.*, 2019)
			Flowers, Leaves	Decoction, Infusion	Cold, flu	(Kılıç & Bağcı, 2013)

continued on following page

Table 5. Continued

Botanical names*	Turkish names	Common names	Used parts	Usage forms	Uses	References
Salvia tomentosa Mill.	Şalba, Çalba, Yakı otu, Ciğer otu, Rus çayı, Calba, Hava otu, Sabala, Ada çayı, Hoşaflama, Moşafla, Moşapla, yakı şalbası, sancı otu, ellik otu, kancık şalba, Boş yaprağı, Adaçayı, Şalba, Büyük Çiçekli Ada Çayı, yakı şablası	Balsamic sage	Aerial parts	Decoction	Stomach ache, diabetes	(Akyol & Altan, 2013)
			Aerial parts	Decoction	Unspecified cancer	((Tuzlaci, 2016)) (Bozyel *et al.*, 2019)
			Aerial parts	Mordanting	Yellow dye, Green dye	(Ünal & Altundağ Çakır, 2024)
			Aerial parts	Infusion	Abdominal pain	(Bulut *et al.*, 2017) (Bulut & Tuzlaci, 2015)
			Aerial parts	Infusion	Anti-inflammatory, shortness of breath, heart diseases, intestinal system activator, losing weight, antidiabetic	(Erucar, Tan, & Miski, 2023)
			Aerial parts	Infusion	Asthma	(Melikoğlu, Kurtoğlu, & Kültürr, 2015)
			Aerial parts	Infusion	Cold, abdominal pain	(Ozdemir Nath & Kultur, 2022)
			Aerial parts	Infusion	Diarrhea	(Erucar, Tan, & Miski, 2023) (Karahüseyin & Sarı, 2019)
			Aerial parts	Infusion	Head ache	(Erbay, Anil, & Melikoğlu, 2018)

continued on following page

Table 5. Continued

Botanical names*	Turkish names	Common names	Used parts	Usage forms	Uses	References
			Aerial parts	Infusion	Nerves softener, relaxant, nervousness, and tension situations	(Erucar, Tan, & Miski, 2023)
			Aerial parts	Infusion	Stomach ache	(Koyuncu *et al.*, 2010)
			Aerial parts	Infusion	Sore throat	(Bulut, Bozkurt, & Tuzlaci, 2017)
			Aerial parts	Infusion after drying	Immune-Boosting	(Sargin & Dogan, 2023)
			Aerial parts	Tea	Unspecified	(Doğan & Tuzlacı, 2015)
			Aerial parts	Oil	Asthma	(Melikoğlu, Kurtoğlu, & Kültürr, 2015)
			Aerial parts	Gargle with Infusion	Sore throat, toothache	(Erucar, Tan, & Miski, 2023)
			Aerial parts	Infusion with vaporiser	Anti-influenza	(Sargin, 2021)
			Aerial parts	Infusion with vaporiser	Asthma, bronchitis, flu, head ache, cold	(Erucar, Tan, & Miski, 2023)
			Aerial parts	Poultice with Infusion	Analgesic, rheumatism, head ache, abdominal pain, cold, sniffles, flu, bronchitis	(Erucar, Tan, & Miski, 2023)
			Aerial parts	Extract (oil), tea	Asthma, cold, wound healing	(Cinbilgel & Kurt, 2019)
			Aerial parts	Food, Tea	asthma	(Arican, Yeşil, & Ecevit Genç, 2013)
			Aerial parts	Infusion, poultice	Gastric diseases, throat, abdominal pain, spasmolytic	(Erucar, Tan, & Miski, 2023)

continued on following page

Table 5. Continued

Botanical names*	Turkish names	Common names	Used parts	Usage forms	Uses	References
			Aerial parts	Unspecified	Analgesic, antiseptic, antimicrobial, antioxidant, antiseptic, stimulant, stomachic, gas removed, tonic, vasoconstrictor in bleeding, wound healing, bronchitis, dyspepsia, febrifuge, cough, hypoglycemia, kidney stone, laryngitis, pharyngitis, uterine cancer, vaginitis	(Karahan *et al.*, 2023)
			Aerial parts	Unspecified	Kidney stone	(Kültür *et al.*, 2021)
			Aerial parts	Unspecified	Tea	(Tütenocaklı & Uysal, 2014)
			Branches	Infusion	Cold, flu	(Polat, Satil, & Çakılcıoğlu, 2011)
			Flowers	Unspecified	Acne vulgaris	(Sari & Erarslan, 2023)
			Leaves	Decoction	Cold, flu, shortness of breath, sore throat	(Kayabasi, Tümen, & Polat, 2023)
			Leaves	Infusion	Abdominal pain, appetite stimulant, colds, urinary tract disorders	(Güner & Selvi, 2016)
			Leaves	Infusion	Analgesic, antipyretic, cold treatments	(Albayrak & Daskin, 2018)
			Leaves	Infusion	Asthma	(Melikoğlu, Kurtoğlu, & Kültürr, 2015)
			Leaves	Infusion	Carminative, antiseptic, tonic, stimulant	(Ozturk, Altay, & Gönenç, 2017)
			Leaves	Infusion	Cold, flu, tonsilitis	(Polat & Satil, 2012)

continued on following page

Table 5. Continued

Botanical names*	Turkish names	Common names	Used parts	Usage forms	Uses	References
			Leaves	infusion	Cold, flu, tonsillitis, throat diseases, appetizer, dyspepsia	(Deniz, Serteser, & Kargıoğlu, 2010)
			Leaves	Infusion	Medicinal tea, cough, cold, flu, stomach pain	(Güzel & Güzelşemme, 2018)
			Leaves	Infusion	Stomach disorders, cold, upper respiratory infections	(Kalankan, Özkan, & Akbulut, 2015)
			Leaves	Infusion	Stomach ache	(Erbay, Anil, & Melikoğlu, 2017)
			Leaves	infusion	Stomachic, diuretic	(Selvi, Dağdelen, & Kara, 2013)
			Leaves	Infusion	Wound healing	(Ozdemir Nath & Kültürr, 2015)
			Leaves	Infusion, Poultice, Maseration	Unspecified	(Sargin, Akcicek, & Selvi, 2013)
			Leaves	Unspecified	Flu, cold, throat infections	(Tütenocaklı & Uysal, 2014)
			Roots	Tea	Lung diseases, kidney diseases, cramp	(Aksoy, Çelik, & Tunay, 2016)
			Shoots	Infusion	Stomach ulcer	(Kültürr *et al.*, 2018)
			Whole plant	Tea	Sedative	(Sağıroğlu & Aydın, 2024)
			Aerial parts, Leaves	Infusion, Mixture, Cataplasm, Mash, Skin bath, Gargle	Angina, bronchitis, pharyngitis and laryngitis, cold and flu, gall bladder stones, diarrhea, sedative, insomnia, carminative, costiveness and intestinal spasm, dyspepsia, pleasure and medicinal tea	(Sargin, Selvi, & López, 2015)

continued on following page

Table 5. Continued

Botanical names*	Turkish names	Common names	Used parts	Usage forms	Uses	References
			Flowers, Leaves	Infusion	Sore throat, stomach ache	(Fakir, Korkmaz, & Icel, 2016)
			Flowers, Leaves, Shoots	Decoction	Influenza, neurotic, common cold	(Karaköse, 2022)
			Flowers, Leaves, Shoots	infusion	Sore throat, antitussive, stomach cold	(Korkmaz, Fakir, & Guller, 2011)
			Flowers, Leaves, Shoots	Infusion	Sore throat, throat inflammation, antitussive, stomach cold, depression, gynaecological disease, ulcer and intestines spasm, cold, exhaustion, antitussive	(Fakir, Korkmaz, & Güller, 2009)
			Flowers, Leaves, Stems	Unspecified	Tea	(Tütenocaklı, 2023)
			Unspecified	Medical, spice	Cold	(Polat & Satil, 2012)
			Unspecified	Unspecified	Abdominal pain	(Bulut & Tuzlaci, 2009)
			Unspecified	Unspecified	General health, well-being, colds, dental health, sleep disorders	(Korkmaz & Fakir, 2009)
			Unspecified	Unspecified	Medicinal	(Satil, Akcicek & Selvi, 2008)
Salvia verbenaca L.	Elmakekiği, Şalba	Wild clary	Leaves	Infusion	Fungal infections	(Demirci & Özhatay, 2012)
			Leaves	Infusion	Respiratory tract diseases	((Tuzlaci, 2016))
			Leaves	Unspecified	Respiratory tract diseases	(Ozturk, Altay, & Gönenç, 2017)
Salvia verticillata L.	Dadırak, Dut çiçeği, Çıban otu	Whorled clary, Lilac sage	Aerial parts	Crushed	Anticoagulant, Wound healing	(Karakaya *et al.*, 2022)
			Aerial parts	Poultice	Wound healing	(Görhan & Öztürk, 2021)

continued on following page

Table 5. Continued

Botanical names*	Turkish names	Common names	Used parts	Usage forms	Uses	References
			Aerial parts	Unspecified	Catarrah, laxative, nausea, colds, stomach ache	(Terzioğlu & Coşkunçelebi, 2021)
			Flowers	Infusion	Menstrual pain	(Karakaya *et al.*, 2019)
			Leaves	Crushed	Wound healing	(Akbulut & Zengin, 2023)
			Leaves	Infusion	Anti-influenza	(Sargin, 2021)
			Leaves	Infusion	Infertility in women, menstrual pain	(Karakaya *et al.*, 2019)
			Flowers, Leaves	Tea	Unspecified	(Çalışkan, Yıldırım, Şenkardeş, 2020)
Salvia verticillata subsp. *amasiaca* (Freyn & Bornm.) Bornm.	Hart şalbası, Dadirak, Karabaş otu, Yağlıkara, Adaçayı, Kayışkıran, Dadırak, Karabaş,	Amasyan whorled clary, Lilac sage, Whorled clary	Aerial parts	Infusion	Immune-Boosting	(Sargin & Dogan, 2023)
			Aerial parts	Tea	Laxative, cold, abdominal pain, stomach ache, nausea	(Cinbilgel & Kurt, 2019)
			Aerial parts	Tea	Sedative, cold	(Erucar, Tan, & Miski, 2023)
			Aerial parts	Tea	Unspecified	(Doğan & Tuzlacı, 2015)
			Aerial parts	Unspecified	Cold, nausea, stomachic, analgesic, antimicrobial, wound healing, antioxidant, antiseptic, laxative, vasoconstrictor in bleeding, toothache	(Karahan *et al.*, 2023)
			Flowers	Honey	Immune-boosting	((Tuzlaci, 2016))
			Leaves	Infusion	Stomach ache	(Erbay, Anil, & Melikoğlu, 2017)

continued on following page

Table 5. Continued

Botanical names*	Turkish names	Common names	Used parts	Usage forms	Uses	References
			Leaves	Decoction, Infusion	Gastrointestinal disorder	(Görhan & Öztürk, 2021)
			Whole plant	Infusion	Kidney stone	(Kültür *et al.*, 2021)
			Whole plant	Infusion, gargle	Fatigue, cough, stomach pain, antibiotics, flu, kidney stones, body resistance, throat inflammation, pharyngitis, bronchitis	(Korkmaz & Karakurt, 2015)
Salvia verticillata subsp. *verticillata* L.	Dadırak, Adaçayı, Yağlıkara, Karacaabla	Whorled clary	Flowers	Honey	Immune-boosting	((Tuzlaci, 2016))
			Flowers	Unspecified	Purple dye	(Badem *et al.*, 2019)
			Leaves	Decoction	Abdominal pain	(Korkmaz & Demirkus, 2023)
			Leaves	Infusion	Cold	((Tuzlaci, 2016))
			Leaves	Unspecified	Cold, Stomach ache	(Koyuncu *et al.*, 2010)
Salvia virgata Jacq.	Fatmanaotu, Kır kekiği, Ada çayı, Ellik otu, Bares, Dağ çayı, Yılancık, Ballıbaba, Katırtırnağı, Yağlısomara, Eli kanlı, Örükleme otu	Southern meadow sage	Aerial parts	Decoction	Cold	(Korkmaz & Demirkus, 2023)
			Aerial parts	Decoction	Hemorrhoid	(Şahin & Kılıç, 2022)
			Aerial parts	Infusion	Cold, antiinflammatory	(Akan & Ayaz, 2016)
			Aerial parts	Infusion	Cold, medicinal tea, hemorrhoid	(Koyuncu *et al.*, 2010)
			Aerial parts	Infusion	Stomach cramps	(Karakaya *et al.*, 2023)
			Aerial parts	Infusion	Tea	(Şenkardeş & Tuzlacı, 2016)
			Aerial parts	Tea, Spice	Cold, hemorrhoid	(Cinbilgel & Kurt, 2019)

continued on following page

Table 5. Continued

Botanical names*	Turkish names	Common names	Used parts	Usage forms	Uses	References
			Aerial parts	Unspecified	Digestive	(Akan *et al.*, 2013)
			Aerial parts	Unspecified	Wound healing, hemorrhoid	(Terzioğlu & Coşkunçelebi, 2021)
			Leaves	Decoction	Uterus cancer	(Bozyel *et al.*, 2019)
			Leaves	Heated	Analgesic, anti-inflammatory	(Kayabaşıi, Tümen, & Polat, 2023)
			Leaves	Unspecified	Respiratory tract diseases	(Ozturk, Altay, & Gönenç, 2017)
			Leaves	Unspecified	Wound healing	(Uzun & Palabas Uzun, 2011)
			Leaves, Stems	Infusion	Heart diseases	(Güneş & Özhatay, 2011)
			Leaves, Stem barks	Powdered	Hairlessness	(Güler, Erkan, & Uğurlu, 2020)
Salvia viridis L.	Zarif şalba, Ada çayı, Adaçayı, Yeşilbaş, Çoban döşeği, Grip çayı, Çobandöşeği	Annual clary, Horminum sage	Aerial parts	Decoction	Stomach ache	(Erbay, Anıl, & Melikoğlu, 2017) (Akan, Korkut, & Balos, 2008)
			Aerial parts	Infusion	Cold, medicinal tea	(Koyuncu *et al.*, 2010)
			Aerial parts	Tea	Cold, flu	(Cinbilgel & Kurt, 2019)
			Aerial parts	Unspecified	Stomachic, constipant	(Terzioğlu & Coşkunçelebi, 2021)
			Seeds	Eaten	Stomach ache	(Erbay, Anil, & Melikoğlu, 2017)
			Whole plant	Tea	Several disorders	(Kaya, Dağlı, & Tosyagülü Çelik, 2020)
			Flowers, Leaves	Infusion	Anti-influenza	(Sargin, 2021)

continued on following page

Table 5. Continued

Botanical names*	Turkish names	Common names	Used parts	Usage forms	Uses	References
			Flowers, Leaves, Shoots	Infusion	Sore throat, throat inflammation, antitussive, stomach cold, depression, gynaecological disease, ulcer, intestines spasm, cold, exhaustion, antitussive	(Fakir, Korkmaz, & Güller, 2009)
			Unspecified	Food, Beverage, Medicinal	Unspecified	(Demirel & Dutkuner, 2021)
Salvia wiedemannii Boiss. **(End.)**	Sultantacı, Adaçayı	Anatolian lulling sage	Aerial parts	Infusion	Cold	((Tuzlaci, 2016))
			Aerial parts	Infusion	Cold, flu	(Ozturk & Altay, 2017)
			Aerial parts	Infusion	Cold, medicinal tea	(Koyuncu *et al.*, 2010)

"*" (Güner et al., 2012); "**(End.)**" Endemic taxon

Table 6. Multi-herbal formulas of the Salvia genus

Botanical names*	Turkish names	Common names	Used parts	Usage forms	Uses	References
Salvia sp. *Urtica pilulifera*	Adaçayı Dalağan	Sage Roman nettle	Leaves +Fruits	Infusion	Herniated thoracic-lumbar disc	(Bozyel, Merdamert Bozyel, & Canli, 2020)
Salvia sp. *Urtica pilulifera*	Adaçayı Dalağan	Sage Roman nettle	Leaves +Fruits	Infusion	Lower back pain	(Bozyel, Bozyel, & Canli, 2020)
Salvia sp. *Juniperus foetidissima* *J. oxycedrus* *Agropyron* sp.	Adaçayı Kokar ardıç Katran ardıcı Otlakayrığı	Sage Foetid juniper Western prickly juniper Wheatgrass	Aerial parts +Fruits +Fruits +Aerial parts	Decoction	Stomach ache, diabetes, vasodilator, tonic, vaginal white discharge	(Sargın & Büyükcengiz, 2019)
Salvia sp. *Juniperus foetidissima* *J. oxycedrus* *Agropyron* sp.	Adaçayı Kokar ardıç Katran ardıcı Otlakayrığı	Sage Foetid juniper Western prickly juniper Wheatgrass	Aerial parts +Resin +Fruits +Aerial parts	Mash, cataplasm, decoction	Gastro-intestinal pains, vaginal white discharge	(Sargın & Büyükcengiz, 2019)
Salvia absconditiflora *Thymus sipyleus* *Cota austriaca*	Kara şalba Sipilkekiği Babuçça	Turkish black sage Sipylos thyme Austrian chamomile	Aerial parts +Aerial parts +Capitula	Infusion	Tea	(Şenkardeş & Tuzlacı, 2016)

continued on following page

Table 6. Continued

Botanical names*	Turkish names	Common names	Used parts	Usage forms	Uses	References
Salvia absconditiflora *Anthemis fumarifolia*** *Astragalus lycius*** *Medicago rigidula* var. *rigidula* *Thymus sipyleus*	Kara şalba Çorak papatyası Bozkırmumu Kabayonca Sipilkekiği	Turkish black sage Noname Noname Tifton bur-clover Sipylos thyme	Aerial parts +Capitula +Flowering parts +Aerial parts +Aerial parts	Infusion	Cough, asthma, urethritis, expectorant	(Tuzlacı & Şenkardeş, 2011)
Salvia absconditiflora *Anthemis fumarifolia*** *Astragalus lycius*** *Medicago rigidula* var. *rigidula* *Thymus sipyleus*	Kara şalba Çorak papatyası Bozkırmumu Kabayonca Sipilkekiği	Turkish black sage Noname Noname Tifton bur-clover Sipylos thyme	Aerial parts +Capitula +Flowering parts +Aerial parts +Aerial parts	Infusion	Urethritis	((Tuzlaci, 2016))
Salvia aethiopis *Abies nordmanniana* subsp. *equi-trojani***	Habeş adaçayı Kazdağı göknarı	Mediterranean sage Trojan fir	Roots +Resin	Decoction with butter and beeswax	Cut and wound healing	((Tuzlaci, 2016))
Salvia candidissima subsp. *candidissima* *Origanum vulgare* subsp. *gracile*	Galabor Kuşzemulu	Eastern blazing white sage Russian oregano	Leaves +Aerial parts	Infusion with honey	Stomach ache	((Tuzlaci, 2016))
Salvia fruticosa *Malus pumila*	Adaçayı Elma	Turkish sage Apple	Leaves +Vinegar	Decoction and mixed (vinegar)	Sore throat	(Boz, İldeniz, & Cabi, 2022)
Salvia fruticosa *Quercus* sp. *Punica granatum*	Adaçayı Meşe Nar	Turkish sage Oak Pomegranate	Leaves +Galls powder +Young stems and cortex	Boiled with wool yarns of handmade carpet	Red dye	(Ozdemir Nath & Kültürr, 2015)
Salvia fruticosa *Thymus longicaulis* *Matricaria chamomilla*	Adaçayı Dağkekiği Alman papatyası	Turkish sage Thyme Scented mayweed	Leaves +Aerial parts +Flowers	Decoction	Medicinal tea	(Boz, İldeniz, & Cabi, 2022)
Salvia fruticosa *Juglans regia* *Quercus* sp. *Rubia tinctorum* *Rhus coriaria*	Adaçayı Ceviz Meşe Kökboyası Sumak	Turkish sage Persian walnut Oak Madder Tanner's sumac	Leaves +Roots +Galls +Roots +Fruits	Boiled with wool yarns of handmade carpet	Brown dye, black dye	(Ozdemir Nath & Kültürr, 2015)
Salvia fruticosa *Thymus longicaulis* *Citrus limon* *Rosmarinus officinalis* *Rosa canina*	Adaçayı Dağkekiği Limon Biberiye Kuşburnu	Turkish sage Thyme Lemon Rosemary Dog-Rose	Leaves +Aerial parts +Fruits +Aerial parts +Fruits	Decoction	Dyspnea	(Boz, İldeniz, & Cabi, 2022)

continued on following page

Table 6. Continued

Botanical names*	Turkish names	Common names	Used parts	Usage forms	Uses	References
Salvia hydrangea *Urtica dioica* *Malva neglecta*	Koç şalba Isırgan Çobançöreği	Noname Common netle Dwarf mallow	Flowering branches +Leaves +Aerial parts	Infusion	Menstrual pain	((Tuzlaci, 2016))
Salvia officinalis *Tilia* sp. *Teucrium* sp. *Urtica* sp. *Thymus* sp.	Tıbbi adaçayı Ihlamur Kısamahmut Isırgan Kekik	Garden sage Lime Woodsage Nettle Thyme	Aerial parts +Flowers +Flowers +Flowers +Leaves	Infusion with honey	Immune-boosting	(Sargin & Dogan, 2023)
Salvia officinalis *Sambucus nigra* *Melissa officinalis* *Piper nigrum* *Zingiber officinale*	Tıbbi adaçayı Ağaç mürver Oğulotu Karabiber Zencefil	Garden sage Elder Lemon balm Balck pepper Ginger	Aerial parts +Flowers or Fruits +Leaves +Fruits +Tubers	Infusion	Immune-boosting	(Sargin & Dogan, 2023)
Salvia tomentosa *Mentha* sp.	Şalba Nane	Balsamic sage Mint	Aerial Parts +Aerial parts	Infusion (foot bath)	Bad odor and sweating of foot or body	(Erucar, Tan, & Miski, 2023)
Salvia tomentosa *Citrus limon*	Şalba Limon	Balsamic sage Lemon	Aerial parts +Peel (dried together)	Infusion	Head ache, abdominal pain, cold, sniffles, flu, bronchitis	(Erucar, Tan, & Miski, 2023)
Salvia tomentosa *Helleborus orientalis*	Şalba Çöpleme	Balsamic sage Lenten-rose	Aerial parts +Roots	Decoction (Bath)	Rheumatism	((Tuzlaci, 2016))
Salvia tomentosa *Petroselinum crispum*	Şalba Maydanoz	Balsamic sage Garden parsley	Aerial parts +Aerial parts	Infusion	Gallbladder stones	(Erucar, Tan, & Miski, 2023)
Salvia tomentosa *Thymus* sp. *Allium sativum*	Şalba Kekik Sarmısak	Balsamic sage Thyme Garlic	Aerial parts +Aerial parts +Cloves	Infusion/Poultice	Hair loss	(Erucar, Tan, & Miski, 2023)
Salvia tomentosa *Tilia tomentosa*	Şalba Gümüşi ıhlamur	Balsamic sage Silver lime	Aerial parts +Flowers	Infusion	Prophylactic, immune-boosting	((Tuzlaci, 2016))
Salvia tomentosa *Tilia tomentosa* *Teucrium polium* *Urtica dioica* *Thymus longicaulis*	Şalba Gümüşi ıhlamur Acıyavşan Isırgan Dağkekiği	Balsamic sage Silver lime Felty germander Common netle Thyme	Aerial parts +Flowers +Flowers +Flowers +Leaves	Infusion with honey	Immune-boosting	(Sargin & Dogan, 2023)
Salvia tomentosa *Origanum vulgare* *Cistus laurifolius* *Populus alba* *Reseda lutea*	Adaçayı Karakınık Karağan Ak kavak Muhabbetçiçeği	Balsamic sage Wild marjoram Laurel-leaved cistus White poplar Wild mignonette	Aerial parts +Aerial parts +Aerial parts + Sprouts + Aerial parts	Mordanting	Yellow dye	(Ünal & Altundağ Çakır, 2024)

"*" (182); "**(End.)" Endemic taxon

5. CONCLUSION

The intricate relationship between plants and humans represents a profound and enduring aspect of human history, influencing cultural, economic, and health-related facets of life. The utilization of plant resources has been instrumental in fulfilling a myriad of human needs, including sustenance, medicinal compounds, shelter, energy, textiles, and personal care products such as perfumes and cosmetics. The transfer of knowledge regarding these botanical applications has been facilitated through oral traditions and written records, transcending generations and cultures.

In contemporary discourse, there is a marked increase in interest in plant-derived pharmaceuticals, driven by a heightened awareness of the adverse effects commonly associated with synthetic drugs. This burgeoning field, referred to as ethnopharmacology, is dedicated to investigating the potential of plants as sources of novel medicinal compounds. This interest has culminated in the introduction of numerous innovative pharmaceuticals into the market.

The therapeutic efficacy of herbal remedies is significantly underpinned by the presence of secondary metabolites, which play a crucial role in their pharmacological activities. This study endeavors to provide a comprehensive analysis of the *Salvia* genus, with a focus on its secondary metabolites, associated biological activities, and traditional medicinal applications. The research findings provide compelling evidence that various species of *Salvia* demonstrate significant therapeutic properties, including marked antioxidant, antimicrobial, cytotoxic, and anti-HIV activities.

REFERENCES

Abu-Izneid, T., Rauf, A., Shariati, M. A., Khalil, A. A., Imran, M., Rebezov, M., Uddin, M. S., Mahomoodally, M. F., & Rengasamy, K. R. R. (2020). Sesquiterpenes and their derivatives-natural anticancer compounds: An update. *Pharmacological Research, 161*, 105165. DOI: 10.1016/j.phrs.2020.105165 PMID: 32835868

Akan, H., & Ayaz, H. (2016). The flora and ethnobotany of Gölpınar (Şanlıurfa-Turkey) promenade place and its surroundings. *Bağbahçe Scientific Journal*, *2*(3), 19–56.

Akan, H., Aydoğdu, M., Korkut, M. M., & Balos, M. M. (2013). An ethnobotanical research of the Kalecik mountain area Şanlıurfa, South-East Anatolia. *Biological Diversity and Conservation*, *6*(2), 84–90.

Akan, H., & Bakır Sade, Y. (2015). Investigation of the ethnobotanical aspects of the town Kâhta and village of Narince. *BEU Journal of Science*, *4*(2), 219–248.

Akan, H., & Balos, M. M. (2023). An ethnobotanical investigation on wild edible plants of Karaköprü (Şanlıurfa). *International Journal of Life Science and Biotechnology*, *6*(1), 61–81. DOI: 10.38001/ijlsb.1246913

Akan, H., Korkut, M. M., & Balos, M. M. (2008). An ethnobotanical study around Arat Mountain and its surroundings (Birecik, Şanlıurfa). *Fırat University Journal of Science and Engineering*, *20*(1), 67–81.

Akan, H., Öz, A., & Pekmez, H. (2018). Some of the plant species used among the local people in Ortaca (Muğla). *Turkish Journal of Agriculture - Food Science and Technology*, *6*(9), 1168–1174. DOI: 10.24925/turjaf.v6i9.1168-1174.1981

Akbaş, K., Çıtakoğlu, M., & Davran, S. (2024). Natural plants of the Sandras Mountain (Köyceğiz-Muğla) traditionally employed for therapeutic purposes. *Turkish Journal of Forestry*, *25*(1), 32–40. DOI: 10.18182/tjf.1380456

Akbulut, S. (2021). Medicinal plants preferences for the treatment of COVID-19 symptoms in Central and Eastern Anatolia. *Kastamonu Üniversitesi Orman Fakültesi Dergisi*, *21*(3), 196–207. DOI: 10.17475/kastorman.1048372

Akbulut, S., & Bayramoglu, M. M. (2013). The trade and use of some medical and aromatic herbs in Turkey. *Studies on Ethno-Medicine*, *7*(2), 67–77. DOI: 10.1080/09735070.2013.11886446

Akbulut, S., & Karaköse, M. (2023). An ethnobotanical investigation in Adıyaman (Türkiye). *Journal of Düzce University Botanical Garden and Ornamental Medicinal Plants*, *2*(2), 1–12.

Akbulut, S., Karaköse, M., & Özkan, Z. C. (2019). Traditional uses of some wild plants in Kale and Acıpayam provinces in Denizli. *Kastamonu Üniversitesi Orman Fakültesi Dergisi*, *19*(1), 72–81. DOI: 10.17475/kastorman.543529

Akbulut, S., & Özkan, Z. (2023). Medicinal and aromatic plants use preference against COVID-19 symptoms in Northern Anatolia. *Artvin Çoruh University Journal of Forest Faculty*, *24*(1), 87–95.

Akbulut, S., & Zengin, Z. (2023). Ethnobotanical survey of wild plants used in Gümüşhane province (Turkey). *Boletín Latinoamericano y del Caribe de Plantas Medicinales y Aromáticas*, *22*(2), 237–254. DOI: 10.37360/blacpma.23.22.2.18

Akgul, A., Akgul, A., Senol, S. G., Yildirim, H., Secmen, O., & Dogan, Y. (2018). An ethnobotanical study in Midyat (Turkey), a city on the silk road where cultures meet. *Journal of Ethnobiology and Ethnomedicine*, *14*(1), 1–18. DOI: 10.1186/s13002-017-0201-8 PMID: 29415748

Aksoy, A., Çelik, J., & Tunay, H. (2016). Some plants which are used and sold by the folk in the Bazaar at Gazipaşa (Antalya) district and intended use of them. *Research Journal of Biological Sciences*, *9*(2), 55–61.

Akyol, Y., & Altan, Y. (2013). Ethnobotanical studies in the Maldan Village (Province Manisa, Turkey). *Marmara Pharmaceutical Journal*, *17*(1), 21–25. DOI: 10.12991/201317388

Albayrak, N. B., & Daşkın, R. (2018). Medicinal plants used in Orhaneli and Büyükorhan Districts (Bursa–Northwest Anatolia). *Phytologia Balcanica*, *24*(3), 381–388.

Alkış, A. N., Parmaksız, A., & Akan, H. (2021). Investigation of medicinal plants used for weight loss in herbal markets of Şanlıurfa, birthplace of Abraham, Turkey. *Journal of Medicinal Plants Studies*, *9*(2), 48–58. DOI: 10.22271/plants.2021.v9.i2a.1262

Altay, V., & Çelik, O. (2011). Investigation of some natural plants at the neighborhood markets of Antakya in terms of ethnobotanic. *Research Journal of Biological Sciences*, *4*(2), 137–139. DOI: 10.3923/rjbsci.2011.137.139

Altay, V., & Karahan, F. (2017). Medicinal plants used to sunstroke and sunburn treatment in Anatolian traditional medicine. *Erzincan University Journal of Science and Technology*, *10*(1), 124–137.

Altay, V., Karahan, F., Sarcan, Y. B., & İlçim, A. (2015). An ethnobotanical research on wild plants sold in Kırıkhan district Hatay/Turkey herbalists and local markets. *Biological Diversity and Conservation*, *8*(2), 81–91. DOI: 10.1075/bdc.8.2.03a

Altundağ Çakır, E. (2017). Traditional knowledge of wild edible plants of Iğdır Province (East Anatolia, Turkey). *Acta Societatis Botanicorum Poloniae*, *86*(4), 3568. DOI: 10.5586/asbp.3568

Arican, Y. E., Yeşil, Y., & Ecevit Genç, G. (2013). A preliminary ethnobotanical survey of Kumluca (Antalya). *Journal of the Faculty of Pharmacy. Istanbul University*, *43*(2), 95–102.

Arıtuluk, Z. C., & Ezer, N. (2012). Halk arasında diyabete karşı kullanılan bitkiler Türkiye-II. *Hacettepe University Journal of the Faculty of Pharmacy*, *2*, 179–208.

Aslan, M. (2018). Medical and aromatic plants and their usage in Şanlıurfa province center. *European Journal of Natural Sciences*, *2*(5), 113–120.

Aslan, S., Akan, H., & Pekmez, H. (2020). The ethnobotanical investigation of Yaslıca town and Arıkök neighborhood (Şanlıurfa/Turkey). *Biological Diversity and Conservation*, *13*(1), 44–61. DOI: 10.46309/biodicon.2020.730293

Badem, M., Korkmaz, N., Sener, S. O., Kanbolat, S., Ozgen, U., Sevgi, S., Aliyazicioglu, R., & Coskun, M. (2019). Biological screening of traditional medicinal plants from villages of Akkuş (Ordu) in Turkey on the effects of tyrosinase. *Journal of Pharmaceutical Research International*, *25*(6), 1–10. DOI: 10.9734/jpri/2018/v25i630118

Bağcı, Y., Dural, H., & Savran, A. (2006). Ethnobotanical aspects of some species in Pozantı (Adana) and its vicinity. *Selcuk University Journal of Science Faculty*, *2*(27), 77–82.

Başer, K. H. C., Tümen, G., Malyer, H., & Kirimer, N. (2006). Plants used for common cold in Turkey. In *Proceedings of the IVth International Congress of Ethnobotany (ICEB 2005)* (pp. 133-137).

Baykan, S., Ozturk, B., Sahin, B., & Senol, S. G. (2023). Ethnobotanical study of medicinal plants in Nemrut Mountain, Adiyaman-Turkey. *Journal of Research in Pharmacy*, *27*(6), 2250–2269. DOI: 10.29228/jrp.514

Baytop, T. (1999). *Türkiye'de bitkiler ile tedavi: Geçmişte ve bugün*. Nobel Tıp Kitabevleri.

Berber, İ., Avşar, C., Çine, N., Bozkurt, N., & Elmas, E. (2013). Determination of antibacterial and antifungal activities of methanolic extracts of some plants growing in Sinop. *Karaelmas Science & Engineering Journal*, *3*, 10–16. DOI: 10.7212/zkufbd.v3i1.87

Boz, E., İldeniz, H. K., & Cabi, E. (2022). Some ethnobotanical information from Gönen (Balıkesir) District. *Acta Biologica Turcica*, *35*(4), 1–17.

Bozyel, M. E., Bozyel, E. M., & Canli, K. (2020). Turkish herbal medicine in the treatment of back pain. In *Ethnomedicinal Plant Use and Practice in Traditional Medicine* (pp. 235–251). IGI Global. DOI: 10.4018/978-1-7998-1320-0.ch012

Bozyel, M. E., Canli, K., Benek, A., Simsek, O., Akata, I., & Altuner, E. M. (2023). Biochemical composition, and in vitro antimicrobial and antioxidant activities of *Salvia fruticosa*, an ethnomedicinal plant. *Applied Ecology and Environmental Research*, *21*(4), 3243–3256. DOI: 10.15666/aeer/2104_32433256

Bozyel, M. E., Merdamert Bozyel, E., Canlı, E., & Altuner, E. M. (2019). Anticancer uses of medicinal plants in Turkish traditional medicine. *Kahramanmaras Sütçü Imam Üniversitesi Tarim ve Doga Dergisi*, *22*(Suppl 2), 465–484. DOI: 10.18016/ksutarimdoga.vi.550334

Bozyel, M. E., Merdamert Bozyel, E., & Canli, K. (2020). Ethnobotanical uses of medicinal plants for the treatment of herniated disc in Turkish traditional medicine. In *Ethnomedicinal Plant Use and Practice in Traditional Medicine* (pp. 221–234). IGI Global. DOI: 10.4018/978-1-7998-1320-0.ch011

Bulut, G., Bozkurt, M. Z., & Tuzlacı, E. (2017). The preliminary ethnobotanical study of medicinal plants in Uşak (Turkey). *Marmara Pharmaceutical Journal*, *21*(2), 305–310. DOI: 10.12991/marupj.300795

Bulut, G., Haznedaroğlu, M. Z., Doğan, A., Koyu, H., & Tuzlacı, E. (2017). An ethnobotanical study of medicinal plants in Acipayam (Denizli-Turkey). *Journal of Herbal Medicine*, *10*, 64–81. DOI: 10.1016/j.hermed.2017.08.001

Bulut, G., & Tuzlacı, E. (2009). Folk medicinal plants of Bayramiç (Çanakkale-Turkey). *Journal of the Faculty of Pharmacy. Istanbul University*, *40*, 87–99.

Bulut, G., & Tuzlacı, E. (2015). An ethnobotanical study of medicinal plants in Bayramiç. *Marmara Pharmaceutical Journal*, *19*(3), 268–282. DOI: 10.12991/mpj.201519392830

Cakilcioglu, U., Turkoglu, I., & Kürşat, M. (2007). Ethnobotanical features of Harput (Elazig) and its vicinity. *Research in the East Anatolian Region*, *5*(2), 22–28.

Çakır, D., & Akan, H. (2023). A review on medicinal plants used for women's diseases and health in Anatolia (Turkey). *International Journal of Natural Life Sciences*, *7*(2), 36–54. DOI: 10.47947/ijnls.1329378

Çalışkan, G., Yıldırım, G., & Şenkardeş, İ. (2020). A study on herbs used in food in Rize province within the context of gastronomy tourism. *Journal of Social and Humanities Sciences Research*, *7*(51), 573–583.

Celik, B., & Yesil, Y. (2020). An ethnobotanical study in Pöhrenk village (Çiçekdağı-Kırşehir province/Turkey). *Istanbul Journal of Pharmacy*, *50*(2), 131–141. DOI: 10.26650/IstanbulJPharm.2019.0072

Çinbilgel, İ., & Kurt, Y. (2019). A research on species diversity and ethnobotanical utilization of Lamiaceae family in Southern Turkey. *Süleyman Demirel University Journal of Natural and Applied Sciences*, *23*(1), 90–107.

Çömlekçioğlu, N., & Karaman, Ş. (2008). The medicinal plants found in the local herbal markets in the city of Kahramanmaras in Turkey. *KSU Journal of Science and Engineering*, *11*(1), 23–32.

Dat, N. T., Jin, X., Lee, J. H., Lee, D., Hong, Y. S., Lee, K., Kim, J., & Lee, J. J. (2007). Abietane diterpenes from *Salvia miltiorrhiza* inhibit the activation of hypoxia-inducible factor-1. *Journal of Natural Products*, *70*(7), 1093–1097. DOI: 10.1021/np060482d PMID: 17583950

Demir, İ., & Ayaz, N. (2022). Wild edible plants contributing to the traditional foods of Mardin (Turkey) Province. *Indian Journal of Traditional Knowledge*, *21*(3), 569–582.

Demirci, S., & Özhatay, N. (2012). An ethnobotanical study in Kahramanmaraş (Turkey); wild plants used for medicinal purposes in Andirin, Kahramanmaraş. *Turkish Journal of Pharmaceutical Sciences*, *9*(1), 75–92. DOI: 10.4274/tjps.31992

Demirci Kayıran, S. (2019). Dioscorides'in *De Materia Medica* adlı eserindeki tıbbi bitkilerin Doğu Akdeniz'de günümüzdeki kullanımlarının araştırılması. *Mersin University Medical Faculty Lokman Hekim Medical History and Folk Medicine Journal*, *9*(2), 189–202.

Demirel, O., & Dutkuner, İ. (2021). A study of ethnobotany in Sütçüler (Isparta). In *International Aegean Symposiums on Innovation Technologies & Engineering-IV (September 11-12, 2021)Proceedings Book* (pp. 19–37).

Deniz, L., Serteser, A., & Kargıoğlu, M. (2010). Local names and ethnobotanical features of some plants in Usak University (Usak) and its near vicinity. *Afyon Kocatepe University Journal of Science and Engineering*, *1*, 57–72.

Doğan, A., & Tuzlacı, E. (2015). Wild edible plants of Pertek (Tunceli-Turkey). *Marmara Pharmaceutical Journal, 19*(2), 126–135. DOI: 10.12991/mpj.20151910459

Doğan, G., & Bağcı, E. (2011). The plants benefiting the public in some residential areas of Elazığ (Turkey) using traditional ecological knowledge and their ethnobotanical features. *Fırat University Journal of Science, 23*(2), 77–86.

Doğan, Y., & Ugulu, I. (2013). Medicinal plants used for gastrointestinal disorders in some districts of Izmir province, Turkey. *Studies on Ethno-Medicine, 7*(3), 149–161. DOI: 10.1080/09735070.2013.11886456

Don, M. J., Shen, C. C., Lin, Y. L., Syu, W. J., Ding, Y. H., & Sun, C. M. (2005). Nitrogen-containing compounds from *Salvia miltiorrhiza.Journal of Natural Products, 68*(7), 1066–1070. DOI: 10.1021/np0500934 PMID: 16038550

Don, M. J., Shen, C. C., Syu, W. J., Ding, Y. H., & Sun, C. M. (2006). Cytotoxic and aromatic constituents from *Salvia miltiorrhiza.Phytochemistry, 67*(5), 497–503. DOI: 10.1016/j.phytochem.2005.11.005 PMID: 16368119

Ekren, E., & Çorbacı, Ö. L. (2021). A study on ethnobotanical possibility of uses: The example of Rize urban open green spaces. *Journal of Anatolian Environment and Animal Science, 6*(4), 487–497.

Eksik, C., & Akan, H. (2021). Ethnobotanical evaluation of some plants used by indigenous people in rural villages of Mardin. *Bağbahçe Science Journal, 8*(3), 97–130.

Eminağaoğlu, Ö., Göktürk, T., & Akyıldırım Beğen, H. (2017). Traditional uses of medicinal plants and animals of Hatila Valley National Park, Artvin. *Biological Diversity and Conservation, 10*(3), 33–42.

Er, M., Tugay, O., Özcan, M. M., Ulukuş, D., & Al-Juhaimi, F. (2013). Biochemical properties of some *Salvia* L. species. *Environmental Monitoring and Assessment, 185*(6), 5193–5198. DOI: 10.1007/s10661-012-2935-z PMID: 23064852

Erbay, M. Ş., Anıl, S., & Melikoğlu, G. (2017). Plants used as painkillers in folk medicine in Turkey-I Stomachache. *Marmara Pharmaceutical Journal, 21*(4), 741–755. DOI: 10.12991/mpj.2017.0

Erbay, M. Ş., Anıl, S., & Melikoğlu, G. (2018). Plants used as painkiller in traditional treatment in Turkey-II headache. *Marmara Pharmaceutical Journal, 22*(1), 29–36. DOI: 10.12991/mpj.2018.37

Erbay, M. Ş., & Sarı, A. (2018). Plants used in traditional treatment against hemorrhoids in Turkey. *Marmara Pharmaceutical Journal*, *22*(2), 110–132. DOI: 10.12991/mpj.2018.49

Ergül Bozkurt, A. (2024). Therapeutic uses of the medicinal plants growing in the villages of Yakutiye district, Erzurum, Türkiye. *Journal of Herbal Medicine*, *44*, 100853. DOI: 10.1016/j.hermed.2024.100853

Erucar, F. M., Tan, N., & Miski, M. (2023). Ethnobotanical records of medicinal plants of Turkey effective on stress management compiled with the literature survey in their chemical content and activities. *Records of Natural Products*, *17*(1), 1–92. DOI: 10.25135/rnp.324.2203.2372

Fakir, H., Korkmaz, M., & Güller, B. (2009). Medicinal plant diversity of the western Mediterranean region in Turkey. *Journal of Applied Biological Sciences*, *3*(2), 33–43.

Fakir, H., Korkmaz, M., & Icel, B. (2016). Medicinal plants traditionally used for pain alleviation in Antalya province, Turkey. *Studies on Ethno-Medicine*, *10*(3), 314–324. DOI: 10.1080/09735070.2016.11905503

Görhan, K. Ö., & Öztürk, F. (2021). Ethnopharmacological survey of medicinal and foods plants in Derecik (Hakkari-Turkey). *Indian Journal of Traditional Knowledge*, *20*(2), 416–425.

Gulec, M., Erarslan, Z. B., & Kultur, S. (2023). The medicinal plants traditionally used against cardiovascular diseases in Türkiye. *International Journal of Traditional and Complementary Medicine Research*, *4*(2), 81–96. DOI: 10.53811/ijtcmr.1232190

Güler, B., Erkan, Y., & Uğurlu, E. (2020). Traditional uses and ecological resemblance of medicinal plants in two districts of the Western Aegean Region (Turkey). *Environment, Development and Sustainability*, *22*(3), 2099–2120. DOI: 10.1007/s10668-018-0279-8

Güler, B., Kümüştekin, G., & Uğurlu, E. (2015). Contribution to the traditional uses of medicinal plants of Turgutlu (Manisa–Turkey). *Journal of Ethnopharmacology*, *176*, 102–108. DOI: 10.1016/j.jep.2015.10.023 PMID: 26494509

Güler, B., Manav, E., & Uğurlu, E. (2015). Medicinal plants used by traditional healers in Bozüyük (Bilecik–Turkey). *Journal of Ethnopharmacology*, *173*, 39–47. DOI: 10.1016/j.jep.2015.07.007 PMID: 26188219

Güner, A., Aslan, S., Ekim, T., Vural, M., & Babaç, M. T. (Eds.). (2012). *Türkiye Bitkileri Listesi (Damarlı Bitkiler)*. Nezahat Gökyiğit Botanik Bahçesi ve Flora Araştırmaları Derneği Yayını.

Güner, Ö., & Selvi, S. (2016). Wild medicinal plants sold in Balıkesir/Turkey herbal markets and their usage properties. *Biological Diversity and Conservation*, *9*(2), 96–101.

Güneş, F., & Özhatay, N. (2011). An ethnobotanical study from Kars eastern Turkey. *Biological Diversity and Conservation*, *4*(1), 30–41.

Güzel, Y., & Güzelşemme, M. (2018). Wild plants used as herbal tea in Antakya and Defne provinces of Hatay. *Anadolu Journal of Aegean Agricultural Research Institute*, *28*(1), 1–5.

Güzel, Y., & Kayıkçı, S. (2023). Traditional foraged spice, sauce, and egg-painting plants of Hatay, Türkiye: Bringing the traditional into commerce. *Anadolu Ege Tarimsal Arastirma Enstitüsü Dergisi*, *33*(2), 237–258. DOI: 10.18615/anadolu.1300161

Han, M. İ., & Bulut, G. (2015). The folk-medicinal plants of Kadişehri (Yozgat-Turkey). *Acta Societatis Botanicorum Poloniae*, *84*(2), 237–248. DOI: 10.5586/asbp.2015.021

Hayta, S., Polat, R., & Selvi, S. (2014). Traditional uses of medicinal plants in Elazığ (Turkey). *Journal of Ethnopharmacology*, *154*(3), 613–623. DOI: 10.1016/j.jep.2014.04.026 PMID: 24793217

Horiuchi, K., Shiota, S., Hatano, T., Yoshida, T., Kuroda, T., & Tsuchiya, T. (2007). Antimicrobial activity of oleanolic acid from *Salvia officinalis* and related compounds on vancomycin-resistant enterococci (VRE). *Biological & Pharmaceutical Bulletin*, *30*(6), 1147–1149. DOI: 10.1248/bpb.30.1147 PMID: 17541170

Hussein, A. A., Meyer, J. J., Jimeno, M. L., & Rodríguez, B. (2007). Bioactive diterpenes from *Orthosiphon labiatus* and *Salvia africana-lutea*.*Journal of Natural Products*, *70*(2), 293–295. DOI: 10.1021/np0680376 PMID: 17256988

IARC Working Group on the Evaluation of the Carcinogenic Risk of Chemicals to Humans. (1980). *IARC monographs: Supplement (No. 2-4)*. International Agency for Research on Cancer.

Janicsák, G., Hohmann, J., Zupkó, I., Forgó, P., Rédei, D., & Falkay, G.. (2003). Diterpenes from the aerial parts of *Salvia candelabrum* and their protective effects against lipid peroxidation. *Planta Medica*, *69*(12), 1156–1159. DOI: 10.1055/s-2003-818010 PMID: 14750036

Kabouche, A., Kabouche, Z., Öztürk, M., Kolak, U., & Topçu, G. (2007). Antioxidant abietane diterpenoids from *Salvia barrelieri*.*Food Chemistry*, *102*(4), 1281–1287. DOI: 10.1016/j.foodchem.2006.07.021

Kalankan, G., Özkan, Z. C., & Akbulut, S. (2015). Medicinal and aromatic wild plants and traditional usage of them in Mount Ida (Balıkesir/Turkey). *Journal of Applied Biological Sciences*, *9*(3), 25–33.

Karahan, F., Ozyigit, I. I., Yalcin, I. E., Hocaoglu-Ozyigit, A., Erkencioglu, B. N., & Ilcim, A. (2023). Concentrations of plant mineral nutrients and potentially toxic elements in some medicinal plants in the Asteraceae, Fabaceae, and Lamiaceae families from Southern Turkey: Insights into health implications. *Spectroscopy Letters*, *56*(2), 103–128. DOI: 10.1080/00387010.2023.2181358

Karahüseyin, S., & Sarı, A. (2019). Plants used in traditional treatment against diarrhea in Turkey. *Istanbul Journal of Pharmacy*, *49*(1), 33–44. DOI: 10.26650/IstanbulJPharm.2019.404211

Karakaya, S., Kimişoğlu, Z., Aksakal, Ö., Sümbüllü, Y. Z., İncekara, Ü., & Polat, A. (2023). Plants used in digestive system diseases in traditional medicine (Ardahan, Iğdır, and Kars): Cross-sectional study. *Journal of Traditional Medicine and Complementary Therapies*, *6*(2), 96–104. DOI: 10.5336/jtracom.2023-95342

Karakaya, S., Kımışoğlu, Z., Yılmaz, S. V., Aksakal, Ö., Sümbüllü, Y. Z., İncekara, Ü., & Polat, A. (2022). Traditional medicinal plants used in dermatologic disorders in Ardahan, Iğdır, and Kars. *Sakarya University Journal of Science*, *26*(6), 1142–1158. DOI: 10.16984/saufenbilder.1133853

Karakaya, S., Polat, A., Aksakal, Ö., Sümbüllü, Y. Z., & İncekara, Ü. (2019). Plants used in traditional medicine and other uses in the south of Erzurum (Turkey): An ethnobotanical study. *Ethnobotany Research and Applications*, *18*, 1–18. DOI: 10.32859/era.18.13.1-18

Karaköse, M. (2022). An ethnobotanical study of medicinal plants in Güce district, north-eastern Turkey. *Plant Diversity*, *44*(6), 577–597. DOI: 10.1016/j.pld.2022.03.005 PMID: 36540712

Karaman, Ö., & Elgin Cebe, G. (2016). Diabetes and antidiabetic plants used in Turkey. *Journal of the Faculty of Pharmacy. Ankara University*, *40*(3), 47–61.

Karcı, E., Gürbüz, İ., Akaydın, G., & Günbatan, T. (2017). Folk medicines of Bafra (Samsun-Turkey). *Türk Biyokimya Dergisi*, *42*(4), 381–399. DOI: 10.1515/tjb-2017-0172

Kavaklı, S. A., Kaya, Ö., & Ugurlu, E. (2020). Some medicinal-aromatic plants sold in Eskişehir folk bazaars and usage areas. *Tree and Forest*, *1*(1), 1–11.

Kavaklı, S. A., Yaylacı, Ş. G., & Ugurlu, E. (2020). Some medicinal aromatic plants sold by Kastamonu herbalists and usage areas. *Journal of Institute of Science and Technology*, *10*(4), 2962–2974.

Kaya, A. (2024). Lamiaceae familyasının tüy morfolojisi. *Journal of Faculty of Pharmacy. Ankara University*, *48*(3), 34.

Kaya, Ö. F., Dağlı, M., & Tosyagülü Çelik, H. (2020). An ethnobotanical research in Şanlıurfa central district and attached villages (Turkey). *Indian Journal of Traditional Knowledge*, *19*(1), 7–23.

Kayabaşı, N. P., Tümen, G., & Polat, R. (2023). Ethnobotanical study on the medicinal plants in the Manyas province (Balıkesir, Turkey). *Indian Journal of Traditional Knowledge*, *22*(1), 83–91.

Kılıç, Ö., & Bağcı, E. (2013). An ethnobotanical survey of some medicinal plants in Keban (Elazığ-Turkey). *Journal of Medicinal Plants Research*, *7*(23), 1675–1684.

Kincal, S., Ceylan, O., & Görk, G. (2021). Ethnobotanical features of Ula (Muğla/Turkey) district. *Biological Diversity and Conservation*, *14*(1), 69–81. DOI: 10.46309/biodicon.2021.768665

Kocabas, Y. Z., Erol, A., & Aktolun, O. (2017). Medicinal plants of flora of KSU Avsar campus (Kahramanmaras) and surrounding areas. *Aksaray University Journal of Science and Engineering*, *1*(2), 110–120. DOI: 10.29002/asujse.306972

Korkmaz, E., & Demirkuş, N. (2023). Ethnobotanical therapeutic features of some plants of the vicinity of Bahçesaray (Müküs) in the province of Van/Turkey. *GSC Advanced Research and Reviews*, *15*(3), 178–192. DOI: 10.30574/gscarr.2023.15.3.0231

Korkmaz, M., & Fakir, H. (2009). Determination of final consumer characteristics of non-wood forest products (A case study for Isparta city). *Süleyman Demirel University Faculty of Forestry Journal*, *10*(2), 10–20.

Korkmaz, M., Fakir, H., & Guller, B. (2011). Consumer preferences for medicinal and aromatic plant products: Surveys of urban consumers and sellers in western Mediterranean region of Turkey. *Journal of Medicinal Plants Research*, *5*(10), 2054–2063.

Korkmaz, M., & Karakurt, E. (2014). Medicinal plants sold in the herbal markets in Kelkit (Gümü hane). *Süleyman Demirel University Journal of Natural and Applied Sciences*, *18*(3), 60–80.

Korkmaz, M., & Karakurt, E. (2015). An ethnobotanical investigation to determine plants used as folk medicine in Kelkit Gümüşhane/Turkey district. *Biological Diversity and Conservation*, *8*(3), 290–303.

Koyuncu, O., Yaylaci, O., Öztürk, D., Potoglu Erkara, I., Savaroglu, F., & Akcoskun, O.. (2010). Risk categories and ethnobotanical features of the Lamiaceae taxa growing naturally in Osmaneli (Bilecik/Turkey) and environs. *Biological Diversity and Conservation*, *3*(3), 31–45. DOI: 10.1075/bdc.3.3.03k

Kültürr, Ş., Altınbaşak, O., Anıl, S., & Melikoğlu, G. (2018). Medicinal plants used for gastric ulcer in Turkey. *Marmara Pharmaceutical Journal*, *22*(1), 1–14.

Kültürr, Ş., Gürdal, B., Sari, A., & Melikoğlu, G. (2021). Traditional herbal remedies used in kidney diseases in Turkey: An overview. *Turkish Journal of Botany*, *45*(4), 269–287. DOI: 10.3906/bot-2011-32

Liu, J., Shen, H. M., & Ong, C. N. (2000). Salvia miltiorrhiza inhibits cell growth and induces apoptosis in human hepatoma HepG2 cells. *Cancer Letters*, *153*(1-2), 85–93. DOI: 10.1016/S0304-3835(00)00391-8 PMID: 10779635

Liu, R. H. (2004). Potential synergy of phytochemicals in cancer prevention: Mechanism of action. *The Journal of Nutrition*, *134*(12), 3479S–3485S. DOI: 10.1093/jn/134.12.3479S PMID: 15570057

Lu, Y., & Foo, L. Y. (2001). Antioxidant activities of polyphenols from sage (*Salvia officinalis*). *Food Chemistry*, *75*(2), 197–202. DOI: 10.1016/S0308-8146(01)00198-4

Melikoğlu, G., Kurtoğlu, S., & Kültürr, Ş. (2015). Türkiye'de astım tedavisinde geleneksel olarak kullanılan bitkiler. *Marmara Pharmaceutical Journal*, *19*(1), 1–11. DOI: 10.12991/mpj.2015198604

Miura, K., Kikuzaki, H., & Nakatani, N. (2002). Antioxidant activity of chemical components from sage (*Salvia officinalis* L.) and thyme (*Thymus vulgaris* L.) measured by the oil stability index method. *Journal of Agricultural and Food Chemistry*, *50*(7), 1845–1851. DOI: 10.1021/jf011314o PMID: 11902922

Norouzi, R.I, Babalar, M., & Mirmasoumi, M.III. (2017). Investigation of hairy root induction in some *Salvia* L. species. *Yaftah*, *4*(2), 173–180. DOI: 10.21859/acadpub.nbr.4.2.173

Olcay, B., & Kültürr, S. (2020). Medicinal plants used in traditional treatment of hypertension in Turkey. *International Journal of Science and Technology Research*, *6*(3), 80–95.

Ortega, A., Cárdenas, J., Gage, D. A., & Maldonado, E. (1995). Abietane and clerodane diterpenes from *Salvia regla.Phytochemistry*, *39*(4), 931–933. DOI: 10.1016/0031-9422(95)00083-J

Ötnü, H., & Akan, H. (2020). Plants sold for phytotherapy in pharmacies and herbalists of Şanlıurfa. *KSU Journal of Agricultural and Natural Sciences*, *23*(4), 947–965.

Öz Aydın, S., Dirmenci, T., Tümen, G., & Başer, K. H. C. (2006). Plants used as analgesic in the folk medicine of Turkey. In *Proceedings of the IVth International Congress of Ethnobotany (ICEB 2005)*. Ege Yayınları (pp. 167-171).

Özdemir, E., & Kültürr, Ş. (2017). Wild edible plants of Savaştepe district (Balıkesir, Turkey). *Marmara Pharmaceutical Journal*, *21*(3), 578–589. DOI: 10.12991/marupj.319328

Özdemir Nath, E., & Kültürr, Ş. (2015). Natural dye plants in Kepsut (Balıkesir, Turkey). *IUFS Journal of Biology*, *74*(2), 25–32.

Ozdemir Nath, E., & Kultur, S. (2022). An ethnobotanical study of medicinal plants in Savaştepe (Balikesir-Turkey). *Clinical and Experimental Health Sciences*, *12*(4), 954–980. DOI: 10.33808/clinexphealthsci.1026438

Ozturk, M., & Altay, V. (2017). An overview of the endemic medicinal and aromatic plants of Turkey—conservation and sustainable use. In *International Congress on Medicinal and Aromatic Plants Full Text Proceedings Book* (pp. 11–39).

Ozturk, M., Altay, V., & Gönenç, T. M. (2017). Herbal from high mountains in the East Mediterranean. In *Drug Discovery from Herbs – Approaches and Applications* (pp. 327–367). DAYA Publishing House.

Palasoglu, B., & Eminagaoglu, O. (2022). Folk medicines of Beşpare villages (Artvin-Turkey). *Turkish Journal of Biodiversity*, *5*(1), 1–16.

Plattner, R. D., & Powell, R. G. (1978). A secoisolariciresinol branched fatty diester from *Salvia plebeia* seed. *Phytochemistry*, *17*(1), 149–150. DOI: 10.1016/S0031-9422(00)89701-0

Polat, R., & Satıl, F. (2012). An ethnobotanical survey of medicinal plants in Edremit Gulf (Balıkesir–Turkey). *Journal of Ethnopharmacology*, *139*(2), 626–641. DOI: 10.1016/j.jep.2011.12.004 PMID: 22193175

Polat, R., Satıl, F., & Çakılcıoğlu, U. (2011). Medicinal plants and their use properties of those sold in herbal markets in Bingöl, Turkey. *Biological Diversity and Conservation*, *4*(3), 25–35.

Powell, R. G., & Plattner, R. D. (1976). Structure of a secoisolariciresinol diester from *Salvia plebeia* seed. *Phytochemistry, 15*(12), 1963–1965. DOI: 10.1016/S0031-9422(00)88856-1

Rahmanifar, B., Livadariu, O., & Cornea, C. P. (2023). Review on secondary metabolites in *Salvia* spp. *Scientific Bulletin. Series F. Biotechnologies, 27*(1).

Ren, Y., Houghton, P. J., Hider, R. C., & Howes, M. J. R. (2004). Novel diterpenoid acetylcholinesterase inhibitors from *Salvia miltiorrhiza.Planta Medica, 70*(3), 201–204. DOI: 10.1055/s-2004-815535 PMID: 15114495

Sağıroğlu, M., & Aydın, D. (2024). An ethnobotanical research in Cumalıkızık and its surroundings (Bursa). *Afyon Kocatepe University Journal of Science and Engineering, 24*(4), 758–772.

Sağıroğlu, M., Dalgıç, S., & Toksoy, S. (2013). Medicinal plants used in Dalaman (Muğla), Turkey. *Journal of Medicinal Plants Research, 7*(28), 2053–2066. DOI: 10.5897/JMPR2013.2590

Şahin, T., & Kılıç, Ö. (2022). A review: Some plants used for hemorrhoids in Turkey traditional medicine. *Russian Journal of Biological Research, 9*(1), 8–29. DOI: 10.2138/rjbr.2022.9.1.8

Şahin Fidan, E., & Akan, H. (2019). An ethnobotanical study in some villages around the Tek Tek Mountains National Park, Şanlıurfa (Turkey). *Bağbahçe Science Journal, 6*(2), 64–94.

Sandal Erzurumlu, G. (2021). Use of medicinal plants in landscape architecture design. *Acta Biologica Turcica, 34*(3), 146–156.

Santos-Gomes, P. C., Seabra, R. M., Andrade, P. B., & Fernandes-Ferreira, M. (2002). Phenolic antioxidant compounds produced by in vitro shoots of sage (*Salvia officinalis* L.). *Plant Science, 162*(6), 981–987. DOI: 10.1016/S0168-9452(02)00052-3

Saraç, D. U., Özkan, Z. C., & Akbulut, S. (2013). Ethnobotanic features of Rize/Turkey province. *Biological Diversity and Conservation, 6*(3), 57–66.

Sargin, S. A. (2021). Potential anti-influenza effective plants used in Turkish folk medicine: A review. *Journal of Ethnopharmacology, 265*, 113319. DOI: 10.1016/j.jep.2020.113319 PMID: 32882361

Sargın, S. A., Akçicek, E., & Selvi, S. (2013). An ethnobotanical study of medicinal plants used by the local people of Alaşehir (Manisa) in Turkey. *Journal of Ethnopharmacology, 150*(3), 860–874. DOI: 10.1016/j.jep.2013.09.040 PMID: 24126062

Sargın, S. A., & Büyükcengiz, M. (2019). Plants used in ethnomedicinal practices in Gulnar district of Mersin, Turkey. *Journal of Herbal Medicine*, *15*, 100224. DOI: 10.1016/j.hermed.2018.06.003

Sargin, S. A., & Dogan, Y. (2023). Immune-boosting plants used in Turkish folk medicine and their potential against COVID-19. In *Ethnopharmacology and Drug Discovery for COVID-19: Anti-SARS-CoV-2 Agents from Herbal Medicines and Natural Products* (pp. 479–548). Springer Nature Singapore. DOI: 10.1007/978-981-99-3664-9_18

Sargin, S. A., Selvi, S., & López, V. (2015). Ethnomedicinal plants of Sarıgöl district (Manisa), Turkey. *Journal of Ethnopharmacology*, *171*, 64–84. DOI: 10.1016/j.jep.2015.05.031 PMID: 26026370

Sarı, F., & Erarslan, Z. B. (2023). A scoping review of traditional medicinal plants used to treat acne vulgaris in Turkey. *European Journal of Integrative Medicine*, *64*, 102305. DOI: 10.1016/j.eujim.2023.102305

Sarı, F., Kültürr, Ş., & Koçyiğit, M. (2023). Traditional usages of some medicinal plants for pediatric diseases. *Journal of Faculty of Pharmacy Ankara University*, *47*(3), 1101–1118. DOI: 10.33483/jfpau.1214245

Sarıkaya, A. G., & Karabay, S. (2021). Determination of medicinal and aromatic plants sold by herbalists in Afyonkarahisar province and their usage purposes. *European Journal of Science and Technology*, *23*, 120–125. DOI: 10.31590/ejosat.799168

Sarıkaya, S., Öner, H., & Harput, Ş. (2010). Medicinal plants used for the treatment of diabetes in Turkey. *Journal of the Faculty of Pharmacy. Ankara University*, *39*(4), 317–342.

Satıl, F., Akçiçek, E., & Selvi, S. (2008). An ethnobotanical study in Madra Mountain (Balıkesir–İzmir) and its vicinity. *Research Journal of Biological Sciences*, *1*(1), 31–36.

Selvi, S., Dağdelen, A., & Kara, S. (2013). Medicinal and aromatic plants consumed as herbal tea and collected from Ida Mountains (Balıkesir-Edremit). *Tekirdag Ziraat Fakültesi Dergisi*, *10*(2), 26–33.

Şenkardeş, İ., & Tuzlacı, E. (2016). Wild edible plants of the southern part of Nevşehir in Turkey. *Marmara Pharmaceutical Journal*, *20*(1), 34–43. DOI: 10.12991/mpj.20163435871

Sharma, Y., Fagan, J., & Schaefer, J. (2019). Ethnobotany, phytochemistry, cultivation and medicinal properties of Garden sage (*Salvia officinalis* L.). *Journal of Pharmacognosy and Phytochemistry*, *8*(3), 3139–3148. DOI: 10.22271/jpp.2019.v8.i3l.13767

Sirri, M., Özaslan, C., & Fidan, M. (2021). Some natural and weeds used for food and folk medicine in Eruh District of Siirt/Turkey. *MAS Journal of Applied Science*, *6*(Special issue), 1118–1129.

Sırrı, M., & Sırrı, G. (2020). Current status of wild plant and weed species consumed as food in Hakkâri province. *European Journal of Science and Technology*, *19*, 393–409. DOI: 10.31590/ejosat.697536

Tepe, B., Sökmen, M., Akpulat, H. A., & Sökmen, A. (2006). Screening of the antioxidant potentials of six *Salvia* species from Turkey. *Food Chemistry*, *95*(2), 200–204. DOI: 10.1016/j.foodchem.2004.12.031

Terzioğlu, S., & Coşkunçelebi, K. (2021). Medicinal plants of northeast Anatolia. In *Biodiversity, Conservation and Sustainability in Asia: Volume 1: Prospects and Challenges in West Asia and Caucasus* (pp. 275–337). Springer International Publishing. DOI: 10.1007/978-3-030-59928-7_11

Topçu, G., Altiner, E. N., Gözcü, S., Halfon, B., Aydın, Z., & Pezzuto, J. M.. (2003). Studies on di- and triterpenoids from *Salvia staminea* with cytotoxic activity. *Planta Medica*, *69*(5), 464–467. DOI: 10.1055/s-2003-39705 PMID: 12802732

Topçu, G., Türkmen, Z., Ulubelen, A., Schilling, J. K., & Kingston, D. G. (2004). Highly hydroxylated triterpenes from *Salvia kronenburgii*.*Journal of Natural Products*, *67*(1), 118–121. DOI: 10.1021/np030359b PMID: 14738403

Tütenocaklı, T. (2023). Plants consumed as food in ethnobotanical perspective: The case study of Yenice-Çanakkale-Turkiye. *Current Trends in Natural Sciences*, *12*(23), 224–233. DOI: 10.47068/ctns.2023.v12i23.025

Tütenocaklı, T., & Uysal, I. (2014). An ethnobotanical study in Nevruz Village (Yenice, Çanakkale, Turkey). In *Environment and Ecology in the Mediterranean Region II* (pp. 359-372).

Tuzlacı, E. (2016). *Türkiye Bitkileri Geleneksel İlaç Rehberi* [Traditional Medicinal Plants of Turkey]. İstanbul Tıp Kitabevleri.

Tuzlacı, E., & Şenkardeş, İ. (2011). Turkish folk medicinal plants, X: Ürgüp (Nevşehir). *Marmara Pharmaceutical Journal*, *15*(2), 58–68. DOI: 10.12991/201115432

Ünal, S., & Altundağ Çakır, E. (2024). Natural dye plants in Sındırgı Yağcıbedir Carpets (Balıkesir, Turkey). *Eurasian Journal of Forest Science*, *12*(2), 66–72. DOI: 10.31195/ejejfs.1456411

Uysal, I., Gücel, S., Tütenocakli, T., & Öztürk, M. (2012). Studies on the medicinal plants of Ayvacik-Çanakkale in Turkey. *Pakistan Journal of Botany*, *44*(Suppl 1), 239–244.

Uysal, İ., Onar, S., Karabacak, E., & Çelik, S. (2010). Ethnobotanical aspects of Kapıdağ peninsula (Turkey). *Biological Diversity and Conservation*, *3*(3), 15–22. DOI: 10.1075/bdc.3.3.02u

Uzun, A., & Palabas Uzun, S. (2011). Medicinal and aromatic plant taxa of Altındere Valley (Maçka/Trabzon). In *2nd International Non-Wood Products Symposium* (pp. 269–282).

Uzun, M., & Kaya, A. (2019). Traditional medicinal plants used for oral and dental diseases in Turkey. *Biological Diversity and Conservation*, *12*(1), 138–148. DOI: 10.5505/biodicon.2019.09797

Valeriote, F., Grieshaber, C. K., Media, J., Pietraszkewicz, H., Hoffmann, J., Pan, M., & McLaughlin, S. (2002). Discovery and development of anticancer agents from plants. *Journal of Experimental Therapeutics & Oncology*, *2*(4), 228–236. DOI: 10.1046/j.1359-4117.2002.01038.x PMID: 12416027

Veitch, N. C., Grayer, R. J., Irwin, J. L., & Takeda, K. (1998). Flavonoid cellobiosides from *Salvia uliginosa.Phytochemistry*, *48*(2), 389–393. DOI: 10.1016/S0031-9422(97)01111-4

Wang, X., Morris-Natschke, S. L., & Lee, K. H. (2007). New developments in the chemistry and biology of the bioactive constituents of Tanshen. *Medicinal Research Reviews*, *27*(1), 133–148. DOI: 10.1002/med.20077 PMID: 16888751

Weng, X. C., & Gordon, M. H. (1992). Antioxidant activity of quinones extracted from tanshen (*Salvia miltiorrhiza* Bunge). *Journal of Agricultural and Food Chemistry*, *40*(8), 1331–1336. DOI: 10.1021/jf00020a007

Wu, Y. B., Ni, Z. Y., Shi, Q. W., Dong, M., Kiyota, H., Gu, Y. C., & Cong, B. (2012). Constituents from *Salvia* species and their biological activities. *Chemical Reviews*, *112*(11), 5967–6026. DOI: 10.1021/cr200058f PMID: 22967178

Xu, G., Peng, L. Y., Lu, L., Weng, Z. Y., Zhao, Y., Li, X. L., & Zhang, L. (2006). Two new abietane diterpenoids from *Salvia yunnanensis.Planta Medica*, *72*(1), 84–86. DOI: 10.1055/s-2005-873184 PMID: 16450305

Yalçın, S., Akan, H., & Çakılcıoğlu, U. (2022). Traditional uses of some food plants in Suruç (Şanlıurfa, Turkey). *Turkish Journal of Natural Sciences*, *11*(1), 59–65.

Yapar, Y. (2024). Food plants of Azap Mountain (Türkiye, Erzurum-Horasan) and its surroundings. *Bağbahçe Bilim Dergisi*, *11*(1), 87–96. DOI: 10.24122/bbd.2024.111

Yaşar, H. İ., Koyuncu, O., Koyuncu, F. T., & Kuş, G. (2019). Sale of medicinal and aromatic plants and economic dimensions in Eskişehir herbalist. *Research Journal of Biological Sciences*, *12*(2), 25–28.

Yeşil, Y., Çelik, M., & Yılmaz, B. (2019). Wild edible plants in Yeşilli (Mardin-Turkey), a multicultural area. *Journal of Ethnobiology and Ethnomedicine*, *15*(1), 1–19. DOI: 10.1186/s13002-019-0327-y PMID: 31690334

Yeşil, Y., & İnal, İ. (2019). Traditional knowledge of wild edible plants in Hasankeyf (Batman Province, Turkey). *Acta Societatis Botanicorum Poloniae*, *88*(3), 3633. DOI: 10.5586/asbp.3633

Yeşil, Y., & İnal, İ. (2021). Ethnomedicinal plants of Hasankeyf (Batman-Turkey). *Frontiers in Pharmacology*, *11*, 624710. DOI: 10.3389/fphar.2020.624710 PMID: 33776756

Yeşilada, E., Honda, G., Sezik, E., Tabata, M., Goto, K., & Ikeshiro, Y. (1993). Traditional medicine in Turkey IV. Folk medicine in the Mediterranean subdivision. *Journal of Ethnopharmacology*, *39*(1), 31–38. DOI: 10.1016/0378-8741(93)90048-A PMID: 8331960

Zhang, Z. F., Chen, H. S., Peng, Z. G., Li, Z. R., & Jiang, J. D. (2008). A potent anti-HIV polyphenol from *Salvia yunnanensis.Journal of Asian Natural Products Research*, *10*(3), 252–255. DOI: 10.1080/10286020701605075 PMID: 18335344

Zhang, Z. F., Peng, Z. G., Gao, L., Dong, B., Li, J. R., Li, Z. Y., & Chen, H.-S. (2008). Three new derivatives of anti-HIV-1 polyphenols isolated from *Salvia yunnanensis.Journal of Asian Natural Products Research*, *10*(5), 391–396. DOI: 10.1080/10286020801966591 PMID: 18464075

Chapter 14
The Secondary Metabolites of Bryophytes and Their Therapeutic Applications

Atakan Benek
https://orcid.org/0000-0001-6726-5968
Dokuz Eylül University, Turkey

Dilay Turu
https://orcid.org/0000-0002-8485-0488
Graduate School of Natural and Applied Sciences, Dokuz Eylül University, Turkey

Mustafa Eray Bozyel
https://orcid.org/0000-0001-5556-4880
Dokuz Eylül University, Turkey

Özcan Simsek
https://orcid.org/0000-0002-3210-7641
Yenice Vocational School, Çanakkale Onsekiz Mart University, Turkey

Kerem Canlı
https://orcid.org/0000-0001-6061-6948
Dokuz Eylül University, Turkey

ABSTRACT

Bryophytes, which include about 24,000 taxa and consist of mosses (Bryopsida), liverworts (Hepaticopsida), and hornworts (Anthocerotopsida), are the largest

DOI: 10.4018/979-8-3693-9112-9.ch014

group of secondary terrestrial plants after angiosperms. Indigenous communities globally use bryophytes for various medicinal purposes, including antimicrobial, antipyretic, dermatological, hepatic, cardiovascular, and wound-healing properties. Found in diverse habitats, excluding oceans, bryophytes are significant sources of bioactive compounds, particularly secondary metabolites such as steroids, alkaloids, phenols, coumarins, flavonoids, and tannins. These compounds demonstrate various therapeutic activities, including antimicrobial, antioxidant, anti-inflammatory, antidiabetic, and anti-cancer effects. This study aims to provide a comprehensive review of the ethnomedicinal uses of bryophytes and the therapeutic applications of their secondary metabolites.

1. INTRODUCTION

Bryophytes are “nonvascular plants” also termed “amphibious plants” and the second largest group of terrestrial plants. The Ancient Greek words “φυτόν” (phutón,-phyton) meaning plant and “βρύον” (brúon, bryon) meaning tree moss, liverwort, are the origin of the name “bryophyte’’. The plants have survived in both aquatic and terrestrial environments under a wide range of environmental and climatic conditions and have been evolving for a longer period than other groups of land plants, (Asakawa, Ludwiczuk, & Nagashua, 2013a) (Hanson & Rice, 2013) (Smithsonian Tropical Research Institute, 2021). Comprising three plant phyla, 'bryophytes' are characterized by a common haploid-dominant life cycle and unbranched sporophytes with a sporangium. These groups include mosses (*Bryophyta*), liverworts (*Marchantiophyta*), and hornworts (*Anthocerophyta*), (Shaw & Renzaglia, 2004). There are approximately 23,000 bryophyte taxa worldwide. *Marchantiophyta*, consists of 6000 species, Anthocerotophyta, consists of 300 species, and *Bryophyta* consist of 14,000 species. However, the number of taxa changes almost every year due to synonymization of some species and discovery of new ones, (Sabovljević *et al.*, 2016).

It has been demonstrated that it would be more accurate to examine the three plant classes that make up this group at the division level as a result of research done on the rbcl chloroplast genes of the plants included in the bryophyte group and the analysis of morphological characteristics and rRNA sequences together, (Glime, 2022). Nonetheless, taking into account the conventional application of the term “Bryophyte,” it is acknowledged that the *Bryophyta* division continues to encompass three classes collectively because of the strong ties among the three groups it covers and the fact that some researcher has examined the three groups concurrently, (Canli, 2012). The International Code of Botanical Nomenclature/Vienna Code/ICN (formerly known as the International Code of Botanical Nomenclature/ICBN) suggests using the names *Hepaticopsida*, *Anthoceropsida*, and *Bryopsida*, even though these names are still used in conventional categorization, (Karahan, 2021).

In their life cycle, the dominant part is the green portion of the plant known as the gametophyte, while the brown portion, called the sporophyte, is unbranched and short-lived. For most of their life cycle, bryophytes, which are photosynthetic plants, are dependent on the gametophyte via the seta. During reproduction, biflagellate sperm reach the egg through water to achieve fertilization. The fertilized egg is located within the archegonium, and due to this characteristic, the term archegoniates is also used for bryophytes, (Kirmaci, 2007).

One of the largest groups in the plant kingdom and considered among the primitive plants, the oldest fossil record of bryophytes belongs to *Metzgeriothallus sharonae*. *M. sharonae* is a small leaf-like liverwort thallus from the Late Middle Devonian period. Although the exact ancestor of modern-day bryophytes is unknown, it is thought that they evolved from a common ancestor shared with green algae, (Hernick, Landing, & Bartowski, 2008). There are three widely accepted hypotheses regarding the emergence of bryophytes. The first hypothesis posits that bryophytes originated from primitive vascular plants, suggesting the formation of a radially symmetrical upright gametophore, as well as the possibility of ancestral archegoniate plants persisting from evolutionary lines of leafy and thalloid forms. The second hypothesis proposes that a single-celled green alga could have evolved into a plant adapted to an environment with high moisture content in the soil, and that it could be the ancestor of both *Charophyta* algae and plants with archegonia. The third hypothesis asserts that bryophytes originated from the *Chlorophycean* line, which bears archegonia, within green algae that diverged into two evolutionary lines known as *Charophyceae* and *Chlorophyceae*, (Schofield, 2001).

Like other plants in the plant kingdom, bryophytes have cellulose in their cell walls and produce carotene, chlorophyll a and b, and xanthophyll in their structures. Although these characteristics make them similar to higher plants, they differ from higher plants in that they lack true leaves, stems, and roots, and do not have a developed vascular system. Without true roots, bryophytes attach to the substrate they live on through filamentous structures called rhizoids, which can be unicellular or multicellular. Bryophytes do not absorb the nutrients they need from the soil. Therefore, they perform water and mineral uptake, as well as photosynthesis, through their entire surface. Since bryophytes do not have stomata in their leaves, they cannot regulate gas exchange or control water loss, (Özen, 2017).

Bryophytes are found in microhabitats within most ecosystems. Being part of many cycles within their habitats, bryophytes play an important role in providing shelter for other groups of organisms, helping them survive and reproduce during challenging periods. While some animals consume bryophytes, it is generally accepted that they are largely avoided by herbivorous animals due to their interesting chemical composition, (Ingimundardóttir, Weibull, & Cronberg, 2014).

Although various studies have been conducted and data have been obtained on the presence of bioactive secondary metabolites in flowering plants, very little is known about the secondary metabolites of non-vascular plants within the Bryophyte division. The bryophyte division, which includes mosses, hornworts and liverworts, is the second most diverse plant group in the world after flowering plants. There aren't many studies on the chemistry of bryophytes despite their extensive distribution across such a large geographic area on Earth. According to reports, only 6% of liverworts and 2% of mosses have undergone chemical analysis, (Sahilli & Alataş, 2024). Some researchers think this is because bryophytes are unfit for human consumption. Mosses, hornworts and liverworts are considered by many scientists to be an almost unexplored natural reservoir of new biologically active secondary metabolites, (Frahm, 2004) (Valeeva *et al.*, 2022).

The small size of bryophytes and their adaptation to specific habitat conditions make their collection and identification challenging. As a result, the evaluation of their potential for medicinal use was neglected for a long time. However, recent research has revealed many biologically active molecules and pharmacological activities associated with bryophytes. To date, the major pharmaceutical effects discovered include various properties such as antioxidant, antifungal, anti-inflammatory, antibacterial, antitumor, and antiviral activities, (Cianciullo *et al.,* 2021) (Das *et al.,* 2022) (Marques *et al.,* 2022) (Yayintas, Yilmaz, & Sökmen, 2019) (Negi & Chaturvedi, 2021) (Kim *et al.,* 2021). The main bioactive compounds extracted from different bryophytes are classified among various secondary metabolite groups, such as terpenoids, highly unsaturated fatty acids, alkanones, phytosterols, flavonoids and their glycosides, phenylpropanoids, benzenoids, and bibenzyl derivatives, (Markham & Porter, 2016) (Matos *et al.,* 2021).

Throughout history, one of the key ways humans have utilized plants is in combating diseases. People across different regions have learned about plants' medicinal effects through experience and experimentation. Today, this collective knowledge is widely acknowledged and has given rise to ethnobotany, a field dedicated to substantial research, (Rahman *et al.,* 2019). Apart from ethnobotany, which refers to all plants, bryologist Seville Flowers first used the term "ethnobryology" in 1957 to describe the therapeutic use of bryophytes. Flowers (1957) used the word ethnobryology to refer to the Gosiute people of Utah's usage of bryophytes as medicine. Compared to seed plants, there is less information in the literature regarding the therapeutic use of bryophytes. This is because researchers in the subject of ethnobotany typically focus seed plants, and bryophytes are less frequently utilized medicinally today.

The term ethnobryology encompasses all three subclasses within the division Bryophyta, which includes mosses (Bryophyta), hornworts (Anthocerotophyta), and leafy liverworts (Marchantiophyta). To date, approximately 150 ethnobotanical bryophyte species have been listed. A large majority of these listed species have been reported for their use in traditional Chinese medicine (27%) and by Native Americans (28%). Among bryophytes, the genera *Sphagnum*, *Marchantia*, and *Polytrichum* are known to have the most widespread medicinal use, (Harris, 2008). This study describes the biochemical contents and medicinal uses of mosses (*Bryophyta*), liverworts (*Marchantiophyta*), and hornworts (*Anthocerotophyta*), which together comprise the division *Bryophyta*.

2. MOSSES (BRYOPHYTA)

Mosses (*Bryophyta*) are the largest group of bryophytes, with about 14,000 species. Mosses are generally small plants ranging in size from a few mm to a few cm. The largest recorded moss species are *Dawsonia superba* Grev., which can grow up to 70 cm, and *Fontinalis antipyretica* Hedw., which can grow up to 2 m, (Sabovljević *et al.*, 2016). The terms acrocarp and pleurocarp refer to two morphologically distinct groups of mosses. Acrocarpous mosses grow upright on the surface of the substrate and typically do not branch. In contrast, pleurocarpous mosses grow parallel to the surface of the substrate and usually exhibit branching, (Ginting, Amrul & Susilo, 2021).

Mosses can thrive in a wide range of wet soils and moist environments, from swamps to alpine and Arctic regions; sometimes they are found completely submerged in water, while at other times they grow on soil, rocks, and tree trunks. Some of their important characteristics include serving as a food source for certain animals, their ability to store minerals, and providing egg-laying and sheltering areas for many insect species, (Çetin, 1998). Mosses are organisms capable of surviving under extremely harsh conditions. When the water availability in their environment decreases or the habitat dries out completely, the leaves of mosses curl up and take on a brown appearance, and they completely halt all physiological activities until the water levels return to a life-sustaining level. Thanks to this ability, they can persist in their environment for many years, (Benek, 2020).

One of the most important characteristics of mosses is the presence of hygroscopic peristome teeth, which are seen in most species of this group and are responsible for regulating spore dispersal. Moss capsules typically contain two sets of peristome teeth: an inner and an outer set. The outer peristome teeth are more hygroscopic than the inner ones, (Glime, 2022). The outer peristome teeth close in humid air conditions and open in dry air conditions. In mosses, spore dispersal generally occurs over an extended period of time, (Karaburun, 2012).

When examining the life cycle of mosses, a haplodiplontic alternation of generations is observed. These plants are capable of both sexual and asexual reproduction. In mosses, sexual reproduction occurs in the form of oogamy, and the haploid (n) gametophyte generation is followed by the diploid (2n) sporophyte generation. This process is referred to as heterophasic/antithetic alternation of generations. The gametophyte generation can be monoicous or dioicous. The reproductive organs in females are known as archegonia, while in males, they are referred to as antheridia. Spermatozoids produced in the antheridia reach the archegonia through chemotaxis and water. As a result of fertilization, a diploid (2n) sporophyte plant develops on the gametophyte, forming a structure known as a spore capsule. The sporophyte is nutritionally dependent on the gametophyte. Sporogenous tissue (archesporium), formed through the differentiation of the inner tissue of the sporophyte, undergoes meiosis to produce haploid (n) spore tetrads. These spores germinate to form protonema, which develops into the gametophyte plant. In most mosses, the dispersal of spores from the capsule is facilitated by the operculum at the top of the capsule, the peristome teeth beneath the operculum, and the annulus, (Gürsu, 2012).

2.1 Secondary Metabolites in Mosses

There are more than 14,000 species of mosses worldwide, but only a small group has been chemically analyzed, (Asakawa, 1995). When studies on the secondary metabolites of mosses are examined, it is observed that the presence of anthocyanin pigments in the genus Sphagnum was first demonstrated by Paul in 1908 (Hazer, Çölgeçen, & Uyar, 2017). Carbohydrates constitute the main chemical components of mosses, (Maksimova *et al.,* 2013). In addition to carbohydrates, they contain many different secondary metabolites. Many of these secondary metabolites do not have a clear metabolic function but are thought to have high biological activity, (Asakawa, Ludwiczuk, & Nagashima, 2013a).

2.1.1 Terpenoids

Terpenoids are biologically active compounds commonly found in mosses. The terms 'terpene' and 'terpenoid' are frequently used interchangeably. Terpenes are simple hydrocarbon compounds, while terpenoids are modified terpenes that have undergone structural rearrangements through the addition of one or more oxygen atoms. Terpenoids are classified according to the number of carbon atoms in their structure, with monoterpenoids (C10), sesquiterpenoids (C15), diterpenoids (C20), and triterpenoids (C30) being the most prevalent and distinctive in bryophytes,

(Commisso *et al.,* 2021). Terpenoids in moss structures play roles in adapting to stress conditions, protecting against pathogens, and regulating various environmental interactions. Terpenoids synthesized through unique biosynthetic pathways in mosses are particularly notable for their antioxidant, antimicrobial, and cytotoxic properties, (Sen *et al.,* 2023).

In mosses, the distinctive terpenoid groups are triterpene compounds, which include ursane, fernane, hopane, lupane, cycloartane, friedelane, taraxane, dammarane, polypodane, obtusifolane, and serratane triterpenoids, (Asakawa, Ludwiczuk, & Nagashima, 2013a). Various studies have been conducted by scientists to reveal the terpenoids found in the biochemical structure of mosses. In a study conducted in 1998, the presence of polypoda-7,13,17,21-tetraene was identified in the diethyl ether extract of the moss *Floribundaria aurea* subsp. *nipponica*, as well as in the ether extract. Further purification of the ether extract revealed the presence of dammara-17Z,21-diene in addition to diploptene, (Toyota, Masuda, & Asakawa, 1998).

As a result of the biochemical analyses conducted, the presence of monoterpenes, sesquiterpenes, and diterpenes was commonly identified in the genera *Mnium, Plagiomnium, Homalia, Plagiothecium*, and *Taxiphyllum,* (Asakawa, 1995). The most commonly detected monoterpenoid in mosses is β-sitrositrial. Additionally, compounds such as α-pinene, β-pinene, bornyl acetate, camphene, and limonene have also been identified as frequent components in mosses, (Asakawa, Ludwiczuk, & Nagashima, 2013).

In a study conducted in 2021, the histochemical compartmentalization of terpenes was examined in *Hennediella heimii* (Pottiaceae), *Entosthodon hungaricus* (Funariaceae), and *Physcomitrella patens* (Funariaceae), a species known for its salt tolerance, under salt stress. The study found that terpenoid compounds were predominantly located in the protonemal cells of all three tested moss species and were also present in the phylloids, a distribution shown to be related to the intensity of NaCl stress, (Ćosić *et al.,* 2021).

2.1.2 Flavonoids and Phenolic Compounds

The term 'Polyphenol' or 'Phenolic' is chemically defined as substances that contain a hydroxyl group on their aromatic ring, in addition to various functional groups such as esters, methyl esters, and glycosides, (Özcan, 2010). Various studies have been conducted on the flavonoid and phenolic compound contents of mosses. These studies particularly focus on the antioxidant potential and biological activity of phenolic compounds in mosses. For example, some studies have stated that only

5% of mosses have been chemically analyzed and therefore their phenolic contents represent a large resource open to discovery, (Hazer, Çölgeçen, & Uyar, 2017).

Studies in the literature reveal that moss species exhibit a wide diversity of flavonoids. The first moss species in which a flavonoid was identified is *Plagiomnium cuspidatum* (Hedw.) T.J. Kop., in which saponarin was detected, (Kozlowski, 1921). Three rare flavonoid compounds, including 3-deoxyanthocyanin, luteolinidin 5-O-glucoside, and 5-O-diglucoside, have been isolated from the cell sap of *Bryum cryophilum* Mårtensson, (Bendz, Mårtensson, & Terenius, 1962). *Hedwigia ciliata* (Hedw.) P. Beauv. contains at least twelve different types of flavonoids, (Schofield, 1985). Two new cinnamoyl bibenzyls, pallidisetin A and B, have been isolated from *Polytrichum pallidisetum* Funck, (Zheng *et al.,* 1994). Coumarin has been isolated from the species *Atrichum undulatum* (Hedw.) P. Beauv., *Polytrichum formosum* Hedw., and *Tetraphis pellucida* Hedw, (Jung, Zinsmeister, & Geiger, 1994).

The presence of phenolic acids was first reported in *Aulacomnium androgynum* (Hedw.) Schwägr. In the methanol extract of A. androgynum, four phenolic acids—protocatechuic, p-hydroxybenzoic, vanillic, and trans-cinnamic acids were identified, (Oztopcu-Vatan *et al.,* 2017).

In a study conducted in 2008, the phenolic compositions of *Brachytheciastrum velutinum* (Hedw) Ignatov & Huttunen and *Kindbergia praelonga* (Hedw) Ochyra were revealed for the first time. Methanol extracts of the moss samples were analyzed by HPLC, identifying four phenolic acids—4-O-caffeoylquinic, 5-O-caffeoylquinic, caffeic, and ellagic acids—as well as the flavonoids apigenin-7-O-glucoside, luteolin, and apigenin in the methanol extract of *B. velutinum*. In the methanol extract of *K. praelonga*, 4-O-caffeoylquinic, 5-O-caffeoylquinic, caffeic, p-coumaric, ferulic, and ellagic acids, along with derivatives of caffeic and p-coumaric acids, were detected. Additionally, apigenin-7-O-glucoside, luteolin, apigenin, and an unidentified flavanone were found in the methanol extract of *K. praelonga* (Jocković *et al.,* 2008).

2.1.3 Medical Uses of Mosses

The medicinal use of mosses dates back to ancient times. Mosses are prominent in folk medicine and modern pharmaceutical research for their antimicrobial, antifungal, and cytotoxic properties. They have been used particularly in traditional medical systems of countries like China and India for treating infections, reducing fever, and healing wounds. Native Americans also used moss, mixed with honey, to disinfect wounds, (Motti, Palma, & de Falco, 2023). In regions such as Europe, Africa, and South America, information on the folk therapeutic applications of mosses is quite limited. Compared to the ethnobotanical literature on vascular plants, there are various reasons for the scarcity of knowledge about mosses. Due to their small size, the difficulty of species identification, and the lack of prominent features such as flowers or fruits, many characteristics of mosses remain unexplored, (Stech *et al.,* 2018).

Conducting ethnobotanical research on plants helps preserve traditional knowledge of medicinal plants and provides a foundation for developing new drugs through phytochemical and biochemical studies, (Lubaina *et al.,* 2014). sses are included in traditional Chinese medicine, which is rooted in philosophical principles that later influenced the development of Taoism and Confucianism. Ancient Chinese scholars categorized all natural phenomena as complementary yet opposing forces known as Yin and Yang. In traditional Chinese medicine, Yin represents an organism's physical characteristics, while Yang denotes its physiological functions, (Tang *et al.,* 2008). In traditional Chinese medicine, *Bryum argenteum* Hedw has been used as an antidote, antipyretic, and antifungal; *Dicranum majus* Sm. as a cough suppressant; *Ditrichum pallidum* (Hedw.) Hampe for convulsions in infants; *Fissidens nobilis* Griff. as a diuretic and hair growth stimulant; *Funaria hygrometrica* Hedw. as a hemostatic and sedative; *Mnium cuspidatum* Hedw. as a hemostatic; *Sphagnum sericeum* Müll. Hal. for treating acne, hemorrhoids, and eye diseases; and *Weissia controversa* Hedw. for sinus infections, (Harris, 2008) (Asakawa, 2007) (Chinese Materia Medica Editorial Committee, 1999) (Ding, 1982).

Traditional Indian medicine encompasses thousands of different plants. In India, one of the world's most populous countries, plants are widely utilized in folk medicine across numerous regions and among hundreds of communities. One unique approach in traditional Indian medicine is the Paracelsus doctrine, which is based on the resemblance between parts of plants and the shape or structure of the human or animal organs they are meant to heal, (Benek, Canli, & Altuner, 2022). For instance, *Polytrichum commune* has a hairy calyptra resembling hair, and in ancient times, oil extracted from this moss was used by women as a hair treatment, (Glime, 2007). In traditional Indian medicine, *Barbula indica* (Hook.) Spreng. has been used as an antipyretic; *Brachythecium rutabulum* (Hedw.) Schimp. for the treatment of cuts, burns, and wounds; and *Polytrichum juniperinum* Hedw. as a diuretic and for the treatment of burns and prostate issues, (Lubaina *et al.*, 2014) (Pant & Tewari, 1989) (Karpinski & Adamczak, 2017).

Knowledge of traditional medicine and treatments among Native American communities has been passed down primarily through oral traditions, often involving ceremonial practices. Indigenous people learn and honor these healing methods and materials under the guidance of elders. Much of this knowledge is believed to remain within Native communities as secrets, as most information is shared orally without written records, (Redvers & Blondin, 2020). In traditional American medicine, where numerous bryophytes are utilized, mosses hold significant value. The Gosiute Native Americans in Utah, for example, used various moss genus such as *Philonotis*, *Bryum*, and *Mnium* to alleviate pain from burns (Sabovljević et al., 2016) (Ando

& Matsuo, 1984). In traditional American medicine, *Bryum capillare* Hedw. has been used for the treatment of burns and fungal infections; *Fissidens adianthoides* Hedw. as a diuretic and to stimulate hair growth; and *Thuidium schistocalyx* (Müll. Hal.) Mitt. for relieving headaches, (Sabovljević *et al.,* 2016) (Sturtevant, 1954) (Boom, 1996).

Bryophytes, like other plants, attracted the interest of early modern botanists in the early 16th century. European herbaria created between approximately 1542 and 1577 contain up to 34 identifiable bryophyte species, collected with specific intent, (Stech *et al.,* 2018). During this period, bryophytes were also likely considered as potential medicinal plants. In 1549, Fuchs proposed *Polytrichum*, a newly identified moss species, as a candidate for medicinal use. He described this moss as beneficial for strengthening hair roots, covering baldness in cases of alopecia, aiding in the removal of thick and sticky substances from the lungs, and functioning as a diuretic, (Fuchs, 1990) (Drobnik & Stebel, 2015). In traditional European medicine, *Bryum argenteum* Hedw. and *Ceratodon purpureus* (Hedw.) Brid. were used to treat fungal infections; *Dicranum scoparium* Hedw. was applied for its antimicrobial properties; *Funaria hygrometrica* Hedw. served as a diuretic and for passing kidney stones; and *Polytrichastrum alpinum* (Hedw.) G. L. Sm. was used to alleviate nasal discharge and eye watering, (Frahm, 2004) (Agelet & Valles, 2003) (Pavletić & Stilinović, 1963).

3. LIVERWORTS (MARCHANTIOPHYTA)

Liverworts (*Marchantiophyta*) comprise approximately 8,000 species and are found across all continents, occupying both aquatic and arid niches. Evidence from fossil records and phylogenetic studies indicates that the first land plants, which evolved around 470 million years ago, resembled liverworts. Liverworts are members of the non-vascular plant class, commonly found in moist and shaded habitats. Their small, leaf-like or thallus-like structures are distinct features that differentiate them from other bryophytes. Often the first plants to colonize environments, liverworts play significant roles in ecosystems. They contribute to soil stabilization and the transformation of organic matter. Beyond their ecological functions, liverworts are also noteworthy for their biological diversity and morphological structures. They hold great importance not only for ecosystem health but also in pharmacological research. Certain metabolites found in liverworts, such as *Marchantia polymorpha*, are critical for plant defense mechanisms and have potential medicinal applications, (Asakawa, 2004).

As some of the earliest terrestrial plants, liverworts are notable for their secondary metabolites, which possess significant medicinal potential. Many of these biologically important secondary metabolites are typically stored within oil bodies, which serve as essential markers for classification within *Marchantiophyta*, (Asakawa *et al.*, 2009). The oil bodies of liverworts were first described by Hübener in 1834 as transparent drops with a shiny, membranous texture in *Jungermannia taylorii* (current taxonomic name: *Mylia taylorii*). Through light and electron microscopy, Pihakaski identified the oil body as the primary location of lipids in liverwort cells. Suire et al. confirmed that the oil body serves as the site of intracellular isoprenoid synthesis in liverworts, reinforcing the idea that it is an active cellular compartment, (He, Sun, & Zhu, 2013). Major metabolites produced by liverworts include terpenoids, flavonoids, phenolic compounds, and benzyl derivatives.

3.1 Secondary Metabolites in Liverworts

Nowadays, liverworts are the subject of the majority of bryophyte research because, in contrast to mosses and hornworts, they have cellular oil bodies, (Karim *et al.*, 2014). Many secondary metabolites produced by liverworts, which are significant in terms of biological activity, are typically found within oil bodies and essential oils. Depending on the composition of these secondary metabolites, this can sometimes lead to a pleasant fragrance. However, the scent of bryophytes depends not only on the content of secondary metabolites in their volatile oils but also on the habitat conditions of the plants. For instance, species of *Frullania* are able to produce tamariskol only when cultivated in high mountainous areas. While a species of liverwort, *Cyathodium foetidissimum*, collected in Tahiti was reported to have a pleasant odor, the same species found on Ua Huka in the Marquesas Islands in 2009 was reported to emit scent resembling urine and feces, (Dziwak *et al.*, 2022).

3.1.1 Terpenoids

All living things contain terpenes and terpenoids, a class of naturally occurring, biochemically active compounds. For instance, carotenoids are crucial in photosynthetic species, while steroids are necessary parts of cell membranes in eukaryotic cells. As a result, the biosynthesis of terpenes and terpenoid compounds is thought to be very old, (Lange et al., 2000) (Rao, 2021). Low-molecular-weight, volatile or semi-volatile terpenoids such as isoprene, monoterpenoids, sesquiterpenoids, and diterpenoids found in plants participate in various biotic interactions both above and below ground and protect plants against abiotic stress, (Tholl, 2015).

Terpenoids are an important class of secondary metabolites abundant in liverworts, contributing to their biological activity. The significant abundance of oil bodies, a key cellular compartment of liverworts, may be one factor contributing to the tremendous structural variety of these organisms, which have been estimated to produce about 1600 terpenoids, (He, Sun, & Zhu, 2013). Common terpenoids found in liverworts include sesquiterpenes and diterpenes, which are often known for their antimicrobial, anti-inflammatory, and antioxidant activities.

A study by Stelmasiewicz, Świątek, and Ludwiczuk (2021) focused on *Marchantia polymorpha* L. and its endophytes. Mass spectrometry and gas chromatography (GC-MS) were used to analyze the extracts. The endophyte extract was found to contain compounds with diketopiperazine structures. The volatile extract of the liverwort revealed high amounts of sesquiterpenoids, including cuparane, chamigrane, acorane, and thujopsane types. Ethyl acetate extracts obtained from endophytic bacteria demonstrated strong anticancer potential against cervical adenocarcinoma and hypopharyngeal squamous cell carcinoma in a panel of cancer (FaDu, HeLa, and SCC-25) and normal (VERO) cell lines.

In a publication by Asakawa, Ludwiczuk, and Nagashima (2013) terpenoids in liverworts are examined as an important group of secondary metabolites. The diversity, structures, and classifications of various terpenoids found in liverwort species like Marchantia polymorpha are discussed in detail. Among sesquiterpenes, the significance of compounds such as marchantin A and B, as well as the cuparane-type sesquiterpene alcohol (–)-tamariscol 1, is highlighted. Other cuparane-type sesquiterpenes include compounds such as cuparenediol and 2-hydroxy-4-methoxycuparene. Diterpenoids, particularly in *Jungermannia* species, include compounds like ent-trachyloban-17-al, which are noted for their antimicrobial effects.

3.1.2 Flavonoids and Phenolic Compounds

Flavonoids and phenolic compounds present in liverworts play an essential role in the secondary metabolite profiles of these plants. Flavonoids are compounds known for their antioxidant, antimicrobial, and anti-inflammatory properties, contributing significantly to plant defense mechanisms, (Asakawa et al., 2013). Phenolic compounds, on the other hand, help prevent cellular damage by reducing oxidative stress and typically protect plants against UV radiation, pathogens, and other environmental stressors, (Bié *et al.*, 2023). These compounds are valuable not only for the ecological functions of liverworts but also for their potential medicinal applications. Both flavonoids and phenolic compounds are notable for their role in the biological activities of liverworts, garnering attention in pharmacological research.

Common flavonoids in liverworts and mosses include luteolin, apigenin, and their derivatives. In liverwort species like *Marchantia polymorpha*, luteolin, apigenin, and isoriccardin C are particularly prevalent. The possibility of isolating these compounds suggests their potential as natural products. Existing studies have documented the antioxidant, antimicrobial, and anti-inflammatory properties of these flavonoids, (Horn *et al.*, 2021).

The primary classes of flavonoids in bryophytes include flavones, flavonols, isoflavonoids, aurones, 3-deoxyanthocyanins, anthocyanins, and the recently discovered auronidins unique to liverworts. Red flavonoid pigments bound to the cell wall, such as riccionidin (an auronidin), have been reported from liverworts, (Berland *et al.*, 2019).

In a study conducted by Sharma, Sharma, and Katoch (2013), the extraction of phenolic content was carried out, and the phenolic compounds isolated from the methanolic extract of *Reboulia hemispherica* were evaluated for their antimicrobial properties against a range of microorganisms. The results indicated that *Escherichia coli* exhibited the highest sensitivity to the phenolic compounds, while *Bacillus cereus* and two fungal species, *Aspergillus niger* and *Penicillium notatum*, demonstrated the least sensitivity. Notably, *Staphylococcus aureus, Enterococcus faecalis*, and *B. cereus* showed a decreased response to the phenolic compounds when compared to the crude methanolic extract. On the other hand, *E. coli*, *Pseudomonas aeruginosa, Klebsiella species, B. subtilis,* and *P. notatum* displayed greater sensitivity to the phenolic compounds than to the methanolic extract itself, suggesting that the phenolic compounds may play a significant role in enhancing antimicrobial activity, particularly against gram-negative bacteria.

3.1.3 Bibenzyls and Bis-bibenzyls

Liverworts (*Marchantiophyta*) are prolific producers of bibenzyl and bis-bibenzyl compounds, with 103 such compounds characterized to date. Although the physiological and ecological roles of these compounds are not yet fully understood, they have been widely studied. For example, Marchantin A, one of the best-known bis-bibenzyls specific to liverworts, has been isolated from Marchantia species and is well-documented for its antibacterial and antifungal activities, (Horn *et al.,* 2021).

Bibenzyl derivatives, unique metabolites of liverworts, are highly bioactive compounds. In 1974, the bibenzyl compound lunularin was reported to be isolated from *Marchantia polymorpha* in South Africa. Bibenzyls are particularly noted for their anticancer and antimicrobial activities. Bibenzyl and bis-bibenzyl derivatives isolated from species such as *M. polymorpha* and *Radula perrottetii* have demonstrated various bioactivities. Notably, bis-bibenzyls, aside from their distinctive structures, exhibit a range of biological activities, including antifungal, antimicrobial, antioxidant, antitrypanosomal, antiviral, muscle relaxant effects, and inhibition of NO production and tubulin polymerization, (Asakawa *et al.*, 2021).

3.2 Medical Uses of Liverworts

Liverworts have been used in traditional medicine for centuries. They have found a place in Asian countries, especially in the treatment of conditions such as liver diseases and skin infections. Modern scientific research has revealed that metabolites isolated from these plants exhibit various biological activities.

3.2.1 Antimicrobial Activity

Liverworts have demonstrated significant antimicrobial activity in various studies, highlighting their potential as sources of new bioactive compounds.

Millar *et al.* (2007) conducted a study involving *Blasia pusilla*, *Pallavicinia lyellii*, and *Radula obconica*, revealing that only *R. obconica* exhibited notable antibacterial activity, particularly against *Bacillus subtilis*. This activity was attributed to bibenzyl compounds, which are common in liverworts but rare in other plants. The study underscores the potential of liverworts in developing antibiotics targeting Gram-positive bacteria.

A separate investigation on the liverwort *Mastigophora diclados* identified sesquiterpenoids and bis-bibenzyls as key antimicrobial agents. This study reinforced the unique bioactive properties of liverwort secondary metabolites, showing significant inhibition of bacterial and fungal growth. The compounds exhibited particularly strong effects against pathogens such as *B. subtilis*, (Komala *et al.,* 2010).

In another study by Scher *et al.* (2004) on *Bazzania trilobata*, methanolic extracts were examined and found to have potent antifungal properties. Several compounds isolated from the liverwort extract were identified as potential candidates for treating fungal infections, and the antifungal potential of some isolated compounds was reported for the first time. These findings highlight the therapeutic potential of liverworts.

3.2.2 Anti-Inflammatory Properties

Nine novel pinguisane-type sesquiterpenoids isolated from the liverwort *Trocholejeunea sandvicensis* Mizut (Lejeuneaceae) were tested for their anti-inflammatory effects. Compounds 1, 9, and 10 notably inhibited LPS-induced NO production by 83.15%, 83.54%, and 96.28%, respectively, indicating that *T. sandvicensis* is a valuable source of potential anti-inflammatory compounds, (Zhu *et al.,* 2021).

In another study, the phytochemical content and pharmacological effects of eight liverwort species' extracts were investigated with a focus on their major volatile compounds and their anti-inflammatory and antinociceptive potential. Results showed that liverworts such as *Porella cordaeana*, *Plagiochasma rupestre*, and *Reboulia hemisphaerica* exhibited anti-inflammatory effects in carrageenan-induced edema models, achieving a reduction in inflammatory response by 25-30%, attributed to their sesquiterpene content. These findings scientifically support the traditional medicinal use of liverworts, (Tosun *et al.*, 2013).

Methanolic extract of *Marchantia polymorpha* L. was observed to reduce the production of inflammatory markers such as NO, iNOS, and COX-2 in LPS-stimulated HaCaT cells. The extract also effectively suppressed mRNA levels of pro-inflammatory cytokines IL-6 and IL-1β, highlighting its potential as an anti-inflammatory agent, (Kim *et al.*, 2021).

These studies reveal that liverworts exert anti-inflammatory effects through various mechanisms, underscoring their value as significant natural sources for future drug development.

3.2.3 Antioxidant Activity

A study examined the biochemical, antioxidant, and antimicrobial properties of *Frullania dilatata*. The ethanol extract's antioxidant activity was measured using the DPPH (2,2-diphenyl-1-picrylhydrazyl) radical scavenging method, with ascorbic acid serving as a positive control for comparison. *F. dilatata* exhibited significant antioxidant activity, with an EC50 value of 0.03169 mg/ml. These results indicate that *F. dilatata* could be considered a natural antimicrobial and antioxidant agent, (Simsek *et al.*, 2023).

In a study assessing the biological activities of *Marchantia polymorpha* L. samples successfully grown in vitro, the ethyl acetate fraction showed the highest ferric reducing power and DPPH radical scavenging capacity. Additionally, the n-hexane and chloroform extracts displayed significant tyrosinase inhibition and anti-proliferative activity against MCF-7 cells. This research suggests that *Marchantia polymorpha* can be cultivated in vitro and that this biomass has antioxidant, antibacterial, and anti-proliferative potential, (Quach, 2020).

Another study explored the antioxidant and anti-diabetic properties of *Ptychanthus striatus*, *Pellia epiphylla*, and *Bazzania oshimensis*. Various analyses indicated the anti-diabetic potential of these species through α-amylase and α-glucosidase inhibition. Additionally, their antioxidant activities, assessed by DPPH, metal chelation, and superoxide assays, were found to be high. *B. oshimensis* extract exhibited a strong DPPH radical scavenging activity and also had higher ABTS radical scavenging activity compared to the other two species. Results indicate that these plant extracts provide sufficient hydrogen molecules to reduce DPPH and ABTS radicals. *B. oshimensis* also showed the highest ability to reduce oxidized $Fe3+$ to $Fe2+$ among the plants, while the metal chelation test indicated that *P. epiphylla* exhibited the highest chelation activity. These findings suggest that these liverwort species contain phytochemicals of clinical and cosmetic importance, (Mukhia *et al.,* 2015).

3.2.4 Anticancer Activity

This review, examining the anticancer potential of bryophytes, reveals that this plant group contains compounds demonstrating cytotoxic activity against various cancer cell lines. The most potent of these compounds are primarily terpenoids and bibenzyls, which exert effects mainly through apoptosis induction. Biochemical markers such as DNA fragmentation, proteolysis of polymerase proteins, and caspase activation have been associated with the apoptotic effect of these plants. These findings suggest that bryophytes should be considered a potential source for cancer treatment, (Dey & Mukherjee, 2015).

The series of sesquiterpenes known as plagiochilins, isolated from liverworts of the genus *Plagiochila*, have shown antiproliferative properties and have been particularly effective against prostate cancer cells. Specifically, plagiochilin A exhibits a unique mechanism of action by inhibiting the final stage of cytokinesis (membrane abscission). Due to this distinct mechanism and structure-activity relationship, plagiochilin A emerges as a promising candidate for next-generation cancer drugs targeting the cytokinesis pathway, (Bailly, 2023).

Marchantin C, isolated from liverworts of the genus *Marchantia*, has been identified as a microtubule inhibitor in cancer cells, arresting the cell cycle at the G2/M phase. In A172 and HeLa cells, marchantin C inhibits microtubule polymerization and, in in-vivo studies, suppresses the growth of human cervical cancer xenografts. The potential of marchantin C to induce apoptosis in tumor cells suggests its promise as an antitumor therapeutic agent, (Shi *et al.,* 2009).

4. HORNWORTS (ANTHOCEROTOPHYTA)

Hornworts (*Anthocerotophyta*), a group of non-vascular plants that includes liverworts and mosses, are intriguing due to their unique secondary metabolites and potential medicinal applications. Unlike vascular plants, hornworts lack a true vascular system; however, they possess distinctive features such as a sporophyte that grows from a basal meristem, allowing for continuous growth. Additionally, they play crucial ecological roles, including water regulation, erosion control, nitrogen enrichment, and providing habitats for other organisms, (Vanderpoorten, Papp, & Gradstein, 2010).

Despite their primitive forms, these plants have developed numerous adaptive traits to thrive in terrestrial environments. One of the most significant adaptive features is the production of secondary metabolites. Particularly, in response to biotic and abiotic environmental stressors, bryophytes have produced a diverse range of secondary metabolites, including terpenoids, phenolic compounds, and alkaloids. Due to the substances, they produce, these plants rich in secondary metabolites can protect themselves from competition, microbial attacks, and insect or animal predation. Moreover, these compounds are essential for the bryophytes' ability to withstand drought, protect against UV radiation, and survive freezing temperatures, (Değirmenci & Ezer, 2024).

4.1 Secondary Metabolites in Hornworts

In contrast to many other plant species that have been thoroughly researched, hornworts are known to contain a diverse range of secondary metabolites that are frequently overlooked, yet they may possess significant pharmacological potential. Secondary metabolites are substances produced by plants that do not participate directly in the organism's regular growth, development, or reproduction. Rather, these compounds are typically involved in defense mechanisms or play a role in various ecological interactions. The secondary metabolites found in hornworts can be categorized into several primary groups, such as terpenoids, flavonoids, and phenolic compounds, each contributing to the plant's overall biological activity.

4.1.1 Terpenoids

Terpenoids are a class of secondary metabolites commonly found in plants, including bryophytes. There are approximately 300 species of hornworts; however, only a few have been biochemically studied, and there is very limited data regarding the presence of terpenes in hornworts. According to Xiong *et al.* (2018), common mono- and sesquiterpenoids have been identified in two different species of *Anthoceros*, namely *A. punctatus* and *A. agrestis*. Additionally, Sonwa and König (2003) detected various monoterpenes, including limonene, in another species of *Anthoceros*.

In a study conducted by Sonwa and König (2003), several monoterpenoids were identified in the essential oil of *Anthoceros caucasicus*. Notably, compounds such as myrcene, terpinolene, and limonene were listed as major constituents. A review of existing studies on these substances reveals that terpinolene is known for its antifungal, antibacterial, and antioxidant properties, (Menezes *et al.*, 2021). Limonene, another commonly used monoterpene, is widely employed in cleaning products, food items, and cosmetic formulations, and is one of the most popular fragrances. A large number of studies investigating the medicinal properties of limonene have highlighted its wide range of beneficial health effects, which include anti-inflammatory, antioxidant, antinociceptive, anticancer, antidiabetic, antihyperalgesic, antiviral, and gastroprotective properties, (Vieira *et al.*, 2018). While several terpenes have been identified in hornworts, there have been no reports of bioactive compounds that are unique to hornworts specifically. Considering the identified terpenoids, this situation renders hornworts a promising candidate for pharmaceutical applications. Equally important is the isolatability of these compounds. In this regard, it is promising that a known terpenoid, methyl p-coumarate, has been isolated from the tissues of *Anthoceros laevis* and *A. punctatus*, (Mendez & Sanz-Cabanilles, 1979).

4.1.2 Phenolic Compounds

Anthoceros agrestis (Anthocerotaceae), commonly known as hornwort, is regarded as a model organism for studying the transition of plants from aquatic environments to terrestrial habitats, as well as their associated developmental processes. This species contains the general phenylpropanoid pathway, which plays a role in the synthesis of phenolic compounds such as rosmarinic acid and megacerotonic acid. Rosmarinic acid is a widely recognized natural compound found in higher plants, particularly in species from the Lamiaceae and Boraginaceae families. However, its occurrence in lower plants is less well-documented. Known for its various biological and pharmacological effects, rosmarinic acid possesses antioxidant, anti-inflammatory, antimicrobial, and anticancer properties. Due to these beneficial attributes, it has been highlighted as a key compound in pharmaceutical and clinical research, (Vogelsong, Schneider, & Petersen, 2006) (Pezeshki *et al.,* 2022) (Amoah *et al.,* 2016).

4.1.3 Flavonoids

Hornworts (*Anthocerotophyta*) are distinct from other bryophytes and early-evolving plant groups due to their lack of flavonoids. Flavonoids are generally known for their protective roles against UV radiation and their antioxidant properties. The absence of flavonoids in hornworts may have two main evolutionary explanations. Hornworts may have diverged before the evolution of the flavonoid biosynthetic pathway in plants, suggesting that flavonoids are a later adaptation for UV protection. Alternatively, the early hornwort ancestors possessing the flavonoid biosynthesis pathway may have undergone mutations leading to the loss of flavonoid biosynthesis, resulting in the complete disappearance of these metabolites from this lineage, (Horn *et al.*, 2021) (Soriano *et al.*, 2018).

The absence of flavonoids suggests that hornworts may have developed alternative metabolic pathways or other phenolic compounds for UV resistance and stress response; for instance, compounds unique to hornworts, such as rosmarinic acid and anthocerotonic acid, may play a role in this regard. To better understand this evolutionary distinction, further research comparing the metabolic profiles of hornworts with those of other early land plants is needed.

4.2 Medical Uses of Liverworts

Hornworts have long been used in traditional medicine, but scientific studies on their medicinal applications are still limited compared to other plants. Here, we examine some potential medicinal uses based on their secondary metabolites.

4.2.1 Antimicrobial Activity

A study investigated the antimicrobial activity of certain liverworts and hornworts. The antibacterial effects of the methanol and dichloromethane extracts of *Plagiochasma intermedium*, *Asterella wallichiana*, and *Targionia hypophylla* against three bacterial species were evaluated using the agar well diffusion method. Ampicillin and tetracycline were used as positive controls, while solvents served as negative controls. Notably, *Targionia hypophylla* exhibited the highest antibacterial activity against all tested microorganisms. In contrast, *Cyathodium cavernarum* demonstrated lower antimicrobial activity compared to the other plant species, (Sawant & Karadge, 2010).

The methanolic extracts of the stems and leaves of *Cerathophyllum demersum* were found to exhibit strong antibacterial and antifungal activity against isolated bacteria and fungi. Additionally, treating modern Rakta papers with *C. demersum* extract not only improved the physical and mechanical properties of the paper but also enhanced its resistance to microbial attacks. This study suggests that *C. demersum* can be considered not only as an antimicrobial agent but also as a potential biological preservative in the field of paper protection, (Omar *et al.*, 2017).

Bryophytes, particularly hornworts, have yet to be sufficiently studied for their antimicrobial effects. This gap in research becomes more pronounced despite the evidence that hornworts possess bioactive compounds such as phenolic compounds, due to the limited investigation of their antimicrobial properties. This situation increases the demand for alternative natural antimicrobial sources, especially in today's context where traditional antibiotics are losing their efficacy against resistant microorganisms.

5. CONCLUSION

Mosses (*Bryophyta*) are the largest group of bryophytes, encompassing around 14,000 species that typically range from a few millimeters to a few centimeters in size. The largest species include *Dawsonia superba*, reaching up to 70 cm, and *Fontinalis antipyretica*, which can grow up to 2 m. Mosses are categorized into two groups: acrocarpous, which grow upright and usually do not branch, and pleurocarpous, which grow parallel to the substrate and exhibit branching. They thrive in various moist environments, provide food and shelter for insects, and can endure harsh conditions by halting physiological activities when water is scarce. Key to moss reproduction is the presence of hygroscopic peristome teeth, which regulate spore dispersal. Mosses exhibit haplodiplontic alternation of generations, with both sexual (oogamy) and asexual reproduction. The gametophyte generation can be monoicous or dioicous, producing sperm and eggs in antheridia and archegonia, respectively. Fertilization results in a sporophyte dependent on the gametophyte, with spores that germinate into protonema. While over 14,000 moss species exist, only a few have been chemically analyzed, revealing that carbohydrates are their main components along with various secondary metabolites thought to possess biological activity. Among these metabolites, terpenoids, which include monoterpenoids, sesquiterpenoids, diterpenoids, and triterpenoids, play a critical role in stress adaptation and protection against pathogens. Triterpenes, such as ursane and hopane, are particularly notable for their beneficial properties.

Liverworts (*Marchantiophyta*) encompass around 8,000 species found on every continent in various habitats. Evidence suggests they are among the earliest land plants, evolving roughly 470 million years ago. As non-vascular plants, liverworts thrive in moist, shaded areas and are characterized by small, leaf-like or thallus structures. They play crucial roles in ecosystems by stabilizing soil and transforming organic matter and are also significant in pharmacological research due to their diverse secondary metabolites, particularly in species like *Marchantia polymorpha*. Liverworts are a primary focus in bryophyte research due to their unique cellular oil bodies, which store biologically important metabolites. These metabolites contribute to the plants' fragrances and vary with habitat conditions. For example, certain *Frullania* species produce specific scents only in mountainous regions. Terpenoids, a significant class of secondary metabolites, are prevalent in liverworts. They play essential roles in plant interactions and protection against stress. Approximately 1,600 terpenoids have been identified in liverworts, including sesquiterpenes and diterpenes known for antimicrobial and antioxidant properties. Research indicates that liverworts like *Marchantia polymorpha* produce various terpenoids with potential anticancer effects.

Hornworts (*Anthocerotophyta*) are non-vascular plants known for their unique secondary metabolites that may have medicinal applications. They lack a true vascular system but feature a continuously growing sporophyte and play essential ecological roles, including water regulation and habitat provision. These plants produce a range of secondary metabolites, such as terpenoids and phenolic compounds, which help them defend against competition and environmental stressors. Although often overlooked, hornworts have demonstrated significant pharmacological potential, with compounds like myrcene, limonene, and terpinolene exhibiting beneficial properties. *Anthoceros agrestis* is a model organism for studying plant evolution from aquatic to terrestrial habitats and produces valuable phenolic compounds like rosmarinic acid, known for its antioxidant and anticancer effects. Overall, hornworts present a promising area for further medicinal research.

The objective of this study was to examine the significance and prospective medicinal applications of secondary metabolites in bryophytes. It is established that bryophytes produce a variety of bioactive compounds, including flavonoids, terpenoids, alkaloids and phenolic acids. These exhibit a range of pharmacological properties, including anti-inflammatory, antimicrobial and antioxidant effects. The study investigates the chemical profiles of these secondary metabolites, elucidating their role in plant defence mechanisms and their interactions with biotic and abiotic factors in the environment. Furthermore, this research highlights the traditional and modern medicinal uses of bryophytes and their potential as sources of new therapeutic agents. In conclusion, this study aims to contribute to the understanding of bryophytes not only as ecological actors but also as valuable resources in the field of herbal medicine and natural product research.

REFERENCES

Agelet, A., & Valles, J. (2003). Studies on pharmaceutical ethnobotany in the region of Pallars (Pyrenees, Catalonia, Iberian Peninsula). Part II. New or very rare uses of previously known medicinal plants. *Journal of Ethnopharmacology*, *84*(2-3), 211–227. DOI: 10.1016/S0378-8741(02)00319-7 PMID: 12648818

Amoah, S. K., Sandjo, L. P., Kratz, J. M., & Biavatti, M. W. (2016). Rosmarinic acid—Pharmaceutical and clinical aspects. *Planta Medica*, *82*(5), 388–406. DOI: 10.1055/s-0035-1568274 PMID: 26845712

Ando, H., & Matsuo, A. (1984). Applied bryology. *Advances in Bryology*, *2*, 133–224.

Asakawa, Y. (1995). Chemical constituents of the bryophytes. *Progress in the Chemistry of Organic Natural Products*, •••, 1–562. PMID: 23556317

Asakawa, Y. (2004). Chemosystematics of the Hepaticae. *Phytochemistry*, *65*(6), 623–629. DOI: 10.1016/j.phytochem.2004.01.003 PMID: 15016562

Asakawa, Y. (2007). Biologically active compounds from bryophytes. *Pure and Applied Chemistry*, *79*(4), 557–580. DOI: 10.1351/pac200779040557

Asakawa, Y., Ludwiczuk, A., & Nagashima, F. (2013). Chemical constituents of bryophyta. In Asakawa, Y., Ludwiczuk, A., & Nagashima, F. (Eds.), *Chemical constituents of bryophyta* (pp. 563–605). Springer. DOI: 10.1007/978-3-7091-1084-3_5

Asakawa, Y., Ludwiczuk, A., & Nagashima, F. (2013a). Phytochemical and biological studies of bryophytes. *Phytochemistry*, *91*, 52–80. DOI: 10.1016/j.phytochem.2012.04.012 PMID: 22652242

Asakawa, Y., Ludwiczuk, A., Nagashima, F., Toyota, M., Hashimoto, T., Tori, M., Fukuyama, Y., & Harinantenaina, L. (2009). Bryophytes: Bio- and chemical diversity, bioactivity, and chemosystematics. *Heterocycles*, *77*(1), 99. DOI: 10.3987/REV-08-SR(F)3

Asakawa, Y., Ludwiczuk, A., Novakovic, M., Bukvicki, D., & Anchang, K. Y. (2021). Bis-bibenzyls, bibenzyls, and terpenoids in 33 genera of the Marchantiophyta (liverworts): Structures, synthesis, and bioactivity. *Journal of Natural Products*, *85*(3), 729–762. DOI: 10.1021/acs.jnatprod.1c00302 PMID: 34783552

Bailly, C. (2023). Discovery and anticancer activity of the plagiochilins from the liverwort genus *Plagiochila.Life (Chicago, Ill.)*, *13*(3), 758. DOI: 10.3390/life13030758 PMID: 36983914

Bendz, G., Mårtensson, O., Terenius, L., Block-Bolten, A., Toguri, J. M., & Flood, H. (1962). Moss pigments. I. The anthocyanins of *Bryum cryophilum* O. Mårt. *Acta Chemica Scandinavica (Copenhagen, Denmark)*, *16*(5), 1183–1190. DOI: 10.3891/acta.chem.scand.16-1183

Benek, A. (2020). *Determination of antimicrobial, antioxidant, and antibiofilm activities of some mosses* (Master's thesis). Kastamonu University, Graduate School of Natural and Applied Sciences, Kastamonu, Turkey.

Benek, A., Canlı, K., & Altuner, E. M. (2022). Traditional medicinal uses of mosses. *Anatolian Bryology*, *8*(1), 57–65. DOI: 10.26672/anatolianbryology.1061190

Berland, H., Albert, N. W., Stavland, A., Jordheim, M., McGhie, T. K., Zhou, Y., & Bovy, A. (2019). Auronidins are a previously unreported class of flavonoid pigments that challenge when anthocyanin biosynthesis evolved in plants. *Proceedings of the National Academy of Sciences of the United States of America*, *116*(40), 20232–20239. DOI: 10.1073/pnas.1912741116 PMID: 31527265

Bié, J., Sepodes, B., Fernandes, P. C., & Ribeiro, M. H. (2023). Polyphenols in health and disease: Gut microbiota, bioaccessibility, and bioavailability. *Compounds*, *3*(1), 40–72. DOI: 10.3390/compounds3010005

Boom, B. M. (1996). *Ethnobotany of the Chácobo Indians*. Advances in Economic Botany.

Canlı, K. (2012). *Determination of antimicrobial activity of Akdağ (Amasya) moss (Musci) flora and some moss species collected from the area* (PhD thesis). Ankara University, Graduate School of Natural and Applied Sciences, Ankara, Turkey.

Çetin, B. (1998). Ormanın su deposu. *Yeşil Atlas*, *1*, 92–93.

Chinese Materia Medica Editorial Committee. (1999). *Chinese Materia Medica* [Zhong Hua ben Cao]. Vol. 2). Shanghai Science and Technology Press.

Cianciullo, P., Maresca, V., Sorbo, S., & Basile, A. (2021). Antioxidant and antibacterial properties of extracts and bioactive compounds in bryophytes. *Applied Sciences (Basel, Switzerland)*, *12*(1), 160. DOI: 10.3390/app12010160

Commisso, M., Guarino, F., Marchi, L., Muto, A., Piro, A., & Degola, F. (2021). Bryo-activities: A review on how bryophytes are contributing to the arsenal of natural bioactive compounds against fungi. *Plants*, *10*(2), 203. DOI: 10.3390/plants10020203 PMID: 33494524

Ćosić, M. V., Janošević, D. A., Oaldje, M. M., Vujičić, M. M., Lang, I., Sabovljević, M. S., & Djuric, S. (2021). Terpenoid evidences within three selected bryophyte species under salt stress as inferred by histochemical analyses. *Flora (Jena), 285*, 151956. DOI: 10.1016/j.flora.2021.151956

Das, K., Kityania, S., Nath, R., Das, S., Nath, D., & Talukdar, A. D. (2022). Bioactive compounds from bryophytes. In *Bioactive Compounds in Bryophytes and Pteridophytes* (pp. 1–15). Springer International Publishing., DOI: 10.1007/978-3-030-97415-2_2-1

Değirmenci, U., & Ezer, T. (2024). *Homalothecium philippeanum* (Spruce) Schimp. (Bryophyta) ekstresinin Asetilkolinesteraz enzim aktivitesine etkisi. *Lokman Hekim Dergisi, 14*(3), 587–593. DOI: 10.31020/mutftd.1479130

Dey, A., & Mukherjee, A. (2015). Therapeutic potential of bryophytes and derived compounds against cancer. *Journal of Acute Disease, 4*(3), 236–248. DOI: 10.1016/j.joad.2015.04.011

Ding, H. (1982). *Medicinal spore-bearing plants of China*. Shanghai Science and Technology Press.

Drobnik, J., & Stebel, A. (2015). Central European medicinal bryophytes in the 16th-century work by Caspar Schwenckfeld, and their ethnopharmacological origin. *Journal of Ethnopharmacology, 175*, 407–411. DOI: 10.1016/j.jep.2015.09.033 PMID: 26432352

Dziwak, M., Wróblewska, K., Szumny, A., & Galek, R. (2022). Modern use of bryophytes as a source of secondary metabolites. *Agronomy (Basel), 12*(6), 1456. DOI: 10.3390/agronomy12061456

Flowers, S. (1957). Ethnobryology of the Gosuite Indians of Utah. *The Bryologist, 60*(1), 11–14. DOI: 10.1639/0007-2745(1957)60[11:EOTGIO]2.0.CO;2

Frahm, J. P. (2004). Recent developments of commercial products from bryophytes. *The Bryologist, 107*(3), 277–283. DOI: 10.1639/0007-2745(2004)107[0277:RDOCPF]2.0.CO;2

Fuchs, L. (1990). *De historia stirpium commentarii insignes*. Apud Audoenum Paruum sub Lilio Aureo.

Ginting, N., Amrul, H. M. Z., & Susilo, F. (2021). An overview of bryophytes division. [Jurnal Biologi Lingkungan dan Kesehatan]. *BIOLINK, 8*(1), 10–20. DOI: 10.31289/biolink.v8i1.4294

Glime, J. M. (2007). Economic and ethnic uses of bryophytes. *Flora of North America, 27*, 14–41.

Glime, J. M. (2022). Bryoecol. Retrieved July 21, 2024, from http://www.bryoecol.mtu.edu/

Gürsu, G. (2012). *Karasu (Sakarya) moss (Musci) flora* [Master's thesis, Ankara University, Graduate School of Natural and Applied Sciences].

Hanson, D. T., & Rice, S. K. (2013). What can we learn from bryophyte photosynthesis? In *Photosynthesis in bryophytes and early land plants* (pp. 1–8). Springer Netherlands., DOI: 10.1007/978-94-007-6074-6_1

Harris, E. S. (2008). Ethnobryology: Traditional uses and folk classification of bryophytes. *The Bryologist, 111*(2), 169–217. DOI: 10.1639/0007-2745(2008)111[169:ETUAFC]2.0.CO;2

Hazer, Y., Çölgeçen, H., & Uyar, G. (2017). Briyofitlerden elde edilen fenolik bileşikler. *Karaelmas Fen Mühendislik Dergisi, 7*(1), 333–340.

He, X., Sun, Y., & Zhu, R. L. (2013). The oil bodies of liverworts: Unique and important organelles in land plants. *Critical Reviews in Plant Sciences, 32*(5), 293–302. DOI: 10.1080/07352689.2013.765765

Hernick, L. V., Landing, E., & Bartowski, K. E. (2008). Earth's oldest liverworts—Metzgeriothallus sharonae sp. nov. from the Middle Devonian (Givetian) of eastern New York, USA. *Review of Palaeobotany and Palynology, 148*(2-4), 154–162. DOI: 10.1016/j.revpalbo.2007.09.002

Horn, A., Pascal, A., Lončarević, I., Volpatto Marques, R., Lu, Y., Miguel, S., & Tavares, P. (2021). Natural products from bryophytes: From basic biology to biotechnological applications. *Critical Reviews in Plant Sciences, 40*(3), 191–217. DOI: 10.1080/07352689.2021.1911034

Ingimundardóttir, G. V., Weibull, H., & Cronberg, N. (2014). Bryophyte colonization history of the virgin volcanic island Surtsey, Iceland. *Biogeosciences, 11*(16), 4415–4427. DOI: 10.5194/bg-11-4415-2014

Jocković, N., Andrade, P. B., Valentão, P., & Sabovljević, M. (2008). HPLC-DAD of phenolics in bryophytes *Lunularia cruciata, Brachytheciastrum velutinum*, and *Kindbergia praelonga. Journal of the Serbian Chemical Society, 73*(12), 1161–1167. DOI: 10.2298/JSC0812161J

Jung, M., Zinsmeister, H. D., & Geiger, H. (1994). New three-and tetraoxygenated coumarin glucosides from the mosses *Atrichum undulatum* and *Polytrichum formosum.Zeitschrift für Naturforschung. C, A Journal of Biosciences*, *49*(11-12), 697–702. DOI: 10.1515/znc-1994-11-1201

Karaburun, P. (2012). *Bryophyte flora of Bolu-Yukarı Gerede Valley* [Master's thesis, Bülent Ecevit University, Graduate School of Natural and Applied Sciences].

Karahan, M. (2021). *Moss flora of Köyceğiz Lake (Muğla) and surrounding sweetgum forests* (Master's thesis). Çankırı Karatekin University, Graduate School of Natural and Applied Sciences, Çankırı, Turkey.

Karim, F. A., Suleiman, M., Rahmat, A., & Bakar, M. F. A. (2014). Phytochemicals, antioxidant and antiproliferative properties of five moss species from Sabah, Malaysia. *International Journal of Pharmacy and Pharmaceutical Sciences*, *6*, 292–297.

Karpinski, T. M., & Adamczak, A. (2017). Antibacterial activity of ethanolic extracts of some moss species. *Herba Polonica*, *63*(3), 3. DOI: 10.1515/hepo-2017-0014

Kim, S. Y., Hong, M., Kim, T. H., Lee, K. Y., Park, S. J., Hong, S. H., Sowndhararajan, K., & Kim, S. (2021). Anti-inflammatory effect of liverwort (*Marchantia polymorpha* L.) and racomitrium moss (*Racomitrium canescens* (Hedw.) Brid.) growing in Korea. *Plants*, *10*(10), 2075. DOI: 10.3390/plants10102075 PMID: 34685885

Kırmacı, M. (2007). *Bryophyte flora of Denizli Mountains (Babadag, Honaz Mountain)* (PhD thesis). Adnan Menderes University, Graduate School of Natural and Applied Sciences, Aydın, Turkey.

Komala, I., Ito, T., Nagashima, F., Yagi, Y., & Asakawa, Y. (2010). Cytotoxic, radical scavenging and antimicrobial activities of sesquiterpenoids from the Tahitian liverwort *Mastigophora diclados* (Brid.) Nees (Mastigophoraceae). *Journal of Natural Medicines*, *64*(4), 417–422. DOI: 10.1007/s11418-010-0423-8 PMID: 20458547

Kozlowski, M. A. (1921). Sur la saponarine chez le *Mnium cuspidatum.Comptes Rendus Hebdomadaires des Séances de l'Académie des Sciences*, *173*, 429–431.

Lange, B. M., Rujan, T., Martin, W., & Croteau, R. (2000). Isoprenoid biosynthesis: The evolution of two ancient and distinct pathways across genomes. *Proceedings of the National Academy of Sciences of the United States of America*, *97*(24), 13172–13177. DOI: 10.1073/pnas.240454797 PMID: 11078528

Lubaina, A. S., Pradeep, D. P., Aswathy, J. M., Remya Krishnan, M. K., & Murugan, K. V. (2014). Traditional knowledge of medicinal bryophytes by the Kani tribes of Agasthiyarmalai biosphere reserve, southern western Ghats. *Indo American Journal of Pharmaceutical Research*, *4*, 2116–2121.

Maksimova, V., Klavina, L., Bikovens, O., Zicmanis, A., & Purmalis, O. (2013). Structural characterization and chemical classification of some bryophytes found in Latvia. *Chemistry & Biodiversity*, *10*(7), 1284–1294. DOI: 10.1002/cbdv.201300014 PMID: 23847073

Markham, K. R., & Porter, L. J. (2016). Chemical constituents of bryophytes. In Harborne, J. B., & Swain, T. (Eds.), *Progress in Phytochemistry* (Vol. 5, p. 181). Elsevier., DOI: 10.1016/B978-0-12-706305-7.50012-2

Marques, R. V., Sestito, S. E., Bourgaud, F., Miguel, S., Cailotto, F., Reboul, P., Jouzeau, J.-Y., Rahuel-Clermont, S., Boschi-Muller, S., Simonsen, H. T., & Moulin, D. (2022). Anti-inflammatory activity of bryophyte extracts in LPS-stimulated RAW264.7 murine macrophages. *Molecules (Basel, Switzerland)*, *27*(6), 1940. DOI: 10.3390/molecules27061940 PMID: 35335304

Matos, T. M., Peralta, D. F., Roma, L. P., & Santos, D. Y. A. C. D. (2021). The morphology and chemical composition of cuticular waxes in some Brazilian liverworts and mosses. *Journal of Bryology*, *43*(2), 129–137. DOI: 10.1080/03736687.2020.1859872

Mendez, J., & Sanz-Cabanilles, F. (1979). Cinnamic acid esters in *Anthoceros* species. *Phytochemistry*, *18*(8), 1409–1410. DOI: 10.1016/0031-9422(79)83039-3

Menezes, I. O., Scher, J. R., Martins, A. O. B. P., Ramos, A. G. B., Quintans, J. D. S. S., Coutinho, H. D. M., & Silva, T. S. (2021). Biological properties of terpinolene evidenced by in silico, in vitro, and in vivo studies: A systematic review. *Phytomedicine*, *93*, 153768. DOI: 10.1016/j.phymed.2021.153768 PMID: 34634744

Millar, K. D., Crandall-Stotler, B. J., Ferreira, J. F., & Wood, K. V. (2007). Antimicrobial properties of three liverworts in axenic culture: *Blasia pusilla, Pallavicinia lyellii*, and *Radula obconica.Cryptogamie. Bryologie*, *28*(3), 197–210.

Motti, R., & de Falco, B. (2021). Traditional herbal remedies used for managing anxiety and insomnia in Italy: An ethnopharmacological overview. *Horticulturae*, *7*(12), 523. DOI: 10.3390/horticulturae7120523

Motti, R., Palma, D., & de Falco, B. (2023). Bryophytes used in folk medicine: An ethnobotanical overview. *Horticulturae*, *9*(2), 137. DOI: 10.3390/horticulturae9020137

Mukhia, S., Mandal, P., Singh, D. K., & Singh, D. (2015). Evaluation of anti-diabetic, antioxidant activity, and phytochemical constituents of liverworts of Eastern Himalaya. *Journal of Chemical and Pharmaceutical Research*, *7*(10), 890–900.

Negi, K., & Chaturvedi, P. (2021). Antifungal activity of *Conocephalum conicum* (L) Dumort. (Marchantiophyta) against *Fusarium oxysporum* f. sp. *lycopersici*. *bioRxiv*. https://doi.org/DOI: 10.1101/2021.07.23.453678

Omar, A. M., Salah, T. A., Mohamed, A. A., & Sheded, M. G. (2017). Attenuation of microbial induced deterioration of cellulose fibers by hornwort (*Ceratophyllum demersum* L.) methanolic extract. *International Journal of Biological Research*, *5*(2), 48–58. DOI: 10.14419/ijbr.v5i2.8479

Özcan, H. M. (2010). The preparation of amperometric biosensor for determination of phenolic compounds [PhD thesis, Trakya University, Graduate School of Natural and Applied Sciences].

Özen, Ö. (2017). *Musci flora of Ardahan (Center) and Göle district* (PhD thesis). Karadeniz Technical University, Graduate School of Natural and Applied Sciences, Trabzon, Turkey.

Oztopcu-Vatan, P., Savaroglu, F., Iscen, C. F., Kabadere, S., Ozturk, N., & Ilhan, S. (2017). Screening of antimicrobial, cytotoxic effects and phenolic compounds of the moss *Aulacomnium androgynum* (Hedw.) Schwagr (Bryophyta). *Journal of Animal and Plant Sciences*, *27*(6), 1559–1569.

Pant, G., & Tewari, S. D. (1989). Various human uses of bryophytes in the Kumaun region of Northwest Himalaya. *The Bryologist*, *92*(1), 120–122. DOI: 10.2307/3244026

Pavletić, Z., & Stilinović, B. (1963). Untersuchungen über die antibiotische Wirkung von Moosextrakten auf einige Bakterien. *Acta Botanica Croatica*, *22*(1), 133–139.

Pezeshki, S., Warmbier, I., Busch, T., Bauerbach, E., Szövenyi, P., & Petersen, M. (2022). The first step into phenolic metabolism in the hornwort *Anthoceros agrestis*: Molecular and biochemical characterization of two phenylalanine ammonia-lyase isoforms. *Planta*, *256*(2), 33. DOI: 10.1007/s00425-022-03944-w PMID: 35796843

Quach, P. N. (2020). Biological activities of in vitro liverwort *Marchantia polymorpha* L. extracts. *Notulae Botanicae Horti Agrobotanici Cluj-Napoca*, *48*(2), 826–838. DOI: 10.15835/nbha48211884

Rahman, I. U., Afzal, A., Iqbal, Z., Ijaz, F., Ali, N., Shah, M., Ullah, S., & Bussmann, R. W. (2019). Historical perspectives of ethnobotany. *Clinical Dermatology*, *37*(4), 382–388. DOI: 10.1016/j.clindermatol.2018.03.018 PMID: 31345328

Rao, S. A. (2021). Structural information of natural product metabolites in bryophytes. In *Evolutionary Diversity as a Source for Anticancer Molecules* (pp. 209–231). Academic Press., DOI: 10.1016/B978-0-12-823037-1.00011-3

Redvers, N., & Blondin, B. S. (2020). Traditional Indigenous medicine in North America: A scoping review. *PLoS One*, *15*(8), e0237531. DOI: 10.1371/journal.pone.0237531 PMID: 32790714

Sabovljević, M. S., Sabovljević, A. D., Ikram, N. K. K., Peramuna, A., Bae, H., & Simonsen, H. T. (2016). Bryophytes—An emerging source for herbal remedies and chemical production. *Plant Genetic Resources*, *14*(4), 314–327. DOI: 10.1017/S1479262116000320

Sahilli, Y. Ç., & Alataş, M. (2024). Polytrichum piliferum Hedw. Ekstraktlarının Antioksidan Aktivitesi ve Bazı Kimyasal Bileşimleri. *Anatolian Bryology*, *10*(1), 58–66. DOI: 10.26672/anatolianbryology.1480997

Sawant, U. J., & Karadge, B. A. (2010). Antimicrobial activity of some bryophytes (liverworts and a hornwort) from Kolhapur district. *Pharmacognosy Journal*, *2*(16), 29–32. DOI: 10.1016/S0975-3575(10)80046-X

Scher, J. M., Speakman, J. B., Zapp, J., & Becker, H. (2004). Bioactivity guided isolation of antifungal compounds from the liverwort *Bazzania trilobata* (L.) SF Gray. *Phytochemistry*, *65*(18), 2583–2588. DOI: 10.1016/j.phytochem.2004.05.013 PMID: 15451321

Schofield, W. B. (1985). *Introduction to bryology*. Macmillan.

Schofield, W. B. (2001). *Introduction to Bryology*. The Blackburn Press.

Sen, K., Khan, M. I., Paul, R., Ghoshal, U., & Asakawa, Y. (2023). Recent advances in the phytochemistry of bryophytes: Distribution, structures, and biological activity of bibenzyl and bisbibenzyl compounds. *Plants*, *12*(24), 4173. DOI: 10.3390/plants12244173 PMID: 38140499

Sharma, C., Sharma, A., & Katoch, M. (2013). Comparative evaluation of antimicrobial activity of methanolic extract and phenolic compounds of a liverwort, *Reboulia hemispherica.Archives of Bryology*, *192*, 1–6.

Shaw, J., & Renzaglia, K. (2004). Phylogeny and diversification of bryophytes. *American Journal of Botany*, *91*(10), 1557–1581. DOI: 10.3732/ajb.91.10.1557 PMID: 21652309

Shi, Y. Q., Zhu, C. J., Yuan, H. Q., Li, B. Q., Gao, J., Qu, X. J., & Tan, H. (2009). Marchantin C, a novel microtubule inhibitor from liverwort with anti-tumor activity both in vivo and in vitro. *Cancer Letters*, *276*(2), 160–170. DOI: 10.1016/j.canlet.2008.11.004 PMID: 19095349

Simsek, O., Canli, K., Benek, A., Turu, D., & Altuner, E. M. (2023). Biochemical, antioxidant properties, and antimicrobial activity of epiphytic leafy liverwort *Frullania dilatata* (L.) Dumort. *Plants*, *12*(9), 1877. DOI: 10.3390/plants12091877 PMID: 37176934

Smithsonian Tropical Research Institute (STRI). (2021). Bryophytes: Tiny plants in a big changing world. Retrieved October 10, 2024, from https://stri.si.edu/story/bryophytes

Sonwa, M. M., & König, W. A. (2003). Chemical constituents of the essential oil of the hornwort *Anthoceros caucasicus.Flavour and Fragrance Journal*, *18*(4), 286–289. DOI: 10.1002/ffj.1201

Soriano, G., Del-Castillo-Alonso, M. Á., Monforte, L., Núñez-Olivera, E., & Martínez-Abaigar, J. (2018). First data on the effects of ultraviolet radiation on phenolic compounds in the model hornwort *Anthoceros agrestis.Cryptogamie. Bryologie*, *39*(2), 201–211. DOI: 10.7872/cryb/v39.iss2.2018.201

Stech, M., van Andel, T., Aptroot, A., Bertin, A., & Stefanaki, A. (2018). Bryophytes and lichens in 16th-century herbaria. *Journal of Bryology*, *40*(2), 99–106. DOI: 10.1080/03736687.2018.1447304

Stelmasiewicz, M., Świątek, Ł., & Ludwiczuk, A. (2021). Phytochemical profile and anticancer potential of endophytic microorganisms from liverwort species, *Marchantia polymorpha* L. *Molecules (Basel, Switzerland)*, *27*(1), 153. DOI: 10.3390/molecules27010153 PMID: 35011384

Sturtevant, W. (1954). *The Mikasuki Seminole: Medical beliefs and practices* [PhD thesis]. Yale University.

Tang, J. L., Liu, B. Y., & Ma, K. W. (2008). Traditional Chinese medicine. *Lancet*, *372*(9654), 1938–1940. DOI: 10.1016/S0140-6736(08)61354-9 PMID: 18930523

Tholl, D. (2015). Biosynthesis and biological functions of terpenoids in plants. In *Biotechnology of isoprenoids* (pp. 63–106). DOI: 10.1007/10_2014_295

Tosun, A., Küpeli Akkol, E., Süntar, I., Özenoğlu Kiremit, H., & Asakawa, Y. (2013). Phytochemical investigations and bioactivity evaluation of liverworts as a function of anti-inflammatory and antinociceptive properties in animal models. *Pharmaceutical Biology, 51*(8), 1008–1013. DOI: 10.3109/13880209.2013.774028 PMID: 23768252

Toyota, M., Masuda, K., & Asakawa, Y. (1998). Triterpenoid constituents of the moss *Floribundaria aurea* subsp. *nipponica.Phytochemistry, 48*(2), 297–299. DOI: 10.1016/S0031-9422(97)00902-3

Valeeva, L. R., Dague, A. L., Hall, M. H., Tikhonova, A. E., Sharipova, M. R., Valentovic, M. A., Bogomolnaya, L. M., & Shakirov, E. V. (2022). Antimicrobial activities of secondary metabolites from model mosses. *Antibiotics (Basel, Switzerland), 11*(8), 1004. DOI: 10.3390/antibiotics11081004 PMID: 35892395

Vanderpoorten, A., Papp, B., & Gradstein, R. (2010). Sampling of bryophytes. In *Manual on field recording techniques and protocols for all taxa biodiversity inventories* (pp. 331–345).

Vieira, A. J., Beserra, F. P., Souza, M. C., Totti, B. M., & Rozza, A. L. (2018). Limonene: Aroma of innovation in health and disease. *Chemico-Biological Interactions, 283*, 97–106. DOI: 10.1016/j.cbi.2018.02.007 PMID: 29427589

Vogelsang, K., Schneider, B., & Petersen, M. (2006). Production of rosmarinic acid and a new rosmarinic acid 3′-O-β-D-glucoside in suspension cultures of the hornwort *Anthoceros agrestis* Paton. *Planta, 223*(2), 369–373. DOI: 10.1007/s00425-005-0089-8 PMID: 16133208

Xiong, W., Fu, J., Köllner, T. G., Chen, X., Jia, Q., Guo, H., & Zhou, S. (2018). Biochemical characterization of microbial-type terpene synthases in two closely related species of hornworts, *Anthoceros punctatus* and *Anthoceros agrestis.Phytochemistry, 149*, 116–122. DOI: 10.1016/j.phytochem.2018.02.011 PMID: 29494813

Yayıntaş, O. T., Yılmaz, S., & Sökmen, M. (2019). Determination of antioxidant, antimicrobial, and antitumor activity of bryophytes from Mount Ida (Çanakkale, Turkey). *Indian Journal of Traditional Knowledge, 18*(2), 395–401. https://nopr.niscair.res.in/handle/123456789/46691

Zheng, G. Q., Ho, D. K., Elder, P. J., Stephens, R. E., Cottrell, C. E., & Cassady, J. M. (1994). Ohioensins and pallidisetins: Novel cytotoxic agents from the moss *Polytrichum pallidisetum.Journal of Natural Products, 57*(1), 32–41. DOI: 10.1021/np50103a005 PMID: 7512623

About the Contributors

Athanasios Alexiou is the Head of Research & Education at Funogen Research Company in Greece and AFNP Med Company in Austria, an Adjunct Professor at the University Centre for Research & Development at Chandigarh University in India, and the Department of Science and Engineering at the Novel Global Community Education Foundation (an educational platform registered in Australia). He also collaborates with international research teams (including Yerevan State University, King Abdulaziz University, the University of Sharjah and Damanhour University). His research area is Computational Biomedicine. He also focuses on developing novel mathematical models and algorithms in neurodegenerative diseases, prognostic Bayesian tools for Neurodegenerative disorders, and the ethical implications of scientific research. He serves as an Associate Editor in highly reputed journals like the Frontiers in Genetics, and Pharmacology in the Section of ELSI, the Frontiers in Neuroscience and Psychology Journals, as a Section Editor in the Current Alzheimer Research Bentham Science journal, Associate Editor in the Infectious Medicine Elsevier Journal, Guest Editor in the Biomedicines journal and in the Oxidative Medicine and Cellular Longevity Hindawi Journal etc.; he is the author of more than 250 peer-reviewed articles/chapters/books in high impact publications and 5 filled patents; he is the editor of several books in known publishing houses (Springer); he has delivered many talks and presentations in international conferences and workshops; he participates in several international funded programs; he serves as a Scientific and Program Committee Member in several conferences and as a Reviewer/Member of the Editorial Board of international journals; he is supervising from diploma to Ph.D. theses and internships' programs; he has over 20 years of mentoring and educational experience. Dr. Alexiou is a Fellow of the Institute of Biomedical Science.

Saurabh Kumar Jha is working as an Assistant Professor, Department of Zoology at Kalindi College, University of Delhi, Delhi. He obtained his M.Sc. (Biotechnology) degree from VIT University, Vellore, and Ph.D. Degree in Biotechnology (Neurobiology) was awarded from Delhi Technological University (Formerly Delhi College of Engineering). His areas of interest in Stem Cell and expertise include molecular chaperone and ubiquitin E3 ligase in neurodegenerative disorders along with therapeutics action of biomolecules in aged neurons and muscles. He has published 160 papers in peer-reviewed and high impact factor International Journals such as MC, JCR, ARR, SC, JAR. JNC, JAD, BBA, APCS, GENE & JTM (h-Index 30; i10-index 85; Cumulative impact factors 1000; Citation Index is 4000) and Fifteen books chapters in Springer International publishing AG and Nova. He has also got "Commendable Research Excellence Award DTU 2018" from Delhi Technological University, Delhi. Recently, Dr. Jha has received "Best Stem Cell Researcher Award 2019" by Prof. (Dr). Michele Zocchi, University of Turin, Italy. He has also presented more than 20 papers in international symposium and proceedings. Further, He has also designed and introduced the two new courses at level of B.Tech/M.Sc./PGD in "Stem Cell Technology and Regenerative Medicine" & "Genetic Engineering" in Sharda University. Dr. Jha has excellent track record in Teaching, Research and Placement in term of B.Tech and M.Tech Biotechnology at Sharda University. Until now, he has currently guided 06 Ph.D., 04 M.Tech, 02 M.Sc. and more than 10 BS students. He has also served various committee Members of Department as well as University level. He is the life and regular member of various professional societies across the globe.

Roma Pandey has done her Ph.D. from Bennett University. She holds sound academic credentials and hands-on trainings from renowned institutions like ICGEB, ICMR-NICPR, IIT, Delhi, Teva Pharmaceuticals and many more. During her 5 years of experience in academics and research institutions, she has received fellowships from prestigious institutions like Indian National Science Academy. She also received Doctoral fellowship from RIS-FITM, Ministry of Ayush. She has presented papers and posters in multiple conferences.

***

Selime Deniz Bozkurt graduated from Antalya Aksu Science High School in 2018. She received her bachelor's degree from the Department of Biochemistry at Ege University Faculty of Science in 2024 and began her master's studies in the Department of Biology at Dokuz Eylül University Graduate School of Natural and Applied Sciences the same year. Her research interests include biochemistry and biology.

Mustafa Eray Bozyel currently works as a Postdoctoral researcher in Kerem Canlı's lab. M. Eray research in Botany. His most recent article is 'Chemical composition, antioxidant, antimicrobial and anticancer activities of endemic Cephalaria tuteliana' and his chapter is 'Ocimum basilicum (Basil): A Medicinal Plant with Proven Ethnomedicinal Uses, Chemical Composition, Bioactivities, and Pharmacological Properties'.

Kerem Canli currently works as Associate Professor in Dokuz Eylül university. Kerem research in Botany and Microbiology. His most recent article is 'In vitro antimicrobial activity screening of Heliotropium europaeum against wide range of microorganisms and multi drug resistant (MDR) bacteria.' and conference paper is 'in vitro antimicrobial activity screening of achillea phrygia and determination of the ethanol extract composition by gas chromatography/mass spectrometry'.

Bilal El-Mansoury is a postdoctoral researcher specializing in Neuroscience and Neurology. His previous research focused on the role of glial cell dysfunction in the pathophysiology of hepatic encephalopathy and neurodegenerative disorders, investigating mechanisms such as neuroinflammation, oxidative stress, and neuronal dysfunction. Currently, Dr. El-Mansoury's work is centered on the regulatory roles of microRNAs and their implications in CDKL5 deficiency disorder, aiming to uncover novel therapeutic strategies for this rare neurodevelopmental condition.

Simran Jatwani is a dedicated Ph.D. scholar in Biotechnology at Bennett University, Greater Noida. With a strong educational foundation, she completed her M.Tech. from Doon University, Dehradun, and her B.Tech. from IMS Ghaziabad. Her journey reflects a passion for scientific inquiry and a commitment to advancing knowledge in biotechnology.

K. Kavitha received her Bachelor's degree in Electronics and Communication Engineering from Madurai Kamaraj University, Madurai, India and her Master's degree in Microwave & Optical Engineering from Madurai Kamaraj University, Madurai, India in She completed her doctoral degree at Anna University, Chennai, specializing in Hyperspectral Image Classification. Currently, she holds the position of Professor and Head in the Department of Electronics and Communication Engineering at Velammal College of Engineering and Technology in Madurai, Tamil Nadu. Her career spans over 23 years, during which she has made significant contributions in the realms of teaching and research. Her research interests encompass diverse areas, including Antenna Design, Hyperspectral Image Classification and Optical System Design. She has published and presented over 100 research articles in renowned international journals and international and national conferences. Presently, she is supervising the research works of ten Ph.D. scholars in various areas of her expertise. In recognition of her outstanding contributions to education, Dr.K.Kavitha was honored with Dr.A.P.K Abdul Kalam Teachers Excellence Award.

Jawad Laadraoui (PhD) is a distinguished neuroscientist and neurophysiologist specializing in neurodegenerative diseases with a focus on understanding epilepsy and its underlying mechanisms. As a professor at Hassan II University of Casablanca, Morocco, he has contributed extensively to understanding epilepsy's pathophysiology and the therapeutic potential of natural compounds. His research emphasizes the interplay between neuroinflammation, glial cell dysfunction, and seizure activity, aiming to uncover innovative treatments for epilepsy and related neurological conditions. Pr. Laadraoui has published influential studies in high-impact journals and authored chapters exploring the role of secondary metabolites and nanotechnology in managing epileptic disorders. His work has gained recognition at international conferences, showcasing his leadership in multidisciplinary collaborations. Beyond research, he mentors graduate students and advocates for integrating computational models to enhance therapeutic approaches, further solidifying his role in advancing epilepsy research and treatment strategies.

Vijay M received his bachelor's degree in Electronics and Communication Engineering from Anna University, Chennai, and his master's degree in Communication Systems from the same institution. He completed his doctoral degree from Anna University, India, in 2022, specializing in deep learning. Currently, he serves as an Associate Professor in the Department of Computer Science and Engineering at the Kalasalingam Academy of Research and Education. His career spans over 12 years, during which he has made significant contributions to teaching and research. His academic contributions include publishing extensively in international journals, patents, book chapters, and conference proceedings. He has published over 16 research papers in international journals and presented 24 papers at international conferences. He has also received the award for “Best Outcome in Academic Performance. Dr. Vijay M's research interests encompass Image Processing, Deep Learning, Machine Learning, Network Security, and Artificial Intelligence. He is an active member of prestigious professional organizations, including the Institute of Electrical and Electronics Engineers (IEEE), ISTE & IETE.

Elif Merdamert-Bozyel completed her undergraduate studies at Çanakkale Onsekiz Mart University, Department of Biology. She completed her Master's thesis in Molecular Toxicology at the Biology Department of the same university. She worked as a biologist at the Health Institutes of Turkey (TUSEB) during the Covid-19 pandemic.

Adnane Moutaouakkil, PhD in Biology, speciality: Microbiology, Biotechnology and Environment. He is the author of several publications on the development of biotechnological processes. He currently works as a researcher at the National Centre for Nuclear Energy, Science, and Technology (Rabat, Morocco).

Odangowei Inetiminebi Ogidi is a Lecturer and Acting Head, Department of Biochemistry, Bayelsa Medical University, Yenagoa, Bayelsa State, Nigeria. He holds a Bachelor of Science degree in Biochemistry, Master of Science and Doctor of Philosophy degrees in Biotechnology. He has also served as a Lecturer, Head of Departments of Science Laboratory Technology and Biochemistry, and Deputy Director, Centre for Continuing Education in Federal Polytechnic Ekowe, Bayelsa State. He has authored over 80 peer-reviewed academic articles in reputable local and international journals, published over 40 book chapters and presented over 35 conference papers. He is a member of various Journal Editorial Boards. He is indexed in World Scientist and University Ranking (AD Scientific Index ID 4306173) amongst other international bodies. He have supervised over 30 ND and HND students and currently supervising over 10 undergraduate students. His research interest has been Environmental Biotechnology, Phytomedicine, Phytochemistry, Human and Environmental health risk assessments and ecotoxicology amongst others. He is a member of West Africa Society of Toxicology, Nigerian Society of Biochemistry and Molecular Biology, Foundation for African Development through International Biotechnology and Nigerian Environmental Society.

Mohammed Rhazi his research has focused on the valorization of terrestrial and marine fishing wastes by the production of chitinous derivatives and their applications in various fields (pharmacology, biomedical, agroalimentary and water treatment). He has been working since 1996 on the complexation of metal ions by chitosan and its derivatives and their interest in wastewater treatment.

S. Raj Kumar received his bachelor's degree in Electronics and Communication Engineering from Anna University, Chennai, and his master's degree in VLSI Design from the same institution. He completed his doctoral degree at Anna University, Chennai, specializing in VLSI device modeling. Currently, he serves as an Assistant Professor in the Department of Electronics Engineering (VLSI Design and Technology) at Velammal College of Engineering and Technology, Madurai, Tamil Nadu, India. His career spans over 11 years, during which he has made significant contributions to teaching and research. His research interests include diverse areas such as modeling and simulation of analog VLSI. He has published over 10 research papers in international journals and presented 20 papers at international conferences. He has also received the award for “Best Outcome in Academic Performance”.

Özcan Şimşek serves as a faculty member at Çanakkale Onsekiz Mart University, Yenice Vocational School, Department of Forestry. He earned his undergraduate degree from Ankara University, Faculty of Science, Department of Biology, and his doctorate from Ankara University, Graduate School of Natural and Applied Sciences, Department of Biology. His research specializes in liverworts within forest ecosystems, with a particular focus on examining their ecological and biological characteristics through laboratory investigations. His work in biodiversity-rich regions, including the Kaz Mountains, makes substantial contributions to the scientific understanding of the area's natural heritage.

Rajesh Tiwari is working as Professor and Academic Coordinator in the Department of Management Studies, Graphic Era (Deemed to be University), Dehradun. He has over twenty years of rich experience in academics and industry. He is MBA (Finance), Chartered Financial Analyst (CFA), UGC-NET, PhD in Management. He has previously worked as Director in Indus University, Ahmedabad, United Group-Greater Noida (Affiliated to Guru Gobind Singh Indraprastha University, New Delhi), Sai Balaji Group-Pune. He has been academic coordinator for Management Programmes of Staffordshire University, UK and other reputed B Schools. He has won best paper award two times. He has published research papers in reputed journals indexed in Scopus, Web of Science and presented papers in national and international journals. He is actively involved in Faculty Development Programme and Management Development Programme. He has been engaged in social initiatives through plantation, blood donation, cleanliness drive and functional literacy programmes. He has been associated with Ministry of MSME, Government of India for Management Development Programmes and Entrepreneurship Development Programmes. He has 5 patents under his credit.

Dilay Turu is a microbiology researcher specializing in antibiotic resistance, biofilm studies, and bioactive compound purification. She earned her B.Sc. in Biology from Dokuz Eylül University in 2022, graduating with honors, and is currently pursuing her M.Sc. with a 3.95/4 GPA. Her research focuses on characterizing bioactive compounds from mosses and their antibiofilm activities. She has published in high-impact journals, presented at international conferences, and worked as a researcher at Dokuz Eylül University's Science and Technology Research Center. Awarded the TÜBİTAK 2210-A scholarship, Dilay combines expertise in phytochemistry and microbiology to explore innovative solutions in health and environmental science.

Index

A

B

H

I

L

M

T

W

www.ingramcontent.com/pod-product-compliance
Lightning Source LLC
LaVergne TN
LVHW081320300926
849161LV00008B/1826